Renal Disease

METHODS IN MOLECULAR MEDICINE™

John M. Walker, SERIES EDITOR

Renal Disease

Techniques and Protocols

Edited by

Michael S. Goligorsky, MD, PhD

New York Medical College,
Valhalla, NY

Humana Press ✳ **Totowa, New Jersey**

BS

© 2003 Humana Press Inc.
999 Riverview Drive, Suite 208
Totowa, New Jersey 07512

www.humanapress.com

Production Editor: Mark J. Breaugh.

Cover design by Patricia F. Cleary.

Cover illustration:Scanning electron microscopy image of glomerular capillaries detected using vascular casting (provided by MS Goligorsky).

For additional copies, pricing for bulk purchases, and/or information about other Humana titles, contact Humana at the above address or at any of the following numbers: Tel.: 973-256-1699; Fax: 973-256-8341; E-mail: humana@humanapr.com; Website: http://humanapress.com

Printed in the United States of America. 10 9 8 7 6 5 4 3 2 1

Library of Congress Cataloging in Publication Data

Main entry under title: Methods in molecular medicine™.

Renal disease : techniques and protocols / edited by Michael S. Goligorsky.
     p. cm. — (Methods in molecular medicine ; 86)
  Includes bibliographical references and index.
   ISBN 1-58829-134-0 (alk. paper)   1-59259-392-5 (E-ISBN)
    1. Kidneys—Pathophysiology—Laboratory manuals. I. Goligorsky, Michael S. II. Series.

RC903.9.R464 2003
616.6'107—dc21

          2002192190

8/27/04

Preface

"Rule IV. There is need of a method for finding out the truth.

Rule V. Method consists entirely in the order and disposition of the objects toward which our mental vision must be directed if we would find out any truth. We shall comply with it exactly if we reduce involved and obscure propositions step be step to those that are simpler, and then starting with the intuitive apprehension of all those that are absolutely simple, attempt to ascend to the knowledge of all others by precisely similar steps."

—Rene Descartes, *Rules for the Direction of Mind*

"…Perhaps he would sooner satisfy himself by resolving light into colours as far as may be done by Art, and then by examining the properties of those colours apart, and afterwards by trying the effects of reconjoyning two or more or all of those, and lastly by separating them again to examine what changes that reconjunction had wrought in them. This will prove a tedious and difficult task to do it as it ought to be done but I could not be satisfied till I had gone through it."

—From Newton's letter, quoted in *The Life of Isaac Newton* by Richard Westfall. Cambridge University Press, 1993.

As much as the progress of a discipline depends on the progress of methods it uses, the overall goal of *Renal Disease: Techniques and Protocols* is to provide a comprehensive and balanced account of adequacy, advantages, and potential pitfalls of various modern approaches to study renal function in health and disease. Toward this end, any possible hesitation in selecting the shortest, safest, and most picturesque path to one's research summit should be alleviated by the expert contributors, who have already taken a similar road and are keen to share their observations. It is our sincere hope that this collection of technical approaches should become a *vade mecum*, which will be both a user-friendly guide for the uninitiated and a thoughtful counselor for the experienced scholar of fluid–electrolyte homeostasis and kidney function.

The last few years have witnessed the completion of the human genome project, development of high-throughput techniques for the screening of expressed genes, and the emergence of technological platforms for the next major enterprise—proteomics research. Yet, the basic tenets of approaching the problem at hand have not undergone transformation since the time when

Rene Descartes formulated them. Simplified models, devoid of the complexities and "obscurities" of reality, remain the bedrock of investigation. Lessons learned are further tested in more complex models, ascending ultimately to the organismal level. Therefore, the flow of chapters in this book has been designed to reflect upon this process—from simple models to integrative physiology.

With this in mind, *Renal Disease: Techniques and Protocols* is subdivided into five sections: (I) Optimizing the Usage of Models of Renal Disease, (II) Choices of Imaging Techniques, (III) Studies of Embryonic Development of the Kidney, (IV) Approaches to Study Molecular Mechanisms of Disease, and (V) Technical Means to Assess Functional Correlates of Disease. Though intricately interconnected, such a subdivision should provide an investigator with a possible path to follow in the course of investigation.

Certain technological areas are not represented in this volume (i.e., gene therapy). This does not reflect this editor's negligence, but rather acknowledges that it has become a subject for another volume published in this series and the interested reader is referred to that edition *(1)*.

Methods per se are not science, but mere tools to achieve scientific goals. And yet in this process new techniques are being born or the old ones modified to satisfy the precise goals of a researcher. The intelligent use of the technological armamentarium is a valuable assistant in our inquiries. It is for this reason that philosophers and thinkers of all times have developed a body of literature that summarizes the diversity of scientific approaches. In addition to the reductive and inductive methods, illustrated by the above quotations from Descartes and Newton, approaches to a problem that are based on theoretical predictions initially unsupported by the facts ("dogmatic method"), reliance on a chance discovery ("haphazard experiment"), as well as the "method of contradiction" and the "method of recodification," searching for known patterns in unknown situations (or vice versa), all enrich the repertoire of strategies to be selected by an investigator *(2)*. The advent of high-throughput screening technologies provides, at least at the first glance, a typical example of a shifting paradigm of research strategies. In contrast to the "dogmatic method," these screening approaches are, basically, unbiased and unenlightened by a hypothesis—perfect examples of what one would call "a fishing expedition." When successful however, they offer the researcher a previously concealed and entirely unexpected set of data. These in turn require the engagement of a "reductive method" to try sorting out potential pathways that have led to the fact(s) disclosed in an unbiased fashion and their consequences. Thus, starting with the Newtonian stance of *hypotheses non fingo* (I don't make hypotheses), these high throughput approaches require just the opposite at the stage when the output from the technological platforms reaches the desk of an astonished investigator.

With more than 50,000 scientific periodicals published worldwide that in toto print weekly more than 40,000 scientific articles, the level of informational barrage to which an investigator is exposed has become almost unbearable. No matter which strategic decisions for attacking the problem at hand have been made, the next challenge of selecting the correct tool set confronts every investigator. Under the stress of informational overflow, this selection turns into an overly complex process. Therefore, a manual, guiding investigators among the thicket of available techniques and providing them with expert insights into the advantages and bottlenecks of each, should serve to strengthen the scientific backbone and save time. With these goals in mind, we offer the reader *Renal Disease: Techniques and Protocols.*

Michael S. Goligorsky, MD, PhD

References

1. Morgan, JR. *Methods in Molecular Medicine, Volume 69: Gene Therapy Protocols, 2nd Ed.* Humana Press, Totowa, NJ, 2001.
2. Moles, A. "La Creation Scientifique," Geneva, 1957; quoted from J. Barzun "Science: The Glorious Entertainment," Harper & Row, New York, 1964.

Acknowledgments

I wish to thank all the contributors of the chapters—the real authors of this book.

It is also my pleasant duty to acknowledge the generous contribution of my colleagues to this volume: my assistant, Donna James, who helped a lot in assembling the Index of the book and in constantly communicating with the authors and the publisher and my colleague, Dr. Sergey Brodsky, who has been indispensable in assisting with the electronic conversion of different chapters to a uniform style. My sincere gratitude goes to Craig Adams and Mark Breaugh of Humana Press, who oversaw the highly professional, timely, and efficient production of the book. And last, but not least, I am indebted to Drs. Christopher Wilcox and Jurgen Schnermann, who have shared with me their time and thoughts, thus helping me to shape the scope and the contents of the book, and who suggested potential contributors for different chapters. The efforts of all these people are cordially appreciated.

Contents

Contributors

NADER G. ABRAHAM • *Department of Pharmacology, New York Medical College, Valhalla, NY*

ISAM ABU-AMARAH • *Department of Medicine, Loyola University Medical Center and Hines VA, Maywood, IL*

ATAKAN AYDIN • *Franz Volhard Clinic HELIOS Klinikum and Max Delbrück Center for Molecular Medicine, Berlin, Germany*

SYLVIA BÄHRING • *Franz Volhard Clinic HELIOS Klinikum and Max Delbrück Center for Molecular Medicine, Berlin, Germany*

MICHAEL BALAZY • *Department of Pharmacology, New York Medical College, Valhalla, NY*

SHRINATH BARATHAN • *O'Brien Renal Research Center, Department of Medicine, Case Western Reserve University, Cleveland, OH*

LAURA BARISONI • *National Institute of Diabetes and Digestive and Kidney Diseases, National Institutes of Health, Bethesda, MD*

BRENDAN J. BARRETT • *Patient Research Centre, Health Sciences Centre, Memorial University of Newfoundland, St. John's, Newfoundland, Canada*

P. DARWIN BELL • *Division of Nephrology, University of Alabama, Birmingham, AL*

ANIL K. BIDANI • *Department of Medicine, Loyola University Medical Center and Hines VA, Maywood, IL*

M. DONALD BLAUFOX • *Department of Nuclear Medicine, Albert Einstein College of Medicine and Montefiore Medical Center, Bronx, NY*

ERWIN P. BÖTTINGER • *Departments of Medicine and Molecular Genetics, Albert Einstein College of Medicine, Bronx, NY*

JAMES P. CALVET • *Department of Biochemistry & Molecular Biology, University of Kansas Medical Center, Kansas City, KS*

MAIREAD A. CARROLL • *Department of Pharmacology, New York Medical College, Valhalla, NY*

DANIEL CASELLAS • *Groupe Rein et Hypertension, Institut Universitaire de Rechereche Clinique, Montpellier, France*

PETER L. CHOYKE • *Department of Radiology, National Institutes of Health, Bethesda, MD*

CLEMENS D. COHEN • *Medizinische Poliklinik, University of Munich, Munich, Germany*

MARK CRABTREE • *Department of Pharmacology, Weill Medical College of Cornell University, New York, NY*

BRYAN M. CURTIS • *Patient Research Centre, Health Sciences Centre, Memorial University of Newfoundland, St. John's, Newfoundland, Canada*

DEB DIAMOND • *Ciphergen Biosystems Inc., Fremont, CA*

RAGHU V. DURVASULA • *Division of Nephrology, University of Washington Medical Center, Seattle, WA*

M. ASHRAF EL-MEANAWY • *Department of Medicine, O'Brien Renal Research Center, Case Western Reserve University, Cleveland, OH*

NICHOLAS R. FERRERI • *Department of Pharmacology, New York Medical College, Valhalla, NY*

ULLA G. FRIIS • *Department of Physiology and Pharmacology, University of Southern Denmark, Odense, Denmark*

ERIC FUNG • *Ciphergen Biosystems Inc., Fremont, CA*

MICHAEL S. GOLIGORSKY • *Departments of Medicine and Pharmacology, New York Medical College, Valhalla, NY*

R. ARIEL GOMEZ • *Department of Pediatrics, University of Virginia School of Medicine, Charlottesville, VA*

ALVIN I. GOODMAN • *Department of Medicine , New York Medical College, Valhalla, NY*

KAREN A. GRIFFIN • *Department of Medicine, Loyola University Medical Center and Hines VA, Maywood, IL*

STEVEN S. GROSS • *Department of Pharmacology, Weill Medical College of Cornell University, New York, NY*

GANG HAO • *Department of Pharmacology, Weill Medical College of Cornell University, New York, NY*

PATRICK S. HAYDEN • *Department of Medicine, O'Brien Renal Research Center, Case Western Reserve University, Cleveland, OH*

ROBERT M. HENDERSON • *Department of Pharmacology, University of Cambridge, Cambridge, UK*

SUDHA K. IYENGAR • *Department of Medicine, O'Brien Renal Research Center, Case Western Reserve University, Cleveland, OH*

EDWIN K. JACKSON • *Center for Clinical Pharmacology, University of Pittsburgh School of Medicine, Pittsburgh, PA*

BOYE L. JENSEN • *Department of Physiology and Pharmacology, University of Southern Denmark, Odense, Denmark*

HOULI JIANG • *Department of Pharmacology, New York Medical College, Valhalla, NY*

FUMIHIKO KAJIYA • *Department of Urology and Medical Engineering, Kawasaki Medical School, Okayama, Japan*

MATTHIAS KRETZLER • *Medizinische Poliklinik, University of Munich, Munich, Germany*

ELLEN M. LEVEE • *Department of Comparative Medicine, New York Medical College, Valhalla, NY*

YIYAN LIU • *Department of Nuclear Medicine, Montefiore Medical Center, Bronx, NY*

JOHN N. LORENZ • *Department of Molecular & Cellular Physiology, University of Cincinnati, Cincinnati, OH*

FRIEDRICH C. LUFT • *Franz Volhard Clinic HELIOS Klinikum and Max Delbrück Center for Molecular Medicine, Medical Faculty of the Charité, Humboldt University of Berlin, Berlin, Germany*

BRENDA S. MAGENHEIMER • *Department of Biochemistry & Molecular Biology, University of Kansas Medical Center, Kansas City, KS*

HANI B. MARCOS • *Department of Radiology, National Institutes of Health, Bethesda, MD*

ROBIN L. MASER • *Department of Biochemistry & Molecular Biology, University of Kansas Medical Center, Kansas City, KS*

JOHN C. MCGIFF • *Department of Pharmacology, New York Medical College, Valhalla, NY*

LEON C. MOORE • *Department of Physiology and Biophysics, SUNY Health Science Center, Stony Brook, NY*

WILLIAM T. NOONAN • *Department of Molecular & Cellular Physiology, University of Cincinnati, Cincinnati, OH*

AKIVA NOVETSKY • *Departments of Medicine and Molecular Genetics, Albert Einstein College of Medicine, Bronx, NY*

THOMAS L. PALLONE • *Division of Nephrology, University of Maryland at Baltimore, Baltimore, MD*

PATRICK S. PARFREY • *Patient Research Centre, Health Sciences Centre, Memorial University of Newfoundland, St. John's, Newfoundland, Canada*

ALAN O. PERANTONI • *Laboratory of Comparative Carcinogenesis, National Cancer Institute, Frederick, MD*

JÁNOS PETI-PETERDI • *Division of Nephrology, University of Alabama, Birmingham, AL*

POTHANA SAIKUMAR • *Department of Pathology, University of Texas Health Science Center, San Antonio, TX*

HIROYUKI SASAKI • *Institute of DNA Medicine, The Jikei University School of Medicine, Tokyo, Japan*

JEFFREY R. SCHELLING • *Department of Medicine, O'Brien Renal Research Center, Case Western Reserve University, Cleveland, OH*

JURGEN SCHNERMANN • *National Institute of Diabetes and Digestive and Kidney Diseases, National Institutes of Health, Bethesda, MD*

JOHN R. SEDOR • *O'Brien Renal Research Center, Department of Medicine, Case Western Reserve University, Cleveland, OH*

MARIA LUISA S. SEQUEIRA LOPEZ • *Department of Pediatrics, University of Virginia School of Medicine, Charlottesville, VA*

STUART J. SHANKLAND • *Division of Nephrology, University of Washington Medical Center, Seattle, WA*

ANJA HVIID SIMONSESN • *Ciphergen Biosystems Inc., Fremont, CA*

OLE SKØTT • *Department of Physiology and Pharmacology, University of Southern Denmark, Odense, Denmark*

ROBERT A. STAR • *National Institute of Diabetes and Digestive and Kidney Diseases, National Institutes of Health, Bethesda, MD*

STEVAN P. TOFOVIC • *Center for Clinical Pharmacology, University of Pittsburgh School of Medicine, Pittsburgh, PA*

POORNIMA UPADHYA • *Department of Urologic Surgery, Vanderbilt University Medical Center, Nashville, TN*

VOLKER VALLON • *Department of Pharmacology, University of Tuebingen, Tuebingen, Germany*

JOEL M. WEINBERG • *Division of Nephrology, University of Michigan Medical Center, Ann Arbor, MI*

SCOT R. WEINBERGER • *Ciphergen Biosystems Inc., Fremont, CA*

I. DAVID WEINER • *Nephrology Section, Malcom Randall VA Medical Center, Gainesville, FL*

SIMON J. M. WELHAM • *Nephro-Urology Unit, Institute of Child Health, University College London, London, UK*

CHARLES S. WINGO • *Nephrology Section, Malcom Randall VA Medical Center, Gainesville, FL*

ADRIAN S. WOOLF • *Nephro-Urology Unit, Institute of Child Health, University College London, London, UK*

SHEN-LING XIA • *Nephrology Section, Malcom Randall VA Medical Center, Gainesville, FL*

TOKUNORI YAMAMOTO • *Department of Urology and Medical Engineering, Kawasaki Medical School, Okayama, Japan*

JIRI ZAVADIL • *Departments of Medicine and Molecular Genetics, Albert Einstein College of Medicine, Bronx, NY*

YANTIAN ZHANG • *Department of Radiology, National Institutes of Health, Bethesda, MD*

CHRISTOPHER A. ZIEN • *Department of Biochemistry & Molecular Biology, University of Kansas Medical Center, Kansas City, KS*

I

OPTIMIZING THE USAGE OF MODELS OF RENAL DISEASE

1

Standards of Animal Care in Biological Experiments

Ellen M. Levee

1. Introduction

The use of animals is a necessary component of experimentation. The utilization of animals is a privilege not a right. Therefore, certain guidelines must be maintained in order to ensure their humane care and use. This chapter includes the basic principles of animal care and use, and reviews various procedures that are specific to renal experimentation. Our goal is also to provide guidance to the knowledgeable neophyte and serve as a refresher for the seasoned researcher. Individuals who are conducting research that involves animal use should enlist the help and guidance of the laboratory animal professional(s) at their respective institutions. Guidance may be provided by an institutional program or individual mentoring, but is a regulatory requirement that must be fulfilled. Proper care and use of animals will provide the investigator with the best scientific results. Unwanted variables in experimental procedures may result from improper care and use, and may confound results. Rodents are the most commonly used animal for experimental procedures. In light of the evolving transgenic technology, this trend will most likely continue.

The use of animals in research is closely regulated by various government and granting agencies. Standards of appropriate animal care and use are set forth in the *Guide for the Care and Use of Laboratory Animals*, commonly known as the *Guide*, and the Animal Welfare Act. The Institutional Animal Care and Use Committee (IACUC) must approve any work involving the use of animals. The IACUC is the oversight committee mandated by law to ensure the humane care and use of animals at each institution (*see* **Note 1**).

2. Materials
2.1. Rodent Survival Surgery

Sterile surgical instruments (depending on the surgery) and suture and hemostatic materials.

From: *Methods in Molecular Medicine, vol. 86: Renal Disease: Techniques and Protocols*
Edited by: M. S. Goligorsky © Humana Press Inc., Totowa, NJ

2.2. Anesthetics

2.2.1. Preemptive and Postoperative Analgesics Available for Rodents

1. Morphine: 10 mg/kg SQ q 6–12 h.
2. Buprenorphine: 1 mg/kg SQ q 12 h.
3. Meperidine: 20 mg/kg SQ or im q 8–12 h.
4. Acetaminophen: 100–300 mg/kg PO q 4 h.

2.2.2. Commonly Used and Approved Anesthetics for Rodents

1. Pentobarbital sodium: 35–45 mg/kg intraperitoneal (ip) or intravenous (iv) for rats and guinea pigs; 60–90 mg/kg ip or iv for mice, gerbils and hamsters.
2. Ketamine HCL: 60–90 mg/kg im in all rodents but requires the addition of xylazine (4–8 mg/kg im) or acepromazine (1–2.5 mg/kg im) for anesthetic plane.
3. Inhalant anesthetic agents (isoflurane, halothane) may be used to effect in a properly vented hood.

3. Methods

3.1. Housing

The proper housing of laboratory animals is important in order to eliminate the effects of unwanted variables and to maintain animals in a disease-free state. In today's animal research environment, the quality of laboratory animals is such that most rodent pathogens and genetic manipulation cause little overt clinical signs but may have profound or unexpected effects on research outcome. The *Guide* addresses the appropriate standards of animal care for many of the species used in research. Cage size, bedding material, cage sanitation, temperature, relative humidity, and photoperiod are all parameters that must be controlled in order to produce sound scientific results. All animal room lights should be on a timer. Light:Dark cycles may be either 12:12 or 14:10, depending upon the type of animal work being done. Reversed light cycles are indicated at times. Species-specific metabolism caging may be used for the collection of urine and feces. The principle of the metabolism cage is to house the animal in a cage with a wire grid floor. The cage is set on a funnel device so that the urine falls onto the sides of the funnel and is channeled into a collection container. The feces drop into a collecting jar. Feeding and watering compartments are constructed in a way that prevents the food and water from significantly contaminating the urine or feces. For collection of small amounts of urine in rodents, it may suffice to rapidly remove the rodent and place the urethral opening over a collecting tube. Rodents frequently urinate upon being handled. Gentle manual expression of the bladder may also be employed.

3.2. Fasting and Water Restriction

The practices of fasting or water restriction may be required for some experimental protocols. These states must be scientifically justified in the animal use proposal. All animals that undergo water restriction or fasting must be closely monitored by the investigator. Behavioral and physiological parameters that will be recorded must be established by the research team before the onset of the experiment. Hydration levels and weight loss should be closely followed (*see* **Note 2**).

3.3. Blood Collection

Blood collection in the rodent may be performed from various sites. The volume of blood in all animals is 60–80 mL/kg. Ten percent of the total volume can be removed from the animal without causing any detrimental effects. As a general rule, the smallest volume possible should be removed. The frequency of the removal of blood is another consideration that should be addressed in the experimental design. Sterile technique and proper training of the animal handler are essential for a successful outcome. Light anesthesia must be employed in the collection of blood from all sites except the tail vein. The method of cardiac puncture should be reserved for terminal bleeds. Indwelling catheters may be used for serial blood withdrawals. The following are acceptable sites for blood withdrawal in the lightly anesthetized rodent: retro-orbital sinus (mouse) or ophthalmic venous plexus (rat), the jugular vein (rat), and nail clipping.

3.4. Protocols

Because the majority of animal models in research are rodents, the remainder of this chapter focuses on procedures that utilize rodents in general, as well as renal-based investigations.

3.4.1. Rodent Survival Surgery

This should be carefully planned in order to ensure adequate time for both the procedure and postoperative recovery time. All materials should be prepared in advance. Rodents should undergo an acclimation period upon arrival to the facilities before any manipulations are performed. Animals should be acquired from approved sources and should be free of disease. The personnel performing the surgical procedures should be well-trained in the technique as well as proper handling of the animal in general. A balanced anesthetic regimen should allow for an appropriate surgical plan, yet should not interfere with the experiment being carried out. Preemptive and postoperative analgesia should be considered as part of the surgical plan and IACUC review process, and should be tailored to the procedure involved. It is imperative to maintain sufficient animal records, including anesthetic doses, intra-operative notes, and postoperative care. It is generally unnecessary to withhold food and water pre-operatively from rodents.

A model protocol for survival rodent surgery, which is consistent with interpretation of the guidelines and which provides satisfactory aseptic conditions, is indicated here:

1. Surgery should be conducted on a clean, uncluttered lab bench or table surface. The surface should be wiped with a disinfectant before and after use, and/or covered with a clean drape.
2. Hair should be removed from the surgical site with clippers or a depilatory. The surgical site should be treated first with an antiseptic scrub and then with an antiseptic solution (chlorhexidine or povidone iodine scrub and solution).
3. All instruments should be sterilized, but the surgical instruments or devices being used may determine the method of choice. Fine-gauge catheters may be sterilized with ethylene oxide. Acceptable techniques for cold sterilization include soaking in 2% glutaraldehyde for 10 h, in 8% formaldehyde and 70% alcohol for 18 h, or in 6% stabilized hydrogen peroxide for 6 h *(2)*. Glass bead sterilizers may be used to maintain instrument sterility in multiple rodent surgery or after cold sterilization.
4. The surgeon should wash his hands with an antiseptic surgical scrub preparation and then aseptically put on gloves. If working alone, the surgeon should have the animal anesthetized and positioned, and have the first layer of the double-wrapped instrument pack opened before putting on sterile gloves.
5. The surgeon should wear a face mask. A cap and sterile gown are recommended, but not required.
6. Multiple surgeries present special problems. After the first surgery, the sterilized instruments may be kept in a sterile tray containing cold sterilizing agent or in an ultrasonic sterilizer or a bead sterilizer (the preferred method). The sterilizing agent should be replaced when contaminated with blood or other body fluids. Sterile gloves should be changed between surgeries.
7. The abdominal or thoracic body wall should be closed with absorbable suture material. The skin should be closed with staples, a nonabsorbable suture material, or the newer absorbable skin sutures in a simple interrupted pattern. Skin sutures or staples should be removed 7–10 d after surgery.
8. Rodents should be recovered from anesthesia in a warmed environment. Antibiotics should not be given routinely after surgery unless justified by the specific procedure.

3.5. Specific Survival Surgical Procedures

3.5.1. Chronic Catheterization of Blood Vessels

Chronic catheterization of blood vessels is often necessary in order to administer test materials or obtain serial blood samples. The jugular vein, carotid artery, tail vein, and femoral artery all lend themselves to chronic catheterization (*see* **Note 3**).

3.5.1.1. JUGULAR VEIN CATHETERIZATION

1. The rat is anesthetized and placed on its back with its head toward the surgeon. The surgical site is prepared as previously described.
2. An incision is made parallel to and on one side of the midline in the neck of the rat.
3. The jugular vein is located (right external jugular vein) and is gently cleaned of fat and tissue using blunt dissection. The vein should be cleared of extraneous tissue of a length of at least 1.5 cm leading to the point where it passes underneath the pectoral muscle. Care must be taken not to handle the vein in order to prevent tearing and spasms from occurring.
4. A pair of small or jeweler's forceps is passed under the vein, and a doubled piece of suture is passed beneath the vein and cut into two pieces.
5. The anterior tie is gently moved cranially as far as possible along the "cleaned" vessel. The suture is then tied to occlude the vessel.
6. The posterior tie is moved gently toward the pectoral muscle, allowing several millimeters between it and the anterior ligature. The first throw of the posterior ligature is done, but it is left loosely around the vein.
7. Next, the jugular vein is lightly lifted by using an opened small or jeweler's forceps under it, or gently lifting the ends of the posterior ligature vertically.
8. A small incision is made in the vein to allow introduction of the catheter (i.d. ~0.5 mm and o.d. ~0.6–1 mm) toward the heart. The opening may be enlarged with a forceps, or a catheter introducer may be employed. If blood is to be withdrawn or blood pressure measured via the catheter, then the tip of the catheter should be advanced until it lies within the superior vena cava or right atrium. If test materials are to be injected, then only a few millimeters of catheter are needed to lie within the vein.
9. The catheter is tested for patency by withdrawing a small amount of blood via a syringe filled with saline. If the catheter is patent, the blood is flushed back into the catheter and the catheter is filled with the heparin/saline lock solution (20 U heparin/1 mL saline). A stainless steel pin is placed in the end of the catheter. Care must be taken to avoid introducing air into the catheter or vein. The posterior ligature is then tied around the vein and catheter.
10. The catheter is fixed to the fascia with a suture. A tension or stress loop should be placed, allowing slack in order to compensate for the animal's movements. This loop helps avoid the catheter from being displaced.
11. The rat is then placed in lateral recumbency, and the dorsal nape of the neck is aseptically prepared.
12. A small incision is made in the nape of the neck. A 16 gauge trocar or a straight forceps is passed through the incision which travels subcutaneously down the side of the neck and exits anterior to the site of entry of the catheter into the jugular vein. The end of the catheter is then grasped by the forceps or passed through the trocar, and passed subcutaneously to the incision at the nape of the neck.

13. The catheter exits outside the incision at the nape of the neck, and is either stoppered or attached outside the cage to an infusion pump. The two skin incisions are then closed using interrupted sutures.
14. Proper catheter maintenance requires daily flushing with fresh heparin/saline solution.

3.5.1.2. CAROTID ARTERY CATHETERIZATION

1. The rat is anesthetized and placed on its back with its head toward the surgeon. The surgical site is prepared as previously described.
2. An incision is made parallel to and on one side of the midline in the neck of the rat.
3. The carotid artery is located medial to and below the jugular vein. The carotid artery (left carotid artery) is gently cleaned of fat and tissue using blunt dissection between the omohyoid, sternomastoid, and sternohyoid muscles. Care should be taken to avoid damaging the vagus nerve. The artery should be cleared of extraneous tissue of a length of at least 1.5 cm.
4. A pair of small or jeweler's forceps is passed under the artery, and a doubled piece of suture is passed beneath the vessel and cut into two pieces.
5. The anterior tie is gently moved cranially as far as possible along the "cleaned" vessel. The suture is then tied to occlude the vessel.
6. The posterior tie is moved gently several millimeters from the anterior ligature. The first throw of the posterior ligature is done, but it is left loosely around the artery.
7. The vessel is then lightly lifted, either by using an opened small or jeweler's forceps under it or gently lifting the ends of the posterior ligature vertically. An aneurysm clamp is used to occlude the carotid at the most distal point.
8. A small stab incision is made in the artery to allow the catheter to be gently forced through it.
9. The posterior ligature is then tied around the carotid artery and catheter. The catheter is advanced toward the heart after removing the aneurysm clamp. The tip of the catheter should lie in the aortic arch.
10. The catheter is then fixed to the fascia via suture. A tension or stress loop should be placed, allowing slack in order to compensate for the animal's movements. This loop helps avoid displacement of the catheter.
11. The catheter is exteriorized through the dorsal nape of the neck as described for the jugular vein catheterization prepared.

3.5.1.3. FEMORAL ARTERY CATHETERIZATION

1. The rat is anesthetized and placed on its back with its head toward the surgeon. The surgical site is prepared as previously described.
2. An incision is made on the proximal medial surface of the hind limb, extending into the groin area.
3. The femoral artery is located in the groin region. The femoral artery is gently separated from the femoral vein and nerve by blunt dissection. The artery should be cleared of extraneous tissue for several millimeters.

4. A pair of small or jeweler's forceps is passed under the artery, and a doubled piece of suture is passed beneath the vessel and cut into two pieces.
5. The posterior tie is gently moved distally as far as possible along the "cleaned" vessel. The suture is then tied to occlude the vessel.
6. The anterior tie is moved gently several millimeters from the anterior ligature. The first throw of the anterior ligature is done, but it is left loosely around the artery.
7. An aneurysm clamp is used to occluded the artery anterior to the ligature.
8. A small stab incision is made in the artery to allow the catheter to be gently forced through it.
9. The anterior ligature is then tied around the artery and catheter. The catheter is advanced toward the body after removing the aneurysm clamp. The tip of the catheter should lie in the dorsal aorta.
10. The catheter is then fixed to the fascia via suture. A tension or stress loop should be placed, allowing slack in order to compensate for the animal's movements. This loop helps to avoid the catheter from being displaced.
11. The catheter is passed subcutaneously along the body and exteriorized through the dorsal nape of the neck as described for the jugular-vein catheterization.

3.5.2. Nephrectomy

3.5.2.1. UNILATERAL NEPHRECTOMY

Nephrectomized rats normally do well with one kidney. The remaining kidney undergoes hypertrophy.

1. The rat is anesthetized and placed in ventral recumbency. The surgical site is prepared as previously described.
2. A dorsoventral incision is made posterior to the costal border of the thorax. This incision should penetrate the abdominal cavity.
3. Using the perirenal fat in order to grasp the kidney, it is freed of its connective tissue and exteriorized from the abdominal cavity.
4. The adrenal gland is located at the anterior pole of the kidney, is detached from the kidney by blunt dissection of its attachments, and is replaced in the abdominal cavity.
5. A suture is placed around the renal vessels and ureter as far as possible toward the midline without occluding any collateral vessels. The suture is securely tied around the vessels and the ureter.
6. The vessels and ureter are transected next to the kidney. The kidney is removed and discarded.
7. The incision is closed in layers, using a simple interrupted suture pattern.

3.5.2.2. 5/6 NEPHRECTOMY

This technique is used to induce a model of chronic renal failure.

1. The rat is anesthetized and placed in ventral recumbency. The surgical site is prepared as previously described.

2. A dorsoventral incision is made posterior to the costal border of the thorax. This incision should penetrate the abdominal cavity.
3. Using the perirenal fat in order to grasp the kidney, it is freed of its connective tissue and exteriorized from the abdominal cavity.
4. The adrenal gland is located at the anterior pole of the kidney, is detached from the kidney by blunt dissection of its attachments, and is replaced in the abdominal cavity.
5. The anterior and posterior poles, along with much of the cortical tissue, are removed using a scalpel.
6. The remaining renal tissue is wrapped in hemostatic gauze and returned to the abdominal cavity. The remaining kidney tissue hypertrophies.
7. The incision is closed in layers, using a simple interrupted suture pattern.
8. Two weeks following the initial surgery, the contralateral kidney is removed following the procedure described for the unilateral nephrectomy.

4. Notes

1. The CEO or Institutional Official following membership guidelines promulgated by regulations appoints the IACUC members. The IACUC reviews, approves, requests modifications, or denies approval of all proposals for laboratory use of animals. The IACUC also reviews the institution's program of care and use on a semi-annual basis and inspects the animal facilities. The animal use proposal must address specific concerns including rationale for the use of animals, as well as the chosen species; justification of the proposed number of animals to be used; a detailed description of the all procedures to be performed; the qualifications and training of personnel; a literature search for alternatives to procedures that may potentially cause pain or distress; the method of euthanasia, and the use of appropriate anesthetics and analgesics when indicated. A program of Animal Care and Use must involve a veterinarian with specific training and experience in the use of animals for research purposes. The investigator should solicit the help of the attending veterinarian in developing an accurate, thorough animal use proposal. The role of the laboratory animal facility staff and the IACUC is that of facilitator, and their collective knowledge should be drawn upon.
2. In water restriction studies, states of dehydration may lead to decreased consumption of food and should be considered in the experimental design.
3. Consideration regarding the choice of catheter should include thromboresistant construction, readily sterilized to reduce the chance of infection, easily inserted, stable longevity, and expediency factors. Bonding techniques to impregnate the catheter with anticoagulants and/or antibiotics may be employed. A heparin/saline lock will further diminish the chance of a thrombus block of the catheter.

Acknowledgment

Special thanks to Mark M. Klinger, DVM, DipACLAM, for his review and suggestions to this chapter.

References

1. Guide for the Care and Use of Laboratory Animals, U.S. Dept. of Health and Human Services, Public Health Service, National Institutes of Health, Publication No. 85–23, Revised 1996.
2. Simmons, B. P. (1983) CDC guidelines for the prevention and control of nosocomial infections. *Am J. Infect. Control* **11(13)**.
3. Wyatt, J. (1989) An institutional protocol for aseptic technique on survival surgery of rodents. *Synapse* **22(1),** 10–14.
4. Waynforth, H. B. and Flecknell, P. A. (1992) *Experimental and Surgical Techniques in the Rat*, 2nd ed., Academic Press Limited, San Diego, CA, pp. 212–233.

2

Models of Polycystic Kidney Disease

Poornima Upadhya

1. Introduction

Polycystic kidney disease (PKD) is a potentially life-threatening disorder that affects both adult and pediatric patients. PKD can be either inherited as a dominant (ADPKD) or a recessive trait (ARPKD) or acquired. The disease is characterized by massive renal enlargement associated with the growth of fluid-filled intrarenal cysts. ADPKD, the most common cystic disease, is caused by mutations at three distinct loci: *PKD1*, *PKD2*, and *PKD3*. The *PKD1* locus was mapped to human Chr 16p13.3, and the *PKD2* locus was mapped to human Chr 4q21–23. The *PKD3* locus has not yet been mapped. *PKD1* is the most commonly inherited mutation. Patients with ADPKD develop renal, hepatic, and pancreatic cysts, abdominal and inguinal hernias, heart-valve defects, and aortic and cerebral aneurysms *(1)*. ARPKD is encountered less frequently. *PKHD1*, a locus on human Chr 6p21-cen that predisposes individuals to develop ARPKD, has been reported. ARPKD patients primarily develop cysts in the collecting ducts, with hepatic fibrosis as an associated extrarenal manifestation *(2)*.

Genetic studies have identified the normal products of the *PKD1*, *PKD2*, and *PHKD1* loci *(3–5)*. Efforts are underway to decipher the functions of the normal protein encoded by each of these three loci. However, the detailed understanding of cystogenesis caused by ADPKD and ARPKD is complicated by their variability with respect to age of onset and extra-renal manifestations *(6,7)*. This variation suggests that other genes modulate the clinical manifestation of PKD caused by any of the previously identified *PKD1*, *PKD2*, *PKD3*, or *PKHD1* disease loci. Because of the uncontrollable genetic variability between human patients, identification of the genes that modulate disease severity in the human population is currently an insuperable problem. Animal models on defined genetic backgrounds substantially simplify the identification of these modifying factors.

From: *Methods in Molecular Medicine, vol. 86: Renal Disease: Techniques and Protocols*
Edited by: M. S. Goligorsky © Humana Press Inc., Totowa, NJ

There are a number of animal models for PKD *(8,9)*. In some of the models, the severity of the disease resulting from the main mutation varies with the genetic background of the mouse *(10–12)*. Characterization studies in the various animal models of PKD will help us gain a fuller comprehension of the clinical manifestations of the disease in humans. This chapter reviews the characteristic morphological features and biochemical and molecular alterations in the common rodent models for PKD.

2. Inherited Models of PKD

2.1. cpk *Mouse*

The *cpk* mutation on mouse Chr 12 arose spontaneously in the C57BL/6J strain *(13)*. PKD in *cpk* homozygotes is aggressive, and its rapid progression to terminal stages leads to death at approx 3 wk of age. Although renal abnormalities are limited to the homozygous *cpk* animals, hepatic cysts have been reported in older heterozygotes. On the DBA/2J background, in addition to the renal phenotype, the *cpk* mutation produces pancreatic and hepatic fibrosis and dilation, making this an attractive animal model for the study of human ARPKD. Light and transmission electron microscopy studies have shown that renal abnormalities appear in the earliest stages within the proximal tubules. However, the site of involvement shifts to cortical and collecting ducts as the disease progresses. Death is most probably the result of end-stage renal failure, since blood-urea nitrogen and serum creatinine levels are elevated at approx 3 wk of age *(14)*.

Biochemical and molecular studies have led to the identification of several cellular and extracellular matrix (ECM) abnormalities in the *cpk* model. Enhanced expression of the proto-oncogenes such as c-myc, c-fos, and c-Ki-ras in the homozygous *cpk/cpk* mutants may reflect epithelial hyperplasia. In addition, the increased level of epidermal growth factor (EGF) in the renal cystic fluid, coupled with the apical mis-localization of the EGF receptor (EGFR), is believed to have mitogenic effects on the cystic epithelium. The epithelial cells of *cpk* homozygotes also show some features of dedifferentiation. Although apical and basolateral localization of Na^+-K^+ATPase expression is a normal transient feature during early renal tubule development, the pump is restricted to the basolateral side later in terminally differentiated cells. However, in some of the cystic collecting tubules the apical membrane expression of Na^+-K^+ATPase remains significantly increased, suggesting the loss of differentiated phenotype. Further evidence for the loss of differentiation comes from the presence of abnormally high levels of sulphated glycoprotein. This suggests that PKD in the *cpk* mice may be caused in part by defective terminal differentiation of the tubular epithelial cells. Additional abnormalities reported in the *cpk* kidneys include increased expression of basement-membrane constituents and remodeling enzymes, matrix metalloproteinases (MMPs), and their specific tissue inhibitors, TIMPs.

Recently, a novel gene, *cystin*, which is disrupted in *cpk* mice was cloned by positional cloning. When expressed exogenously in polarized renal epithelial cells, cystin was detected in cilia, and its expression overlapped with *polaris*, another PKD-related protein. Cystin expression appears to be enriched in the ciliary axoneme. This has led to the speculation that the cystin bound to the axonemal membrane functions as part of a molecular scaffold that stabilizes microtubule assembly within the ciliary axoneme *(14)*. This speculation is supported by the observation of Woo et al. that weekly injections of taxol to the *cpk* mice was able to prolong the survival of the *cpk* mice to more than 200 d with a remarkable reduction in the number of cysts in the taxol-treated animals *(16)*.

2.2. pcy *Mouse*

Takahashi et al. reported a spontaneous occurrence of a recessive form of PKD in the KK strain of the diabetic mouse. Genetic linkage analysis showed that the *pcy* mutation is located on mouse Chr 9 *(17)*. Kidney malformation and progression of PKD in inbred DBA/2-*pcy/pcy* mice has been characterized in detail. Renal cysts develop in all segments of the nephron, and progressively enlarge with age eventually severely distorting the entire kidney in adult animals. Hallmark features of cystic changes similar to those in human polycystic kidney epithelia such as renal tubular apoptosis, cellular hyperplasia, and abnormal basement membrane were observed. However, unlike the apical mislocalization of the Na^+-K^+ATPase in the cystic epithelial cells from some of the human ADPKD patients and the *cpk* mouse, only basolateral localization of the sodium pump was identified in *pcy* renal tubular epithelial cells. The mRNA levels encoding for growth-related proteins, such as TGF-β, PDGF-α, PDGF-β, IGF-1, basic FGF, and cyclin mRNA showed progressive increase with the age of animals. However, since the changes in expression of these genes did not take place in the earliest stages of the renal disease, but followed the progression of the disease, it is unlikely that they are key initiating players of renal cyst development *(18,19)*.

2.3. bpk/jcpk *Mouse*

The *bpk* mutation arose spontaneously in the inbred Balb/c strain. The mutation is autosomal recessive and maps to mouse Chr 10. Cysts develop predominantly in proximal tubules of the kidney in the earliest stages of PKD, and homozygous mutants die at about 1 mo of age. Another mutation, *jcpk* was induced by chlorambucil mutagenesis. The renal disease caused by this mutation is extremely aggressive, and homozygotes survive for less than 2 wk. Cysts appear in all segments of the nephron, including the glomerulus. Because the *bpk* and *jcpk* mutations were mapped close to each other on Chr 10, a complementation test was performed. The complementation test demonstrated that these two mutations were allelic. This was surprising, since despite their distinctly different PKD phenotypes, the *bpk* and *jcpk* mutations appeared to disrupt the same gene. However, since *jcpk* is a chlorambucil mutation that generally involves large deletions or chromosomal rearrangements, it is likely that *jcpk* involves a significantly larger genomic alteration involving two closely linked genes, one of which is *bpk*. These two possibilities can be distinguished once the molecular nature of mutations is determined *(20)*.

2.4. kat *Mouse*

The *kat* mutation arose spontaneously on the RBF/Dn background. The mutation is autosomal recessive, and maps to mouse Chr 8 *(21)*. Cysts appear in all segments of the nephron, including the glomerulus. The homozygous mutant mice exhibit a latent-onset slowly progressing form of PKD with renal pathology similar to human ADPKD. In addition, the *kat* mutation causes pleiotropic effects that include facial dysmorphism, dwarfism, male sterility, anemia, and cystic choroid plexus *(22)*. The gene altered by the *kat* mutation was cloned by positional cloning. The gene altered is *Nek1* (NIMA-related kinase-1) that encodes for a dual-specificity protein kinase. The kinase domain is most similar to NIMA, a protein kinase that controls initiation of mitosis in *Aspergillus nidulans*. The complex pleiotropic phenotypes seen in the homozygous mutant animals suggest that the NEK1 protein participates in different signaling pathways to regulate diverse cellular processes. It has been hypothesized that in the kidney, NEK1 protein belongs to a signaling pathway that promotes the full maturation of renal tubular epithelial cells, suggesting that the loss of NEK1 function traps these tubular epithelial cells in a state of permanent immaturity and growth *(23)*.

During the mapping studies, it was noted that the genetic background or modifier genes alter the severity of PKD caused by the mutation. Genome scans using molecular markers revealed three modifier loci that affect the severity of the PKD caused by the mutation. Additional modifier loci that interact with and modulate the effects of these three modifier loci were also identified. The mapping of these modifier genes, and their eventual identification, will help to reveal factors that can delay disease progression *(12)*.

2.5. jck *Mouse*

The *jck* mutation arose spontaneously in the Tg.ple transgenic line and did not segregate with the transgene. This mouse mutation is inherited as an autosomal recessive trait, and maps to Chr 11. The progression of PKD in this mouse model is slower than that seen in the *cpk* model. Cystic kidneys are detected by 6 wk, and animals survive until 20–25 wk of age. Histological analysis shows cysts predominating in the outer medulla and cortex. Very little is known about the cascade of events that leads to the clinical manifestation of the disease in this model and the role of growth hormones, ECM alterations, proto-oncogene expression, cell proliferation and differentiation *(11,24)*.

2.6. cy *Rat*

The *cy* mutation occurred spontaneously in Han:SPRD rats. Genetic analysis showed that the mutation was inherited as a dominant trait. Heterozygous rats develop a slowly progressing cystic disease that is accompanied with interstitial fibrosis and thickened basement membrane. In this animal model there are extrarenal manifestations besides PKD; these include hyperparathyroidism, osteodystrophia fibrosa, and metastatic calcification of the lungs, stomach, and heart. Histological analysis of the cystic kidney showed gender dimorphism that was more pronounced than in humans: females survive considerably longer than males. Taking the gender difference into account, Zeier et al. tested the impact of castration on progression. A significant slowing of progression occurred in the castrated rats, although the serum urea concentrations were still higher than usually seen in the female rats *(25)*. Similar beneficial effects were also seen in male mutants treated with methylprednisolone, which could reduce the interstitial inflammation and fibrosis, a common feature of PKD. However, mutant female animals did not respond to methylprednisolone treatment. The Han:SPRD cy/+ rat represents a well-documented rat model of ADPKD, with a number of features that resemble the human disease. Thus, this model has been extensively used for studying the pathophysiological events and evaluation of therapeutic interventions *(26)*.

2.7. pck *Rat*

The *pck* rat is a recently identified model of PKD that developed spontaneously in the rat strain Crj:CD/SD *(27)*. The *pck* mutation is inherited as an autosomal recessive trait. The *pck* rats develop liver cysts and progressive cystic enlargement of the kidneys after the first week of life. The renal cysts develop as focal process from thick ascending loops of Henle, distal tubules, and collecting ducts in the corticomedullary and outer medulla region. Apoptosis is common, and affects normal as well as dilated tubules. The basement membranes of the cyst walls exhibited a variety of alterations, including thinning, lamellation, and thickening. Segmental glomerulosclerosis, focal interstitial fibrosis, and inflammation are evident in 2-mo old mutant animals. The PKD is more severe in male than in female *pck* rats, as reflected by the higher kidney weights, although there is no gender difference in the severity of the cystic liver disease.

This *pck* rat is a valuable animal model of ARPKD. Recent genetic analysis of the ARPKD region in humans, identified a candidate gene, *PKHD1*. The *pck* mutation was found to be a splicing defect in the rat ortholog of this candidate gene. The *PKHD1* gene is predicted to encode a large novel protein, fibrocystin, with multiple copies of a domain shared with plexins and transcription factors. Based on its structural features, fibrocystin is believed to be a receptor protein that acts in collecting-duct and biliary differentiation. Interestingly, although the same gene is mutated in both the *pck* rat model and the human ARPKD patients, the *pck* rat model shows some phenotypic differences from the human disease, including the degree of hepatic cyst development, predominant development of renal cysts in the outer medullary-collecting ducts, and mild portal fibrosis in the liver, without formation of fibrous septa or development of portal hypertension *(5)*. This suggests that molecular nature of the mutation at the *PKHD1* locus may partially account for phenotypic variability seen among ARPKD patients.

3. Transgenic Models of PKD

3.1. orpk *Mouse*

The *orpk* transgenic line was developed as a part of a large-scale insertional mutagenesis program. The mutation maps to mouse Chr 14 and is inherited as a recessive trait. The homozygous mutant animals on the FVB/N inbred background have pre-axial polydactyly on all limbs, PKD, and abnormalities of the intrahepatic biliary tract, and are severely growth-retarded. Most of the *orpk*-mutant mice on the FVB/N inbred background die during the first week of life. However, on the C3H inbred genetic background, the mutant mice live longer, have polydactyly that is more variable, develop renal cysts at a slower rate, and have a less aggressive liver lesion. In the kidney, large cysts form in the collecting tubules, yet in the liver there is a consistent biliary hyperplasia and bile ductule ectasia, along with portal fibrosis. These lesions in the kidney and liver are remarkably similar to those seen in human ARPKD. Like human patients with ADPKD or ARPKD, the homozygous mutants exhibit increased expression and apical mis-localization of EGFR. These changes in EGFR were shown to be of physiological relevance, since genetic or pharmacological inhibition of EGFR activity results in a significant improvement in the renal pathology and function *(28,29)*.

Using the integrated transgene as a molecular marker, the mutated gene was cloned. In both multi- and mono-ciliated epithelium and in sperm, polaris, the protein encoded by the mutated gene was localized to the basal bodies and in the axoneme. A cortical collecting duct cell line has been derived from *orpk* mice. These cells were found to be devoid of cilia, but the defect could be corrected by re-expression of the wild-type polaris gene. These data suggest that the primary cilia are important for normal renal function and/or development and that the ciliary defect may be a contributing factor to the cystic disease in *orpk* mice. Further characterization of these cells will be important in elucidating the physiological role of renal cilia and their relationship to cystic disease *(30)*.

3.2. SBM *Mouse*

The *SBM* transgenic mice carry a fusion gene that includes the SV40 enhancer, the β-globin promoter, and the c-myc coding region, which is expressed at high levels in the renal tubular epithelium. These transgenic mice develop markedly enlarged kidneys, runting, and muscular atrophy. The cysts are scattered throughout the cortex and medulla, and the transgenic animals die from renal failure by 5 mo of age. In a large number of SBM transgenic mice, the kidneys contain focal interstitial aggregates of atypical plasma cells. The specific elevated expression of c-myc in hyperplastic renal tubular cyst epithelium of the *SBM* and *cpk* mice, suggests that cyst formation can arise through the deregulation of tubular epithelial cell proliferation *(31)*.

3.3. bcl-2–/– *Knockout*

bcl-2 is distinguished from other proto-oncogenes by its death-repressor activity and intracellular localization. Apoptosis is known to occur in both the nephrogenic and medullary region of the developing kidney, and follows a distinct developmental time-course. The Bcl-2 protein is expressed in the developing human and murine kidney. *bcl-2–/–* mice complete embryonic development, but display growth retardation and early mortality. Veis et al. found that hematopoiesis—including lymphocyte differentiation—was initially normal, but the thymus and spleen underwent massive apoptotic involution. The early mortality of the mutants was caused by renal failure resulting from a severe PKD. The presence of dilated proximal and distal tubular segments and hyperproliferation of epithelium and interstitium characterized the renal cystic disease *(32)*. Cystic kidneys from *bcl-2–/–* mice displayed nuclear localization of β-catenin and a loss of apical brush-border actin staining. However, the protein levels of α-catenin, β-catenin, actin, and E-cadherin were not altered in cystic kidneys compared with normal kidneys. Recently, the expression and activity of focal adhesion tyrosine phosphatases Src homology-2 domain phosphatase (SHP-2), protein tyrosine phosphatase (PTP 1B), and PTP-proline, glutamate, serine, and threonine sequences (PEST) during normal nephrogenesis and in cystic kidneys from *bcl-2–/–* mice were examined. Cystic kidneys from *bcl-2–/–* mice demonstrated a reduced activity, expression, and altered distribution of SHP-2 and PTP 1B. The altered regulation of PTP 1B and SHP-2 in kidneys from *bcl-2–/–* mice correlated with sustained phosphorylation of FAK and paxillin. Taken together, the renal cyst formation in the *bcl-2–/–* mice is believed to be a result of improper cell–cell interactions that interferes with renal maturation by continued activation of growth processes, including activation of FAK and paxillin *(33)*.

4. Transgenic Models Involving Polycystins

Polycystins are a family of transmembrane proteins. As mentioned earlier, two of the polycystin family members, polycystin-1 and -2, are mutated in human ADPKD patients. Polycystin-1 is a 4302 amino acid (aa) glycoprotein. Important features of polycystin-1 include several transmembrane segments and a cytoplasmic C-terminal domain containing potential phosphorylation sites. Polycystin-2 is a 968-aa protein, with a predicted structure that includes two intracellular domains flanking six transmembrane segments. The protein has homology to the voltage-activated Ca^{2+} channel a_{1E} and Na^+ voltage-dependent channels, as well as to the trp family of Ca^{2+} channels. In addition, there is a 29-aa EF hand motif involved in Ca^{2+} binding in the intracellular, C-terminal portion of the protein. The C-terminal tail of polycystin-1 interacts with that of polycystin-2, resulting in the formation of calcium-permeable nonselective cation channels in vitro, suggesting that extracellular signals can be transduced by the polycystin complex to regulate diverse cellular processes. Indeed, the cytoplasmic tail of polycystin-1 has been shown to signal via the G proteins, and its signaling pathway was shown to intersect with that of Wnts, a family of secreted signaling molecules. Polycystin-2 alone also mediates cation currents and functions as a Ca^{2+}-permeable nonselective cation channel *(34,35)*. Both proteins are expressed during renal development, but their exact role in cyst formation and in other disease manifestation is unclear.

4.1. Pkd1-*Targeted Knockout*

None of the genetic animal models of PKD map to the murine *Pkd1* locus. In order to decipher the normal function of polycystin-1, Zhou et al. first introduced into mice by homologous recombination a *Pkd1* truncation mutation. The homozygous mutant mice carrying a deletion of exon 34 (*Pkd1*[del34]) of *Pkd1* developed a severe PKD and pancreatic disease and died during the perinatal period *(36)*.

Since the *Pkd1*[del34] mutation is a truncation mutation, it was not clear whether the phenotype of the animals carrying the mutant allele was the result of the altered function of the truncated form of polycystin-1 or caused by haploinsufficiency. In order to address this, Zhou et al. generated, by homologous recombination, a second targeted mouse mutant with a null mutation (*Pkd1⁻*) in *Pkd1*. The null homozygotes (*Pkd1⁻/⁻*) developed more aggressive but similar renal and cystic disease as the *Pkd1*$^{del34/del34}$ homozygotes. It was also reported that both the *Pkd1⁻/⁻* and *Pkd1*$^{del34/del34}$ homozygotes developed polyhydramnios, hydrops fetalis, occult spina bifida, and osteochondro-dysplasia *(36)*. Interestingly, homozygous mutants with another mutant allele, *Pkd1*^{L}, which produces mutant polycystin-1 protein that is 478 aa longer than that encoded by the *Pkd1*^{del34} mutant allele, show a more severe phenotype, as judged by embryonic lethality at E15.5, and also display a major vascular phenotype *(37)*. Studies of these various knockouts have shown that normal polycystin-1 is required for maintaining the structural integrity of the vasculature and in epithelial and chondrocyte development. The studies also suggest that the molecular nature of mutation at the PKD1 locus may partly account for the phenotypic variability seen in ADPKD *(37)*.

Interestingly, heterozygous *Pkd1*$^{+/del34}$ mice progressively developed scattered renal and hepatic cysts. Cysts were seen from the cortex to the inner medulla. Glomerular cysts were common. Cysts were often surrounded by atrophic parenchyma with interstitial fibrosis and inflammation. EGFR was mislocalized to apical membranes in cysts and some slightly dilated tubules, suggesting that EGFR mis-localization may serve as an early marker of cystic transformation in polycystin-1 deficiency. Liver cysts were filled with clear or dark-brown fluid, which represents the bile salt-independent fraction of bile, indicating that the cyst epithelia, although originating from biliary ductule epithelia, had altered secretory function. This is similar to the human condition, and supports the hypothesis that fluid accumulation in the cysts is primarily the result of increased secretion from the cystic epithelia. The prominent liver changes, combined with the absence of liver cysts in perinatal homozygotes, suggest that polycystin-1 is required in the maintenance—but not the formation—of biliary ducts. The gradual recruitment of cysts and the absence of polycystin-1 in some renal cysts in the *Pkd1*$^{+/del34}$ heterozygous animals are consistent with clinical progression in man *(38)*. It is also consistent with the "two hit" model for cyst development. According to this theory, the germline mutation is insufficient to initiate cyst formation; however, if the wild-type allele required to generate the normal protein is altered by somatic mutation, then the affected cell initiates the cyst phenotype *(39)*.

4.2. Pkd1 *Transgenic Mice*

Two transgenic lines, each with 30 copies of a 108-kb human genomic fragment containing the entire *Pkd1* gene plus the tuberous sclerosis gene, have been established. Transgenic animals often show hepatic cysts, bile-duct proliferation, and renal cystic phenotype, with multiple cysts that are mainly of glomerular origin. Both transgenic lines were found to rescue the embryonic lethal phenotype of the homozygous $Pkd1^{del34/del34}$ animals, demonstrating that the human polycystin-1 can complement for the loss of the endogenous murine protein. The rescued animals were viable into adulthood, although more than one-half of them developed hepatic cystic disease in later life. Studies from this transgenic model of PKD suggest that the level of polycystin-1 may be an important parameter in regulating renal cyst formation *(40)*.

4.3. Pkd2-*Targeted Knockout*

Wu et al., using embryonic stem-cell technology, introduced mutant exon 1 in tandem with the wild-type exon 1 at the mouse *Pkd2* locus. This resulted in an unstable allele ($Pkd2^{WS25}$) that underwent somatic inactivation by intragenic homologous recombination to produce a true null allele. Mice that were heterozygous ($Pkd2^{+/WS25}$) and homozygous ($Pkd2^{WS25/WS25}$) for this mutation developed polycystic kidney and liver lesions that were indistinguishable from human ADPKD. However, the kidneys from the $Pkd2^{WS25/WS25}$ mice showed a more severe but considerably heterogeneous renal phenotype when compared to the kidneys from the $Pkd2^{+/WS25}$ mice. Renal cysts arose from renal tubular cells that lost the capacity to produce Pkd2 protein. Somatic loss of *Pkd2* expression in heterozygous animals was both necessary and sufficient for renal cyst formation, suggesting a cellular recessive mechanism of cyst formation. Wu et al. also introduced a true null ($Pkd2^-$) mutation. The $Pkd2^{-/-}$ mice, which died in utero between embryonic d E 13.5 and parturition, had structural defects in cardiac septation and cyst formation in maturing nephrons and pancreatic ducts. Despite the absence of cystic disease, the adult $Pkd2^{+/-}$ mice had a shorter lifespan compared to their wild-type litter-mates, suggesting the deleterious effect of polycystin-2 haploinsufficiency on long-term survival. These two models have shown that in addition to the role of polycystin-2 in maintenance of renal function, the protein is also essential for the normal development of the interventricular and interatrial septa and the pancreatic duct *(41)*.

5. Molecular Mechanisms of PKD

PKD has puzzled the scientific community for many years. Recent work on the various forms of animal and human PKD by different groups with expertise in diverse fields have clearly shown the multifactorial nature of this disease. Strikingly, although caused by different gene defects, the phenotype involves three central elements (**Fig. 1**). First, there is abnormal epithelial cell proliferation of the epithelial lining around the cyst lumen that accounts for the progressive increase in the surface area of the cyst. Second, epithelial cells lining the macroscopic cysts, which are predominant in PKD, show a net trans-epi-

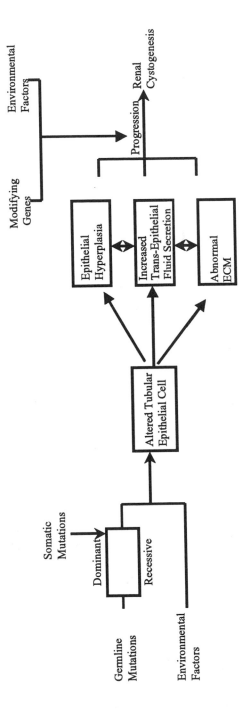

Fig. 1. A schematic representation of the factors that affect the etiology of polycystic kidney disease.

23

thelial fluid secretion (directed toward the cyst lumen) resulting from a faulty signaling that accounts for the fluid accumulation within the cysts. Third, changes in the tubular basement membrane and the extracellular matrix (ECM) of the expanding cyst could result in the disruption of the cytoskeletal-ECM and the cell-matrix interactions.

As mentioned previously, one of the common features in the various animal models of PKD is the augmented expression of several genes such as c-myc, c-fos, and c-ki-ras which are associated with cellular proliferation. In addition, renal cystic changes occur in transgenic mice that express activated proto-oncogenes (c-myc) and growth factors (hGF), which suggests that cellular proliferation may be the central driving force in cyst formation in PKD.

The factors that convert normally reabsorptive renal epithelial cells into the secretory cells responsible for cyst fluid accumulation have not yet been elucidated. It has been proposed that the epithelial cells of the cyst mimic the behavior of the epithelial cells derived from the intestine, where changes in the state of cellular differentiation may account for the functional differences between secretory and absorptive phenotype. It has therefore been suggested that the Cl⁻ and fluid secretion by the cystic cells may be the direct result of the inability of tubular epithelial cells to terminally differentiate rather than the presence of abnormal transport mechanism *(42)*.

ECM composition is known to be important in regulating the growth, shape, and state of differentiation of the overlying epithelial cells. In turn, the state of differentiation of the overlying epithelial cell influences the pattern of ECM synthesis. It has therefore been proposed that defective interactions between the tubular epithelial cells and the ECM may be the initiating event in cyst formation. It is evident that the three central pathogenic characteristics seen in the various animal and human forms of the cystic disease—increased cell proliferation, altered ECM composition, and fluid accumulation—might influence each other and therefore cannot be studied as independent features.

Kidney development begins with the reciprocal interactions between the ureteric bud and the metanephric mesenchyme that lead to condensation of the metanephric mesenchyme, which then aggregates into pretubular clusters and undergoes epithelialization to form renal tubules. Subsequent morphogenesis and differentiation of the tubular epithelium lead to the establishment of a functional nephron *(43)*. Grantham et al. have suggested that the continued proliferation of the cystic epithelium may be a consequence of the failure of renal tubular epithelial cells to terminally differentiate *(42)*. This state of immaturity of the renal epithelial cells may either be the result of an arrest in its maturation during renal development or the permanent de-differentiation state of the normal tubular epithelium, acquired as a result of an environmental insult such as an injury. Many of the genes whose mutation lead to PKD in the various animal models may act in common or interrelated pathways involved in the formation or maintenance of renal tubules.

Future research should be focused on a better understanding of the cascade of pathological events and the normal function of the gene mutated in each of these rodent models of PKD. Deciphering the interrelationship between the various models of PKD will help us deduce biological pathways that are important in maintaining the function/stability of the kidney. Generation and analysis of compound homozygous and heterozygous mutant animals by intercrossing the various mutant models will provide answers regarding the interrelationship between the various models. In addition, modifier genes and environmental factors that are known to alter the severity of the renal disease in some of the animal models can also be used as additional determinants to further define the interrelationship between the various models. These studies will help in the identification of pathways and cellular processes involved in the normal interaction between epithelial cells and their environment and will provide additional avenues to develop therapeutic interventions to treat this devastating human disease.

References

1. Harris, P. C., Ward, C. J., Peral, B., and Hughes, J. (1995) Autosomal dominant polycystic kidney disease: molecular analysis. *Hum. Mol. Genet.* **4**, 1745–1749.
2. Sessa, A., Meroni, M., Righetti, M., Battini, G., Maglio, A., and Puricelli, S. L. (2001) Autosomal recessive polycystic kidney disease. *Contrib. Nephrol.* **136**, 50–56.
3. Hughes, J., Ward, C. J., Peral, B., Aspinwall, R., Clark, K., San Millan, J. L., et al. (1995) The polycystic kidney disease 1 (PKD1) gene encodes a novel protein with multiple cell recognition domains. *Nat. Genet.* **10**, 151–160.
4. Mochizuki, T., Wu, G., Hayashi, T., Xenophontos, S. L., Veldhuisen, B., Saris, J. J., et al. (1996) PKD2, a gene for polycystic kidney disease that encodes an integral membrane protein. *Science* **272**, 1339–1342.
5. Ward, C. J., Hogan, M. C., Rossetti, S., Walker, D., Sneddon, T., Wang, X., et al. (2002) The gene mutated in autosomal recessive polycystic kidney disease encodes a large, receptor-like protein. *Nat. Genet.* **30**, 259–269.
6. Peters, D. J. and Breuning, M. H. (2001) Autosomal dominant polycystic kidney disease: modification of disease progression. *Lancet* **358**, 1439–1444.
7. Zerres, K., Rudnik-Schoneborn, S., Steinkamm, C., Becker, J., and Mucher, G. (1998) Autosomal recessive polycystic kidney disease. *J. Mol. Med.* **76**, 303–309.
8. McDonald, R. A. and Avner, E. D. (1996) Mouse models of polycystic kidney disease, in *Polycystic Kidney Disease* (Watson, M.L., and Torres, V.E., eds.), Oxford University Press, Oxford, pp. 63–87.
9. Schieren, G., Pey, R., Bach, J., Hafner, M., and Gretz, N. (1996) Murine models of polycystic kidney disease. *Nephrol. Dial. Transplant.* **11** (**Suppl. 6**), 38–45.

10. Woo, D. D., Nguyen, D. K., and Khatibi, N., and Olsen, P. (1997) Genetic identification of two major modifier loci of polycystic kidney disease progression in pcy mice. *J. Clin. Invest.* **100**, 1934–1940.

11. Iakoubova, O. A., Duskin, H., and Beier, D. R. (1995) Localization of a murine recessive polycystic kidney disease mutation and modifying loci that affect disease severity. *Genomics* **26**, 107–114.

12. Upadhya, P., Churchill, G., Birkenmeier, E. H., Barker, J. E., and Frankel, W. N. (1999) Genetic modifiers of polycystic kidney disease in intersubspecific KAT2J mutants. *Genomics* **58**, 129–137.

13. Davisson, M., Guay-Woodford, L., Harris, W., and D'Eustachio, P. (1991) The mouse polycystic kidney disease mutation (cpk) is located on proximal chromosome 12. *Genomics* **9**, 778–781.

14. Gattone, V. H., MacNaudhton, K. A., and Kraybill, A. L. (1996) Murine autosomal recessive polycystic kidney disease with multiorgan involvement induced by the cpk gene. *Anat. Rec.* **245**, 488–499.

15. Hou, X., Mrug, M., Yoder, B. K., Lefkowitz, E. J., Kremmidiotis, G., D'Eustachio, P., et al. (2002) Cystin, a novel cilia-associated protein, is disrupted in the cpk mouse model of polycystic kidney disease. *J. Clin. Invest.* **109**, 533–540.

16. Woo, D. D., Miao, S. Y., Pelayo, J. C., and Woolf, A. S. (1994) Taxol inhibits progression of congenital polycystic kidney disease. *Nature* **368**, 750–753.

17. Nagao, S., Watanabe, T., Ogiso, N., Marunouchi, T., and Takahashi, H. (1995) Genetic mapping of the polycystic kidney gene, pcy, on mouse chromosome 9. *Biochem. Genet.* **33**, 401–412.

18. Takahashi, H., Calvet, J. P., Dittemore-Hoover, D., Yoshida, K., Grantham, J. J. and Gattone, V. H. (1991) A hereditary model of slowly progressive polycystic kidney disease in the mouse. *J. Am. Soc. Nephrol.* **1**, 980–989.

19. Nakamura, T., Ebihara, I., Nagaoka, I., Tomino, Y., Nagao, S., Takahashi, H., et al. (1993) Growth factor gene expression in kidney of murine polycystic kidney disease. *J. Am. Soc. Nephrol.* **3**, 1378–1386.

20. Guay-Woodford, L. M., Bryda, E. C., Christine, B., Lindsey, J. R., Collier, W. R., Avner, E. D., et al. (1996) Evidence that two phenotypically distinct mouse PKD mutations, bpk and jcpk, are allelic. *Kidney Int.* **50**, 1158–1165.

21. Janaswami, P. M., Birkenmeier, E. H., Cook, S. A., Rowe, L. B., Bronson, R. T., and Davisson, M. T. (1997) Identification and genetic mapping of a new polycystic kidney disease on mouse chromosome 8. *Genomics* **40**, 101–107.

22. Vogler, C., Homan, S., Pung, A., Thorpe, C., Barker, J., Birkenmeier, E. H., et al. (1999) Clinical and pathologic findings in two new allelic murine models of polycystic kidney disease. *J. Am. Soc. Nephrol.* **10**, 2534–2539.

23. Upadhya, P., Birkenmeier, E. H., Birkenmeier, C. S., and Barker, J. E. (2000) Mutations in a NIMA-related kinase gene, Nek1, cause pleiotropic effects including a progressive polycystic kidney disease in mice. *Proc. Natl. Acad. Sci. USA* **97**, 217–221.

24. Atala, A., Freeman, M. R., Mandell, J., and Beier, D. R. (1993) Juvenile cystic kidneys (jck): a new mouse mutation which causes polycystic kidneys. *Kidney Int.* **43**, 1081–1085.

25. Zeier, M., Pohlmeyer, G., Deerberg, F., Schonherr, R., and Ritz, E. (1994) Progression of renal failure in the Han: SPRD polycystic kidney rat. *Nephrol. Dial. Transplant.* **9**, 1734–1739.

26. Griffin, M. D., Torres, V. E., and Kumar R. (1997) Cystic kidney diseases. *Curr. Opin. Nephrol. Hypertens.* **6**, 276–283.

27. Lager, D. J., Qian, Q., Bengal, R. J., Ishibashi, M., and Torres, V. E. (2001) The pck rat: a new model that resembles human autosomal dominant polycystic kidney and liver disease. *Kidney Int.* **59**, 126–36.

28. Moyer, J. H., Lee-Tischler, M. J., Kwon, Heajoon-Y., Schrick, J. J., Avner, E. D., Sweeney, W. E., et al. (1994) Candidate gene associated with a mutation causing recessive polycystic kidney disease in mice. *Science* **264**, 1329–1333.

29. Murcia, N. S., Sweeney, W. E., Jr., and Avner, E. D. (1999) New insights into the molecular pathophysiology of polycystic kidney disease. *Kidney Int.* **55**, 1187–1197.

30. Yoder, B. K., Tousson, A., Millican, L., Wu, J. H., Bugg, C. E. Jr., Schafer, J. A., et al. (2002) Polaris, a protein disrupted in orpk mutant mice, is required for assembly of renal cilium. *Am. J. Physiol. Renal. Physiol.* **282**, F541–F552.

31. Trudel, M., Barisoni, L., Lanoix, J., and D'Agati, V. (1998) Polycystic kidney disease in SBM transgenic mice: role of c-myc in disease induction and progression. *Am. J. Pathol.* **152**, 219–229.

32. Veis, D. J., Sorenson, C. M., Shutter, J. R., and Korsmeyer, S. J. (1993) Bcl-2-deficiency mice demonstrate fulminant lymphoid apoptosis, polycystic kidneys, and hypopigmented hair. *Cell* **75**, 229–240.

33. Sorenson, C. M. and Sheibani, N. (2002) Altered regulation of SHP-2 and PTP 1B tyrosine phosphatases in cystic kidneys from bcl-2 -/- mice. *Am. J. Physiol. Renal. Physiol.* **282**, F442–F450.

34. Somlo, S. and Markowitz, G. S. (2002) The pathogenesis of autosomal dominant polycystic kidney disease: an update. *Curr. Opin. Nephrol. Hypertens.* **4**, 385–394.

35. Calvet, J. P. and Grantham, J. J. (2001) The genetics and physiology of polycystic kidney disease. *Semin. Nephrol.* **21**, 107–123.

36. Lu,W., Shen, X., Pavlova, A., Lakkis, M., Ward, C. J., Pritchard, L., et al. (2001) Comparison of Pkd1-targeted mutants reveals that loss of polycystin-1 causes cystogenesis and bone defects. *Hum. Mol. Genet.* **10**, 2385–2396.

37. Kim, K., Drummond, I., Ibraghimov-Beskrovnaya, O., Klinger, K., and Arnaout, M. A. (2000) Polycystin 1 is required for the structural integrity of blood vessels. *Proc. Natl. Acad. Sci. USA* **97**, 1731–1736.

38. Lu, W., Fan, X., Basora, N., Babakhanlou, H., Law, T., Rifai, N., et al. (1999) Late onset of renal and hepatic cysts in Pkd1-targeted heterozygotes. *Nat. Genet.* **21**, 160–161.

39. Qian. F., Watnick, T. J., Onuchic, L. F., and Germino, G. G. (1996) The molecular basis of focal cyst formation in human autosomal dominant polycystic kidney disease type I. *Cell* **87**, 979–987.

40. Pritchard, L., Sloane-Stanley, J. A., Sharpe, J. A., Aspinwall, R., Lu, W., Buckle, V., et al. (2000) A human PKD1 transgene generates functional polycystin-1 in mice and is associated with a cystic phenotype. *Hum. Mol. Genet.* **9**, 2617–2627.

41. Wu, G., Markowitz, G. S., Li, L., D'Agati, V. D., Factor, S. M., Geng, L., et al. (2000) Cardiac defects and renal failure in mice with targeted mutations in Pkd2. *Nat. Genet.* **24**, 75–78.
42. Sullivan, L. P., Wallace, D. P., and Grantham, J. J. (1998) Epithelial transport in polycystic kidney disease. *Physiol. Rev.* **78**, 1165–1191.
43. Lechner, M. S. and Dressler, G. R. (1997) The molecular basis of embryonic kidney development. *Mech. Dev.* **62**, 105–120.

3

Rat Models of the Metabolic Syndrome

Stevan P. Tofovic and Edwin K. Jackson

1. Introduction

For some diseases, a line of causality exists in which a given antecedent elicits a particular disorder, which can be treated by interrupting a specific pathway of events. Most biomedical scientists have uncritically adopted the "line-of-causality" metaphor, and have therefore selected for study animal models of disease in which this metaphor by design must work because the models are chosen accordingly. Although peer review rewards the use of such models, and research with linear models of disease is often intellectually satisfying, it is doubtful that such an approach in the end will lead to breakthroughs for the treatment of the major diseases facing humankind today, such as cancer and cardiovascular disease.

Perhaps a more appropriate metaphor for the pathophysiology of diseases such as cancer and cardiovascular disease is a "web of causality"—an intermingling set of causes that reinforce one another through a network of highly complex interactions. Frustratingly, the outcome of pharmacologically manipulating a web of causality is much less predictable, and in some cases simply unknowable. For this reason, it is critical to have animal systems at hand that accurately model the web-of-causality diseases. With such models, hypotheses regarding how to effectively intervene in the causal network can be accurately, rapidly, and relatively inexpensively tested in preclinical studies.

The purpose of this chapter is to describe several web-of-causality rat models for the metabolic syndrome. The metabolic syndrome is characterized by the deadly triad of hypertension, insulin resistance, and hyperlipidemia (1), and is often accompanied by obesity (2,3). We selected the metabolic syndrome because: i) the metabolic syndrome is a prototypical web-of-causality disease; ii) the metabolic syndrome is a leading cause of morbidity and mortality in

From: *Methods in Molecular Medicine, vol. 86: Renal Disease: Techniques and Protocols*
Edited by: M. S. Goligorsky © Humana Press Inc., Totowa, NJ

modern societies *(3,4)*; iii); the metabolic syndrome carries a high risk for renal disease *(5,6)* and iv) rat models of the metabolic syndrome are now readily available and reasonably well-described.

2. A Brief History of the Development of Rat Models of the Metabolic Syndrome

2.1. Obese and Lean Zucker Rat

In 1961, Zucker and Zucker *(7)* at the Laboratory of Comparative Pathology in Stow, Massachusetts noticed a spontaneous mutation in an outbred stock of rats that produced obesity in homozygotes with only mild insulin resistance and normoglycemia (pre-diabetic state). Homozygotes for the mutation are now referred to as "obese Zucker rats," and heterozygotes for the mutation or homozygous normal are known as "lean Zucker rats." Heterozygous, lean Zucker rats are not obese or pre-diabetic. It was not until 1996 that Chua et al. *(8)* demonstrated this mutation to be caused by a single nucleotide substitution (A to C transition) at position 880 of the leptin-receptor gene, resulting in an amino acid substitution (Gln to Pro) at position 269. This single amino acid substitution eventuates a leptin-receptor that has a greatly reduced binding affinity for leptin *(9)*. This allelic variant of the leptin receptor gene has been variously referred to as *fa*, Lepr^{fa}, or Ob-R^{fa}, but usually just *fa*.

2.2. Obese and Lean Zucker Diabetic Fatty (ZDF) Rat

The Zuckers distributed Zucker rats to a number of laboratories, including the laboratory of Dr. Walter Shaw at Eli Lilly. In 1977, Dr. Shaw transferred some of his Zucker rats to Dr. Julia Clark at the Indiana University School of Medicine, and Dr. Clark noted that some of the male obese Zucker rats were diabetic *(10)*, although the expression of this trait was inconsistent. Dr. Richard Peterson at Indiana acquired the Clark colony, re-derived the diabetic lineage, and inbred the diabetic trait in the obese males *(11,12)*, thus establishing the ZDF rat.

Like obese Zucker rats, obese ZDF rats are homozygous for the *fa* allele. Male obese ZDF rats express a number of abnormalities including: i) glucose intolerance that worsens with age; ii) hyperglycemia that develops between 7 and 10 wk of age; iii) early hyperinsulinemia that quickly decreases as the β-cells fatigue; iv) hyperlipidemia; v) mild nephropathy with hydronephrosis; vi) impaired wound healing; and vii) hyperleptinemia *(12)*. Female obese ZDF rats do not express the diabetic phenotype on regular rat chow, but develop the diabetic phenotype when consuming a diabetogenic diet *(12)*. Lean ZDF rats, whether male or female and whether heterozygous or homozygous, do not express the diabetic phenotype.

2.3. Spontaneously Hypertensive Rat (SHR) and Wistar-Kyoto (WKY) Rat

In the early 1960s, Drs. Aoki and Okamoto at Kyoto University developed the SHR by breeding an outbred Wistar male with spontaneous hypertension and a female with slightly higher than normal blood pressure *(13)*. The offspring were inbred (brother × sister) by careful selection for the hypertensive phenotype. At F13, Aoki and Okamoto supplied a breeding stock of SHR to the NIH, and this strain is now designated SHR/N. In 1971, the NIH established normotensive "control" rats by inbreeding (brother × sister) a colony of Wistar rats from which the SHR were derived. These normotensive control rats are now referred to as WKY rats.

The cause of hypertension in SHR is polygenic, but not yet understood. Hypertension develops beginning at approx 6 wk of age. There are considerable genetic differences between SHR and WKY rats, and, therefore, no ideal control exists for SHR *(14)*. Nonetheless, the SHR is a very useful model of genetic hypertension because drugs that lower blood pressure in SHR also decrease blood pressure in humans with essential hypertension. Investigators have used SHRs extensively (more than 12,000 articles in Medline) and for more than 30 yr to test antihypertensive drugs and to examine mechanisms of genetic hypertension *(14)*. SHR generally do not evolve either renal failure or heart failure, although a stroke-prone substrain has been developed *(15)*.

2.4. Obese and Lean Koletsky Rat

Dr. Richard Koletsky and colleagues developed the Koletsky rat in 1969 *(16)*. In 1968, these investigators obtained a female SHR/N from the NIH colony and crossed this female with a male Sprague-Dawley rat. They then inbred the offspring with a hypertensive phenotype. Importantly, after several generations of inbreeding, an obese phenotype appeared among some of the litters, and thus began the Koletsky strain. Investigators at Case Western Reserve University School of Medicine have continuously inbred (brother × sister) lean heterozygous Koletsky rats that carry the obesity gene from 1971 to the present (>60 generations of inbreeding).

In 1996, Takaya et al. *(17)* determined that obese Koletsky rats have a nonsense mutation in the leptin-receptor gene (T to A transition at position +2289) which codes for a premature stop codon in the extracellular domain of the leptin receptor (position 763). This mutated allele for the leptin receptor is variably known as cp, k, fa^{cp}, fa^k, Lepr^k, or Ob-R^k. If homozygous for the fa^{cp} allele, the animal is an obese Koletsky rat, and if not, the animal is a lean Koletsky rat.

Obese Koletsky rats have an interesting phenotype which includes: i) severe hypertension (similar to SHR in this regard); ii) hyperlipidemia (markedly elevated triglycerides and moderately elevated cholesterol); iii) fasting hyperinsulinemia, insulin resistance, but normal fasting glucose levels; iv) severe nephropathy (proteinuria and focal segmental glomerulosclerosis); v) high circulating levels of leptin; and vi) death at 225–375 d as a result of renal failure. Before 1980, obese Koletsky rats expressed vascular pathology; however, since that time this phenotype has disappeared *(18)*.

2.5. Obese and Lean Spontaneously Hypertensive and Heart Failure (SHHF/Mcc-fa^{cp}, SHR/N-cp, SHR/N:Mcc-cp, SHHF/Mcc-cp) Rat

The obese Koletsky rat was backcrossed for seven generations onto the SHR/N, and then transferred to Dr. Sylvia McCune's facility at Ohio State University *(19)*. Dr. McCune conducted selective breeding to reduce the incidence of spontaneous tumors and to decrease the age at which animals develop congestive heart failure (CHF). Today, obese males that are fed a diet containing 0.001% estrone (to render them able to breed) are bred with heterozygous females so that all offspring possess the *fa^{cp}* gene. The offspring that are obese homozygotes are known as obese SHHF/Mcc-*fa^{cp}*, and those that are heterozygotes are called lean SHHF/Mcc-*fa^{cp}*.

Obese males have overt diabetes, and obese females have insulin resistance, yet heterozygotes have normal insulin sensitivity. All SHHF/Mcc-*fa^{cp}*, regardless of genotype or gender, eventually develop spontaneous dilated cardiomyopathy (subcutaneous edema, dyspnea, cyanosis, lethargy, piloerection, cold tails, enlarged hearts, thickened ventricles, dilated heart chambers, hepatomegaly, ascites, pulmonary edema, and pleural effusions). However, the age of expression of overt symptoms of CHF is highly dependent on both genotype and gender. Obese male SHHF rats develop CHF at 10–13 mo of age, obese females and lean heterozygote males at 14–18 mo, and lean heterozygote females at about 2 yr. Animals are severely hypertensive until the onset of severe CHF, and then blood pressure falls to normotensive levels. Proteinuria also develops with the same genotype and gender dependency as described for CHF, and renal histopathology is consistent with diabetic nephropathy. The obese animals have elevated triglycerides and cholesterol.

2.6. Obese and Lean ZSF$_1$ Rats

The ZSF$_1$ (previously ZDF × SHHF, ZSF1) rat is the most recently produced rat strain for the metabolic syndrome *(20)*, and contains genes from all of the rat strains described here. It is generated by crossing a female heterozygous lean ZDF rat with a male heterozygous lean SHHF/Mcc-*fa^{cp}* rat. Obese ZSF$_1$ are *fa/fa^{cp}* at the leptin receptor gene locus, and lean ZSF$_1$ are either +/*fa*, +/*fa^{cp}* or +/+ at the leptin-receptor gene locus. We have extensively character-

Table 1
Cholesterol and Triglyceride Levels
in Male Lean and Obese ZSF$_1$ Rats (n = 6 to 10) at Various Ages

Strain	Age	Cholesterol (mg/dL)	Triglycerides (mg/dL)
Obese ZSF$_1$	12 wk	196 ± 8	970 ± 6
	14 wk	248 ± 12	
	19 wk	286 ± 8	5200 ± 72
	29 wk	632 ± 39	4351 ± 550
	38 wk	1199 ± 172	390 ± 101
	47 wk	320 ± 41	
Lean ZSF$_1$	12 wk	93 ± 4	104.6 ± 7.2
	14 wk	84 ± 4	
	19 wk	81 ± 6	194 ± 23
	29 wk	109 ± 4	

Data were obtained in conscious animals from tail-vein blood samples.

ized the male obese ZSF$_1$ rat in our laboratories at the University of Pittsburgh, and have utilized this animal model to investigate the cardiorenal protective effects of several drugs. In our view, the male obese ZSF$_1$ rat represents the most useful model to date of the metabolic syndrome. In the following section, we summarize our experience with this model.

3. Phenotype of Male Obese ZSF$_1$ Rats
3.1. Dyslipidemia

An important feature of the metabolic syndrome and a cardinal phenotype of the male obese ZSF$_1$ rat is abnormally high plasma levels of cholesterol and triglycerides. In this regard, male obese ZSF$_1$ rats are similar to male obese SHHF/Mcc-*fa*[cp] rats, and both of these strains have much higher cholesterol and triglyceride levels compared with male SHR, WKY, lean SHHF/Mcc-*fa*[cp] or lean ZSF$_1$ rats *(20)*. **Table 1** compares plasma lipid levels in male obese ZSF$_1$ vs male lean ZSF$_1$ at various ages. As illustrated, hyperlipidemia is present in male obese ZSF$_1$ rats at least by 12 wk of age, and progressively worsens until approx 38 wk of age. By 47 wk of age, cholesterol and triglyceride levels are reduced from the peak levels observed at 38 wk of age, but remain markedly elevated. The reduction in plasma lipids in obese ZSF$_1$ at 47 wk of age is most likely a result of the fact that the animals become very susceptible to developing chronic renal failure, which causes them to reduce their food intake and lose body wt (**Table 2**).

Table 2

Metabolic and Renal Excretory Function Parameters in Male Adult (24–36 wk) and Aged (46–48 wk) WKY, SHR, Lean (Ln) or Obese (Ob) SHHF/Mcc-fa^{cp} and Obese ZSF$_1$ Rats (n = 6 to 10)

Parameters	WKY		SHR		Ln-SHHF	Ob-SHHF		Ob-ZSF$_1$	
	36 wk	47 wk	36 wk	47 wk	36 wk	24 wk	47 wk	36 wk	47 wk
Body wt (g)	634 ± 11.3	645 ± 14.4	413 ± 5.8	407 ± 9.5	440 ± 10.2	558 ± 11	672 ± 40	747 ± 12	654 ± 46
Food intake (g/kg/d)	35.7 ± 2.8	41.7 ± 1.3	43.9 ± 3.2	51.4 ± 2.1	61.1 ± 4.1	59.5 ± 1.9	40.6 ± 3.9	59.8 ± 4.1	35.1 ± 3.6
Fluid intake (mL/kg/d)	71.0 ± 3.8	73.0 ± 5.9	94.9 ± 2.7	109.8 ± 7.7	93.8 ± 6.7	142.7 ± 9.4	108.2 ± 14.6	109.9 ± 11.2	138.2 ± 13.5
Urine volume (mL/kg/d)	30.2 ± 4.4	46.0 ± 7.6	33.6 ± 4.4	47.3 ± 6.4	43.8 ± 3.6	81.1 ± 16.2	84.2 ± 10.2	94.0 ± 11.7	125.0 ± 12.7
Sodium excretion (mEq/kg/d)	2.0 ± 0.2	3.51 ± 0.25	2.3 ± 0.22	3.33 ± 0.26	3.2 ± 0.23	ND	3.18 ± 0.36	3.94 ± 0.43	3.37 ± 0.37
Potassium excretion (mEq/kg/d)	5.1 ± 0.44	10.5 ± 0.56	5.3 ± 0.30	10.5 ± 0.88	9.3 ± 0.41	ND	9.6 ± 0.87	10.7 ± 1.03	8.1 ± 0.83
Urinary protein (mg/kg/d)	58.2 ± 8.7	44.5 ± 7.6	93.1 ± 8.2	109.0 ± 21.0	572 ± 58.1	260.4 ± 27.8	2335 ± 427	782 ± 52	1668 ± 208
Plasma creatinine (mg/dL)	0.41 ± 0.03	0.66 ± 0.03	0.5 ± 0.07	0.97 ± 0.07	0.63 ± 0.06	0.44 ± 0.03	1.03 ± 0.3	0.83 ± 0.04	3.62 ± 0.59
Creatinine Clearance (L/kg/d)	7.2 ± 0.82	5.73 ± 0.34	5.7 ± 0.62	3.89 ± 0.39	3.3 ± 0.4	6.2 ± 0.27	2.41 ± 0.78	2.65 ± 0.35	0.67 ± 0.1

Data were obtained in conscious animals placed in metabolic cages for 48 h.

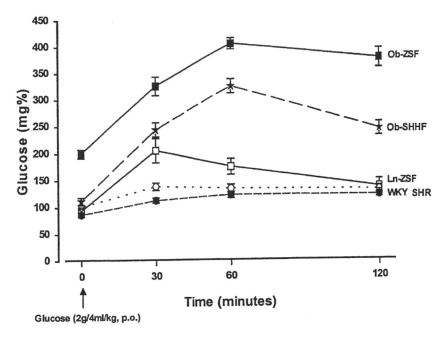

Fig. 1. Plasma glucose levels following an oral glucose challenge (2 g glucose per kg) in 16-wk-old normotensive Wistar Kyoto (WKY), Spontaneously Hypertensive rats (SHR), 19-wk-old lean ZSF$_1$ rats (Ln-ZSF) and obese ZSF$_1$ rats (Ob-ZSF) and obese SHHF/Mcc-*fa*^{cp} rats (Ob-SHHF).

3.2. Insulin Resistance and Type II Diabetes

Another defining characteristic of the metabolic syndrome is insulin resistance progressing to type II diabetes, and male obese ZSF$_1$ rats strongly display this phenotype. As shown in **Fig. 1**, the oral glucose tolerance test is impaired in 19-wk-old male obese ZSF$_1$ rats compared with 19-wk-old male lean ZSF$_1$, lean or obese SHHF/Mcc-*fa*^{cp}, SHR, or WKY rats. As illustrated in **Fig. 2**, 16-wk-old male obese ZSF$_1$ rats are hyperinsulinemic and respond to an oral glucose challenge with a larger increase in plasma insulin compared with the age-matched male lean ZSF$_1$ rats. Type II diabetes persists in older male obese ZSF$_1$ rats. In both the fasted and fed state, plasma glucose and insulin levels are higher in 38-wk-old male obese, compared with lean ZSF$_1$ rats (**Fig. 3**). Moreover, male obese ZSF$_1$ rats are more glucosuric compared with male lean ZSF$_1$ rats (**Fig. 4**) and more polyuric compared with age-matched male WKY, SHR, and lean and obese SHHF/Mcc-*fa*^{cp} (**Table 2**).

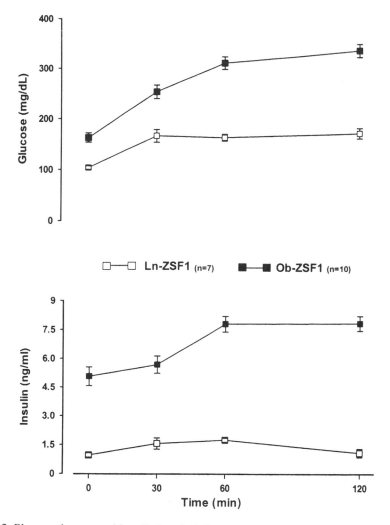

Fig. 2. Plasma glucose and insulin levels following an oral glucose challenge (2 g glucose per kg) in 16-wk-old lean ZSF_1 rats (Ln-ZSF1) and obese ZSF_1 rats (Ob-ZSF1).

3.3. Hypertension

The third component of the "deadly triad" is hypertension, and as illustrated in **Tables 3** and **4**, male obese ZSF_1 rats are hypertensive compared with WKY rats and have similar levels of mean arterial blood pressure and ventricular peak systolic pressure compared with male SHR, lean ZSF_1, and obese SHHF/Mcc-fa^{cp} rats.

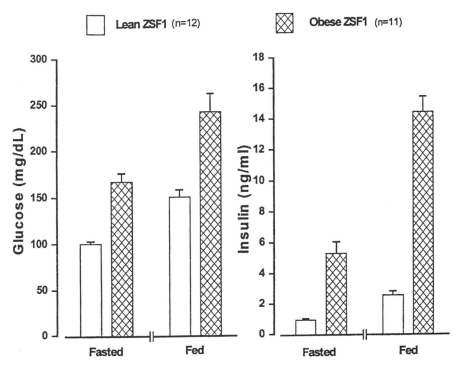

Fig. 3. Glucose and insulin levels in 38-wk-old lean and obese ZSF₁ (ZSF1) rats.

3.4. Obesity

In humans, the metabolic syndrome is usually, although not always, associated with obesity. Male obese ZSF₁ rats are hyperphagic compared to age-matched WKY and SHR rats (**Table 2**) and, at most ages, have a body wt greater than age-matched male WKY, SHR, lean and obese SHHF/Mcc-*fa*ᶜᵖ and lean ZSF₁ rats (**Tables 2, 3**). Very old, obese ZSF₁ begin to lose weight as they become seriously ill, so that by 47 wk of age, obese ZSF₁ may have the same body wt as WKY rats (**Table 2**). However, the fat distribution is strikingly different in old obese ZSF₁ (pear-shaped body structure with large deposits of fat in the abdominal cavity) compared with old WKY (more even distribution of body fat).

3.5. Left Ventricular Dysfunction

Obese ZSF₁ rats are derived from SHHF/Mcc-*fa*ᶜᵖ rats, and therefore some degree of left ventricular dysfunction would be expected. As shown in **Table 4**, compared with 47-wk-old male SHR, +dP/dtᵐᵃˣ (index of systolic function)

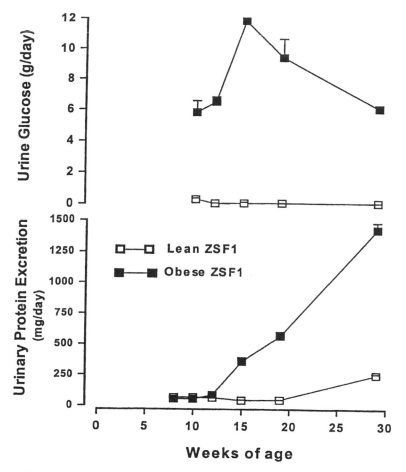

Fig. 4. Age-related changes in urinary glucose and protein excretion in lean and obese ZSF₁ (ZSF1) rats.

and –dP/dt^{max} (index of diastolic function) are mildly decreased and left-ventricular-end diastolic volume is increased in male obese ZSF₁ rats and are similar to levels observed in age-matched male lean and obese SHHF/Mcc-fa^{cp} rats. In evaluating left ventricular performance parameters, it is important to compare ZSF₁ and SHHF/Mcc-fa^{cp} rats to SHR, rather than WKY, because hypertension markedly influences the absolute values of +dP/dt^{max} and –dP/dt^{max}.

3.6. Nephropathy

Male obese ZSF₁ rats develop severe renal disease, and this is the usual cause of death in these animals. As shown in **Table 3**, renal blood flow and

Table 3

Renal Function in Male WKY, SHR, Lean (Ln) or Obese (Ob) ZSF$_1$ Rats and Obese SHHF/Mcc-fa^{cp} Rats (n = 8 to 10)

Parameter	WKY 14 wk	SHR 14 wk	Ob-SHHF 24 wk	Ln-ZSF$_1$ 16 wk	Ob-ZSF$_1$ 16 wk
Body wt (g)	412 ± 21	309 ± 10	558 ± 11	482 ± 5	626 ± 6
Total kidney weight (g)	3.29 ± 0.15	2.40 ± 0.12	3.35 ± 0.09	2.4 ± 0.06	4.16 ± 0.11
Kidney/body wt ratio (g/kg)	7.98 ± 0.4	7.76 ± 0.31	6.0 ± 0.27	4.96 ± 0.24	6.64 ± 0.31
Mean arterial blood pressure (mmHg)	112.9 ± 2.3	142.6 ± 4.8	143.2 ± 3.3	133.4 ± 1.9	151.4 ± 2.5
Renal blood flow (mL/min/g kidney)	5.76 ± 0.61	3.52 ± 0.53	4.93 ± 0.87	6.12 ± 0.4	2.11 ± 0.2
Renal plasma flow (mL/min/g kidney)	3.04 ± 0.33	1.62 ± 0.23	2.66 ± 0.41	2.62 ± 0.2	1.01 ± 0.08
Renal vascular resistance (mmHg/mL/min/g kid)	23.9 ± 2.3	48.6 ± 6.6	35.6 ± 5.5	23.2 ± 1.5	79.7 ± 6.8
Urine volume (mL/min/g kidney)	6.3 ± 1.4	4.4 ± 1.1	7.72 ± 1.7	19.1 ± 1.5	19.4 ± 1.6
Glomerular filtration rate (mL/min/g kidney)	1.41 ± 0.16	1.71 ± 0.4	0.95 ± 0.07	1.38 ± 0.1	0.77 ± 0.04
Sodium excretion (mEq/min/g kidney)	0.83 ± 0.33	0.42 ± 0.19	N.D.	0.66 ± 0.12	0.43 ± 0.15
Potassium excretion (mEq/min/g kidney)	1.01 ± 0.14	0.73 ± 0.22	N.D.	1.11 ± 0.10	0.79 ± 0.16

Data were obtained in anesthetized rats. Renal blood flow and glomerular filtration rate were measured using transit-time flowmetry and inulin clearance, respectively.

Table 4
Heart Function in Male Adult (24–36 wk of age) and Aged (47–56 wk of age) WKY, SHR, Lean (Ln) and Obese (Ob) SHHF/Mcc-fa^{cp} and Obese ZSF$_1$ Rats (n = 6 to 10)

Parameters	WKY 36 wk	WKY 47 wk	SHR 36 wk	SHR 47 wk	Ln-SHHF 36 wk	Ln-SHHF 56 wk	Ln-SHHF 24 wk	Ln-SHHF 47 wk	Ob-ZSF$_1$ 36 wk	Ob-ZSF$_1$ 47 wk
Heart rate (beats/min)	345 ± 15	345 ± 14	389 ± 10	379 ± 10	349 ± 9.3	362 ± 10	358 ± 9	358 ± 16	363 ± 4	349 ± 9
VPSP (mmHg)	158.7 ± 6.5	125.5 ± 4.4	201 ± 5.0	252 ± 15.8	202 ± 4.8	169.6 ± 10.1	174.2 ± 6.1	195 ± 15.3	188.6 ± 4.8	169.8 ± 17.7
+dP/dt^{max} (mmHg sec^{-1})	10452 ± 943	7651 ± 1319	14607 ± 1594	13551 ± 1505	13135 ± 1112	9834 ± 1482	10741 ± 920	11219 ± 1068	14539 ± 692	10153 ± 2074
–dP/dt^{max} (mmHg sec^{-1})	7079 ± 563	4642 ± 756	8991 ± 707	10103 ± 599	7844 ± 741	6410 ± 898	8303 ± 932	7690 ± 1217	7633 ± 293	5200 ± 1258
VEDP (mmHg)	6.6 ± 1.34	6.90 ± 1.87	6.6 ± 3.59	2.98 ± 2.42	6.37 ± 1.1	15.9 ± 1.93	2.21 ± 2.7	10.85 ± 3.77	2.98 ± 1.37	7.12 ± 2.30
VMDP (mmHg)	–6.8 ± 2.70	–1.90 ± 1.79	–6.1 ± 3.4	–9.23 ± 4.04	–2.3 ± 2.1	3.9 ± 1.36	–4.64 ± 3.97	–4.55 ± 3.33	–2.68 ± 1.81	–2.06 ± 0.94

VPSP, ventricular peak systolic pressure; +dP/dt^{max}, maximum dP/dt during ventricular contraction; –dP/dt^{max}, maximum –dP/dt during the ventricular relaxation; VEDP, ventricular end diastolic pressure; VMDP, ventricular minimum diastolic pressure. Data were obtained in anesthetized rats using a digital heart performance monitor.

glomerular filtration rate are decreased and renal vascular resistance is increased even in young adult (16-wk-old) male obese ZSF_1 rats compared with either male WKY, SHR, lean ZSF_1, or obese SHHF/Mcc-fa^{cp} rats. Proteinuria is much worse in male obese ZSF_1 rats compared with either male WKY, SHR, lean SHHF/Mcc-fa^{cp} or lean ZSF_1 rats (**Table 2, Fig. 4**). Histological analysis reveals that male obese ZSF_1 rats have worse glomerulosclerosis, tubular atrophy, tubular dilatation, cast formation, interstitial inflammation, interstitial fibrosis, medial hypertrophy, and arteriolar sclerosis compared with either SHR or WKY rats (*20*).

4. Response of Male Obese ZSF₁ Rats to Pharmacological Interventions

Our laboratory has begun to examine the effects of pharmacological interventions on the natural history of the metabolic syndrome in male obese ZSF_1 rats. The purpose of these studies is to identify promising pharmacological strategies for reducing cardiovascular/renal morbidity and mortality in human beings.

4.1. Angiotensin Converting Enzyme Inhibitors

The HOPE study has identified angiotensin-converting enzyme (ACE) inhibitors as drugs that reduced cardiovascular disease deaths, myocardial infarction, stroke, and overall mortality in patients at high risk for cardiovascular disease (*21*). Therefore, ACE inhibitors may have beneficial effects on the metabolic syndrome. To test this hypothesis, we treated 18-wk-old male obese ZSF_1 rats for 8 wk with enalapril (0.03% in the drinking water). Although enalapril significantly reduced blood pressure and glomerulosclerosis, it did not improve the dyslipidemia, type II diabetes, or obesity (*22*). In contrast, early (8 wk of age), long-term (30 wk) treatment with captopril (0.5% in the drinking solution) not only reduced blood pressure (–10%), proteinuria (–40%), glomerulosclerosis and renal tubulointerstitial changes, but also ameliorated the type II diabetes and lowered total cholesterol levels (–20%) (*23*). Body wt was unchanged. These studies indicate that ACE inhibitors may be useful for the metabolic syndrome; however, it may be necessary to initiate treatment when the patient is relatively young, and ACE inhibitors will not correct the obesity.

4.2. Estradiol Metabolites

In general, female rats of any of the previously described strains have a less severe phenotype compared to males. This gender dimorphism suggests that estradiol may significantly attenuate the metabolic syndrome. However, estradiol cannot be used in male patients with the metabolic syndrome because of the feminizing effects of estadiol and would have limited utility in female patients because of increased risk of cancer in hormone-sensitive tissues (e.g., breast and uterus).

Our recent in vitro studies suggest that non-estrogenic metabolites of estradiol, specifically 2-hydroxyestradiol and 2-methoxyestradiol, markedly inhibit the migration of, proliferation of, and extracellular matrix (ECM) production by vascular smooth-muscle cells, cardiac fibroblasts, and glomerular mesangial cells (24). These in vitro studies suggest that estadiol metabolites are useful in the metabolic syndrome.

To test this hypothesis, we treated male obese ZSF$_1$ rats for 24 wk with either 2-hydroxyestradiol or vehicle. Relative to the vehicle group, 2-hydroxyestradiol reduced food consumption, decreased body wt, lowered plasma levels of cholesterol, improved the oral glucose tolerance test, reduced glycated hemoglobin levels, attenuated glucosuria, polyuria, and polydipsia, reduced proteinuria, attenuated glomerulosclerosis, improved vascular endothelial function, and lowered arterial blood pressure (25). In summary, 2-hydroxyestradiol improved almost all aspects of the metabolic syndrome phenotype. These results demonstrate the utility of obese ZSF$_1$ rats and the promise of estradiol metabolites for the treatment of the metabolic syndrome.

4.3. Caffeine

A reduced rate of energy expenditure may contribute to the development of obesity, and a defect in energy expenditure occurs in obese rats with the *fa* mutation (26). This is most likely the result of leptin's inability—because of a mutated leptin receptor in the hypothalamus—to increase energy expenditure (27). The use of ephedrine-caffeine mixtures to increase energy expenditure may cause weight reduction in both humans and obese rats (28). Although caffeine is widely used, little attention has been payed to its metabolic and renal effects in the settings of obesity, hypertension, and insulin resistance.

Recently, we conducted short-term (8 wk) and long-term (30 wk) studies on the effects of caffeine consumption in adult (16 wk of age) and young (8 wk of age) obese male ZSF$_1$ rats, respectively (29,30). In both adult and young animals, caffeine reduced body wt, reduced glucosuria, improved insulin sensitivity, had no effects on triglycerides and glycerol levels, and significantly increased total cholesterol levels. Despite improved glucose control, caffeine augmented proteinuria and reduced the glomerular filtration rate in both age groups, and increased blood pressure, and induced more severe glomerular and tubulointerstitial changes in young animals. These experiments imply that the health consequences of chronic caffeine consumption may depend strongly on the underlying pathophysiology. They also confirm the utility of obese ZSF$_1$ rats, and warrant further studies of caffeine's effects in nephropathy associated with the metabolic syndrome.

Table 5
Phenotypes of Male Rat Models of the Metabolic Syndrome

	Hypertension	Dyslipidemia	Type II Diabetes	Obesity	Left Ventricular Dysfunction	Glomerulosclerosis
Lean Zucker	No	No	No	No	No	No
Obese Zucker	No	No	No	Yes	No	No
Lean ZDF	No	No	No	No	No	No
Obese ZDF	No	Yes	Yes	Yes	No	No (Hydronephrosis)
WKY	No	No	No	Yes (aged only)	No	No
SHR	Yes	No	No	No	No	No
Lean Koletsky	Yes	No	No	No	No	No
Obese Koletsky	Yes	Yes	No	Yes	No	Yes
Lean SHHF	Yes	No	No	No	Yes	No
Obese SHHF	Yes	Yes (Severe)	Yes	Yes	Yes (Severe)	Yes
Lean ZSF_1	Yes	No	No	No	No	No
Obese ZSF_1	Yes	Yes (Severe)	Yes (Severe)	Yes (Severe)	Yes	Yes (Severe)

5. Conclusion

Table 5 provides a direct phenotype comparison of the animal models discussed in this chapter. Of these animal systems, only four would qualify as models for the metabolic syndrome—male obese ZDF, obese Koletsky, obese SHHF/Mcc-fa^{cp}, and obese ZSF$_1$ rats. Obese ZDF rats have dyslipidemia, type II diabetes, and obesity. On the down side, obese ZDF rats are not truly hypertensive and do not express target-organ sequelae, such as left ventricular dysfunction and glomerulosclerosis. Moreover, obese ZDF rats usually express hydronephrosis *(31)*. Obese Koletsky rats express hypertension, dyslipidemia, obesity, and glomerulosclerosis, but do not have type II diabetes and have preserved left ventricular function. Both obese SHHF/Mcc-fa^{cp} and obese ZSF$_1$ rats exhibit hypertension, severe dyslipidemia, type II diabetes, obesity, left ventricular dysfunction, and glomerulosclerosis. Type II diabetes, obesity, and glomerulosclerosis are more severe in obese ZSF$_1$ compared with obese SHHF/Mcc-fa^{cp}, and obese ZSF$_1$ rats usually die of end stage renal disease. In contrast, SHHF/Mcc-fa^{cp} usually have more severe left ventricular dysfunction and usually die of congestive heart failure. The obese ZSF$_1$ rat is a genetic blend of all of the rats discussed in this chapter, and has the most severe metabolic syndrome. The decision to use obese ZSF$_1$ or obese SHHF/Mcc-fa^{cp} depends on the researcher's goal. If the researcher's objective requires the most severe type of metabolic syndrome or requires an animal model of the metabolic syndrome with severe renal disease, the obese ZSF$_1$ is most appropriate. However, if the research's goal is best achieved with a milder form of metabolic syndrome or if left ventricular dysfunction is particularly important, then the obese SHHF/Mcc-fa^{cp} is the more appropriate model system.

References

1. Reaven, G. M. (1988) Role of insulin resistance in human disease. *Diabetes* **37,** 1595–1607.
2. Rocchini, A. P. (1995) Insulin resistance, obesity and hypertension. *Am. J. Nutr.* **125,** 1718S–1724S.
3. Vega, G. L. (2001) Obesity, the metabolic syndrome, and cardiovascular disease. *Am. Heart J.* **142,** 1108–1116.
4. Isomaa, B., Almgren, P., Tuomi, T., Forsen, B., Lahti, K., Nissen, M., et al. (2001) Cardiovascular morbidity and mortality associated with the metabolic syndrome. *Diabetes Care* **24,** 683–689.
5. Marks, J. B. and Raskin, P. (1988) Nephropathy and hypertension in diabetes. *Med. Clin. N Am.* **82,** 877–907.
6. Sowers, J. R. and Epstein, M. (1995) Diabetes mellitus and associated hypertension, vascular disease and nephropathy. An update. *Hypertension* **26,** 869–879.
7. Zucker, L. M. and Zucker, T. F. (1961) Fatty, a new mutation in the rats. *J. Hered.* **52,** 275–287.

8. Chua, S. C., Jr., White, D. W., Wu-Peng, X. S., Liu, S. M., Okada, N., Kershaw, E. E., et al. (1996) Phenotype of fatty due to Gln269Pro mutation in the leptin receptor (Lepr). *Diabetes* **45**, 1141–1143.
9. White, D. W., Wang, Y., Chua, S. C., Jr., Morgenstern, J. P., Leibel, R. L., Baumann, H., et al. (1997) Constitutive and impaired signaling of leptin receptors containing the Gln → Pro extracellular domain *fatty* mutation. *Proc. Natl. Acad. Sci. USA* **94**, 10657–10662.
10. Clark, J. B., Palmer, C. J., and Shaw, W. N. (1983) The diabetic Zucker fatty rat. *Proc. Soc. Exp. Biol. Med.* **173**, 68–75.
11. Peterson, R. G., Shaw, W. N., Neel, M.-A., Little, L. A., and Eichberg, J. (1990) Zucker diabetic fatty rats as a model for non-insulin-dependent diabetes mellitus. *ILAR News* **32**, 16–19.
12. Peterson, R. G. (2000) The Zucker diabetic fatty (ZDF) rat, in *Animal Models of Diabetes: A Primer* (Sima, A. A. F. and Shafrir, E., eds.), Taylor and Francis, London, UK, pp. 109–128.
13. Okamoto, K. and Aoki, K. (1963) Development of a strain of spontaneously hypertensive rats. *Jpn. Circ. J.* **27**, 282–293.
14. Pinto, Y. M., Paul, M., and Ganten, D. (1998) Lessons from rat models of hypertension: from Goldblatt to genetic engineering. *Cardiovas. Res.* **39**, 77–88.
15. Yamori, Y., Tomimoto, K., Ooshima, A., Hazama, F., and Okamoto, K. (1974) Proceedings: developmental course of hypertension in the SHR-substrains susceptible to hypertensive cerebrovascular lesions. *Jpn. Heart J.* **15**, 209–210.
16. Koletsky, S. (1972) New type of spontaneously hypertensive rats with hyperlipemia and endocrine gland defects, in *Spontaneous Hypertension: Its Pathogenesis and Complications* (Okamoto, K., ed.), Igaku Shoin Ltd., Tokyo, Japan, pp. 194–197.
17. Takaya, K., Ogawa, Y., Hiraoka, J., Hosoda, K., Yamori, Y., Nakao, K., et al. (1996) Nonsense mutation of leptin receptor in the obese spontaneously hypertensive Koletsky rat. *Nat. Genet.* **14**, 130–131.
18. Koletsky, R. J., Friedman, J. E., and Ernsberger, P. (2000) The obese spontaneously hypertensive rats (SHROB, Koletsky rats): A model of metabolic syndrome X, in *Animal Models of Diabetes: A Primer* (Sima, A. A. F. and Shafrir, E., eds.), Taylor and Francis, London, UK, pp. 109–128.
19. McCune, S. A., Baker, P. B., and Stills, H. F. Jr. (1990) SHHF/Mcc-cp rat: model of obesity, non-insulin-dependent diabetes, and congestive heart failure. *ILAR News* **32**, 23–27.
20. Tofovic, S. P., Kusaka, H., Kost, C. K. Jr., and Bastacky, S. (2000) Renal function and structure in diabetic, hypertensive, obese, ZDFx SHHF-hybrid rats. *Renal Fail.* **22**, 387–406.
21. Yusuf, S., Sleight, P., Pogre, J., Bosch, J., Davies, R., and Dagenais, G. (2000) Effects of an angiotensin-converting-enzyme inhibitor, ramipril, on cardiovascular events in high-risk patients. *N. Engl. J. Med.* **342**, 145–153.
22. Tofovic, S. P., Kusaka, H., Jackson, E. K., and Bastacky, S. I. (1999) Renal function and structure in obese ZDFxSHHF (hybrid)fa/fa^{cp} rats treated with caffeine or enalapril. *J. Am. Soc. Nephrol.* **10**, 672A.

23. Kost, K. C., Jr., Bastacky, S. I., Jackson, E. K., and Tofovic, S. P. (2001) Renoprotective effects of angiotensin converting enzyme inhibition in an animal model of renal disease characterized by multiple risk factors. *J. Am. Soc. Nephrol.* **12,** 839A.

24. Dubey, R. K. and Jackson, E. K. (2001) Cardiovascular protective effects of 17β-estradiol metabolites. *J. Appl. Physiol.* **91,** 1868–1883.

25. Tofovic, S. P., Dubey, R. K., and Jackson, E. K. (2001) 2-Hydroxyestradiol attenuates the development of obesity, metabolic syndrome, and vascular and renal dysfunction in obese ZSF1 rats. *J. Pharmacol. Exp. Therap.* **299,** 973–977.

26. Planche, E., Joliff, M., de Gasquet P., and Leliepvre X. (1983) Evidence of a defect in energy expenditure in 7-day-old Zucker rat (fa/fa). *Am. J. Physiol.* **245,** E107–E113.

27. Meister, B. (2000) Control of food intake via leptin receptors in the hypothalamus. *Vitam. Horm.* **59,** 265–304.

28. Dulloo, A. G. and Miller, D. S. (1987) Reversal of obesity in the genetically obese fa/fa Zucker rat with ephedrine/methylxanthines thermogenic mixture. *J. Nutr.* **117,** 383–389.

29. Tofovic, S. P., Kost, C. Jr., Jackson, E. K., and Bastacky, S. I. (2002) Long-term caffeine consumption exacerbates renal failure in obese, diabetic, ZSF1 (fa/fa [cp]) rats. *Kidney Int.* **61,** 1433–1444.

30. Tofovic, S. P., Kusaka, H., Jackson E. K., and Bastacky, S. I. (2001) Renal and metabolic effects of caffeine in obese (fa/fa [cp]), diabetic, hypertensive, ZSF1 rats. *Renal Failure* **23,** 159–173.

31. Vora, J. P., Zimsen, S. M., Houghton, D. C., and Anderson, S. (1996) Evolution of metabolic and renal changes in the ZDF/Drt-fa rat model of type II diabetes. *J. Am. Soc. Nephrol.* **7,** 113–117.

4

Models of Glomerulonephritis

Raghu V. Durvasula and Stuart J. Shankland

1. Introduction

Understanding the mechanisms of glomerular injury is critically dependent on the histologic assessment of cellular responses, immune processes, and ultrastructural changes. However, studies of human disease have been limited by a relative lack of tissue sampling. Renal biopsy is often performed only when the diagnosis of glomerular disease cannot be determined based on clinical grounds or in conjunction with indirect markers such as serologies, complement levels, and urine microscopy. Furthermore, a biopsy is typically undertaken upon clinical presentation, thereby providing a mere "snapshot" of the disease. In the absence of serial histologic evaluation, the opportunity to delineate mechanisms of disease progression is limited. However, the use of animal models has overcome a number of these hurdles, thereby advancing our current knowledge and understanding of the pathogenesis of glomerular disease. Animal studies afford the opportunity to study the development, progression, and resolution of disease over time. Furthermore, the host response to injury may be deliberately modified, either generally (as with nonspecific immunosuppressants) or selectively (as with target gene deletions or neutralizing antibodies), thereby providing further insight into pathogenetic mechanisms that cannot be undertaken in man.

Animal models have not been without criticism. The induction of disease often requires the administration of antigens such as bovine serum albumin (BSA) or antibodies derived from an entirely different species. Alternatively, other models require that pharmacologic agents be repeatedly administered in supraphysiologic doses as in puromycin aminonucleoside nephrosis. As a result, it has been argued that such models are largely contrived, and bear little resemblance to human disease. Although the inciting events in such models often have no counterpart in human disease, the subsequent mechanisms of injury and mediators of disease progression are often common across species, and therefore very relevant to an understanding of human processes.

From: *Methods in Molecular Medicine, vol. 86: Renal Disease: Techniques and Protocols*
Edited by: M. S. Goligorsky © Humana Press Inc., Totowa, NJ

A wide variety of animal species have been used in the establishment of glomerular disease models. Rodent models are preferred for a number of reasons, including costs, low maintenance requirements for upkeep, proliferative capacity with short gestational periods, and ease of handling. Among rodents, most models are established in the rat species, perhaps because of their larger size and general susceptibility to renal injury. Mice have posed unique challenges related to species-specific inherent resistance to certain forms of injury, particularly complement-mediated immune processes. However, with recent advances in biogenetic engineering, it is now possible to create transgenic strains in which the function of specific genes may be selectively altered, either through overexpression or targeted deletion. As a result, there is renewed interest in established murine models of renal disease which afford the unique opportunity to decipher the specific role a particular gene plays in mediating disease progression *(1)*.

Animal models of glomerular disease have previously been classified based on mechanisms of immune injury *(2)* and relevance to human disease counterparts *(3)*. In this chapter, we have chosen to discuss models based on the glomerular cell that is the primary target of injury, recognizing that injury may not be limited to a single cellular constituent or structure, such that overlap may occur. Although a number of animal models have been summarized and referenced in **Table 1**, a detailed discussion will focus on the most established models that have made the greatest contribution to our present understanding of mechanisms of glomerular disease. Models of diabetic nephropathy are the focus of other chapters in this text. Similarly, models of lupus nephritis are beyond the scope of this chapter. For a detailed discussion, the reader is referred to recent reviews by Foster *(4)* and Peutz-Koostra et al. *(5)*.

2. Models of Visceral Epithelial-Cell (Podocyte) Injury

2.1. Puromycin Aminonucleoside Nephrosis

Since the first description by Frenk et al. almost 50 years ago, puromycin aminonucleoside (PAN) nephrosis has become one of the most widely studied models of glomerular disease. Considered by many to be an accurate experimental model of minimal-change disease, PAN nephrosis has fueled a large body of research into mechanisms of proteinuria.

2.1.1. Disease Induction

Although puromycin (an antibiotic derivative from *Streptomyces alboniger*) by itself does not cause nephrosis, PAN results in a toxic injury of the visceral glomerular epithelial cell, also known as the podocyte, with ensuing proteinuria. Rats are uniquely susceptible to this toxic effect, and attempts at establishing the PAN nephrosis model in other species have been largely disappointing. Many dosing regimens have been studied, ranging from daily low-dose subcutaneous (sc) injections (1.67 mg per 100 g body tissue) to single high-dose intraperito-neal (ip) injections (15 mg per 100 g body tissue) *(6,7)*.

2.1.2. Disease Course and Pathogenesis

Although the onset of disease varies depending on the species of rat and dos-ing regimen *(8)*, within a given species with constant dosing parameters, disease progresses in a very predictable manner. The abrupt onset of proteinuria occurs on d 5, and peaks by d 12, with eventual resolution by d 28. As with minimal-change disease in man, light microscopy is largely unrevealing in the first few days, although electron micrographs show podocyte vacuolization and foot-pro-cess effacement. Focal areas of epithelial detachment result in exposed glomeru-lar basement membrane (GBM) immediately prior to the development of severe proteinuria *(6)*. In vitro studies with cultured human podocytes revealing decreased α-3, β-1 integrin levels, and impaired cellular attachment in response to PAN exposure are consistent with the primary role of cellular detachment in the pathogenesis of proteinuria in this disease model *(9)*.

2.1.3. Relevance and Implications for Human Disease

Similar to minimal-change disease in humans, PAN nephrosis is associated with a selective increase in fractional clearance of albumin (relative to other proteins), suggesting that altered-charge selectivity of the glomerular capillary wall plays a role in proteinuria *(10)*. Although studies of the anionic sites of the GBM and levels of heparan sulfate have not been revealing *(11)*, a dramatic reduction in the podocyte polyanion podocalyxin has been demonstrated in PAN nephrosis, with associated impairment in sialylation *(12)*.

However, discrepancies exist between this animal model and minimal-change disease. Unlike the human counterpart, PAN nephrosis is associated with a marked tubulo-interstitial infiltrate of mononuclear cells, consisting initially of T-lymphocytes with the subsequent influx of macrophages by the second wk *(13)*. These histologic changes are often accompanied by a reduction in the glomerular filtration rate. Furthermore, over time (and especially with repeated administration of PAN), rats may develop chronic injury with histologic fea-tures of focal segmental glomerulosclerosis (FSGS). Nonetheless, the rat model of PAN nephrosis has contributed dramatically to our understanding of the podocyte response to injury and cell biology, including the identification of the novel protein *podoplanin (14)*, which may play a critical role in maintaining the structural integrity of foot processes and glomerular permeability *(15)*.

2.2. Adriamycin Nephropathy

Adriamycin nephropathy represents another model of podocyte injury resulting from a toxic insult. Unlike PAN nephrosis, in which repeated injec-tions are needed to induce chronic injury, the adriamycin nephropathy model

Table 1
Commonly Used Animal Models of Glomerular Disease

Model name	Primary site of injury	Species	Mechanism of injury	Characteristics	Refs.
PAN nephrosis	Podocyte	Rat	Direct cellular toxicity of aminonucleoside	Proteinuria caused by selective podocyte injury. Typically self-limited disease. Resembles minimal-change disease.	6,7
Adriamycin nephropathy	Podocyte	Rat, mouse	Direct cellular toxicity of adriamycin	Proteinuria caused by selective podocyte injury. Progressive renal insufficiency. Resembles focal sclerosis.	17
Heymann nephritis	Podocyte	Rat	Immune complex-mediated with complement activation	Subepithelial immune deposits with membrane attack complex-induced podocyte injury and progressive renal insufficiency. Resembles membranous nephropathy.	24,84
Polycation-induced nephrosis	Podocyte	Rat	Impairment in charge selectivity of capillary membrane following infusion of polycation (protamine sulfate, poly-L-lysine)	Podocyte swelling with retraction of foot processes accompanied by a reduction in stainable glomerular anionic sites	89,90

50

Thy.1 nephritis	Mesangial cell	Rat	Antibody-mediated with complement activation	Mesangiolysis with subsequent mesangial proliferative response and matrix accumulation. Disease self-limited.	34
Habu venom nephritis	Mesangial cell	Rat, mouse, rabbit	Proteolytic effect of venom on mesangial matrix	Matrix dissolution and micro-aneurysmal changes with subsequent mesangioproliferative response. Disease self-limited.	47
Anti-endothelial cell antibody	Endothelial cell	Rat	Antibody-mediated with complement activation	Mesangiolysis with features of thrombotic microangiopathy. Disease self-limited.	54
Concanavalin A (ConA) model	Endothelial cell	Rat	Antibody-mediated	Antibody reaction against planted exogenous (lectin) antigen resulting in exudative and proliferative glomerulonephritis	88
Anti-GBM disease	Glomerular basement membrane (GBM)	Rat, dog, cat, mouse, sheep, rabbit	Antibody-mediated with complement activation Role for cell-mediated immunity suggested.	Linear binding of antibody to GBM with inflammatory response. GBM disruption with crescentic formation and progressive renal impairment.	61
Murine crescentic nephrotoxic glomerulonephritis	Visceral and parietal epithelial cells	Mouse	Antibody-mediated	Crescentic glomerulonephritis with epithelial-cell proliferation, progressing to glomerulosclerosis with tubulointerstitial fibrosis	85

(continued)

51

Table 1 (continued)

Remnant kidney	Glomerulus	Rat, mouse, cat, goat	Hemodynamic and nonhemodynamic processes	Glomerular hypertrophy with increased Pgc and snGFR. Macrophage influx and cytokine activation with progressive glomerulosclerosis and tubulo-interstitial fibrosis	*69,70*
Spontaneously hypertensive rat (SHR)	Glomerulus	Rat	Hemodynamic	Increased Pgc associated with mesangial expansion and glomerulosclerosis	*86,87*

Pgc, intraglomerular capillary pressure; snGFR, single nephron glomerular filtration rate.

is largely self-perpetuating following a single dose, and thus is regarded as an animal model of FSGS (*16*).

2.2.1. Disease Induction

Bertani et al. demonstrated that the administration of a single intravenous (iv) dose of adriamycin (7.5 mg/kg of body wt) in rats reliably produces podocyte injury (*17*). Although most established in the rat, adriamycin nephropathy has also been reproduced in mice (*18*), specifically the Balb/c strain.

2.2.2. Disease Course and Pathogenesis

Abrupt onset of proteinuria is typically seen by 7–10 d (*17*). It has been speculated that the delayed onset of proteinuria (compared to PAN nephrosis) is a consequence of the different cellular targets (adriamycin targets DNA; PAN impairs ribosomal function) (*19*). Over the course of the next 5 wk, the magnitude of proteinuria progressively increases, with the development of nephrotic syndrome. Micropuncture studies performed by Odonnell et al. demonstrated significant reductions in glomerular filtration rate and renal plasma flow, accompanied by a decrease in ultrafiltration coefficient and an increase in glomerular capillary pressure (*20*). These early studies failed to demonstrate loss of renal function or the development of glomerulosclerosis, casting doubt as to the potential causal role of glomerular capillary hypertension in mediating glomerulosclerosis. However, subsequent studies with longer follow-up periods indeed demonstrated an inexorable decline in renal function with associated uremic manifestations by 6 mo (*21*).

Similar to PAN nephrosis, ultrastructural studies performed early in the disease course during the first 10 d identify the podocyte as the primary target of injury, with disruption of the interdigitating architecture of the foot processes. The mesangial and endothelial cells are largely unaffected (*17*). Histologic assessment beyond 14 wk revealed progressive podocyte injury with extensive foot-process effacement and vacuolization, associated with widespread glomerulosclerosis. Tubulo-interstitial damage includes tubular atrophy with patchy fibrosis and mononuclear-cell infiltrate.

2.2.3. Relevance and Implications for Human Disease

Although the mechanisms that mediate progressive injury in adriamycin nephropathy have not been completely elucidated, recent studies have confirmed the important roles of reactive oxygen intermediates and hyperlipidemia in accelerating the disease process (*22,23*). Therefore, although the cause of initial renal injury is markedly different from focal segmental glomerulosclerosis in man, both processes show similarities with respect to the progressive deterioration in renal function.

2.3. Heymann Nephritis

In 1959, Heymann et al. first described their model of an indolent form of immune complex-mediated glomerular injury. Considered by many to be indistinguishable from human membranous nephropathy, Heymann nephritis has been the subject of intense research over the past 40 yr and has provided valuable insight into mechanisms of immune-mediated glomerular injury.

2.3.1. Disease Induction

There are two forms of Heymann nephritis—active and passive. In the active form of Heymann nephritis, immunization of rats with crude kidney extracts, enhanced with complete Freund's adjuvant, results in the insidious onset of proteinuria by 4–6 wk. Subsequent studies successfully utilized a refined extract of the proximal tubular brush border (termed fx1A). Immunizing rats with anti-sera from sheep generated against the fx1A fraction reproduced disease in an accelerated fashion—a variant commonly referred to as passive Heymann nephritis (PHN).

2.3.2. Disease Course and Pathogenesis

Serial histologic analysis reveal the early binding of anti-fx1A antibodies with subsequent shedding of immune complexes into the subepithelial space by as early as 24 h. Indeed, immunofluorescence confirms immunoglobulin (IgG) deposition of the capillary wall in a fine granular pattern *(24)*. By d 4, podocyte foot-process effacement occurs, corresponding with the onset of proteinuria. Although renal function is preserved initially, progressive deterioration with glomerulosclerosis occurs over time. Much attention has been focused on determining the pathogenic antigen of the fx1A fraction. The large membrane glycoprotein gp330 plays a critical role, as selective removal of anti-gp330 antibody from anti-fx1A sera prevents the formation of immune deposits in PHN *(25)*. gp330, also known as megalin, has been characterized as a polyspecific receptor that structurally resembles lipoprotein receptor-related protein (LRP). Its family of ligands includes calcium, apolipoprotein E and J, and urinary plasminogen-activator inhibitor, as well as certain aminoglycosides. In addition to the tubular-brush border, megalin is also expressed along the clathrin-coated pit of podocyte foot processes. Upon antibody recognition, the resulting immune complex undergoes internalization prior to shedding into the subepithelial space, where it becomes fixed to the GBM *(26)*. It is interesting to note that although monoclonal antibodies (MAbs) directed against gp330 mediate immune-deposit formation, proteinuria does not ensue. This important observation reveals that despite its critical role, gp330 is not the only antigen involved in disease induction.

The membrane-attack complex of complement also colocalizes to immune deposits, and has been shown to play a critical role in mediating injury in both active and passive forms of Heymann nephritis *(27)*. C6-deficient rats, which are unable to assemble C5b-9, fail to develop proteinuria despite IgG and c3 deposition *(28)*. Inhibiting the activation of the alternative pathway with cobra venom factor also prevents podocyte injury *(29)*. Mounting evidence suggests that in order to cause podocyte injury, polyclonal anti-sera in PHN must target specific complement regulatory proteins. CD59, an inhibitor of c8-c9 insertion, and crry, an inhibitor of c3 and c5 convertases, are both widely expressed in renal tissue of the rat, including the podocyte *(30)*. Rats immunized with anti-fx1a antibody that are selectively depleted of IgG recognize crry form immune deposits but fail to develop proteinuria *(31)*. Furthermore, when monoclonal anti-gp330 antibodies are combined with anti-crry and CD59 F(ab')$_2$ fragments, proteinuria results *(32)*. Indeed urinary levels of c5b-9 have been shown to parallel immunologic disease activity experimentally, and portend the onset of proteinuria *(27)*. Taken together, these studies suggest that complement regulatory proteins, which normally prevent c5b-9-mediated injury, become overwhelmed in PHN *(32)*.

The subsequent sublytic injury of the podocyte results in the activation of a number of cellular processes, including induction of proteases, generation of reactive oxygen species (ROS), and lipid peroxidation, which has been shown to play a role in mediating tissue injury *(29)*. We have recently shown that despite engaging the cell cycle in response to c5b-9 induced injury in vivo and in vitro, podocytes are unable to progress beyond the G2-M checkpoint, because of the activation of specific cell-cycle regulatory proteins *(32a)*.

2.3.3. Relevance and Implications for Human Disease

Although frequently referred to as "experimental membranous nephropathy," differences exist between PHN and its human counterpart. Perhaps the biggest shortcoming and criticism has been the inability to demonstrate gp330, or an equivalent antigen, in human disease. Nonetheless, Heymann nephritis has been studied intensively over the past four decades, and has contributed greatly to our understanding of immune complex-mediated renal disease. Specifically, this model provided the first demonstration that immune complexes in the kidney may not originate from passive trapping of circulating complexes, but may form *in situ* in response to cell-membrane antigens *(33)*. Furthermore, a pathogenic role for the complement-membrane attack complex has been demonstrated in antibody-mediated glomerular disease.

3. Models of Mesangial-Cell Injury
3.1. THY-1 Nephritis

Thy-1 nephritis is a model of mesangioproliferative glomerulonephritis in the rat. Thy-1 antigen is an 18 kDa glycosylated phosphatidylinositol membrane protein, which is ubiquitously expressed on thymocytes. However, it is also uniquely expressed on the cell surface of mesangial cells in the rat, where its exact function remains unknown.

3.1.1. Disease Induction

The administration of a single iv injection (typically 20 mg per 100 g body wt) of monoclonal or polyclonal antibodies directed against the Thy-1 antigen predictably results in mesangial-cell injury *(34)*.

3.1.2. Disease Course and Pathogenesis

Intense mesangiolysis occurs within the first 48 h, with a selective depletion of mesangial cells (to 10% of normal numbers) and dissolution of mesangial matrix *(34)*. The structural support of neighboring capillary loops becomes compromised, resulting in segmental microaneurysmal changes. The complement dependence (and specifically the critical role of the membrane-attack complex) has been underscored by studies performed in c-6 deficient rats, which displayed marked attenuation of mesangiolysis following administration of anti-thymocyte serum *(35)*.

Beginning as early as d 3 post-injection of anti-thy 1 antibody, an intense mesangial response is observed, with initial influx of extraglomerular mesangial cells and subsequent mesangial cell proliferation, so that by d 5, mesangial cell counts may be up to 3× greater than normal values. The proliferative response has been correlated with changes in specific cell cycle regulatory proteins *(36)*. Selective inhibition of CDK2 with the purine analog Roscovitine significantly reduces mesangial-cell proliferation, which in turn causes a decrease in extracellular matrix (ECM) proteins, and preservation of renal function *(37)*. Platelets and macrophages are increased in the glomerulus *(38)*. Mesangial cells increase the synthesis and release of a number of mitogens including platelet-derived growth factor (PDGF), basic fibroblast growth factor (bFGF), and endothelin, and selectively blocking these reduces mesangial-cell proliferation *(39–42)*. In addition to an absolute increase in cell number, mesangial cells undergo a transformation to myofibroblasts. Mesangial expansion is accompanied by matrix accumulation (including *de novo* expression of the interstitial collagens type I and III), largely because of the effects of transforming growth factor (TGF)-β1 *(43)*.

By 6–8 wk, spontaneous recovery ensues with mesangial cell number restored to baseline in an apoptotic-dependent manner, and normalization of ECM *(44)*. Although residual mesangiosclerosis is not typical, if repeated courses of anti-Thy-1 antibody are administered, chronic scarring may result.

3.1.3. Relevance and Implications for Human Disease

Although there may not be a human counterpart to the mechanism of initial injury in Thy-1 nephritis, this model has provided valuable insight into the mesangial response in a number of clinical conditions, including lupus nephritis, IgA nephropathy, diabetes mellitus, and membranoproliferative glomerulonephritis.

3.2. Habu Venom Nephritis

Although venom from of a number of snake species has been reported to cause glomerular injury, the best-characterized model remains habu venom nephritis.

3.2.1. Disease Induction

Successfully induced in both rabbit and mouse species (45,46), this model has been most widely studied in the rat. Following the iv injection of a near-lethal dose of venom (2–4 mg/kg) from the pit viper *Trimeresurus flavoviridis*, subjects develop intense mesangiolysis within hours.

3.2.2. Disease Course and Pathogenesis

Unlike the thy-1 nephritis model, the principal target appears to be mesangial matrix (presumably caused by the proteolytic activity of venom), and not the mesangial cell *per se* (45). Consequently, mesangial cell necrosis is not a prominent feature, and an early reduction in cell number is not seen. In addition to mesangial damage, endothelial cell injury is an early feature of habu venom nephritis, with resultant cystic dilatation of capillary loops. These microaneurysms become engorged with blood elements, including platelets, fibrin, and erythrocytes (47). By d 3 following disease induction, an intense mononuclear cell infiltrate is noted, caused mainly by a mesangioproliferative response. Macrophage recruitment seems to play a much lesser role. A pathogenic role for platelets (48) and macrophages (49) in mediating the mesangial cell response, through the release of various mitogens including PDGF and fibronectin, has been postulated. Pharmacologic inhibition of platelet secretory function has been shown to attenuate the extent and severity of glomerular injury by some groups (50), but not others (51).

3.2.3. Relevance and Implications for Human Disease

Similar to the thy-1 model, glomerular injury in habu venom nephritis is typically self-limited, with gradual resolution over the course of several weeks. However, when the two models are induced concurrently, severe mesangiolysis ensues, with marked destruction of the capillary network and progression to global sclerosis by 8 wk. However, treatment with vascular endothelial growth factor (VEGF), an endothelial-specific mitogen, significantly increased endothelial-cell proliferation with resultant capillary repair and improvement in renal function, thereby underscoring the importance of angiogenesis in the recovery process of severe glomerulonephritis (52).

4. Models of Endothelial-Cell Injury

Endothelial injury underlies vasculitis and allograft rejection. Within the glomerulus, endothelial damage and the consequent activation of the coagulation cascade is central to the development of thrombotic microangiopathy (TMA). TMA may be secondary to systemic processes (thrombotic thrombocytopenic purpura [TTP], malignant hypertension, or collagen vascular disease), or is renal-limited in hemolytic uremic syndrome (causes including verotoxin-associated, human immunodeficiency virus [HIV], radiation, oral contraceptives, calcineurin inhibitors, or heredity) *(53)*. We have developed a rat model of glomerular endothelial injury that resembles TMA.

4.1. Disease Induction

Antibodies against glomerular endothelial cells are generated by immunizing a goat with cultured rat glomerular endothelial cells. Selective renal or systemic perfusion with purified anti-GEN IgG results in acute renal insufficiency in a dose-dependent fashion.

4.2. Disease Course and Pathogenesis

Within hours after antibody administration, there is a reduction in platelet counts and evidence of intravascular hemolysis *(54)*. Histologic evaluation reveals immediate and widespread platelet aggregation within capillary loops, associated with endothelial swelling and areas of denuded basement membrane. A mesangial response is seen, with features of mesangiolysis and mild expansion. Although leukocytes are not seen in the glomeruli, polymorphonucleocyte infiltration of the interstitium occurs, with significant tubular injury. By d 10, glomerular thrombosis and mesangiolysis resolve, as does the initial endothelial proliferative response.

4.3. Relevance and Implications for Human Disease

The importance of the membrane-attack complex c5b-9 in mediating injury in this model has been confirmed by neutralizing the complement regulatory protein CD59, with resultant worsening severity of injury *(55)*. The beneficial roles of nitric oxide and VEGF in protecting against injury in this model of thrombotic microangiopathy has been demonstrated *(56,57)*. Further studies with this model will likely shed insights into the important role of the endothelial cell in glomerular disease *(58)*.

5. Models of GBM Injury

First described over 100 yr ago, anti-GBM disease represents the oldest experimental model of kidney disease. Although a number of different variations have been reported, including Masugi nephritis, nephrotoxic serum nephritis, and experimental autoimmune glomerulonephritis *(59,60)*, they all share the common feature of circulating auto-antibodies, which recognize and bind the GBM, resulting in complement-mediated glomerular injury.

5.1. Disease Induction

Disease has been successfully induced in a variety of mammalian species, including the dog, rat, monkey, and sheep, although rabbits seem to develop the most aggressive disease *(2)*. Repeated injections of a heterologous crude extract of glomerular protein results in the production of immunogenic antibodies, which mediate injury. Although active forms of disease are studied, more often the pathogenic antibodies are isolated and purified from the immunized "reservoir" host and then passively administered.

5.2. Disease Course and Pathogenesis

Following the iv injection of antibodies, an initial *heterologous phase* of injury ensues, notable for the rapid binding of antibody to the GBM in a linear distribution. Over the next several h, complement fixation results in an influx of polymorphonucleocytes, with a subsequent proliferative response (largely consisting of macrophages) *(61)*, disruption of the basement membrane, and early crescent formation. By d 10, the host has mounted an immune response against the foreign antibody bound to the GBM, which further drives glomerular damage and proteinuria in what is known as the *autologous phase* of disease. Over the course of the next several wk, the crescentic response continues, with progressive deterioration in renal function, typically resulting in death caused by uremic complications.

5.3. Relevance and Implications for Human Disease

Decades of research in anti-GBM experimental models led to the eventual characterization of Goodpasture's disease in man and identification of the target antigen, namely the NC-1 domain of the $\alpha 3$ chain of type IV collagen. However, studies of early experimental models revealed that eluates from nephritic animals contained antibodies that reacted with a number of additional targets, including antigens of Bowman's capsule and tubular basement membranes *(62)*. Attempts to duplicate human nephritis in animals with purified antibodies that are specific for the a3COL(IV) antigen have been largely unsuccessful. Therefore, although circulating anti-GBM antibodies may be the hallmark of this disease, other factors must also be at play. The finding that more aggressive injury in the active model of disease may be induced by immunizing concurrently with complete Freund's adjuvant has implicated the cellular immune response in the pathogenesis of glomerular injury *(63)*. In a series of elegant studies, Kalluri et al. demonstrated that although different strains of inbred mice injected with purified antibody against the Goodpasture antigen all displayed a linear binding pattern of the GBM on immunofluorescence, the development of glomerular injury was largely determined by the MHC class II background, suggesting a possible T cell-dependent response *(64)*. The authors subsequently demonstrated that passive transfer of activated lymphocytes from a nephritic strain to a syngeneic recipient could reproduce glomerular injury in the new host. Furthermore, the passive transfer of anti-a3(iv) antibodies into syngeneic mice with intact T cell receptors resulted in disease, whereas syngeneic recipients devoid of T cell receptor remained resistant to disease. Indeed, subsequent studies by Reynolds et al. in which T cell activation was inhibited by administration of blocking antibodies confirmed a critical role for cellular immune response in mediating renal injury *(65,66)*.

Recent studies with transgenic knockout mice have provided the opportunity to study specific aspects of the immune response, including the role of complement activation *(67)* as well as signaling and adhesion molecules *(68)*. Therefore, although differences may exist between experimental forms of anti-GBM disease and its counterpart in man, these models have provided valuable insight into the pathogenesis of immune-mediated glomerular injury.

6. Models of Global Sclerosis
6.1. Remnant Kidney Model

Once renal function has deteriorated to levels below 50% of baseline, a progressive loss of renal reserve will typically follow, despite removal of the inciting event. This observation has formed the basis for the establishment of the remnant kidney model, the most widely studied animal model of progressive renal failure. Although successfully induced in a variety of animal species—including cats, goats, and mice—the "five-sixths" remnant kidney model has been best-characterized in rats.

6.1.1. Disease Induction

Disease is induced by unilateral surgical nephrectomy, followed by selective ablation of the upper and lower poles of the remaining kidney. The result is hypertrophy of the remaining glomeruli, with associated glomerulosclerosis and interstitial fibrosis *(69,70)*. The method of renal ablation of the remaining kidney has been implicated in determining disease progression in the remnant kidney *(71)*. Infarction (through ligation of the posterior and anterior branches of the renal artery) results in progressive renal insufficiency. In contrast, excision of the upper and lower poles (polectomy) results in glomerular hypertrophy, but this is not accompanied by a loss of renal function. It has been theorized that hypertension, seen only with the infarction method, is the critical determinant in mediating renal injury, because of the transmission of systemic pressure to the glomerulus.

6.1.2. Disease Course and Pathogenesis

Micropuncture studies have demonstrated that in response to reduced renal mass, the remaining nephrons undergo a series of adaptive hemodynamic responses, including hypertrophy (increased glomerular volume), hyperfiltration (increased single-nephron glomerular filtration rate), and hypertension (increased glomerular capillary pressure) *(72,73)*. The reduction of intraglomerular capillary pressure and filtration rate through dietary (low-protein diet) or pharmacologic (ACE inhibitors, antihypertensives) interventions has confirmed that these hemodynamic responses are maladaptive, and promote progressive renal injury *(74)*.

Although capillary hypertension may play a key role, it appears that nonhemodynamic processes are similarly involved in mediating injury in the remnant kidney model. Serial histologic evaluation reveals an early mesangioproliferative response within the first few days, followed by an influx of macrophages *(75)*. This cellular response results in the release of a number of cytokines and growth factors, including PDGF, endothelin-1, angiotensin II, and TGF-β, all of which have been implicated in ECM expansion and sclerosis *(75,76)*. Selective blocking studies of angiotensin II or endothelin-1 have both proven effective in ameliorating proteinuria and glomerulosclerosis *(76,77)*.

A pathogenic role for infiltrating mononuclear cells has been demonstrated by studies involving the antiproliferative agent mycophenolate (MMF), which selectively targets lymphoid cells. Although glomerular hypertrophy remained unaffected, MMF therapy in rats with remnant kidney disease blunted the mononuclear-cell influx and preserved renal function while dramatically reducing glomerulosclerosis and tubulointerstitial fibrosis *(78)*. Furthermore, injury mediated by oxygen radicals as a result of increased oxygen consumption in remaining nephrons has been suggested *(79)*.

6.1.3. Relevance and Implications for Human Disease

Taken together, studies performed with the remnant kidney disease model have revealed numerous hemodynamic and nonhemodynamic mechanisms of progressive renal damage. These findings have had a dramatic impact on the clinical management of chronic renal insufficiency, including the widespread use of angiotensin II blockade, protein restriction, and blood pressure control as measures to retard the rate of disease progression.

7. Conclusion

Although the classic animal models described in this chapter have provided tremendous insight into the *general* mechanisms and consequences of glomerular injury, progress has been steady, representing collective research efforts over the past several decades. However, many questions remain unanswered. It is the authors' belief that knowledge and insight into mechanisms of glomerular injury will take a quantum leap over the next 10–15 yr. The advent of transgenic and knockout murine models will greatly advance our level of understanding by allowing manipulation of the host response to disease induction in a *specific* and targeted manner. Furthermore, with the recent introduction of microarray *(80,81)* and proteomic *(82)* methodologies in nephrology research, novel proteins that are critical to glomerular structure and function will likely be discovered. Such novel proteins may then be deleted or selectively inactivated. An example is the model of monoclonal antibodies against nephrin protein, which has led to a greater understanding of the complex ultrastructure of the podocyte *(83)*. Ultimately, it is the hope that a better understanding of cellular function and mechanisms of glomerular injury will translate into potential avenues for therapeutic options to aid in the clinical management of glomerular disease.

Acknowledgments

This work was supported by Public Health Service grants (DK34198, DK52121, DK51096, DK56799) and a George O'Brien Kidney Center Grant (DK47659). Stuart J. Shankland is an Established Investigator of the American Heart Association.

References

1. Anders, H. J. and Schlondorff, D. (2000) Murine models of renal disease: possibilities and problems in studies using mutant mice. *Exp. Nephrol.* **8,** 181–193.
2. Wilson, C. B. (1997) Immune models of glomerular injury, (Neilson, E. G. and Couser, W. G., eds.), Lippincott-Raven Publishers, Philadelphia, pp. 729–773.
3. Hoedemaeker, P. J. and Weening, J. J. (1989) Relevance of experimental models for human nephropathology. *Kidney Int.* **35,** 1015–1025.
4. Foster, M. H. (1999) Relevance of systemic lupus erythematosus nephritis animal models to human disease. *Semin. Nephrol.* **19,** 12–24.
5. Peutz-Koostra, C. J., et al. (2001) Lupus nephritis: lessons from experimental animal models. *J. Lab. Clin. Med.* **137,** 244–260.
6. Ryan, G. B. and Karnovsky, M. J. (1975) An ultrastructural study of the mechanisms of proteinuria in aminonucleoside nephrosis. *Kidney Int.* **8,** 219–232.
7. Messina, A., et al. (1987) Glomerular epithelial cell abnormalities associated with the onset of proteinuria in aminonucleoside nephrosis. *Am. J. Pathol.* **126,** 220–229.
8. Grond, J., et al. (1988) Differences in puromycin aminonucleoside nephrosis in two rat strains. *Kidney Int.* **33,** 524–529.
9. Krishnamurti, U., et al. (2001) Puromycin aminonucleoside suppresses integrin expression in cultured glomerular epithelial cells. *J. Am. Soc. Nephrol.* **12,** 758–766.
10. Osicka, T. M., Hankin, A. R., and Comper, W. D. (1999) Puromycin aminonucleoside nephrosis results in a marked increase in fractional clearance of albumin. *Am. J. Physiol.* **277,** F139–F145.
11. Groggel, G. C., et al. (1987) Changes in glomerular heparan sulfate in puromycin aminonucleoside nephrosis. *Am. J. Pathol.* **128,** 521–527.
12. Kerjaschki, D., Vernillo, A. T., and Farquhar, M. G. (1985) Reduced sialylation of podocalyxin—the major sialoprotein of the rat kidney glomerulus—in aminonucleoside nephrosis. *Am. J. Pathol.* **118,** 343–349.
13. Eddy, A. and Michael, A. F. (1988) Acute tubulointerstitial nephritis associated with aminonucleoside nephrosis. *Kidney Int.* **33,** 14–23.
14. Breiteneder-Geleff, S., et al. (1997) Podoplanin, novel 43-kd membrane protein of glomerular epithelial cells, is down-regulated in puromycin nephrosis. *Am. J. Pathol.* **151,** 1141–1152.

15. Matsui, K., et al. (1999) Podoplanin, a novel 43-kDa membrane protein, controls the shape of podocytes. *Nephrol. Dial. Transplant.* **14,** S9–S11.
16. Chen, A., et al. (1998) Experimental focal segmental glomerulosclerosis in mice. *Nephron* **78,** 440–452.
17. Bertani, T., et al. (1982) Adriamycin-induced nephrotic syndrome in rats: sequence of pathologic events. *Lab. Investig.* **46,** 16–23.
18. Wang, Y., et al. (2000) Progressive adriamycin nephropathy in mice: sequence of histologic and immunohistochemical events. *Kidney Int.* **58,** 1797–1804.
19. Whiteside, C., et al. (1989) Glomerular epithelial cell detachment, not reduced charge density, correlates with proteinuria in adriamycin and puromycin nephrosis. *Lab. Investig.* **61,** 650–660.
20. O'Donnell, M. P., et al. (1985) Adriamycin-induced chronic proteinuria: a structural and functional study. *J. Lab. Clin. Med.* **106,** 62–67.
21. Okuda, S., et al. (1986) Adriamycin-induced nephropathy as a model of chronic progressive glomerular disease. *Kidney Int.* **29,** 502–510.
22. Song, H., et al. (2000) Glomerulosclerosis in adriamycin-induced nephrosis is accelerated by a lipid-rich diet. *Pediatr. Nephrol.* **15,** 196–200.
23. Van den Branden, C., et al. (2000) Renal antioxidant enzymes and fibrosis-related markers in the rat adriamycin model. *Nephron* **86,** 167–175.
24. Salant, D., Darby, C., and Couser, W. G. (1980) Experimental Membranous Glomerulonephritis in Rats. *J. Clin. Invest.* **66,** 71–81.
25. Kerjaschki, D. and Neale, T. J. (1996) Molecular mechanisms of glomerular injury in rat experimental membranous nephropathy (Heymann nephritis). *J. Am. Soc. Nephrol.* **7,** 2518–2526.
26. Kerjaschki, D., et al. (1989) Transcellular transport and membrane insertion of the c5b-9 membrane attack complex of complement by glomerular epithelial cells in experimental membranous nephropathy. *J. Immunol.* **143,** 546–552.
27. Couser, W. G., Schulze, M., and Pruchno, C. J. (1992) Role of c5b-9 in experimental membranous nephropathy. *Nephrol. Dial. Transplant.* **Suppl 1,** 25–31.
28. Baker, P. J., et al. (1989) Depletion of c6 prevents development of proteinuria in experimental membranous nephropathy in rats. *Am. J. Pathol.* **135,** 185–194.
29. Salant, D., et al. (1980) A new role for complement in experimental membranous nephropathy in rats. *J. Clin. Invest.* **66,** 1339–1350.
30. Quigg, R. J., et al. (1995) Crry and CD59 regulate complement in rat glomerular epithelial cells and are inhibited by the nephritogenic antibody of passive Heymann nephritis. *J. Immunol.* **154,** 3437–3443.
31. Schiller, B., et al. (1998) Inhibition of complement regulation is key to the pathogenesis of active Heymann nephritis. *J. Exp. Med.* **188,** 1353–1358.
32. Cunningham, P. N., et al. (2001) Glomerular complement regulation is overwhelmed in passive Heymann nephritis. *Kidney Int.* **60,** 900–909.
32a. Pippin, J. W., Durvasula, R. V., et al. (2003) Complement (C5b-9) induces DNA damage in podocytes *in vitro* and *in vivo*: A novel response to sublytic injury. *J. Clin. Invest.*, in press.
33. Couser, W. G., et al. (1978) Experimental glomerulonephritis in the isolated perfused rat kidney. *J. Clin. Investig.* **62,** 1275–1287.

34. Jefferson, J. A. and Johnson, R. J. (1999) Experimental mesangial proliferative glomerulonephritis (the anti-Thy-1. 1 model). *J. Nephrol.* **12,** 297–307.

35. Brandt, J., et al. (1996) Role of complement membrane attack complex (C5b-9) in mediating experimental mesangioproliferative glomerulonephritis. *Kidney Int.* **49,** 335–343.

36. Shankland, S. J., et al. (1996) Changes in cell-cycle protein expression during experimental mesangial proliferative glomerulonephritis. *Kidney Int.* **50,** 1230–1239.

37. Pippin, J., et al. (1997) Direct in vivo inhibition of the nuclear cell cycle cascade in experimental mesangial proliferative glomerulonephritis with roscovitine, a novel cyclin-dependent kinase antagonist. *J. Clin. Investig.* **100,** 2512–2520.

38. Johnson, R. J., et al. (1990) Platelets mediate glomerular cell proliferation in immune complex nephritis induced by anti-mesangial cell antibodies in the rat. *Am. J. Pathol.* **136,** 369–374.

39. Johnson, R. J., et al. (1992) Inhibition of mesangial cell proliferation and matrix expansion in glomerulonephritis in the rat by antibody to platelet-derived growth factor. *J. Exp. Med.* **175,** 1413–1416.

40. Fukuda, K., et al. (1996) Role of endothelin as a mitogen in experimental glomerulonephritis in rats. *Kidney Int.* **49,** 1320–1329.

41. Haseley, L. A., et al. (1999) Dissociation of mesangial cell migration and proliferation in experimental glomerulonephritis. *Kidney Int.* **56,** 964–972.

42. Johnson, R. J., et al. (1991) Expression of smooth muscle cell phenotype by rat mesangial cells in immune complex nephritis. *J. Clin. Invest.* **87,** 847–858.

43. Border, W. A., et al. (1990) Suppression of experimental glomerulonephritis by antiserum against transforming growth factor β1. *Nature* **346,** 371–374.

44. Shimizu, A., et al. (1995) Apoptosis in the repair process of experimental proliferative glomerulonephritis. *Kidney Int.* **47,** 114–121.

45. Morita, T., Yamamoto, T., and Churg, J. (1998) Mesangiolysis: an update. *American Journal of Kidney Diseases* **31,** 559–573.

46. Nakao, N., et al. (1998) Tenascin-C promotes healing of Habu–Snake venom-induced glomerulonephritis. *Am. J. Pathol.* **152,** 1237–1245.

47. Cattell, V. and Bradfield, J. W. (1977) Focal mesangial proliferative glomerulonephritis in the rat caused by Habu snake venom. *Am. J. Pathol.* **87,** 511–524.

48. Barnes, J. L. and Abboud, H. E. (1993) Temporal expression of autocrine growth factors corresponds to morphological features of mesangial proliferation in habu snake venom-induced glomerulonephritis. *Am. J. Pathol.* **143,** 1366–1376.

49. Barnes, J. L., Hastings, R. R., and De La Garza, M. (1994) Sequential expression of cellular fibronectin by platelets, macrophages, and mesangial cells in proliferative glomerulonephritis. *Am. J. Pathol.* **145,** 585–597.

50. Barnes, J. L. (1989) Amelioration of Habu venom-induced glomerular lesions: Potential role for platelet secretory proteins. *J. Lab. Clin. Med.* **114,** 200–206.

51. Cattell, V. and Mehotra, A. (1980) Effect of anti-platelet medications on Habu snake venom nephritis. *Br. J. Exp. Pathol.* **61,** 310–314.

52. Masuda, Y., et al. (2001) Vascular endothelial growth factor enhances glomerular capillary repair and accelerates resolution of experimentally induced glomerulonephritis. *Am. J. Pathol.* **159,** 599–608.

53. Nangaku M, et al. (1998) A new model of renal microvascular injury. *Curr. Opin. Nephrol. Hypertens.* **7,** 457–462.
54. Nangaku, M., et al. (1997) A new model of renal microvascular endothelial injury. *Kidney Int.* **52,** 182–194.
55. Nangaku, M., et al. (1998) CD59 protects glomerular endothelial cells from immune-mediated thrombotic microangiopathy in rats. *J. Am. Soc. Nephrol.* **9,** 590–597.
56. Shao, J., et al. (2001) Protective role of nitric oxide in a model of thrombotic microangiopathy in rats. *J. Am. Soc. Nephrol.* **12,** 2088–2097.
57. Suga, S., et al. (2001) Vascular endothelial growth factor (VEGF 121) pro-tects rats from renal infarction in thrombotic microangiopathy. *Kidney Int.* **60,** 1297–1308.
58. Kang, D. H., et al. (2002) Role of microvacular endothelium in progressive renal disease. *J. Am. Soc. Nephrol.* **13,** 806–816.
59. Allison, M. E., Wilson, C. B., and Gottschalk, C. W. (1974) Pathophysiology of experimental glomerulonephritis in rats. *J. Clin. Invest.* **53,** 1402–1423.
60. Germuth, F. G., et al. (1978) Antibasement membrane disease. II. Mechanism of glomerular injury in an accelerated model of Masugi nephritis. *Lab. Investig.* **39,** 421–429.
61. Lan, H. Y., et al. (1997) Local macrophage proliferation in the pathogenesis of glomerular crescent formation in rat anti-glomerular basement membrane (GBM) glomerulonephritis. *Clin. Exp. Immunol.* **110,** 233–240.
62. Steblay, R. and Rudofsky, U. (1968) In vitro and in vivo properties of autoantibodies eluted from kidneys of sheep with autoimmune glomerulonephritis. *Nature* **218,** 1269–1271.
63. Moorthy, A. V. and Abreo, K. (1983) potentiation of nephrotoxic serum nephritis in Lewis rats by Freund's complete adjuvant—possible role for cellular immune mechanisms. *Clin. Immunol. Immunopathol.* **28,** 383–394.
64. Kalluri, R., et al. (1997) Susceptibility to anti-glomerular basement membrane disease and Goodpasture syndrome is linked to MHC class II genes and the emergence of T cell-mediated immunity in mice. *J. Clin. Investig.* **100,** 2263–2275.
65. Reynolds, J., et al. (2000) CD28-B7 blockade prevents the development of experimental autoimmune glomerulonephritis. *J. Clin. Invest.* **105,** 643–651.
66. Reynolds, J., et al. (2002) Anti-CD8 monoclonal antibody therapy is effective in the prevention and treatment of experimental autoimmune glomerulonephritis. *J. Am. Soc. Nephrol.* **13,** 359–369.
67. Quigg, R. J., et al. (1998) Transgenic mice overexpressing the complement inhibitor crry as a soluble protein are protected from antibody-induced glomerular injury. *J. Exp. Med.* **188,** 1321–1331.
68. Janssen, U., et al. (1998) Improved survival and amelioration of nephrotoxic nephritis in intercellular adhesion molecule-1 knockout mice. *J. Am. Soc. Nephrol.* **9,** 1805–1814.
69. Shimamura, T. and Morrison, A. B. (1975) A progressive glomerulosclerosis occurring in partial five-sixths nephrectomized rats. *Am. J. Pathol.* **79,** 95–106.
70. Faraj, A. H. and Morley, A. R. (1992) Remnant kidney pathology after five-sixth nephrectomy in rat. *APMIS* **100,** 1097–1105.
71. Griffin, K., Picken, M., and Bidani, A. K. (1994) Method of renal mass reduction is a critical modulator of subsequent hypertension and glomerular injury. *J. Am. Soc. Nephrol.* **4,** 2023–2031.

72. Hostetter, T., et al. (1981) Hyperfiltration in remnant nephrons: a potentially adverse response to renal ablation. *Am. J. Physiol.* **241**, F85–F93.
73. Brown, S. A. and Brown, C. A. (1995) Single nephron adaptation to partial renal ablation in cats. *Am. J. Physiol.* **269**, R1002–R1008.
74. Brenner, B. M., Lawler, E. V., and Mackenzie, H. S. (1996) The hyperfiltration theory: a paradigm shift in nephrology. *Kidney Int.* **49**, 1774–1777.
75. Floege, J., et al. (1992) Glomerular cells, extracellular matrix accumulation, and the development of glomerulosclerosis in the remnant kidney model. *Lab. Investig.* **66**, 485–496.
76. Brochu, E., et al. (1999) Endothelin ET-A receptor blockade prevents the progression of renal failure and hypertension in uraemic rats. *Nephrol. Dial. Transplant.* **14**, 1881–1888.
77. Junaid, A., Hostetter, T., and Rosenberg, M. E. (1997) Interaction of angiotensin II and TGF-β1 in the rat remnant kidney. *J. Am. Soc. Nephrol.* **8**, 1732–1738.
78. Romero, F., et al. (1999) Mycophenolate mofetil prevents the progressive renal failure induced by 5/6 renal ablation in rats. *Kidney Int.* **55**, 945–955.
79. Schrier, R. W., et al. (1994) Increased nephron oxygen consumption: Potential role in progression of chronic renal disease. *American Journal of Kidney Diseases* **23**, 176–182.
80. Yano, N., et al. (2000) Genomic repertoire of human mesangial cells: comprehensive analysis of gene expression by cDNA array hybridization. *Nephrology* **5**, 215–223.
81. Kurella, M., et al. (2001) DNA microarray analysis of complex biologic processes. *J. Am. Soc. Nephrol.* **12**, 1072–1078.
82. Knepper, M. A. (2002) Proteomics and the kidney. *J. Am. Soc. Nephrol.* **13**, 1398–1408.
83. Topham, P. S., et al. (1999) Nephritogenic mAb 5-1-6 is directed at the extracellular domain of rat nephrin. *J. Clin. Invest.* **104**, 1559–1566.
84. Edgington, T. S., Glassock, R. J., and Dixon, F. J. (1968) Autologous immune complex nephritis induced with renal tubular antigen. *J. Exp. Med.* **127**, 555–572.
85. Ophascharoensuk, V., et al. (1998) Role of intrinsic renal cells versus infiltrating cells in glomerular crescent formation. *Kidney Int.* **54**, 416–425.
86. Dworkin, L. D. and Feiner, H. D. (1986) Glomerular injury in uninephrectomized spontaneously hypertensive rats: a consequence of glomerular capillary hypertension. *J. Clin. Invest.* **77**, 797–809.
87. Martinez-Maldonado, M., et al. (1987) Pathogenesis of systemic hypertension and glomerular injury in the spontaneously hypertensive rat. *Am. J. Cardiol.* **60**, 471–521.
88. Golbus, S. M. and Wilson, C. B. (1979) Experimental glomerulonephritis induced by in situ formation of immune complexes in glomerular capillary wall. *Kidney Int.* **16**, 148–157.
89. Seiler, M. W., Venkatachalam, M. A., and Cotran, R. S. (1975) Glomerular epithelium: structural alterations induced by polycations. *Science* **189**, 390–393.
90. Seiler, M. W., et al. (1977) Pathogenesis of polycation-induced alterations ("fusion") of glomerular epithelium. *Lab. Investig.* **36**, 48–61.

II

CHOICES OF IMAGING TECHNIQUES IN STUDIES OF RENAL DISEASE

5

Functional Studies of the Kidney with Magnetic Resonance Imaging

Hani B. Marcos, Yantian Zhang, and Peter L. Choyke

1. Introduction

The measurement of renal function by imaging techniques is an important clinical and research tool. Early and reliable detection of changes in renal function are used to evaluate prognosis and the therapeutic approach to patients, and can be used to influence patient management. One intrinsic limitation of laboratory methods of evaluation is that they provide only a global evaluation of renal function with little anatomic information. Radionuclide methods of evaluation offer an advantage to biochemical methods because they can demonstrate side-to-side differences in renal function *(1)*. However, radionuclide methods are limited by spatial resolution, as well as the exposure to radioactive contrast agents that accumulate in the bladder and thus disproportionately irradiate the gonads.

Magnetic resonance imaging (MRI) of the kidneys has been investigated as an alternative to existing imaging methods *(2)*. Advantages include the ability to image in any plane, higher spatial resolution, absence of ionizing radiation, and a safe contrast agent to use as a filtration marker *(3)*. The recent development of fast pulse sequences and the ability to compensate for respiratory motion, as well as new analytic methods, make MRI even more appealing as a method of evaluating renal function *(4,5)*. The purpose of this chapter is to review the current status of functional imaging of the kidney with MRI.

1.1. Principles and Techniques

1.1.1. Physical Basis

MRI generates images by applying a magnetic field to the body and stimulating protons with radiofrequency waves. As they relax back toward their

From: *Methods in Molecular Medicine, vol. 86: Renal Disease: Techniques and Protocols*
Edited by: M. S. Goligorsky © Humana Press Inc., Totowa, NJ

ground state, a small signal is induced in radiofrequency receivers. This signal can then be used to generate a complete two- or three-dimensional image.

1.1.2. T1 and T2 Relaxation

After radiofrequency irradiation and displacement from their normal alignment with the main magnetic field, protons relax in two distinct but simultaneous ways. The protons, which can be envisioned as small bar magnets, will attempt to realign with the main magnetic field after excitation. This process of longitudinal relaxation is known as T1 relaxation. At the same time, the individual protons dephase with respect to each other. This process of transverse relaxation is known as T2 relaxation. Transverse relaxation occurs more rapidly if the local magnetic field is heterogeneous, and this process is known as T2* relaxation *(6)*.

2. Materials

2.1. Contrast Agents

Contrast agents are used in MRI to change the T1 and T2 relaxation rates that are normally found in tissues. The currently approved gadolinium (Gd) chelates are small molecules, less than 1000 Daltons, which are in widespread clinical use. These agents primarily affect the T1 of tissue by accelerating the process of longitudinal relaxation *(7)*. At high concentrations they also affect T2 and T2*. To avoid the competing effects of T1 shortening (which brightens the image) and T2/T2* shortening (which darkens the image), gadolinium chelates are used in low concentrations. Thus, for functional imaging of the kidney, a low dose of Gd chelate is used (.01–.05 mmol/kg).

2.2. Gd Chelates

Gd chelates are relatively safe, and do not injure the kidney. Several large studies have shown no effect of Gd chelates on renal function, even at doses of 0.3 mmol/kg *(8)*. Gd chelates also have a low rate of allergic reactions. Serious reactions are seen in approx 1:50,000 to 1:100,000 injections.

3. Methods

3.1. Renal MRI with Gd Chelates

A functional dynamic enhanced MRI is based on the idea that the Gd chelate is filtered by the kidney and is neither secreted nor reabsorbed *(9)*. T1-weighted gradient echo MRI images of the kidney are obtained before and after the injection of the contrast agent. The kidney is monitored periodically for up to 20 min after contrast injections. The coronal plane is usually selected to image the kidneys. Scans are obtained every 30 sec and this allows the generation of time-signal curves over the kidney parenchyma. If low doses are used, this study can be repeated within 20–30 min. A patient undergoing a functional MRI must be adequately hydrated before the test because dehydration will result in hyperconcentration of the Gd chelate, which in turn results in T2* shortening. Since this reduces the signal in the kidney at the same time that the T1 effects are increasing the signal, it leads to a nonlinear relationship between Gd concentration and the MR signal, which is undesirable for a functional test.

3.2. Renal MRI with Captopril

The time-signal excretion curve of Gd chelates can be manipulated by the use of an angiotensin-converting enzyme (ACE) inhibitor such as captopril *(10)*. In the presence of renal artery stenosis, captopril will decrease the compensatory efferent arteriolar vasoconstriction, leading to a decreased pressure drop across the glomerulus. This will lead to decreased excretion of the Gd chelate. By comparing the excretion curve before and after captopril, it is possible to evaluate the likelihood of physiologically significant renal artery stenosis leading to renovascular hypertension.

The time-signal profiles of dynamic MRIs allow the differentiation between normal and abnormal patients with a variety of renal diseases. Evaluation of renal perfusion with MRI has become more feasible with the development of rapid data acquisition methods that allow the collection of an image in less than 1 sec. The study is also greatly aided by surface coils placed over the kidney, which improve signal reception.

3.3. MR Renography (Fig. 1)

The pattern of enhancement within the kidney can be divided into several different phases. The vascular phase begins about 10–30 sec after injection, and is characterized by the intense enhancement of the renal cortex, reflecting glomerular filtration, while the medulla remains unenhanced. During the tubular phase that follows, contrast enters the medulla, first descending the loop of Henle and then ascending it to the collecting ducts. During the excretory phase, contrast is excreted into the renal pelvis and ureters *(11)*.

A normal time-signal curve from a cursor placed over the cortex reveals a rapid rise in signal after injection, followed by a slow fall in signal that reflects gradual clearance. The medullary curve is similar, except the onset of the rise in signal is delayed by several seconds, and the rate of decline in signal is often less because the tubules concentrate the residual Gd chelate. If the patient is dehydrated or a high dose of contrast is used, the medullary signal may actually become stronger (darker) with time, reflecting T2* changes.

Changes in MR renograms reflect glomerular filtration. The initial slope of the contrast uptake as well as the rate of decline of signal can be measured.

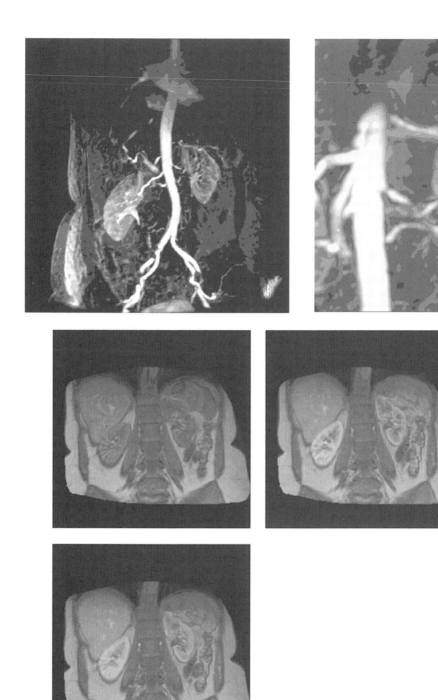

Fig. 1.

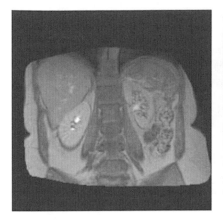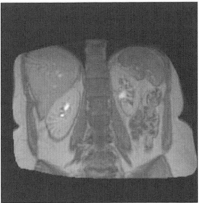

Fig. 1. *(continued)* A 60-yr-old female with a history of renovascular hypertension who underwent contrast-enhanced MRA of renal arteries. There is a significant stenosis of the left renal artery. The right renal artery shows normal caliber. MR renography time-series images over 20 min show a delay and decrease in signal intensity enhancement in the left renal parenchyma compared to the right kidney.

The time between the arrival of contrast and the first appearance of enhanced urine (renal transit time) can also be evaluated.

3.4. Arterial Spin Labeling

Arterial Spin Labeling (ASL) is another method of evaluating renal function. Instead of employing an exogenous contrast agent, this technique tags the blood upstream of the kidney with a radiofrequency pulse that can then be measured downstream within the kidney. Thus, if a tag is placed over the abdominal aorta cephalad to the kidneys, the spin labeling effect can be measured over the kidneys as a reduction in signal that is proportional to the blood flow. By continuously applying the tag, a steady-state magnetization will be reached in the kidney tissue *(12)*. These images must be adjusted for artifacts caused by magnetization transfer, an MR artifact induced by exchanges between free and bound tissue water. Comparison of images obtained before and after the application of the tag allows for quantitative measurement of renal perfusion. The main advantages of this technique are that it uses endogenous contrast, can continuously monitor blood flow, and is potentially quantitative. However, the technique is not yet widely available on clinical scanners.

3.5. Diffusion Imaging

Thermal-induced molecular motion causes nuclear spins to dephase under a magnetic-field gradient, thereby reducing the MR signal. The signal reduction is proportional to the strength of the applied magnetic-field gradients. In order to generate a diffusion image, motion-sensitizing bipolar magnetic-field gradients are applied. Areas of high water mobility have substantial signal attenuation, and therefore appear darker. The rate at which signal declines is a function of gradient strength and the apparent diffusion coefficient (ADC) *(13)*. Clearly, such diffusion-weighted imaging (DWI) is also sensitive to bulk motion as well as blood flow and tubular transit. By creating ADC maps of the kidney, specific measurements in the region of interest over the cortex and medulla can be obtained. These measurements cannot yet be translated into quantitative blood flow or tubular flow measurements; however, they may be a noninvasive method of detecting changes in these parameters. A major limitation of Diffusion imaging is that the images are sensitive to movement (respiratory or patient movement), and thus must either be obtained very quickly or with a motion-correction algorithm. An interesting application of DWI is that it can reveal non-isotropic motion—e.g., motion that favors one direction over another. This is of a major interest to renal imaging because the geometry of tubular flow is critical to renal function.

3.6. Blood Oxygen Level Determination (Fig. 2)

Blood Oxygen Level Determination (BOLD) imaging has been widely used in brain studies to detect regions of cerebral activation during specific tasks. In these experiments, the patient is asked to perform a specific task (such as finger tapping), and regions of increased blood flow can be detected in the brain, corresponding to the activated regions. This phenomenon is based on changes in the deoxyhemoglobin-to-oxyhemoglobin ratio in a particular tissue. Deoxyhemoglobin is paramagnetic (and thus relaxes more quickly), whereas oxyhemoglobin is diamagnetic (relaxes more slowly). Thus, as fresh oxygenated blood enters a specific part of the brain, it changes the oxy/deoxy hemoglobin ratio, and produces an MR signal increase in T2*-weighted images *(14,15)*.

Relative regional oxygenation can also be measured in the kidney using this technique. Prasad et al. performed BOLD studies in healthy volunteers at different ages. BOLD effects were found when furosemide, but not acetazolamide, was administered to the subjects. Furosemide inhibits active transport and is expected to improve oxygenation in the medulla, whereas acetazolamide, an inhibitor of proximal tubular reabsorption, produces minimal changes in oxygenation *(16)*. These results demonstrate the feasibility of BOLD MR imaging techniques to monitor changes in regional oxygenation. In an unpublished study using the BOLD technique in patients with renovascular hypertension, breathing room air and Carbogen (95% oxygen, 5% carbon dioxide) through a reservoir apparatus demonstrated reversible changes in the hypoxia regions within the kidneys during Carbogen inhalation.

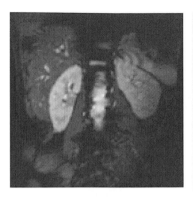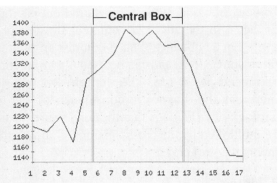

Fig. 2. A 19-yr-old female with elevated blood pressure who underwent a carbogen breathing test. Echo-planar image acquired after carbogen inhalation shows a significant change in signal intensity in inner medullary pixels. This reflects changes of deoxyhemoglobin to oxyhemoglobin ratio in a given tissue. The graph shows the effect of breathing room air then carbogen (central box) and then returning to the room air. Note the rise in signal during carbogen inhalation.

3.7. Magnetic Resonance Angiography (Fig. 1)

Magnetic Resonance Angiography (MRA) is based on the rapid injection of intravenous (iv) Gd chelate during the acquisition of a heavily T1-weighted three-dimensional (3D) sequence. If the scanning is timed properly (using a test bolus or an automated bolus detection method), only the aorta and renal arteries will be seen. This provides for noninvasive method of evaluating renal arteries for stenosis *(17)*. As scanning times have decreased, it has become possible to use very thin slices with high resolution to more accurately measure the degree of stenosis and detect other pathology such as fibromuscular hyperplasia and renal artery aneurysm. This technique has been widely adopted, and has proven to be highly accurate when compared to conventional angiography. Nonetheless, angiography retains a higher spatial resolution, and MRA tends to slightly overestimate the degree of stenosis.

Of course, an MRA simply displays the anatomy and does not provide information about the functional significance of the anatomic lesion. Thus, MRA can be combined with the functional MRI techniques previously described. Specifically, captopril can be administered before the dynamic MR sequence to detect changes in renal function in the affected kidney *(10)*.

Another method of evaluating renal arterial blood flow is phase-contrast angiography. This technique makes use of the fact that as protons move in the direction of a magnetic gradient they gain phase with respect to protons in stationary tissue. The accrued phase gain of moving protons is related to the velocity of blood. If the applied gradient is properly scaled to the peak velocity expected in the artery, a complete flow velocity waveform over the cardiac cycle can be obtained. Phase-contrast angiography can be performed in two or three dimensions, and can be used in conjunction with a conventional contrast-enhanced MRA *(18)*. The combined information from both techniques increases the diagnostic confidence of the test. Moreover, phase-contrast angiography (PCA) is quantitative, since mean velocity within the vessel can be multiplied by the cross-sectional diameter to obtain flow-volume measurements (cc/sec) *(19)*.

4. Notes

1. Currently, there are a number of techniques that can measure renal function noninvasively with MRI. Compared to nuclear medicine techniques, MRI offers the advantages of higher spatial resolution and absence of radiation.
2. However, if too high a dose of contrast is given or if the patient is dehydrated, spurious results may be obtained because of the nonlinear relationship between signal intensity and Gd concentration at high Gd concentrations.
3. Also limiting the use of MRI is the absence of user-friendly software analysis packages for renal function.
4. However, as MRI technology progresses, clinicians will become more interested in using a single test to obtain necessary information to manage patients. Functional imaging of the kidney with MRI is a versatile and accurate method for measuring renal functions in vivo.

References

1. Taylor, A. (1999) Radionuclide renography: a personal approach. *Semin. Nucl. Med.* **29(2),** 102–127. Review.
2. Bennett, H. F. and Li, D. (1997) MR imaging of renal function. *Magn. Reson. Imaging Clin. N. Am.* **5(1),** 107–126.
3. Choyke, P. L., Frank, J. A., Girton, M. E., Inscoe, S. W., Carvlin, M. J., Black, J. L., et al. (1989) Dynamic Gd-DTPA-enhanced MR imaging of the kidney: experimental results. *Radiology* **170,** 713–720.
4. Lee, V. S., Rusinek, H., Johnson, G., Rofsky, N. M., Krinsky, G. A., and Weinreb, J. C. (2001) MR renography with low-dose gadopentetate dimeglumine: feasibility. *Radiology* **221(2),** 371–379.
5. de Priester, J. A., Kessels, A. G., Giele, E. L., den Boer, J. A., Christiaans, M. H., Hasman, A., et al. (2001) MR renography by semiautomated image analysis: performance in renal transplant recipients. *J. Magn. Reson. Imaging* **14(2),** 134–140.
6. Taylor, J., Summers, P. E., Keevil, S. F., Saks, A. M., Diskin, J., Hilton, P. J., et al. (1991) Advances in contrast-enhanced MR imaging. Principles. *AJR Am. J. Roentgenol.* **156(2),** 236–239.
7. Nelson, K. L., Gifford, L. M., Lauber-Huber, C., Gross, C. A., and Lasser, T. A. (1995) Clinical safety of gadopentetate dimeglumine. *Radiology* **196,** 439–443.

8. Prince, M. R., Arnoldus, C., and Frisoli, J. F. (1996) Nephrotoxicity of high-dose gadolinium compared to iodinated contrast. *JMRI* **6,** 162–166.

9. Frank, J. A., Choyke, P. L., Austin, H. A., 3rd, Girton, M. E., and Weiss, G. (1991) Gadopentetate dimeglumine as a marker of renal function. Magnetic resonance imaging to glomerular filtration rates. *Invest. Radiol.* **26 Suppl 1,** S134–S136; discussion S137–S138.

10. Grenier, N., Trillaud, H., Combe, C., et al. (1996) Diagnosis of renovascular hypertension: feasibility of captopril-sensitized dynamic MR imaging and comparison with captopril scintigraphy. *AJR* **166,** 835–843.

11. Taylor, J., Summers, P. E., Keevil, S. F., Saks, A. M., Diskin, J., Hilton, P. J., et al. (1997) Magnetic resonance renography: optimisation of pulse sequence parameters and Gd-DTPA dose, and comparison with radionuclide renography. *Magn. Reson. Imaging* **15(6),** 637–649.

12. Berr, S. S., Hagspiel, K. D., Mai, V. M., Keilholz-George, S., Knight-Scott, J., Christopher, J. M., et al. (1999) Perfusion of the kidney using extraslice spin tagging (EST) magnetic resonance imaging. *J. Magn. Reson. Imaging* **10(5),** 886–891.

13. Siegel, C. L., Aisen, A. M., Ellis, J. H., Londy, F., and Chenevert, T. L. (1995) Feasibility of MR diffusion studies in the kidney. *J. Magn. Reson. Imaging* **5(5),** 617–620.

14. Prasad, P. V., Edelman, R. R., and Epstein, F. H. (1996) Noninvasive evaluation of intrarenal oxygenation with BOLD MRI. *Circulation* **15;94(12),** 3271–3275.

15. Prasad, P. V., Chen, Q., Goldfarb, J. W., Epstein, F. H., and Edelman, R. R. (1997) Breath-hold R2* mapping with a multiple gradient-recalled echo sequence: application to the evaluation of intrarenal oxygenation. *J. Magn. Reson. Imaging* **7(6),** 1163–1165.

16. Prasad, P. V., Epstein, F. H., Li, W., et al. (1996) Intrarenal oxygenation with BOLD MRI: effects of diuretics, In *Proceedings of the International Society of Magnetic Resonance in Medicine*, New York, p. 9.

17. Schoenberg, S. O., Knopp, M. V., Londy, F., Krishnan, S., Zuna, I., and Lang, N. (2002) Morphologic and functional magnetic resonance imaging of renal artery stenosis: a multireader tricenter study. *J. Am. Soc. Nephrol.* **13(1),** 158–169.

18. Dong, Q., Schoenberg, S. O., Carlos, R. C., Neimatallah, M., Cho, K. J., Williams, D. M., et al. (1999) Diagnosis of renal vascular disease with MR angiography. *Radiographics* **19(6),** 1535–1554.

19. Marcos, H. B. and Choyke, P. L. (2000) Magnetic resonance angiography of the kidney. *Semin. Nephrol.* **20(5),** 450–455.

6

Use of Radionuclides to Study Renal Function

Yiyan Liu and M. Donald Blaufox

1. Introduction

1.1. Measurement of Glomerular Filtration Rate (GFR)

Radionuclides have been used to study renal function clinically since the introduction of the radioisotope renogram by Taplin *(1)* and Kimball *(2)*. This use is mainly directed at the excretory functions of the kidney that involve glomerular filtration and tubular secretion. Glomerular filtration is a process that may be quantified by the measurement of the rate of renal clearance of a particular substance in the blood. The indicator must meet the following criteria: i) free filtration through the glomerular capillary membranes; ii) no secretion or absorption by the renal tubules; iii) no metabolism by the kidney; iv) no binding to plasma proteins; v) nontoxic and inert; and vi) measurable with high accuracy. Radiochemical purity is an additional requirement when radiolabeled agents are used.

The clearance of insulin is accepted as the standard for the determination of the glomerular filtration rate (GFR). Its accurate measurement is difficult for routine clinical use because it is expensive, time-consuming, and requires a steady-state plasma concentration and multiple urine samples for the greatest accuracy. This has been compounded by the fact that it no longer is readily available.

Endogenous creatinine clearance is used as a more convenient index of GFR, but it is inaccurate. Results depend on a complete and accurately timed urine collection, which is difficult to achieve. In pathologic states, its validity as a glomerular filtration marker is limited *(3–5)*. The creatinine clearance can vary in an individual by as much as 25% because of methodological errors *(6)*. Serum creatinine is a good index of renal function, but its relationship to clearance is dependent on muscle mass, so that it is difficult to define normal values.

Radionuclide techniques have been developed in an effort to overcome these limitations and to help serve the need to evaluate renal function in clinical

From: *Methods in Molecular Medicine, vol. 86: Renal Disease: Techniques and Protocols*
Edited by: M. S. Goligorsky © Humana Press Inc., Totowa, NJ

practice. The chemical properties of inulin do not allow for easy labeling with radioactive nuclides, although carbon-14, iodine-125, iodine-131 and chromium-51 have been used with varying degrees of success. Radiolabeled vitamin B12 has also been used in attempts to measure GFR, but the lack of predictability of the exact amount of protein binding is a serious drawback. Radiographic contrast agents labeled with either I-125 or I-131 are used to measure GFR, but they are not ideal for renal imaging and thus individual renal GFR cannot be calculated *(7)*. ^{125}I-Iothalamate has been widely used to measure total renal clearance *(8,9)*. Ethylenediaminetetraacetic acid (EDTA) labeled with Cr-51 yields a plasma clearance that correlates very well with insulin clearance *(10)*, but it is not suitable for imaging available in the United States.

Since its introduction in early the 1970s, diethylenetriaminepentaacetic acid (DTPA) labeled with Technitium-99 has been a primary choice for clinical GFR measurement in the United States. Tc-99m-DTPA satisfies the requirements of a suitable clearance agent for GFR measurement, and is discussed in detail in the following section.

Various techniques have proven valuable in the measurement of GFR with radionuclides. The general principles of these techniques follow.

1.1.1. Continuous Infusion Techniques
With or Without Urine Collection

This method requires a continuous intravenous (iv) infusion to maintain a constant plasma concentration while collecting several consecutively timed urine samples (bladder catheterization may be necessary for accurate collections). Clearance is calculated from the formula *UV/P* (where *U* and *P* are urine and plasma concentrations of radioactivity, respectively, and *V* is the urine volume per min). This clearance is equivalent to the total urinary excretion divided by the integral of plasma concentration for any given interval.

The constant-infusion technique alternatively may be performed without urine collection. After the intravenously infused substance reaches equilibrium in its total volume of distribution, the rate of disappearance of the tracer via glomerular filtration is equivalent to the rate of infusion. Equilibrium can be determined with external counting. Clearance is then calculated by dividing the rate of infusion by the plasma level. One potential source of error in this method is the accumulation of tracer metabolites that are cleared at a slower rate than the radiotracer. This may artificially overestimate the plasma concentration of tracer and then underestimate clearance *(11)*.

Generally, these constant-infusion techniques offer little advantage over nonradioactive methods other than simplification of the measurement because of the ease of quantitating radioactivity. Radionuclide determinations of GFR are usually performed with single-injection techniques.

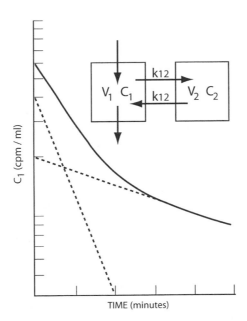

Fig. 1. A two-compartment plasma-clearance curve. The dose (D) is injected into the plasma. Throughout the study, it is excreted by renal clearance (Cl). It distributes in the central compartment whose volume is V1 at a changing concentration (C1). The direction of diffusion into the second compartment (V2) at rate K_{12} or K_{21} depends upon the concentration gradient (C2). Clearance values can be calculated from this curve.

1.1.2. Urinary Clearance with Single Injection

The ability to measure plasma concentrations of radiotracers at either very high or very low levels enables one to determine clearance after a single iv injection. Several plasma samples are taken during the entire clearance period, and a semilog plot is made of their radionuclide concentrations. The individually collected urine samples are also measured and counted. The standard formula UV/P can then be applied to each clearance sample. These clearances are usually determined after the disappearance of activity from the plasma has began to approach a single exponential.

1.1.3. Single Injection with a Dual-Compartmental Analysis

The most popular model of the excretion of a GFR tracer is a dual-compartmental model that is described by a biexponential curve (**Fig. 1**). The initial phase of the curve is rapid, and is primarily affected by the redistribution of radiotracer into the extracellular space. The second portion of the curve is much slower, and results primarily from the elimination of the tracer by glomerular filtration once distribution in the extracellular space is complete. Both processes occur throughout the study. A complete plasma-clearance curve must be obtained to represent activity in the two compartments accurately. This requires multiple blood samples (at least six). Then a multicompartmental analysis of the tracer-disappearance curve can be used to estimate GFR with a formula based on a two-compartment model *(12)*.

Russell et al. *(13)* evaluated the optimal sample timing following a single injection for GFR measurements, assuming the two-compartment model. The results showed that for the most accurate values, sample times must begin by 10 min and continue for at least 240 min. Six blood samples were recommended and the duration of sampling should be at least 3 h, since the slow compartment of excretion accounted for the majority of the clearance. Modification of these times results in some loss of accuracy, but the error with a 120-min sampling time is usually acceptable clinically (<5%).

1.1.4. Single Injection with Single-Compartment Analysis

A desire for simplification has led to the replacement of multi-compartmental models with single-compartment models that need only two or three blood samples **(Fig. 2)**. Further simplified techniques requiring only one blood sample also have been developed *(14,15)*. Blood samples are drawn after equilibration of the injected radiotracer with extracellular fluid (ECF) is complete. Thus, the assumption is made that the clearance agent is distributed in a single compartment, from which it is eliminated exclusively by the kidneys. The model curve would then be similar to the second, slower exponential of the two-compartment model. These methods disregard the initial fast component of the plasma-concentration curve, and measured GFR values usually are greater than the true GFR because of overestimation of the volume of distribution *(11)*.

Several studies have compared the two-sample method with the two-compartmental model for GFR measurement. Waller et al. *(15)* found that the correlation was excellent ($r = 0.996$) between the clearance obtained from 2- and 4-h plasma samples and a seven-plasma-sample technique. Another method requires samples between 1 h and 3 h after injection, and yields results comparable to the multiple sample techniques ($r = 0.962$) *(16)*. It is recommended that sampling times should start 1 h after injection because complete equilibration is not to reached at the earlier times. Most investigators wait 2 h. It is important to note that although the correlation is very good, the values are not identical.

The one-sample technique obviously is the simplest in vitro method for the measurement of GFR. The technique basically measures the plasma concentration of radiotracer at the time the sample is drawn, and compares it to the amount of tracer injected using carefully calibrated standards. Although its application is limited in some clinical situations, the one-sample method is generally considered to be accurate enough for routine clinical use.

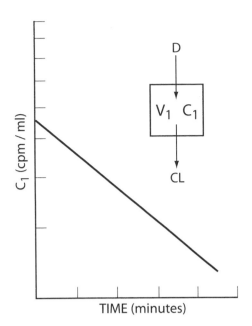

Fig. 2. A single-compartment model. The dose (D) is injected into a single compartment (V1), and the curve obtained is a single compartment. In order to obtain a single-compartment curve, a predetermined portion of the complete curve must be sampled. The time relationships will vary depending upon the tracer used.

1.1.5. Other Techniques

GFR can be estimated based on the rate of tracer appearance within the urine. Jackson et al. *(17)* described a method that corrected excreted activity in the bladder 30 min after tracer injection for postvoiding bladder residual urine volume and compared it with a plasma-activity curve obtained by using a single blood sample at 30 min and a gamma camera-generated blood-pool time-activity curve from the heart. The GFR was calculated from the terminal slope of the plasma-disappearance curve. This technique was found to have a good correlation with 24-h creatinine clearance ($r = 0.968$). However, as stated previously, urinary methods are inconvenient, and are prone to collection errors.

Bianchi has described a similar technique that permits individual renal clearance to be calculated *(18)*.

Measurement of GFR is considered by nephrologists to be the most useful test of renal function because a reduction in GFR is an accurate index in most pathological states. The selected protocols and choice of methods are discussed in the following section. Measurements of renal function using tubular secreted agents are generally preferred by nuclear medicine practitioners because these agents have superior imaging characteristics.

1.2. Measurement of Effective Renal Plasma Flow (ERPF)

Among patients who are studied by imaging techniques, the preferred radiopharmaceuticals are usually excreted by the renal tubules. Renal plasma flow is estimated from the clearance of a compound that is almost completely extracted from the renal blood. Since no compound is totally extracted in a single pass through the kidney, the measurement of renal plasma flow realistically falls slightly below the true renal plasma flow, and thus is known as effective renal plasma flow.

Paraminohippuric acid (PAH) is used as the standard for ERPF measurement because its clearance most closely approximates total renal plasma flow. Although the measurements of PAH clearance are very accurate, this method requires constant infusion and urine collection, is inconvenient, and lacks precision. For these reasons, PAH clearance is now rarely used to measure renal function in humans (43,44). Chemical methods are not suitable for single injection because the amounts used may exceed Tm.

The introduction of radionuclides and their use in monitoring renal function has made ERPF measurement convenient and less time-consuming. Many methods of ERPF measurement with radionuclides have been reported in the literature. Most of the variety is between the number of plasma samples and the timing of these samples.

The most common technique is a single bolus administration of the radiotracer followed by either one- or two-plasma samples. Both methods assume that the material is distributed in a single compartment and is excreted only by the kidney.

In 1963, Blaufox et al. (45) demonstrated the inverse relation of the specific plasma concentration of I-131-OIH (orthoiodohippuric acid) to the ERPF after a single injection, and presented this method to calculate an index for estimation of renal function. They showed that an OIH-clearance technique requiring only two-plasma samples (more than 20 min after injection) leads to results with a good correlation to PAH clearance ($r = 0.90$), but their values were generally 10–15% higher (46) (Fig. 3). The rate of disappearance of isotope is used to estimate renal clearance, which is calculated from the product of the slope of the exponential disappearance and the volume of distribution (46). The single sample method requires only a single blood sample at about 44 min (for hippuran). This sample is assumed to fit to a known parabolic or exponential function to calculate the clearance (47). ERPF also can be measured in vivo by an imaging method. Studies have shown that a one-sample method with I-131-OIH is more accurate than the gamma camera in vivo method (48).

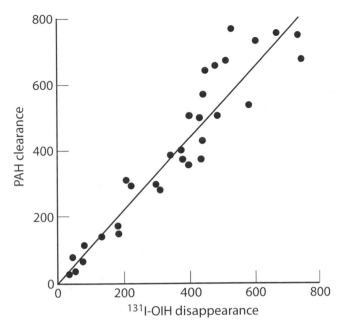

Fig. 3. The continuous-infusion clearance of PAH vs a single-injection clearance of I-131-OIH. The excretion ratio of Hippuran is slightly lower than that of PAH, resulting in a systematic underestimate. However, the extraction is high enough to provide a useful estimate of the ERPF.

1.3. Determination of Individual Renal Function

It is imperative that unilateral renal function can be measured, because total renal function may be nearly normal even in the presence of functional loss of one kidney. Gamma camera techniques have been developed to measure both global and differential GFR and ERPF.

In most cases, the injected tracer leaves the kidney within the first 3 min. Relative renal uptake of the radiopharmaceutical is proportional to the contribution of each kidney to total renal function before there is any significant excretion into the collecting system. The most commonly used approach is to compare counts summed over a 1 min period, from 1–2 or 2–3 min after radionucleotide administration. Later time periods should be avoided because the radiotracer is present in significant amounts in the collecting system after this time. Differential GFR can be determined from the net counts accumulated by each kidney during the first few min of the study. Correction can be made for tissue attenuation and background. Although several techniques utilize one blood sample for multiple corrections of the GFR calculation (*62*), most do not require blood or urine samples. The obvious advantage of gamma camera tech-

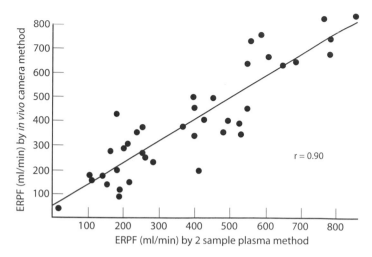

Fig. 4. The correlation between the ERPF measured with I-131-OIH by in vitro two-sample method and in vivo camera method. The correlation coefficient was 0.90.

niques is speed, ease of performance, and suitability for simultaneous clinical renography. However, gamma camera techniques are considerably less accurate in estimating GFR than in vitro measurement (**Fig. 4**).

Of all of the commercially available radiopharmaceuticals for renography, Tc-99m-DTPA is widely used for GFR andTc-99m-MAG3 for ERPF. The accumulation of Tc-99m-DTPA within each kidney at the 2–3 min time interval following tracer arrival is proportional to GFR *(63)*. Linear regression analysis of the percent uptake of Tc-99m-DTPA with a 24-h creatinine clearance showed an excellent correlation of these two variables *(64)*. Delpassand et al. *(65)* also found an excellent correlation between GFR estimated using the dual-detector gamma camera and GFR measured using the plasma clearance of Tc-99m DTPA with multiple blood samples. GFR can be estimated by determining the absolute amount of Tc-99m-DTPA in the kidney at 1–2 or 2–3 min after injection and expressing this amount as a fraction of the injected dose *(66)*. The determination of the absolute amount in the kidneys requires a knowledge of the exact amount of activity injected, correction for any residual activity in the syringe or in the patient's arm, the conversion factor from counts to uCi (kBq), and kidney depth correction. A similar technique can be used to calculate ERPF from the Tc-99m-MAG3 uptake at 1–2 or 2–3 min after injection. Although these techniques for in vivo measurement of total function are reproducible in an individual, they are not very accurate, with errors up to 25%. Estimation of relative individual function has a much smaller error of about 5%.

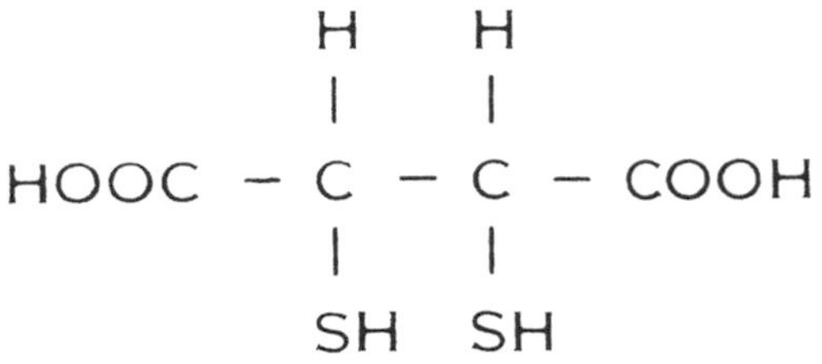

$$
\begin{array}{ccccc}
& H & & H & \\
& | & & | & \\
HOOC & - \ C & - \ C & - \ COOH \\
& | & & | & \\
& SH & & SH &
\end{array}
$$

DMS (MW 182)

Fig. 5. The structure formula of DMSA (dimercapto-succinic acid).

Another useful radiopharmaceutical for split kidney function is Tc-99m-DMSA (dimercapto-succinic acid) (**Fig. 5**). A chelate of DMSA with Tc-99m was found to accumulate in the kidneys, and was introduced as a substitute for organomercurial substances in renal parenchymal imaging. Tc-99m-DMSA is 90% protein-bound, and peritubular uptake accounts for about 65% of its excretion. Glomerular filtration accounts for about 35% (*67*). It has been reported to be localized in the proximal tubule of the cortex, with only negligible activity in the papilla and medulla (*67*). However, Yee et al. reported a significant effect of urinary PH on DMSA excretion, suggesting a significant role for the distal tubule (*68*). Regardless of its actual mechanism of excretion, Tc-99m-DMSA is a cortical scanning agent, and an indicator of functional tubular renal mass. The precise mechanism of tubular uptake remains unknown. The specific cortical uptake of DMSA yields a high sensitivity for detecting defects and scars in the renal cortex. Tc-99m-DMSA has also been used to evaluate renal function by SPECT quantitation (*69*).

1.4. Radionuclide Renogram

Series images of the kidney may be obtained following bolus injection of a renally excreted radionuclide. Regions of interest are then drawn around the kidneys, and a time-activity curve is generated from the renal activity at 15-sec intervals. This time-activity curve is known as a renogram. The rengogram was the earliest routine clinical application of radionuclides in clinical evaluation of renal function (*1,2*). In current practice, renograms are derived from dynamic renal imaging studies by drawing kidney regions of interest on the computer.

The renogram represents several different components of radionuclide distribution: the appearance of radionuclide in the renal area (first phase), accumulation in the kidney prior to significant excretion (second phase), and the

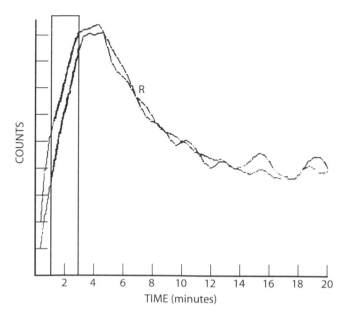

Fig. 6. The normal renogram with three phases of radionuclide distribution: appearance of tracer in the kidney at the first min, accumulation in the kidney by 3–5 min and dominant excretion after about 5 min.

third phase in which excretion is the dominant effect (**Fig. 6**). Since the kidneys receive approx 20% of the cardiac output, the first phase of the curve is rapidly up-sloping, with the sudden appearance of tracer. This begins about 15–20 sec after injection and reaches an inflection point at 30–50 sec. Renal tubular function and background activity also affect the initial slope. The second phase of the renogram is represented by a less rapid increase in activity, which usually reaches a peak at 3–5 min. This portion of the curve represents accumulation prior to significant emptying of the collecting system. By about 3–5 min, in normally hydrated, normally functioning kidneys, the renal activity begins to leave the kidney via the collecting system and reaches the bladder. The curve thereafter is represented by a rapid falling slope. A curve can then be generated that primarily represents perfusion. Rapidly acquired frames immediately following the bolus of either Tc-99m-MAG3 or Tc-99m-DTPA (2–3 sec each) delineate the aorta and the kidneys. Normally, activity is seen in the kidneys with 3.5 sec of being seen in the aorta (*76,77*).

The slope of the renogram curve is affected by many factors. Pre-renal insults affect the first portion of the curve. Renal diseases such as glomerulonephritis and obstruction will delay reaching the bladder, and affect the third portion of the curve (*76*).

Conventional radionuclide renograms may be modified to include the administration of a potent diuretic—for example, lasix—for the study of urinary tract obstruction. The prolonged retention of radioactivity in a nonobstructed, dilated system is caused by a reservoir effect. Increased urine flow produced by lasix results in a prompt washout of activity in a dilated, nonobstructed system. In cases of mechanical obstruction, the capacity of washout is much less, resulting in prolonged retention of tracer proximal to the obstruction *(60,78)*.

Renograms are used to diagnose renal arterial stenosis (RAS) with pharmacological intervention of angiotensin-converting enzyme inhibitor (ACEI). Glomerular filtration is driven by pressure across the renal glomerulus. When perfusion pressure drops in the presence of RAS, renal filtration also decreases. The normal compensatory response from the renin-angiotensin system produces constriction of the efferent arterioles of the glomerulus and raises the filtration pressure. ACEIs block the conversion of angiotensin I to angiotensin II, preventing this normal compensatory mechanism, which is mediated by angiotensin II. Glomerular filtration falls in the involved kidney because of a decrease of post-glomerular resistance. This decrease in renal glomerular filtration can be assessed noninvasively evaluated with renal scintigraphy and the renogram, using captopril as an ACE inhibitor. The definitive pattern with renin-dependent renovascular hypertension is an abnormal ACE inhibition study after a normal baseline study without ACE inhibition. In normal subjects and patients with hypertension that is unrelated to renal artery stenosis, the renogram curve remains unchanged compared with baseline after administration of the ACE inhibition.

1.5. PET in the Evaluation of Renal Function

Positron emission tomography (PET) is a nuclear medicine technique that lends itself to high resolution and accurate quantitation. A positron emitter ejects a positively charged electron from its nucleus during decay. The positron promptly collides with a negatively charged electron, and the two are annihilated with the emission of two 511 KeV gamma rays at 180° to each other. This double simultaneous emission allows highly accurate reconstruction of the original event by a ring detector and computer software. A more detailed description of the basic principles of PET imaging is readily found in the literature.

PET has recently emerged as an important diagnostic modality in clinical medicine. F-18 fluorodexyglucose (FDG)-PET has become an established imaging approach in oncology *(81,82)*. PET is also employed in the evaluation of CNS disorders (such as Alzheimer's and Parkinson's disease) and in vivo myocardial perfusion and metabolism *(83,84)*. Since PET involves cross-sectional imaging of a particular organ through quantitation of the distribution of a radioactive indicator, its clinical usefulness in evaluation of the perfusion and function would appear to be in those organ systems most intimately regulated by blood flow—for example, the heart, brain, or kidney. However, in contrast to the heart and brain, the use of PET in the kidney has not been well-defined. There is some limited experimental application of PET in determination of renal blood flow (RBF). To validate dynamic PET imaging as an estimate of RBF, the radioactive microsphere (MS) method in animals is usually cited as standard comparison for quantitative measure of the regional perfusion. Limited preliminary data show a good correlation between RBF measured by PET and RBF measured by MS, and a constant agreement between those two methods over a wide range of RBF *(85,86)*. However, to date, despite the potential benefits of renal hemodynamic studies, RBF measurement by PET in humans has not been validated.

Another potential application of PET in the kidney is the investigation of receptors. One of these is the angiotensin II (ANG II) receptor. ANG II is the biologically active component of the renin-angiotensin system, and it plays a pivotal role in the regulation of cardiovascular, renal, and endocrine function *(87)*. ANG II receptors are specific, membrane-bound, and concentrated in a variety of tissues and organs. Two distinct subtypes of the ANG II receptors have been separated based on their different affinities for nonpeptide antagonists. They are designated as AT1 and AT2, respectively *(88)*. The ANG II-AT1 receptor mediates all known physiological effects of ANG II, including renal blood flow, glomerular filtration, aldosterone secretion, and sodium and water reabsorption *(89)*. Szabo et al. radiolabeled a series of nonpeptide AT1 antagonists with ^{11}C and quantitated AT1 receptors in vivo with PET imaging *(90–92)*. Preliminary results demonstrated excellent PET images of AT1 receptors in dog kidneys with a high radioligand accumulation in the renal cortex. The specific binding of a selective AT1 antagonist is suitable for quantitative PET imaging of ANG II-AT1 receptors.

PET has also been used for the study of endothelin (ET) receptors. ET is a peptide with potent vasoactive properties, and is involved in several pathologic states, including renal, pulmonary, cardiovascular diseases, and angiogenesis. Thus, the study of expression of ET receptors is of clinical significance. Szabo et al. used ^{11}C-labeled ET-receptor antagonist for ET-receptor imaging in vivo, and found a wide expression of the receptors in various organs, including the kidney *(93)*.

Compared with traditional and more advanced receptor assay techniques in vitro, such as receptor-ligand binding assays, receptor autoradiography, PCR, and *in situ* hybridization, a significant advantage of the receptor quantitative imaging with PET is evident: it allows in vivo, noninvasive, and easily repeated or follow-up studies. All of these studies are still preliminary and experimental. Their application in humans has not yet been confirmed.

2. Materials

2.1. Measurement of GFR

Several radioactive agents labeled with gamma emitters are readily available for clinical GFR measurement. Radiolabeled insulin derivatives and vitamin B12 have been used with varied success, but are rarely used in recent times *(19–22)*.

I-131-Diatrizoate (DZT) has been used for GFR measurements. Plasma-protein binding of this agent is low, and tubular reabsorption and secretion of the tracer has not been observed. Determination of GFR by a single-plasma sample technique with single injection of I-131-DZT has been reported to yield accurate GFR values *(14)*.

I-125-Iothalamate is commercially available and has been successfully used for clearance measurement in several clinical series in adults and children in a number of recent clinical trials *(8,9)*.

EDTA is a chelating agent eliminated by glomerular filtration without undergoing metabolic change and very little tubular secretion. Chromium-51-EDTA is commercially available, and is widely used for GFR measurement in Europe but not in the United States. Binding to serum proteins has been reported to be low, and extrarenal elimination of the tracer is insignificant *(23)*. Cr-51-EDTA exhibits a high degree of radiochemical stability. A good correlation has been obtained between Cr-51-EDTA and insulin clearance, both by continuous infusion and single-sample techniques *(24,25)*. Cr-51 is not suitable for external imaging.

Tc-99m-DTPA is the most popular choice for clinical GFR measurement. DTPA complexes are stable, have low protein binding, are cleared by glomerular filtration, and are not reabsorbed or secreted. In man, about 4–5% of the administered dose is widely distributed in various tissues at 24 h which probably represents non-chelated activity. Biliary excretion and GI elimination are negligible *(26)*.

The ideal physical properties of Tc-99m for noninvasive external imaging and the ready commercial availability of high purity-labeled DTPA make it convenient and inexpensive to use clinically for GFR measurement. DTPA clearance is slightly lower compared to insulin *(27)* (**Fig. 7**). Strict quality control and checking for protein binding of the preparation are very important.

2.2. Measurement of Effective Renal Plasma Flow (ERPF)

Ideally, an agent for the measurement of renal plasma flow must have an extraction efficiency of 100%. PAH is the nearest, with an extraction efficiency

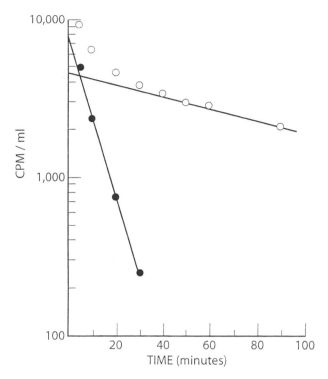

Fig. 7. Tc-99m-DTPA plasma clearance.

of about 90%. The two radiopharmaceuticals that most closely resemble the PAH are I-131-OIH and Tc-99m-MAG3 (Mercaptoacetyl triglycine) **(Fig. 8)**.

The clearance values with hippuran have been reported to be lower than those of PAH by about 15% **(Fig. 9)**, probably because of free iodine, different tubular transport, and plasma-protein-binding characteristics. Non-ionic diffusion of hippuran in the distal tunbule has been reported. The free iodine content in clinical preparations should not exceed 2%. Currently, I-131-Hippuran is being used less often for determination of the ERPF, since this I-131 labeled agent yields images of poor quality with the gamma camera system.

Tc-99m-MAG3 has become the clinical renal radiopharmaceutical agent of choice for imaging since its introduction in 1986. Tc-99m-MAG3 combines the advantages of the favorable imaging characteristics of a Tc-99m label with the favorable biologic properties of a compound that is cleared by tubular secretion *(49)*. The plasma clearance of Tc-99m-MAG3 is lower than that of I-131-OIH, with a ratio of about 75% *(49)* **(Fig. 10)**. This is attributed to very high protein binding, which makes its glomerular filtration negligible and also may limit

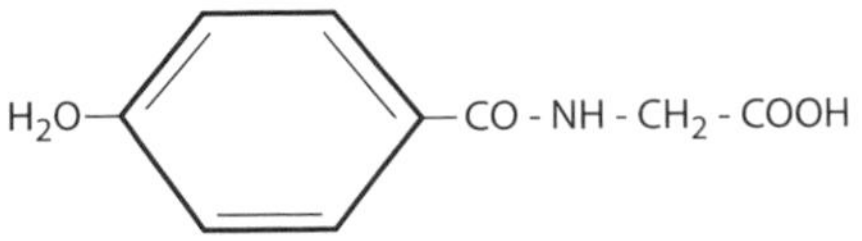

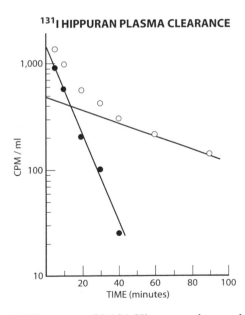

H₂O— ⟨benzene ring⟩ —CO - NH - CH₂ - COOH

Paraminohippuric acid

I— ⟨benzene ring⟩ —CO - NH - CH₂ - COOH

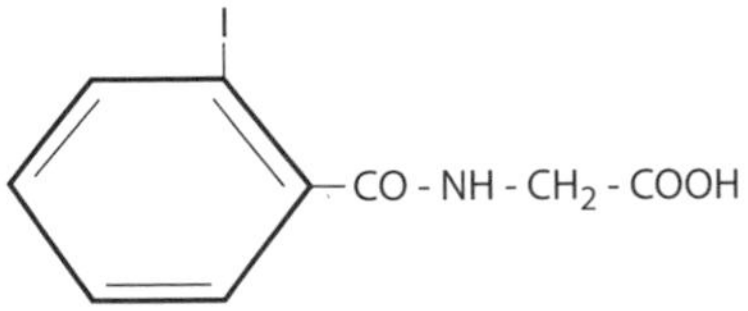

Orthoiodohippurate

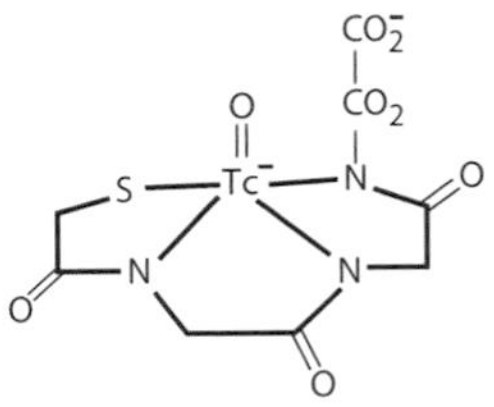

Mercaptoacetyl triglycine

Fig. 8. The structure formulas of the ERPF agents. PAH, paraminohippuric acid; OIH, orthoiodohippurate; MAG3, mercaptoacetyl triglycine.

^{131}I HIPPURAN PLASMA CLEARANCE

Fig. 9. The curve of I-131-Hippuran plasma clearance.

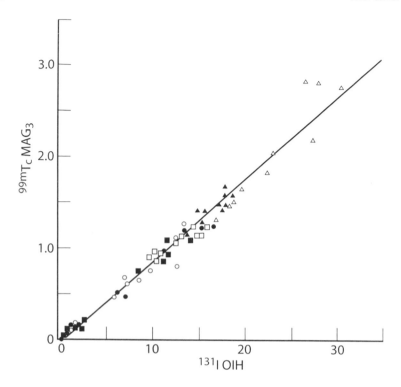

Fig. 10. Tc-99m-MAG3 plasma clearance vs I-131-OIH plasma clearance. The plasma clearance of Tc-99m-MAG3 is lower than that of I-131-OIH, with a ratio of approx 75%.

tubular extraction *(49,50)*. Bubeck et al. *(51)* proposed to describe the clearance of MAG3 as the tubular extraction ratio (TER) to emphasize the potential role of this agent in the follow-up of renal diseases in which tubular function is impaired, and also because of its lower estimate of renal plasma flow.

Another Tc-99m-labeled agent N,N-ethlenedicysteine (Tc-99m-EC) has been introduced as an alternative to MAG3 *(52)*. EC has a lesser degree of protein binding and a more rapid plasma-clearance rate that approaches that of hippuran. Preliminary clinical studies indicate a close similarity between EC and MAG3, both in renographic curves and renal imaging quality *(52)*.

2.3. Determination of Individual Renal Function

1. Gamma camera: Large field of view.
2. Collimator: Low energy, high resolution, parallel hole.
3. Energy window: 20% window centered at 140 keV.
4. Tc-99m-DTPA 3 mCi (for GFR) and Tc-99m-MAG3 10 mCi (for ERPF).

Table 1
Relative Clearance Values and Extraction Ratio

Compound	Clearance, mL/min (Normal adult)	ER	References
Inulin	100–125	25%	*59,61*
Tc-99m-DTPA	100–120	20%	*36,37,60*
Cr-51-EDTA	100–125	25%	*59,61*
PAH	550–600	90%	*43,49*
I-131-Hippuran	500–550	80–85%	*46,60*
Tc-99m-MAG₃	300–400	40–50%	*49,58,60*
Tc-99m-EC	350–400	40–50%	*52,60*

DTPA, diethylenetriaminepentaacetic acid; MAG3, mercaptoacetyl triglycine; EDTA, ethylenediaminetetraacetic acid; PAH, paraminohippuric acid; EC, N,N-ethlenedicysteine.

2.4. Radionuclide Renogram

Radiopharmaceutical: 1 mCi of Tc-99m-MAG3 or 3 mCi of Tc-DTPA. Because of resultant higher signal-to-noise ratio, the first-choice radiopharmaceuticals are those with a high extraction fraction, such as Tc-99m-MAG3 or I-123-OIH. Tc-99m-DTPA is a secondary choice for renogram, particularly in patients with impaired renal function.

Instrumentation:

1. Camera: Large field of view gamma camera.
2. Collimator: Low energy, all purpose, parallel hole.
3. Photopeak: 15% to 20% window center over 140 Kev.

2.5. PET in the Evaluation of Renal Function

There are two fundamental approaches to the measurement of tissue perfusion with PET: dynamic imaging following bolus injection and static imaging at steady state. Two types of tracers can be used for the bolus injection technique, either highly extracted with retention in tissue *(85,94)* or highly diffusible tracers with perfusion—limited transport between tissue and blood *(95,96)*. The steady-state technique must use an ultra-short-lived tracer *(97)*.

Highly extracted blood-flow tracers used in the single bolus technique include rubidium-82 *(98)* and nitrogen-13-ammonia *(85,94)*. Rubidium-82 is a potassium analog, which is taken up via the Na^+/K^+ pump. The half-life of Rb-82 is 76 sec. This very short half-life allows the performance of multiple sequential studies before and after various pharmacological interventions. Nitrogen-13 ammonia has a physical half-life of 10 min and a higher extraction than Rb-82. The N-13 label remains fixed in the heart or kidney with a longer biological residence time than Rb-82 because ammonia is metabolically changed to glutamine. For both Rb-82 and N-13 ammonia, extraction efficiency drops at higher rates of flow, but they provide a useful map of regional perfusion over a range of flow rates.

The measurement of tissue perfusion in a steady state makes use of ultrashort-lived tracers such as oxygen-15-labeled water, which has a half life of 2 min *(86,99)* and Rb-82. The labeled water is delivered continuously at a constant concentration to all the tissues of the body at equilibrium. The concentration of radioactivity in the tissue and in arterial blood becomes constant, and is proportional to input and inversely proportional to the sum of washout and decay. Oxygen-15-water is diffusable, and compared with ammonia, is not extracted or metabolized in the kidney. Oxygen-15-water kinetics can be described by a simple monocompartmental model that is more accurate for high flows typically measured in the kidney *(94)*. But Nitzsche et al. compared RBF measured by PET using oxygen-15-water and nitrogen-13-ammonia, and found a good correlation between the two methods in normal human volunteers *(100)*.

For the evaluation of ANG II-AT1 receptors with PET, ^{11}C-labeled selective AT1 antagonists is used *(91)*. The drug MK-996 is a potent nonpeptide AT1 selective antagonist that has been applied for treatment of essential hypertension. Szabo et al. labeled an analog of MK-996, a substituted benzoyl sulfonamide (L-159,884), for PET imaging *(90,91)*. It yielded a rapid, specific, and saturable binding with good PET imaging.

3. Methods

3.1. Measurement of Glomerular Filtration Rate (GFR) (see Notes 1–5)

3.1.1. Urinary Clearance Method (UV/P)

1. Patient preparation:
   The patient is hydrated with 3–5 glasses of water 30 min prior to the test. The patient must not void during the study unless instructed. No breakfast or coffee, tea, or orange juice is allowed on the day of the test, but a light lunch is permitted.
2. D5W at 125 mL per h for a normal patient or saline 0.9% at 125 mL per h for a diabetic patient is infused in one arm and blood drawing via heplock is performed in the opposite arm.
3. The patient is asked to void, and then 1 mCi Tc-99m-DTPA (1 mL in 5-mL syringe) is injected via the iv line. The exact time of injection will correspond to time zero.
4. 1 mCi Tc-99m-DTPA is retained for use as a standard.
5. The patient is asked to void at 1 h post injection, and the urine is discarded.
6. At 2 h after the DTPA injection, withdraw 6 mL of blood from the arm and transfer it into a test tube with heparin. **Caution:** Do not sample from the arm into which the injection was made.

7. The patient voids, the volume is recorded, and a 10-mL sample is transferred into a test tube. Pre-voiding activity over the bladder may be measured for residual urine determination *(28)*.
8. Measure and record the residual urine volume, if applicable, immediately after voiding. This step can be omitted in most patients with normal lower-urinary-tract function.

   If residual urine is determined, the patient is placed in the supine position, and a 2 × 2 in NaI crystal with a 5-inch cylindrical collimator is positioned directly over the bladder. Pre and post-void Tc-99m activity over the bladder and thigh are counted 3× for 1 min each. The final bladder activity counting rate is determined after subtracting the thigh count as a bladder background count. Residual volume is estimated as:

$$\text{Residual volume} = \frac{(\text{voided volume}) \times (\text{residual count})}{(\text{initial count}) - (\text{residual count})}$$

9. **Steps 7, 8,** and **9** are repeated at 3 and 4 h post-tracer injection.
10. Duplicate plasma and urine samples and a diluted Tc-99m-DTPA standard are counted in a gamma-well counter.
11. Determination of renal clearance:

    The Tc-99m-DTPA renal clearance can be calculated both with and without correction for residual urine volume in the bladder. The clearance can be calculated from a variation of the standard, *UV/P* method.

    The final clearance (2–4 h) is calculated as the average of the clearance at 2–3 h and 3–4 h using the formula:

$$\text{GFR} = \underline{\quad} \times \left(\frac{UV\ (2\text{–}3\ \text{h})}{P\ (2.5\ \text{h})} + \frac{UV\ (3\text{–}4\ \text{h})}{P\ (3.5\ \text{h})} \right)$$

Where U = Urine (cpm/mL)
$\quad V$ = Voided urine (mL)
$\quad P$ = Mid-point plasma (cpm/mL)

Correction for the residual urine volume in the bladder may be calculated using the formula:

$$\text{GFR}\ (2\text{–}3\ \text{h}) = UV/P\ (2.5\ \text{h})$$

Where $UV = B - A$ (corrected for the residual urine volume)
$\quad A = U\ (1\text{–}2\ \text{h, cpm/mL}) \times \text{Residual Volume}\ (1\text{–}2\ \text{h, mL})$
$\quad B = U\ (2\text{–}3\ \text{h, cpm/mL}) \times (\text{Voided Volume} + \text{Residual Volume}\ 2\text{–}3\ \text{h, mL})$

The 3–4 h collection is corrected in the same manner using the residual activity from 2–3 h.

3.1.2. Slope Method

As described previously, the slope method assumes that the radiopharmaceutical is distributed in a single compartment and excreted only by the kidney. This is obviously an oversimplification of the actual physiologic events following a single iv injection. In order to obtain a single-component curve, a predetermined portion of the complete curve must be sampled. The time relationship will vary depending upon which agent is being used (**Fig. 2**).

1. Inject 1 mci of Tc-99m-DTPA (all doses should be adjusted by body wt in children).
2. Obtain blood samples at 2, 3, and 4 h after administration of Tc-99m-DTPA.
3. Count radioactivity (cpm) for each plasma sample.
4. The clearance (GFR) is calculated from the slope of the line calculated from a semi-logarithmic plot of the three samples here. The formula is:

$$\text{Clearance or GFR} = \frac{\text{Dose injected (cpm)}}{A_0 \text{ (cpm/mL)}} \times \text{Slope}$$

Where A_0 is the intercept at time 0.

5. The result may be corrected by the Brochner-Mortensen formula to reduce the overestimation of GFR in the monoexponential model (*29*):

$$Cl_1 = 0.99 \times Cl_2 - 0.0012 \times Cl_2^2$$

Where Cl_1 is the clearance corrected for the first exponential and Cl_2 is the noncorrected clearance.

3.1.3. One-Plasma-Sample Method (No Urine Collection)

A blood sample is drawn at 180–240 min after the iv administration of 1 mCi Tc-99m-DTPA. Plasma radioactivity is determined.

There are many formulas for single plasma sample GFR measurement:

1. Christensen and Groth's method modified by Watson (*30*):

$$\text{GFR (mL/min)} = [-b + (b^2 - 4ac)^{1/2}]/2a$$

Where $a = t \times (0.0000017 \times t - 0.0012)$
$b = t \times (-0.000775 \times t + 1.31)$
$c = ECV \times \ln (ECV/V_t)$
ECV = extracellular volume (mL) = $8116.6 \times BSA - 28.2$
V_t = tracer apparent volume (mL) of distribution at time t
t = sample time (min)
BSA = body surface area (m²).

For a 3-h plasma sample:

$$A = -0.1609;\ b = 210.7;\ c = ECV \times \ln (ECV/V_{180})$$

Where V_{180} = tracer apparent volume (mL) of distribution at 180 min.

For a 4-h plasma sample:

$$A = -0.1901;\ b = 269.8;\ c = ECV \times \ln (ECV/V_{240})$$

Where V_{240} = tracer apparent volume (mL) of distribution at 240 min.

The formula can be corrected for the exact sampling time by substituting it for t.

2. Groth and Aasted's method *(31)*:

$$GFR\ (mL/min/1.73\ m^2) = (0.213 \times T - 104) \times \ln (Y_t \times A/Q_o) + 1.88 \times T - 928$$

Where T = sample time (min); T = 180 for 3-h method;
T = 240 for 4-h method.
Y_t = the activity counts of 180-min or 240-min plasma sample (cpm /mL)
A = body surface area (m^2)
Q_o = total injected dose counts (cpm)

3. Russell's method *(32)*:

$$GFR\ (mL/min) = A \times \ln (D/P) + B$$

Where $A = -0.278 \times T + 119.1 + 2450/T$
$B = 2.886 \times T - 1222.9 - 16820/T$
D = total injected dose counts (cpm)
P = plasma activity (cpm/mL)
T = sampling time (180 min)

3.2. Measurement of Effective Renal Plasma Flow (ERPF) (see Notes 6–8)

The following protocols are for both two- and single-sample method with I-131-OIH.

3.2.1. Blood Sampling

1. Insert an iv line for drawing blood.
2. Draw 300 uCi of I-131-OIH into a 10-mL syringe with normal saline and bring the total vol of 5.0 mL and mix.
3. Obtain a 10-µl aliquot in duplicate from the 5-mL dose and measure in the well counter as the standard.
4. Inject the patient with the 5-mL dose (the injection site should not be used to obtain the blood sample).
5. Draw 5-mL blood samples into heparinized syringes at 20 and 45 min after the OIH injection for the two-sample method. One 44-min sample alone is used for the one-sample method.

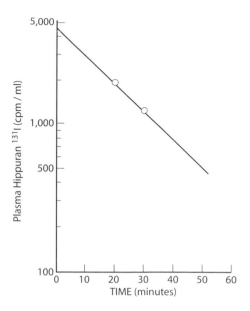

Fig. 11. The simplified one-compartment method for calculating I-131-OIH clearance (slope/intercept method).

6. Pipet 1.0 mL of the plasma after centrifuging into the counting vial with an Eppendorf pipet. Do not disturb the interface between the plasma and the red cell.

3.2.2. Complete Plasma Curve

The complete plasma concentration can be plotted when multiple blood samples are obtained over approx 60 min.

1. Prepare a standard of the radiopharmaceutical to be used.
2. Inject a known amount of radioactivity into the patient's arm.
3. Draw blood samples for the opposite arm at 5, 10, 15, 20, 30, 40, and 60 min post-injection.
4. Separate the plasma by centrifuging and withdraw 2 mL for counting with an automatic well-type counter.
5. Plot net counts against time on semilogarithmic paper and derive a biexponential curve. The terminal segments are extrapolated, and the rate constant and intercept A are determined.

3.2.3. Calculation

1. In the two-sample method, the ERPF is calculated from the slope of a line calculated from two plasma samples taken at predetermined intervals *(46)* (**Fig. 11**).

$$\text{Clearance} = V_D \times K$$
$$V_D = \text{Dose injected/t}_0 \text{ intercept}$$
$$K = 0.693/\text{t}_{1/2}$$

2. In the single-sample method, the concentration of OIH in the plasma at a given time after injection is inversely related to the ERPF *(53)*. Tauxe et al. *(47)* investigated the time relationship of this reciprocal concentration. They determined that a correlation of the observed data points with ERPF may be approximated by either quadratic or exponential curves with fitted parameters. The quadratic fit has the equation: $\text{ERPF} = A + Bx + Cx^2$ with coefficients A, B, and C. These coefficients are dependent on the time chosen for obtaining the plasma sample. The lowest standard error of the estimate is obtained for blood sampled at 44 min or 45 min after injection of IOH. At 45 min $A = -51.1$, $B = 8.21$, and $C = -0.019$ and the standard error of the estimate is 32.44 mL/min.

3.2.4. Tubular Extraction Ratio with MAG3

The specific plasma concentration measured at a certain time postinjection of a substance eliminated by the kidney depends on renal function as well as on the distribution volume and plasma volume. Because the plasma volume has a linear dependence on the body surface (BS) area *(54)*, the plasma concentration is reciprocal to the BS, which in turn is representative of the body dimensions. Bubeck *(55,56)* developed a new principle for determination of tubular extraction ratio (TER) with Tc-99m-MAG3 that allows the universal application of known algorithms by normalizing the plasma concentration with respect to individual body dimensions of adults as well as children.

Blood sampling is performed between 25 and 40 min post-injection in children and between 20 and 50 min post-injection in adults. Bubeck's formula *(55)* is as follows:

$$\text{TER (MAG3)} = a + b \ln (\text{ID/Cn}_t) \text{ mL/min/1.73m}^2$$

where ID = injected activity dose (cps); C = time-specific plasma concentration (cps/L); Cn = C × BS/1.73 m^2 = normalized plasma concentration (cps/L/1.73m^2); t = time of blood sampling post-injection; $a = -517\,e^{-0.011t}$; $b = 295e^{-0.016t}$.

An alternative is the use, in children more than 1 yr of age, of a specific pediatric algorithm, developed by the European Pediatric Task Group *(57)*:

$$\text{Tc-99m-MAG3 clearance} = A/(P(t) \times e^{-a(t-35)}) + B$$

Where $A = 665.89$; $P(t)$ = plasma concentration (%ID/L); $a = 0.0298512$; t = any time between 30 and 40 min; $B = 1.89$.

The result of the clearance must be corrected for body surface area.

3.3. Determination of Individual Renal Function (see Notes 9–11)

3.3.1. Quantitation of GFR

1. The patient should be hydrated by drinking at least one large glass of water 30 min prior to the study. The patient should void before beginning the study.
2. Before injection, obtain a 1-min count of the syringe with the gamma camera by placing it 30 cm in front of the center of the camera.
3. Position the patient supine on the imaging table with the detector positioned posteriorly.
4. Place a 21-gauge butterfly needle and tubing set in an antecubital vein. Inject 3 mCi Tc-99m-DTPA, and flush the butterfly tubing with saline.
5. Acquire a quantitative renal study: Acquire serial 1-sec images for 60 sec, then a 1-min image.
6. Obtain an image of the injection site to detect infiltration.
7. Obtain a 1-min count of the residual radiopharmaceutical in the syringe, again with the syringe 30 cm in front of the center of the camera.
8. Place a region of interest around both kidneys and below both kidneys for background.
9. Determine the counts in the four regions of interest from 2–3 min post-injection.
10. Calculate the global and fractional right and left GFR using the GFR Worksheet provided here.

If ERPF measurement is required, protocols and acquisition steps for Tc-99m-MAG3 are identical to those for Tc-99m-DTPA.

3.3.2. Data Processing

1. Place regions of interest over the cortex of each kidney (excluding the calyces) and lateral to or around each kidney for background subtraction.
2. Generate 20-min renal cortex and background curves.
3. Subtract the background curves from the corresponding renal cortex curves. Be sure that curves are normalized for area—e.g., per pixel, before subtraction.
4. Display curves with "Time" on the X-axis and "Counts" on the Y-axis.

3.3.3. Glomerular Filtration Rate Worksheet

1. Calculate the net injected dose from the syringe image:

Net injected Dose (cts) = Pre-injection (cts) – Post-injection (cts)

2. Calculate the renal depth of both kidney using the following equations *(70)*:

Right kidney depth = 13.3 (weight/height) + 0.7

Left kidney depth = 13.2 (weight/height) + 0.7

Omission of kidney depth correction results in a negligible error. Measurement of kidney depth with ultrasound or using a geometric mean of the count rate is preferable to formula correction.

3. Calculate the percent uptake of the injected dose in each kidney at 2–3 min using the equation:

$$K_U = \frac{(A - B) \times P \times 100\%}{(E \exp - uY) \times D}$$

Where:

   K_U = Percent uptake (%)
   A = Counts per pixel right or left kidney (cts/px)
   B = Counts per pixel corresponding background (cts/px)
   P = Pixels in kidney region of interest (px)
   E = Natural log = 2.718
   u = Attenuation coefficient for Tc-99m = 0.153
   Y = Kidney depth (mm)
   D = Net counts for syringe containing dose (cts)
   exp = Exponent

4. Calculate the GFR for each kidney using the equation:

   Right Kidney GFR (mL/min) = U (%) × 9.75621 – 6.19843

   Left Kidney GFR (mL/min) = U (%) × 9.75621 – 6.19843

5. Add the GFRs for the two kidneys together to obtain the global GFR.

3.4. Radionuclide Renogram (see Notes 12–15)

3.4.1. General Renogram

1. Hydration. The patient should drink 300–500 mL of water by mouth before the study. For children, iv hydration may be necessary, with 5% dextrose in water, 15 mL/kg over 30 min.
2. Intravenous dose injection and the computer acquisition: 1 frame/sec for 60 sec, then 15-sec frames for 20–30 min.
3. Processing: Draw regions of interest on computer for kidneys and background. Generate time-activity curve for 60-sec flow phase (optional) and 20–30 min dynamic study using 15- or 30-sec frames.

3.4.2. Diuretic Renogram

This procedure will usually follow a baseline study with no intervention.

1. Hydrate the patient as described in **Subheading 3.4.1.**
2. Bladder catheter is optional. If catheter is not used, complete bladder emptying is necessary before diuretic injection and after 20 min study.
3. Furosemide dose: Adult: 40 mg iv., adjusted based on the patient's creatinine. Children: 1 mg/kg to a maximum of 40 mg.
4. Imaging procedure: (a) Start computer and run for at least 60 sec before diuretic injection; (b) acquire for 20–30 min on computer after injection of furosemide; and (c) obtain post-void image in the patients without catheter.

There are many suggested variations of this procedure. The reader is referred to the references for more detail.

3.4.3. Captopril Renogram

This procedure will usually follow a baseline study with no intervention.

1. No ACE inhibitor for 3–5 d before study. Avoid diuretics if possible. Provide hydration as in **Subheading 3.4.1.**
2. Administer ACE inhibitor. 25 mg Captopril orally 1 h before starting the radionuclide study. The dose for children is 0.3–0.5 mg/kg with a maximum of 25 mg. Measure the patient's BP before administration of Captopril. Monitor BP and record every 15 min before and during study. A symptomatic decrease in BP may require saline infusion and may yield a false-positive result.
3. Inject radiopharmaceutical (Tc-99m-MAG3) intravenously and start image as in **Subheading 3.4.2.**

3.5. PET In the Evaluation of Renal Function (see Note 16)

Currently no established protocols are available for RBF measurement with PET. Only limited studies were done on an experimental basis. The following protocols are from Juillard et al. *(86)* who used oxygen-15-water for RBF measurement in PET. The study was based on a one-compartment model. The mono-compartmental model described by Kety and Smith has been validated for the measurement of myocardial and cerebral blood flow by PET *(84,101)*.

Briefly, about 10 mci of oxygen-15-water is injected intravenously. Starting simultaneously, a dynamic series of images is acquired using PET. Photon attenuation is corrected using a transmission scan obtained with a germanium source. A region of interest is drawn automatically around the aorta on a static image as a line limited by 80% of the maximum activity for the aorta. ROIs are drawn manually around the renal cortex on static images. Time activity curves are generated for the aorta and each renal cortex. Renal blood flow, delay between aortic and kidney perfusion by oxygen-15-water, and vascular fraction in the kidney are fitted with a nonlinear regression module of a software.

4. Notes

1. Quality control and protein binding of the radionuclides:
   a. Adequate quality control of the Tc-99m-DTPA preparation must be emphasized *(33,34)*. None of the procedures for measuring GFR will yield accurate results if the DTPA being used is associated with high protein binding. Protein binding and impurities vary among different preparations.
   b. When Tc-99m-DTPA is administered intravenously, a small fraction of activity is bound to plasma protein. The protein-bound fraction is believed to represent an impurity. Clearance is reduced by binding of the radionuclide to serum protein. Stabilized preparations must be used for accurate GFR estima-

tion, and protein binding must be checked before a specific preparation is used. The amount of impurity varies with the manufacturer of the agent. Differences in protein-binding characteristics of various commercial forms of Tc-99m-DTPA have been postulated as the possible cause of differences in GFR determined using the different preparations. Carlsen et al. *(35)* evaluated four different commercially available Tc-99m-DTPA products and correlated their clearance with simultaneous Cr-51-EDTA clearance. Two of these were produced in the United States, one from France, and a fourth from Switzerland. Plasma clearances of Tc-99m-DTPA correlated highly with Cr-51-EDTA, but accuracy varied. The final disappearance-rate constants of all four Tc-99m-DTPA products were lower than those of Cr-51-EDTA, with a net effect of underestimation of the Cr-51 GFR at high clearance levels. Protein binding was suggested as the likely explanation for the slower disappearance-rate constants of Tc-99m-DTPA compared with Cr-51-EDTA at high clearance values, since the influence of protein binding increases at high clearance values as the protein-bound fraction accumulates.

  c. The most significant potential errors caused by protein binding occur when using procedures that require the evaluation of the plasma-disappearance curve over a period of several hours because the small amount of radiotracer that is protein-bound after bolus injection becomes relatively more significant as the unbound component is cleared.

   The amount of impurity also may depend on the time interval between kit preparation and injection. Although package inserts usually advocate prompt use, the impurities have been reported to decrease with time for a few h after preparation *(33)*.

  d. Purity of the radiopharmaceutical can be monitored by laboratory tests. However, it can change with any change in the source or handling of the radionuclides or with any change in the time interval between kit preparation and usage. Therefore, Russell et al. *(36)* routinely used ultrafiltered plasma for correction of protein binding prior to counting. Clinically, this is cumbersome, but not necessarily impractical. Many laboratories accept the small error, and do not correct for protein binding.

2. Choice of methods: The spectrum of accuracy varies widely based on the method chosen to calculate GFR. Unfortunately, most studies perform correlations but avoid the more critical paired t-test. The complete plasma-clearance curve is the most accurate method, but requires multiple blood samples. The one-sample method is accurate enough for routine clinical work, whereas the two-sample technique is generally recommended for either investigational use or circumstances requiring special accuracy (**Fig. 12**). Urinary clearance techniques provide the most accurate results.

   Among a variety of single-blood-sample methods available, Li and Blaufox *(37)* reported that the Groth 4-h sample method had the best value of both absolute difference and percent absolute difference, and provided a better estimation of GFR than other single-plasma-sample methods when compared to a urinary clearance method as the standard.

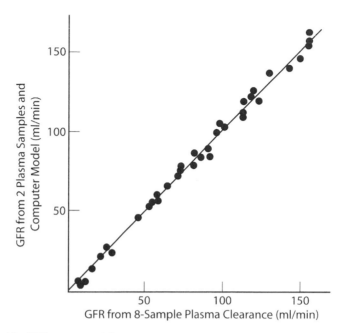

Fig. 12. GFR measured from two-plasma samples vs reference GFR calculated from eight-point plasma clearance with Tc-99m-DTPA. The correlation coefficient was 0.998. Reproduced with permission from Russell et al. (1985) Single-injection plasma-clearance method without urine collection. *J. Nucl. Med.* **26**, 1244.

The level of renal function is an important determination of the overall accuracy in each method. Most single-sample GFR methods are reliable, and yield a small percent of absolute difference when they are used for those patients with GFR >30 mL/min *(37)*. But single-sample methods tend to be increasingly inaccurate when the GFR is less than 30 mL/min *(38,39)*, at which point the exponential slope of the plasma curve is slow. Multiple-sample plasma clearance also overestimates GFR because of the substantial and variable extrarenal clearance *(40)*. In the presence of overt renal insufficiency, the method of choice remains the calculation of urinary clearance *(41)*. However, the accuracy of any method at very low levels of renal function is questionable. Delayed single-sample methods as alternatives to urine collection may be used as follows *(3)*:

Estimated GFR 15–30 mL/min—
Blood sampling between 3 and 5 h post-injection

Estimated GFR <15 mL/min—
Blood sampling between 5 and 24 h or only 24 h post-injection

If a one-sample method is used in renal insufficiency, the ideal sampling time would appear to vary inversely with GFR level *(14)*, but any result may be questioned. The single-sample methods have found a more limited application in children for whom different equations should theoretically be used, taking into account the variations in anatomic and biologic factors with age. Ham and Piepsz *(42)* reported a new method for estimating GFR in children using Cr-51-EDTA and a single-sample technique. The Cr-51-EDTA clearance obtained in children of various ages by the two-sample method (2–4 h) closely correlated with the 2-h distribution volume. They showed that a linear regression equation converting 2 h vol of distribution data into GFR estimates was valid in infants and children with a wide range of renal function. These results are similar to those of Tauxe *(7)* who used 91-min data and I-131-DZT clearance with a single blood sample.

Work is continuing to develop a bloodless method for estimating renal function but, as with in most clinical situations, increasing the simplicity of the technique leads to an increasing error of the estimate.

3. Choice of sampling times: It is more important to cover a wide time interval than to have a large number of samples to calculate clearance from multiple plasma samples. When measuring GFR with DTPA, it is recommended to continue data collection for at least 3 h and preferably 4 h *(13)*, since the slow component contributes most of the calculated clearance.

The accuracy is improved for two- or single-sample techniques by using the later blood samples. Several studies showed that two blood samples, obtained at 2 and 4 h after Tc-99m-DTPA injection, allowed for good GFR estimation *(15)*, but Russell et al. *(32)* reported that a 1- and 3-h sample method was nearly as accurate as a 5-h method.

The optimal sampling time for a single-sample method ranges from 180–240 min after the radionuclide injection. The best sampling time for an individual patient depends on the underlying renal function.

4. Urine collection techniques: Determination of urinary clearance requires adequate urine collection. For the greatest accuracy of measurement, the following protocols must be followed:

   a. Hydration

      High urine flow rates are critical. The patients should be well-hydrated before the study. The patients are encouraged to drink several glasses of water and are hydrated with at least 500 mL of fluid 30 min prior to the test. The specific gravity of the urine can be measured and a specific gravity of less than 1.020 is the goal.

   b. Accurate timing of urine collection and careful measurement of urine samples.

   c. Correction for residual urine. Precise measurement of urine volume requires correction for residual urine volume in the bladder. In most patients this is not necessary. Bladder residual urinary volume can be estimated accurately and noninvasively during a radionuclide clearance from the radioactivity that remains in the bladder after voiding. A study of patients with reduced renal function reported that the GFR corrected for residual urine is very reliable, and is the most accurate measurement of GFR in patients with mild to severe

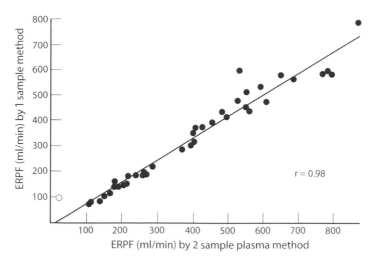

Fig. 13. The correlation between ERPF measured with I-131-OIH by one-sample method and two-sample method. The correlation coefficient was 0.98.

renal insufficiency. Estimation of residual urine is usually indicated in studying patients with reduced renal function *(28)*. This may also be true for diabetics and patients with BPH or other lower-urinary-tract problems.

5. Radioactivity counting: Well counters can be easily saturated by the levels of radioactivity used for imaging techniques. This must be avoided by diluting the sample, delaying counting, or using small aliquots. Depending to some extent on the instrument, no more than approx 0.3 uCi should be placed in the counter. One way to achieve this is to dilute a duplicate of the dose to 100 mL in a volumetric flask, transfer 1 mL of that to a second 100-mL volumetric flask, and then count 0.1 mL of both the twice diluted dose and the patient's plasma.

6. Choice of methods: Both single-sample and two-sample methods are technically simple. The correlation between the two methods is excellent, supporting their close relationship *(48)* (**Fig. 13**). Generally, the two-sample method is more accurate than the one-sample method. For example, Russell et al. *(58)* compared the two methods for ERPF evaluation and found that the one-sample method resulted in an error of 19 mL/min, and 7 mL/min for the two-sample method. Therefore, Blaufox *(59)* and Russell *(58)* recommended a single-sample method for routine clinical ERPF measurement and the two-sample method for research purposes when higher accuracy is essential.

The two-sample method provides accurate measurement of ERPF in adults, but it may not be reliable in children because of the rapidly changing relationship of body compartments, body size, and renal function. The assumptions needed for a single-sample technique may be erroneous unless a curve is constructed for every age or level of renal function. Therefore, in studies with children, the two-sample method remains the technique of choice.

7. Sample Timing: A blood sample should be drawn at 44 or 45 min after OIH injection because the best correlation between ERPF and plasma concentration and the lowest standard error of the estimate are obtained at this time *(47)*. Russell et al. *(58)* found that the 43-min sample time was optimal with MAG3 over a large range of renal function. Later sample times can be used in poor renal function, and shorter sample times in good renal function.

There is some controversy about the timing of sampling for the two-sample method. I-131-OIH distribution and secretion can be described by a biexponential decay approximating a two-compartment model. The first portion of the decay curve is affected primarily by the distribution of I-131-OIH in the extracellular fluid that dominates the initial 10–15 min after injection. The second portion of the curve, which lasts about 15–20 min, is dominated by the intravascular clearance of I-131-OIH by the kidney. Two samples are usually used to estimate the terminal portion of the decay curve, and like the single-sample method, it disregards the extracellular equilibration. This results in a small error from an early loss of tracer. Several correction equations have been proposed *(3,58)*. Consequently, two samples are drawn between 20–60 min. Blaufox *(46)* obtained one sample at 30 min and another at 40 min for I-131-OIH. Russell *(58)* used 12 and 94 min for sampling times with Tc-99m-MAG3. Based on the slope-intercept method for calculation, these sampling techniques yielded varied ERPF results. Hippuran underestimates PAH clearance, and MAG$_3$ is even lower (**Table 1**). Both methods are reproducible in a given individual.

8. Choice of radionuclides: Both I-131-OIH and Tc-99m-MAG3 may be used for ERPF determination. Normal ERPF values are approx 600 mL/min with I-131-OIH, and 370 mL/min for Tc-99m-MAG$_3$. Taylor has proposed a correction factor for MAG$_3$ *(60)*. The obvious advantage of the superior dosimetry of Tc-99m-MAG3 over I-131-OIH makes Tc-99m-MAG3 the ideal agent for clinical studies.

9. Background correction: Background correction may be particularly critical in some methods with the gamma camera, because intra- and extravascular activity is changing rapidly (in opposite directions) during the time when individual kidney function is usually calculated. The contribution of each type of activity varies within different regions of interest *(71)*. The liver, spleen, adrenals, renal hilar vessels, intestine, and soft tissue all contribute to background. No single area accurately represents the intravascular and extravascular components of background. No general consensus has been reached on a method of background subtraction. Delpassand *(65)* selected a ring-shaped background region of interest surrounding the kidney as the most representative background region. Gates *(63)* tested both rings (nearly circumferential background area around the kidney, avoiding the anticipated location of the renal arteries and veins) and semilunar regions (the area adjacent to inferior and lower lateral kidney margin, avoiding the region of the liver and spleen), and found the semilunar area to be slightly better. Piepsz et al. *(72)* found that a double background correction was best. This method combined an area-ratio method (subrenal area that corrects for interstitial background) with a linear-fit method (eliminating residual vascular activity).

Overall, the background correction is a major source of error in the gamma-camera method. The results should be carefully tracked to determine if the background subtraction technique being used is providing appropriate data *(59)*.

10. Time-course of relative uptake: The relative renal uptake of each radiopharmaceutical provides a measure of relative function and is an important parameter in the interpretation of most studies. The measurement is usually made in the 1–2, 1–2.5, or 2–3-min period post-injection for DTPA, MAG3 and OIH. Blaufox et al. *(3)* recommended that any activity lasting less than 1 min should not be included in the determination of individual renal function, since this represents a significant amount of nonrenal radioactivity.

Measurement of relative renal function in patients with renal insufficiency can be misleading because of elevated background activity and reduced renal concentration of radiotracer. When there is delayed excretion of the tracer and obvious splenic or hepatic activity superimposed over one of the kidneys, it often is advantageous to delay the differential uptake measurement to allow renal activity to increase and background activity to decrease rather than use the standard 1–2 or 2–3-min interval after radiotracer injection *(38)*.

11. Determination of kidney depth: Accurate measurement of absolute renal function by the gamma-camera technique requires correction for soft-tissue attenuation, which in turn requires a knowledge of kidney depth. Most investigators strongly suggest consideration of renal depth in calculating camera-based GFR *(73)*. Accuracy in kidney-depth estimation is important for the calculation formula. GFR formulas are suitable for normally positioned kidneys, either upright or supine, but may be incorrect in cases of nephroptosis and some other relatively rare situations.

Although several investigators have used lateral scintigraphy to measure renal depth *(74)*, most authors recommend the formula of calculation for kidney depth based on the patient's height, weight, and age. Gates et al. *(64)* reported a good correlation between renal uptake of DTPA and renal function, using height and weight to measure renal depth. Renal depth was determined by CT in 201 patients without abdominal pathology *(75)*. The difference in renal depth was less than 2.0 cm in 99% of the patients. A difference in 2.0 cm would change the relative uptake from 50/50 to 56/44. Based on these data, Taylor et al. *(60)* defined a relative uptake from 50/50 to 56/44 as normal, 57/43 to 59/41 as borderline, and 60/40 or greater as abnormal. A more flexible and generally accepted range is 60/40, which is less sensitive but more specific for abnormal renal function.

For patients with renal transplantation, depth presents less of a problem because the kidney is relatively superficial, with little intervening tissue.

12. Patient hydration: Patients should be well-hydrated for routine renograms. Dehydration can prolong the excretory phase of the renogram curve. Prior to the test, patients should be instructed to drink plenty of fluids. The nursing staff should be requested to hydrate inpatients. The state of hydration can be evaluated when the patient arrives by collecting a urine sample and measuring the specific gravity. A specific gravity greater than 1.020 suggests some dehydration.

Because a full bladder may affect the drainage of the pelvicaliceal system, voiding before image data acquisition is important.

13. Region of interest selection: Proper ROI selection is very important, and depends on the information needed. Whole-kidney ROIs can be used for function curves if collecting-system activity clears promptly. With collecting system retention, however, the renogram represents a summation of cortical function and collecting system activity. The ability to distinguish cortical function is thus hindered. In these cases two-pixel-wide peripheral cortical ROIs may more accurately represent parenchymal function. Calculation of differential renal function requires ROIs that include the entire kidney, because exclusion of the pelvis and calyces will inevitably exclude some cortex, making quantification erroneous *(77,78,80)*.

14. Quantification: The renograms have been used for various physiological and pathological renal functional evaluation. The different quantitative parameters of function can be derived from the TACs, including the time to peak activity, uptake slope, rate of clearance, and percent clearance at a given time. The parameters used depend on the individual study; no general standard exists. Personal preference and experience also determine the use of quantitative parameters.

15. Background selection: Proper selection of background ROIs is important for accurate quantification. Since there is intervening soft-tissue background both anterior and posterior to the kidney, it is difficult to determine true background. Different methods for background selection are applied in the various nuclear medicine departments, and no universally accepted protocol exists. Regions adjacent to the kidney should be used for background subtraction *(79)*. Typically, two-pixel semilunar ROIs adjacent and inferolateral to the kidneys are chosen. Caution is needed when the liver and spleen overlap the kidneys. This is a special problem with Tc-99m-MAG3 because of its alternative heptobiliary route of excretion. Generally, the accuracy of background subtraction decreases with worsening renal function *(60,79,80)*.

16. The determination of RBF may be useful in clinical and experimental circumstances to evaluate vascular damage to the kidney caused by renal artery stenosis, renal vasculitis, chronic allograft rejection, and nephrotoxic drugs. Based on preliminary studies, PET has the potential to become a valuable noninvasive method for measuring RBF. Advantages of RBF evaluation by PET include the possibility of sequential measurements, a comparison between measurements, and reduced irradiation to the patient *(86)*.

Limitations of the method include the cost of the procedure and the lack of availability of PET facilities, which resolve rapidly. The limited resolution of a PET scan may induce error in external measurement of true activity *(86)*. Among these errors, the partial volume effect (PVE) corresponds to the inaccurate measured activity in a small-size structure. The PVE results in underestimation of true activity, depending on the ratio between the studied structure's size and the size of region of interest. Another potential source of error is the spillover effect (SOE) between two adjacent structures, which is quantitatively more important if structures are closer and have different activities. The evaluation of the PVE and the SOE is an important task for quantitation in PET.

References

1. Taplin, G. V., Meredith, O. M., Kade, H., et al. (1956) The radioisotope renogram. An external test for individual kidney function and upper urinary tract patency. *J. Lab. Clin. Med.* **48,** 886.
2. Kimbel, K. H. (1956) Discussion of paper by W. Schlungbaum and H. Billion, in: Radioaktive isotope in Klinik und Forschung. *Vortrage Geisteiner Int Symp*, Vol. 2 Urban Schwartzenburg, Berlin.
3. Blaufox, M. D., Aurell, M., Bubeck, B., Fommei, E., Piepsz, A., Russell, C., et al. (1996) Report of the radionuclides in nephrourology committee on renal clearance. *J. Nucl. Med.* **37,** 1883–1890.
4. Bueschen, A. J. and Witten, D. M. (1979) Radionuclide evaluation of renal function. *Urol. Clin. North Am.* **6,** 307.
5. Jone, J. and Burnett, P. C. (1974) Creatinine metabolism in human with decreased renal function. *Clin. Chem.* **20,** 1204.
6. Schrier, R. W. (1982) Acute renal failure. *JAMA* **247,** 2515–2518
7. Tauxe, W. N., Bagchi, A., Tepe, P. G., et al. (1987). Single-sample method for the estimation of GFR in children. *J. Nucl. Med.* **28,** 366–371.
8. Odlind, B., Hallgren, R., Sohtell, M., et al. (1985) Is I-125 iothalamate an ideal marker for glomerular filtration. *Kidney Int.* **27,** 9–16
9. Robin, H. A., Hall, R. (1984) Inaccuracy of estimated creatinine clearance for iothalamate GFR. *Amer. J. Kidney Disease* **4,** 48–54
10. Hell, J. E., Guyton, A. C., and Farr, B. M. (1977) A single-injection method for measuring GFR. *Am. J. Physiol.* **232,** F72–F76.
11. Peter, A. M. (1991) Quantification of renal hemodynamics with radionuclides. *Eur. J. Nucl. Med.* **18,** 274–286.
12. Fine, E. J., Axelrod, M., and Blaufox, M. D. (1985) Physiologic aspects of diagnostic renal imaging. *Semin. Nephro.* **5,** 188–207.
13. Russell, C. D. (1993) Optimum sample times for single-injection, multisample renal clearance methods. *J. Nucl. Med.* **34,** 1761–1765.
14. Tauxe, W. N. (1986) Determination of GFR by single plasma sampling technique following injection of radioiodinated diatrizoate. *J. Nucl. Med.* **27,** 45–50.
15. Waller, D. G., Keast, C. M., and Fleming, J. S, et al. (1987) Measurement of GFR with technetium-99m-DTPA: comparison of plasma clearance techniques. *J. Nucl. Med.* **28,** 372–377.
16. Mulligan, J. S., Blue, P. W., and Hasbargen, J. A. (1990) Methods for measuring GFR with Tc-99m-DTPA: An analysis of several common methods *J. Nucl. Med.* **31,** 1211–1219.
17. Jackson, J., Blue, P. W., and Ghead, N. (1985) GFR determined in conjunction with routine renal scanning. *Radiol.* **154,** 203–205.
18. Bianchi C. (1972) Measurement of glomerular filtration rate. *Prog. Nucl. Med.* **2,** 21–53.
19. Marlow, C. G. and Sheppard, G. (1970) Labeled tracer of inulin for physiological measurement. *Clin. Chim. Acta.* **28,** 469.

20. Summer, R. E., Concannon, J. P., and Well, C., et al. (1967) Determination of simultaneous effective renal plasma flow and GFR with I-131-oiodohippurate and I-125 allyl inulin. *J. Lab. Clin. Med.* **69,** 919.

21. Tubis, M., Persons, K., and Rawalay, S. S., et al. (1966) The preparation of labeled carbohydrates for biochemical uses. *J. Nucl. Med.* **7,** 338.

22. Foley, T. H., Jones, N. F., and Clapham, W. F. (1966) Renal clearance of Co-57-cyanocobalamine: importance of plasma protein binding. *Lancet* **2,** 86.

23. Garnett, E. S., Parsons, V., and Veall, N. (1967) Measurement of GFR in man using a Cr-51 edetic acid complex. *Lancet* **3,** 818.

24. Favre, H. R. and Wing, A. T. (1968) Simultaneous Cr-51 edetic acid, insulin and endogeneous creatinine in 20 patients with renal diseases. *Br. Med. J.* **1,** 84.

25. Chantler, C, Garnett, E. S., and Parson, V. (1969) GFR measurement in man by the single injection method using Cr-51-EDTA. *Clin. Sci.* **37,** 169.

26. McAfee, T. G., Gagne, G., and Atkin, H. L, et al. (1979) Biological distribution and excretion of DTPA labeled with Tc-99m and In-111. *J. Nucl. Med.* **20,** 1273.

27. Barbour, G. L., Crumb, K., and Boyd, M., et al. (1976) Comparison of inulin, iothalamate and Tc-99m-DTPA for measurement of GFR. *J. Nucl. Med.* **17,** 317.

28. Fotopolos, A, Blaufox, MD, Lee, H, et al. (1994) Effect of residual urine on apparent renal clearance in patients with reduced function, in O'Reilly, P. H.

29. Brochner-Mortensen, J. (1972) A simple method of estimating GFR. *Eur. J. Nucl. Med.* **19,** 827.

30. Watson, W. S. (1992) A simple method of estimating GFR. . *Eur. J. Nucl. Med.* **19,** 827.

31. Groth, S. and Aasted, M. (1981) Chromium-51 EDTA clearance determined by one plasma sample. *Clin. Physiol.* **1,** 417–425.

32. Russell, C. D., Bischoff, P. G., and Kintzen, F. N., et al. (1985) Measurement of GFR: single injection plasma clearance method without urine collection. *J. Nucl. Med.* **26,** 1243–1247.

33. Russell, C. D., Rowell, K., and Scott, J. W. (1986) Quality control of Tc-99m-DTPA: correlation of analytic test with in vivo protein binding in man. *J. Nucl. Med.* **27,** 560–562.

34. Hosain, F. (1974) Quality control of Tc-99m-DTPA by double tracer clearance technique. *J. Nucl. Med.* **15,** 442.

35. Carlsen, J. E., Moller, M. L., and Lund, J. O., et al. (1980) Comparison of four commercial Tc-99m-DTPA preparations used for the measurement of GFR: concise communication. *J. Nucl. Med.* **21,** 126–129.

36. Russell, C. D., Bischoff, P. G., and Rowell, K. L., et al. (1983) Quality control of Tc-99m-DTPA for measurement of glomerular filtration. *J. Nucl. Med.* **24,** 722–727.

37. Li, Y., Lee, H. B., and Blaufox, M. D. (1997) Single-sample methods to measure GFR with Technetium-99m-DTPA. *J. Nucl. Med.* **38,** 1290–1295.

38. Seanewald, K. and Taylor, A. (1993) A pitfall in calculating differential renal function in patients with renal failure. *Clin. Nucl. Med.* **18,** 377–381.

39. Chatterton, B. E. (1978) Limitations of the single sample tracer method for determining GFR. *Br. J. Radiol.* **51,** 981–985.

40. Israelit, A. H., Long, D. C., White, M. G., et al. (1973) Measurement of GFR utilizing a single subcutaneous injection of I-125-iothalamate. *Kidney Intern.* **4,** 346–349.
41. LaFrance, N. D., Drew, H. H., and Walser, M. (1988) Radioisotopic measurement of GFR in severe chronic renal failure. *J. Nucl. Med.* **29,** 1927–1930.
42. Ham, H. R. and Piepsz, A. (1991) Estimation of GFR in infants and children using a single sample method. *J. Nucl. Med.* **32,** 1294–1297.
43. Blaufox, M. D. (1989) Method for measurement of the renal blood flow, in Evaluation of Renal Function and disease with radionuclides, Blaufox, M. D. ed., Karger, Basel, pp. 84–97.
44. Russell, C. D. and Dubovsky, E. V. (1989) Measurement of renal function with radionuclides. *J. Nucl. Med.* **30,** 2053–2057.
45. Blaufox, M. D., Frohmuller, H. G. W., and Campbell J. C., et al. (1963) A simplified method of estimate renal function with I-131-iodohippurate. *J. Surg. Res.* **3,** 122–125.
46. Blaufox, M. D. and Merrill, J. P. (1966) Simplified hippuran clearance measurement of renal function in man. *Nephron* **3,** 274–281.
47. Tauxe, W. H., Dubovsky, E. V., Kidd, T., et al. (1982) New formulas for the calculation of ERPF. *Eur. J. Nucl. Med.* **7,** 51–54.
48. Fine, E. J., Axelrod, M., Gorkin, J., et al. (1987) Measurement of ERPF: a comparison of methods. *J. Nucl. Med.* **28,** 1393–1400.
49. Eshima, D. and Taylor, A. (1991) Tc-99m MAG3: uptake on the new Tc-99m renal tubular function agent. *Semin. Nucl. Med.* **22,** 61.
50. Bubeck, B., Brandau, W., Weber, E, et al. (1990) Pharmacokinetics of Tc-99m-MAG3 in human. *J. Nucl. Med.* **31,** 1285–1293.
51. Bubeck, B., Brandau, W., Weber, E, et al. (1987) The tubular extraction rate of Tc-99m-MAG3: a new quantitative parameter of renal function. *Nucl. Med. Compact* **18,** 260–267.
52. Ozker, K, Onsel C, Kabasakal, L., et al. (1994) Tc-99m-EC. A comparative study of renal scintigraphy with Tc-99m-MAG3 and I-131-OIH in patients with obstructive renal disease. *J. Nucl. Med.* **35,** 840–845.
53. Blaufox, M. D. (1989) Measurement of renal function with radioactive materials. In Evaluation of Renal Function and Disease with Radionuclides, Blaufox, M. D., ed., Karger, Basel, pp. 12–27.
54. Boer, P. (1984) Estimated lean body mass as an index for normalization of body fluid volumes in humans. *Am. J. Physiol.* **247,** F634–F636.
55. Bubeck, B., Piepenburg, R., Grethe, U., et al. (1992) A new principle to normalize plasma concentrations allowing single-sample clearance determinations in both children and adults. *Eur. J. Nucl. Med.* **19,** 511–516.
56. Bubeck, B. (1993) Renal clearance determination with one blood sample: improved accuracy and universal applicability by a new calculation principle. *Semin. Nucl. Med.* **23,** 73–86.
57. Peipsz, A., Gordon, I., Han, K., et al. (1993) Determination of Tc-99m-MAG3 plasma clearance in children by means of a single blood sample: a multicenter study. *Eur. J. Nucl. Med.* **20,** 244–248.

58. Russell, C. D., Taylor, A., and Eshima, D. (1989) Estimate of Tc-99m-MAG3 plasma clearance in adults from one or two blood samples. *J. Nucl. Med.* **30,** 1955–1959.
59. Blaufox, M. D. (1991) Procedures of choice in renal nuclear medicine. *J. Nucl. Med.* **32,** 1301–1309.
60. Taylor, A. (1998) Radionuclide renography: a personal approach. *Semin. Nucl. Med.* **29,** 102–127.
61. Stacy. B. D. and Thorburn, G. D. (1966) Cr-51-EDTA for estimate of GFR. *Science* **1076,** 152–155.
62. Piepsz, A., Denis, R., and Ham, H. R. (1978) A simple method for measuring separate GFR using a single injection of Tc-99m-DTPA and scintillation camera. *J. Pediatr.* **93,** 769–774.
63. Gates, G. F. (1983) GFR: estimate from fractioned renal accumulation of Tc-99m-DTPA. *Am. J. Roentgenol.* **138,** 565–570.
64. Gates, G. F. (1983) Split renal function testing using Tc-99m-DTPA: a rapid technique for determining differential glomerular filtration. *Clin. Nucl. Med.* **8,** 400–407.
65. Delpassand, E. S., Homayoon, K., Madden, T, et al. (2000) Determination of GFR using dual-detector gamma camera and the geometric mean of renal activity. *Clin. Nucl. Med.* **25,** 258–262.
66. Nielsen, S. P., Moller, M. L., and Trap-Jensen, J. (1997) Tc-99m-DTPA scintillation camera renography: a new method of estimation of single kidney function. *J. Nucl. Med.* **38,** 112–116.
67. DeLange, M. J., Piers, D. A., Kosteerink, J. W. W., et al. (1989) Renal handling of Tc-99m-DMSA: evidence for glomerular filtration and peritubular uptake. *J. Nucl. Med.* **32,** 766–768.
68. Yee, C. A., Lee, H. B., and Blaufox, M. D. (1981) Tc-99mDMSA renal uptake: Influence of biochemical and physiologic factors. *J. Nucl. Med.* **22,** 1054–1058.
69. Groshar, D., Embon, O. M., Frenkel, A., et al. (1991) Renal function and Tc-99m-DMSA uptake in single kidney: the value of in vivo SPECT quantitation. *J. Nucl. Med.* **32,** 766–768.
70. Tonnesen, K. H., Munck, O., Hold, T., et al. (1976) Influence on the radio-renogram of variation in skin to kidney distance and the clinical importance. *J. Urol.* **116,** 282–285.
71. Peter, A. M., Bell, S. D., Gordon, I., et al. (1991) Effective background correction on separate Tc-99m-DTPA renal clearance. *J. Nucl. Med.* **32,** 362–363.
72. Piepsz, A., Dobbeleir, A., and Ham, H. R. (1990) Effect of background correction on separate Tc-99m-DTPA renal clearance. *J. Nucl. Med.* **31,** 430–435.
73. Steinmetz, A. P., Zwas, S. T., and Macadziob, S. (1998) Renal depth estimation to improve the accuracy of GFR. *J. Nucl. Med.* **39,** 1822–1826.
74. Gruenwald, S. M., Collins, C. T., and Fawdry, R. M. (1985) Kidney depth measurement and its influence on quantitation of function from gamma camera renography. *Clin. Nucl. Med.* **10,** 398–392.
75. Taylor, A., Lewis, C., and Giacometti, A. (1993) Improved formulas for the estimation of renal depth in adults. *J. Nucl. Med.* **34,** 1766–1769.

76. Mettler, F. A. and Guiverteau, M. J., eds. (1999) Essentials of nuclear medicine imaging, 4th ed., W. B. Saunders, Philadelphia.

77. Gonzalez, A., Puchal, R., Bajen, M. T., et. al. (1994) Tc-99m-MAG3 renogram in normal subjects and in normalfunctional kidney graft. *Nucl. Med. Commun.* **15,** 680–684.

78. Tomaru, Y., Inoue, T., Oriuchi, N., et al. (1998) Semi-automated renal region of interest selection method using the double threshold technique: inter-operator variability in quantitating Tc-99m-MAG3 renal uptake. *Eur. J. Nucl. Med.* **25,** 55–59.

79. Prigent, A., Cosgriff, P., Gates, G. F., et al. (1999) Consensus report of quality control of quantitative measurement of renal function obtained from the renogram: international consensus committee from the scientific committee of radionuclides in nephrourology. *Semin. Nucl. Med.* **29,** 146–159.

80. Thrall, J. H. and Ziessman, H. A., eds. (2001) Nuclear Medicine. The Requisites, 2nd ed, Mosby Inc., St. Louis.

81. Ramdave, S., Thomas, G. W., Salvatore, T., et al. (2001) Clinical role for F-18 FDG PET for detection and management of renal cell carcinoma. *J. Urol.* **166,** 825–830.

82. Delbeke, D. (1999) Oncological application of FDG PET imaging: brain tumors, colorectal cancer, lymphoma and melanoma. *J. Nucl. Med.* **40,** 591.

83. Choi, Y., Huan, S., Hawkins, R., et al. (1993) A simplified method for the quantification of myocardial blood flow using N-13 ammonia and dynamic PET. *J. Nucl. Med.* **34,** 488.

84. Raichle, M. E., Martin, W. R. W., Herscovitch, P., et al. (1983) Brain blood flow measured with intravenous H2(15)O. Implementation and validation. *J. Nucl. Med.* **24,** 790–798.

85. Killion, D., Nitzsche, E., Choi, Y., et al. (1993) A new method for determination of renal function. *J. Urol.* **150,** 1064–1068.

86. Juillard, L., Janier, M. F., Fouque, D., et al. (2000) Renal blood flow measurement by PET using O-15-labelled water. *Kidney Int.* **57,** 2511–2518.

87. Griendling, K. K., Murphy, T. J., and Alexander, R. W. (1993) Molecular biology of the renin-angiotensin system. *Circulation* **87,** 1816–1828.

88. Bumpus, F. M., Catt, K. J., Chiu, A. T., et al. (1991) Nomenclature for angiotensin receptors. A report of the Nomenclature committee of the Council for High Blood Pressure Research. *Hypertension* **17,** 720–721.

89. Bernstein, K. E. and Alexander, E. W. (1992) Counterpoint: molecular analysis of the angiotensin II receptor. *Endocr. Rev.* **13,** 381–386.

90. Kim, S. E., Scheffel, U., Szabo, Z., et al. (1996) In vivo labeling of angiotensin II receptors with a carbon-11-labeled selective nonpeptide antagonist. *J. Nucl. Med.* **37,** 307–311.

91. Szabo, Z., Kao, P. F., Burns, H. D., et al. (1998) Investigation of angiotensin II / AT1 receptors with carbon-11-L-159,884: A selective AT1 antagonist. *J. Nucl. Med.* **39,** 1209–1213.

92. Szabo, Z., Speth, R. C., Brown, P. R., et al. (2001) Use of PET to study AT1 receptor regulation in vivo. *J. Am. Soc. Nephrol.* **12,** 1350–1358.

93. Aleksic, S., Szabo, Z., Scheffel, U., et al. (2001) In vivo labeling of endothelin receptors with C-11-L-753,037: studies in mice and a dog. *J. Nucl. Med.* **42,** 1274–1280.

94. Chen, B. C., Germano, G., Huan, S. C., et al. (1992) A new non-invasive quantification of renal blood flow with N-13 ammonia, dynamic PET and a two-compartmental model. *J. Am. Soc. Nephrol.* **3,** 1295–1306.

95. Middlekauf, H. R., Nitzsche, E. U., Hamilton, M. A., et al. (1995) Evidence for preserved cardiopulmonary baroreflex control of renal cortical blood flow in humans with advanced heart failure. A PET study. *Circulation* **92,** 395–401.

96. Middlehauff, H. R., Nitzsch, E. U., Nguyen, A. H., et al. (1997) Modulation of renal cortical blood flow during static exercise in humans. *Circ. Res.* **80,** 62–68.

97. Tamaki, N., Alper, N. M., Rabito, C. A., et al. (1988) The effect of captopril on renal flow in renal artery stenosis assessed by PET with rubidum-82. *Hypertension* **11,** 217–222.

98. Mullani, N. A., Ekas, R. D., Marani, S., et al. (1990) Feasibility of measuring first pass extraction and flow with rubidium-82 in the kidneys. *Am. J. Physiol. Imaging* **5,** 133–140.

99. Araiyo, L., Lammertsma, A., Khodes., C., et al. (1986) Noninvasive quantification of regional myocardial blood flow in coronary artery disease with oxygen-15-labelled carbon dioxide inhalation and PET. *Circulation* **83,** 875–885.

100. Nitzsche, E. U., Choi, Y., Killion, D., et al. (1993) Quantification and parametric imaging of renal cortical blood flow in vivo based on Patlak graphical analysis. *Kidney Int.* **44,** 985–996.

101. Kety, S. S. and Smith, S. (1960) Measurement of local blood flow by the exchange of an inert, diffusible substance. *Methods Med. Res.* **8,** 228–236.

7

Intravital Videomicroscopy

Tokunori Yamamoto and Fumihiko Kajiya

1. Introduction

The assessment of single-nephron glomerular function is essential for understanding the fundamental regulatory mechanisms of renal hemodynamics (*1*). In earlier studies, special tracer techniques using fluorescence-labeled erythrocytes, radiolabeled microspheres, and dye solutions were used for analysis of renal hemodynamics. However, it was extremely difficult to perform direct in vivo observation of renal microcirculation. Recently, glomerular function has been directly evaluated with the use of the isolated perfused glomerulus (*2–4*), juxtamedullary nephrons (*5*), and hydronephrotic kidneys (*6,7*). These approaches require invasive manipulations and/or some special animal models that may alter physiologic renal vascular responsiveness, and may thus confound the characterization of these renal vessels.

We recently developed a technique to directly visualize the organ microcirculation with an intravital needle lens-probe videomicroscopy (*8–12*). Using this technique, we have succeeded in assessing in vivo and *in situ* coronary microcirculation (*8–12*). Furthermore, this method allows direct visualization of both subendocardial and intramural microvascular behavior in beating porcine and canine hearts (*12*). The direct observation of the microvasculature localized deeper in the myocardium could encourage further application of this technique to the visualization of in vivo and intact intra-organ microcirculation, including renal glomerular microcirculation. With further improvement of this CCD videomicroscopy, we have developed an intravital pencil lens-probe videomicroscope for direct visualization of the glomerular microcirculation of canine (*18,19*) and rodent kidneys (*15–17*).

In this chapter, we introduce our newly developed videomicroscopic technique in which the in vivo, *in situ*, renal microcirculatory behavior was analyzed, and summarize the characteristics of this system that have been elucidated thus far.

From: *Methods in Molecular Medicine, vol. 86: Renal Disease: Techniques and Protocols*
Edited by: M. S. Goligorsky © Humana Press Inc., Totowa, NJ

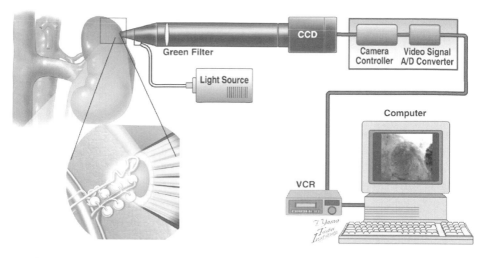

Fig. 1. Illustration of the pencil lens-probe videomicroscope with a charge-coupled device (CCD) camera. The microscope system consists of a pencil lens-probe, camera body containing a monochromatic CCD camera, a cone lens, and a light guide. A pencil-lens probe contains one cone lens with 180 mm in length, and captures the images of glomeruli and the adjoining afferent and efferent arterioles. The images from the CCD camera are converted to digital images, and are recorded with a videocassette recorder (VCR). Intravital pencil lens-probe CCD technique for visualization of renal microcirculation. The tip of the pencil lens-probe was moved carefully with a three dimensional micromanipulator. The probe was pulled back several tens of micrometers to avoid excessive compression on arterioles. IVC, inferior vena cava; Ao, Aorta.

2. Materials

2.1. Principle of Pencil Lens-Probe Videomicroscope System and the Access to Renal Microcirculation (22,23) (Fig. 1)

The system consists of a pencil lens with light guides, a camera body, a control unit, a light source, a monitor, and a videocassette recorder (VCR). The tapered pencil lens (tip diameter: 1 mm) contains a gradient-index (GRIN) lens surrounded by 18 annular optical-fiber light guides. The renal microvasculature and the surrounding tissues are illuminated by a xenon lump (150 W) through a green (complementary color of red) filter to accentuate the contrast between images of the blood-perfused vascular structures and the surrounding tissues. With this visualization system, the images of the erythrocyte are recognized as black, and those of the plasma as white.

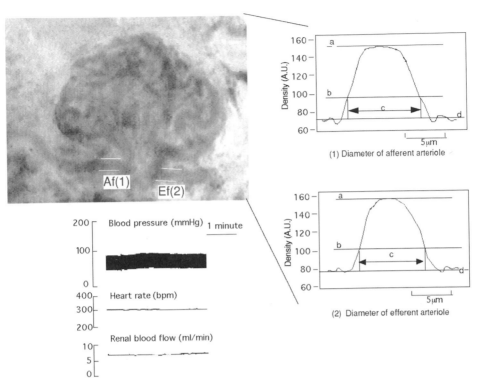

Fig. 2. A representative image of a rat glomerulus and the adjoining afferent and efferent arterioles. The vascular images of the afferent and efferent arterioles were analyzed in a freeze-frame modality. For measurement of vessel diameter, a scanning line was set right across the vessel segment, and the density in a gray-scale mode was counted along the scanning line. The difference in the gray scale between the peak value (a), and the value of mean noise level (d) was divided into quarters. The position with the density of one quarter higher value above the noise level (b) was identified as an inner wall, and the corresponding diameter was recognized automatically (c). Af, afferent arteriole; Ef, efferent arteriole. (From *18*, with permission.)

3. Methods

Under general anesthesia, the probe is introduced into the lateral border of the superficial renal cortex (for visualization of glomerular microcirculation) or brought closely to the surface of the kidney (for visualization of peritubular capillaries). If hemorrhage occurs, the experiment should be discontinued. The pencil lens-probe is manipulated carefully to obtain clear images of renal microvasculature. Video images are continuously recorded on videocassette tapes. The observation of the renal microcirculation is performed during stable hemodynamic conditions (*see* **Notes 1** and **4**).

3.1. Measurement of Microvascular Diameter (22,23) (Fig. 2)

The real-time sequential images of the renal microcirculation are analyzed by a computer system (Power Macintosh G3, Apple Computer, Cupertino, CA); the image size is 640 × 480 pixels, and the pixel size is 0.63 μm.

The images of the renal microvasculature are analyzed in a freeze-frame mode. For measurement of vessel diameter, the images of the vascular segment are rotated to place the segment perpendicular to the scanning line to count the image density. The density in a gray-scale mode along the scanning line is digitized and expressed in arbitrary units. The difference in the gray scale between the peak value (**Fig. 2**, line a), and the value of mean noise level (**Fig. 2**, line d) is divided into quarters. The position with the density of a quarter higher value above the noise level (**Fig. 2**, line b) is identified as an inner wall, and the corresponding diameter is read automatically (**Fig. 2**, line c) (*8–10*). The diameters are determined by averaging at least five measurements during the plateau of the response.

3.2. Analysis of Capillary Erythrocyte Velocity (20)

Video-signals are digitized with an analog-digital converter and fed into a digital video cassette recorder (VCR) (DVCAM, Sony, Japan) interfaced with a computer. Analysis is performed using NIH Image program combined with Matlab or with specifically written programs. Real microvascular blood flow is recorded with a pencil-lens microscope brought into direct contact with the decapsulated renal surface, which has been covered with mineral oil to prevent evaporation. In studies of glomerular microcirculation, a superficial slice through the renal cortex is made to ensure microscope access to glomeruli.

3.3. In Vivo Observation of Canine Renal Microcirculation: Effect of Angiotensin II and Tubuloglomerular Feedback (18) (Fig. 3)

The microcirculation in each glomerulus can be visualized simultaneously with continuous recording of blood pressure and renal blood flow. The administration of angiotensin II (1, 3, 10 and 30 ng/kg/min) produced dose-dependent constriction of afferent (Af) and efferent (Ef) arterioles in similar degrees; at 30 ng/kg/min, angiotensin II elicited $52 \pm 3\%$ ($n = 9$) and $53 \pm 3\%$ decrements in diameter ($n = 9$), respectively. The angiotensin II-induced arteriolar constriction was completely prevented by losartan, an AT1 antagonist. As for the tubuloglomerular feedback, the intrarenal hypertonic saline administration elicited transient increments (from 98 ± 8 to 122 ± 7 mL/min, $n = 6$, $p < 0.05$),

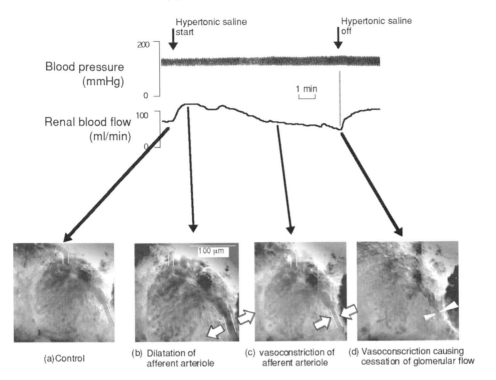

Fig. 3. Hemodynamic tracings (top) and representative images of afferent and efferent arteriolar responses to intrarenal hypertonic saline infusion (bottom). Hypertonic saline elicited a transient increase, followed by a sustained reduction in renal blood flow (RBF). In parallel with the RBF response, an afferent arteriole exhibited a temporary dilation (b) when compared with that under the control condition (a), and a subsequent vasoconstriction (c). Further vasoconstriction caused no visible glomerular capillary flow in some nephrons (d). (From *18*, with permission.)

followed by a marked reduction in renal blood flow (RBF) (78 ± 7 mL/min, $p < 0.05$). This response was accompanied by prominent constriction of Af (from 15.0 ± 1.1 to 8.5 ±1.1 µm, $n = 6$, $p < 0.05$), but not Ef arterioles (from 14.3 ± 1.2 to 13.8 ± 1.0 µm, $n = 3$). Furthermore, this response was completely inhibited by furosemide, a tubuloglomerular feedback inhibitor.

3.4. In Vivo Observation of Rat Renal Microcirculation: Streptozotocin-Induced Diabetic Rats and Spontaneously Hypertensive Rats (17) (Fig. 4)

In normal Wistar-Kyoto (WKY) rats, the diameter of the afferent arterioles (Af) is 11.9 ± 0.7 µm and that of the efferent arterioles (Ef) 8.9 ± 0.7 µm.

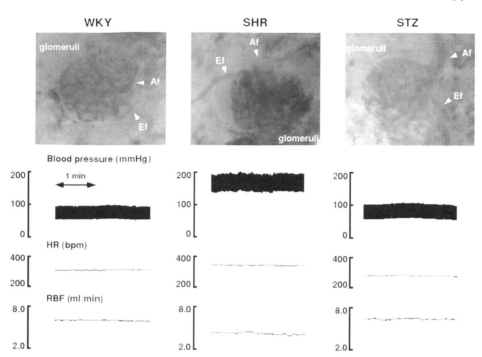

Fig. 4. Typical basal glomeruli and basal hemodynamic status of WKY (left), SHR (center), and STZ (right). Af, afferent arteriole; Ef, efferent arteriole; RBF, renal blood flow. Please note the difference in afferent arteriolar sizes. (From *17*, with permission.)

In SHR, Af diameter was decreased to about 60% of that in WKY. A dose-dependent dilation of both Af and Ef arterioles was observed after administration of barnidipine (1–10 µg/kg iv), a calcium-channel antagonist, in both groups. However, the Af-to-Ef ratios were different among the groups after barnidipine. No change was seen in Af/Ef ratio in WKY. In SHR, the Af/Ef ratio increased significantly because of greater dilation of Af after barnidipine administration. In contrast to SHR, barnidipine dilated Ef markedly in STZ, causing a significant reduction in the Af/Ef ratio.

3.5. RBC Velocity in Peritubular Capillaries After Renal Ischemia (15) *(Fig. 5)*

The peritubular capillary blood flow can be successfully visualized with our microscope. RBC velocity in peritubular capillaries averaged 1069 ± 146 µm/sec (*n* = 15). As expected, clamping the renal artery resulted in a complete cessa-

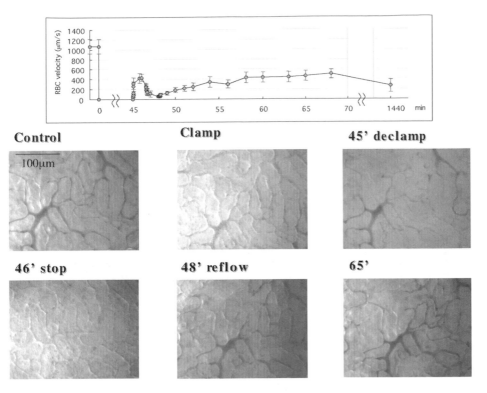

Fig. 5. The time-course of changes in mean RBC velocity and the typical imaging in post-ischemic peritubular capillaries. (From *15*, with permission.)

tion of blood flow accompanied by blanching of the surface, and visualization of individual RBC halted within the vessels. The release of renal artery after 45 min occlusion consistently resulted in an almost instantaneous recovery of blood flow. Surprisingly, within 1–2 min, blood flow became stagnant, and showed only partial recovery by 15–20 min. Twenty-four hours post-ischemia, peritubular capillary blood flow still remained diminished, representing only one-quarter of control level (227 ± 113 μm/sec).

4. Notes

1. Advantages
   a. Several experimental approaches have been developed in the past to characterize the reactivity of renal microvessels to a variety of vasoactive stimuli in vitro or ex vivo, including isolated perfused microvessels (*2–4*), juxtamedullary nephrons (*5*), and hydronephrotic kidneys (*6,7*). Most of these

experimental methods for direct visualization of the renal microcirculation require extensive surgical manipulations, such as isolation of the kidneys or renal microvessels, and induction of hydronephrosis. Our pencil-lens CCD intravital videomicroscopic technique appears to offer several advantages over other methodological approaches. i) Renal microcirculatory (glomerular network and peritubular network) behavior can be evaluated simultaneously with the whole-kidney function (e.g., renal blood flow) as well as systemic hemodynamics (e.g., blood pressure, heart rate, cardiac output) (**Fig. 4**). ii) The *in situ* renal microcirculation is accessible under both physiological *(18)* and pathological *(15,17)* conditions without disrupting the interaction between renal microvessels and perivascular tissues. iii) The tapered and miniature design of the CCD lens in this technique allows us to observe the renal microcirculation not only in large (dog or human *[21]*) but also in small animals (rat and mouse). iv) The experimental preparation for direct visualization of the renal microcirculation is simple *(2–7)*.

Consequently, we believe that this sophisticated technique can offer more substantial information on in vivo renal microcirculation by preserving intact renal vascular responses *(23)*.

2. Disadvantages
   a. A major disadvantage of this technique is the difficulty in establishing the technical stability in the assessment of renal microvascular behavior *(22)*. An extensive training period will be required to acquire skills to obtain clear microvascular images that are suitable for visualizing afferent and efferent arterioles and peritubular capillaries. Additional problems may be related to techniques for the vessel cannulation to administer drugs, especially in small animals.

References

1. Anderson, S. (1994) Relevance of single nephron studies to human glomerular function. *Kidney Int.* **45(1)**, 384–389.
2. Edwards, R. M. (1983) Segmental effects of norepinephrine and angiotensin II on isolated renal microvessels. *Am. J. Physiol.* **244(5)**, F526–F534.
3. Yuan, B. H., Robinette, J. B., and Conger, J. D. (1990) Effect of angiotensin II and norepinephrine on isolated rat afferent and efferent arterioles. *Am. J. Physiol.* **258(3 Pt. 2)**, F741–F750.
4. Ito, S., Johnson, C. S., and Carretero, O. A. (1991) Modulation of angiotensin II-induced vasoconstriction by endothelium-derived relaxing factor in the isolated microperfused rabbit afferent arteriole. *J. Clin. Invest.* **87(5)**, 1656–1663.
5. Carmines, P. K., Morrison, T. K., and Navar, L. G. (1986) Angiotensin II effects on microvascular diameters of in vitro blood-perfused juxtamedullary nephrons. *Am. J. Physiol.* **251(4 Pt. 2)**, F610–F618.
6. Steinhausen, M., Kucherer, H., Parekh, N., Weis, S., Wiegman, D. L., and Wilhelm, K. R. (1986) Angiotensin II control of the renal microcirculation: effect of blockade by saralasin. *Kidney Int.* **30(1)**, 56–61.

7. Loutzenhiser, R., Epstein, M., Hayashi, K., Takenaka, T., and Forster, H. (1991) Characterization of the renal microvascular effects of angiotensin II antagonist, DuP 753: studies in isolated perfused hydronephrotic kidneys. *Am. J. Physiol.* **4(4 Pt. 2),** 309S–314S.

8. Yada, T., Hiramatsu, O., Kimura, A., Goto, M., Ogasawara, Y., Tsujioka, K., et al. (1993) In vivo observation of subendocardial microvessels of the beating porcine heart using a needle-probe videomicroscope with a CCD camera. *Circ. Res.* **72(5),** 939–946.

9. Kajiya, F., Yada T., Kimura, A., Hiramatsu, O., Goto, M., Ogasawara, Y., et al. (1993) Endocardial coronary microcirculation of the beating heart. *Adv. Exp. Med. Biol.* **346,** 173–180.

10. Hiramatsu, O., Goto M., Yada, T., Kimura, A., Tachibana, H., Ogasawara, Y., et al. (1994) Diameters of subendocardial arterioles and venules during prolonged diastole in canine left ventricles. *Circ. Res.* **75(2),** 393–397.

11. Yada, T., Hiramatsu, O., Kimura, A., Tachibana, H., Chiba, Y., Lu, S., et al. (1995) Direct in vivo observation of subendocardial arteriolar response during reactive hyperemia. *Circ. Res.* **77(3),** 622–631.

12. Hiramatsu, O., Goto, M., Yada, T., Kimura, A., Chiba, Y., Tachibana, H., et al. (1998) In vivo observation of the intramural arterioles and venules in beating canine hearts. *J. Physiol.* **509(2),** 619–628.

13. Yamamoto, T., Tanaka, H., Yoshiyuki, J., Ogasawara, Y., and Kajiya, F. (1993) Visualization of intrarenal microvessels and evaluation of the effect of Angiotensin II by a needle probe video microscope with a CCD camera. *J. Am. Soc. Nephrol.* **14,** 574 (abstract).

14. Yamamoto, T., Ogasawara, Y., Nakamoto, H., Eiji, T., Ogasawara, Y., and Kajiya, F. (1997) In-vivo high speed imaging blood flow of canine renal microcirculation by needle-probe CCD microscope with blood flow maker. *Circulation* **96,** I-340 (abstract).

15. Yamamoto, T., Tada, T., Brodsky, S. V., Tanaka, H., Noiri, E., Kajiya, F., et al. Intravital videomicroscopy of peritubular capillaries in renal ischemia. *Am. J. Physiol. Renal Physiol.* Article in Press, published online ahead of print, January 29, 2002.

16. Brodsky, S. V., Yamamoto, T., Tada, T., Kim B., Chen, J., Kajiya, F., et al. Endothelial dysfunction in ischemic acute renal failure: rescue by transplanted endothelial cells. *Am. J. Physiol. Renal Physiol.* Article in Press, published online ahead of print, December 18, 2002.

17. Yamamoto, T., Tomura, Y., Tanaka, H., and Kajiya, F. (2001) In vivo visualization of renal microcirculation in hypertensive and diabetic rats. *Am. J. Physiol. Renal* **281,** F571–F577.

18. Yamamoto, T., Hayashi, K., Matsuda, H., Kubota, E., Tanaka, H., Ogasawara, Y., et al. (2001) In vivo visualization of angiotensin-II and TGF-mediated renal vasoconstriction. *Kidney Int.* **60,** 364–369.

19. Matsuda, H., Hayashi, K., Arakawa, K., Naitoh, M., Kubota, E., Honda, M., et al. (1999) Zonal heterogenecity in action of angiotensin-converting enzyme inhibitor

of renal microcirculation: role of intrarenal bradykinin. *J. Am. Soc. Nephrol.* **10**, 2272–2282.

20. Ogasawara, Y., Takehara, K., Yamamoto, T., Hashimoto, R., Nakamoto, H., Kajiya, F. (2000) Quantitative blood velocity mapping in glomerular capillaries by in vivo observation with an intravital videomicroscopy. *Methods Inf. Med.* **39**, 175–178.

21. Yamamoto, T., Noiri, E., Hayashi, K., Tanaka, H., Ogasawara, Y., and Kajiya, F. (2001) Diagnostic drug for the purpose of single nephron function by the intravenous administration. *Japan Patent* P2001–36, 9037.

22. Yamamoto, T., Hayashi, K., Tomura, Y., Tanaka, H., and Kajiya, F. (2001) Direct in vivo visualization of renal microcirculation by intravital CCD videomicroscopy. *Exp. Nephrol.* **9(2)**, 150–155.

23. Yamamoto, T., Hayashi, K., Matsuda, H. Kubota, E., Ogasawara, Y., Hashimoto, R., et al. (2000) Direct in vivo visualization of glomerular microcirculation by intravital pencil lens probe CCD videomicroscopy. *Clin. Hemorheol. Microcirc.* **23**, 1–6.

8

Confocal and Two-Photon Microscopy

János Peti-Peterdi and P. Darwin Bell

1. Introduction

The majority of renal physiological processes, including glomerular filtrate formation, tubular reabsorption and secretion, and regulation of cortical and medullary blood flow, involve the complex interaction of a number of different cell types. This is exemplified by the juxtaglomerular apparatus (JGA), a highly complex structure that consists of the tubular epithelium; the macula densa (MD); vascular-endothelial, smooth-muscle, and renin granular epithelioid cells; and extra- and intraglomerular mesangial cells. These dissimilar cells interact with each other and form a functional syncitium to control glomerular hemodynamics (tubuloglomerular feedback) and renin release (*1*). Thus far, it has been difficult to visualize certain inaccessible cell types, such as MD cells or renal medullary interstitial cells in native kidney tissue, or to study cellular interactions given the constraints of existing technologies. Recently, multi-photon excitation fluorescence microscopy has been applied to kidney research (*2–4*), and it offers a tremendous increase in optical resolution vs other imaging techniques, even over conventional confocal microscopy. Because of the nature and advantages of two-photon excitation, which are discussed in detail here, multi-photon microscopy is becoming increasingly used in biomedical research particularly for visualization of thick samples of living tissue. To date, two-photon microscopy has been applied in numerous in vivo experimental models, several applications have even used intact conscious whole animals—e.g., in neurobiological research, the mouse brain can be visualized to a depth of 1–2 mm into the cortex (*5*).

We recently demonstrated (*4*) that an entire isolated perfused, living glomerulus (glomerular diameter (100 μm) can be easily optically sectioned, and the complex cell structure and function of the juxtaglomerular apparatus can be visualized in striking detail with two-photon microscopy. Here, we provide

From: *Methods in Molecular Medicine, vol. 86: Renal Disease: Techniques and Protocols*
Edited by: M. S. Goligorsky © Humana Press Inc., Totowa, NJ

detailed information on the principles of multi-photon microscopy, show examples of how to use this technology in renal research, and compare the quality of two-photon imaging with conventional one-photon excitation confocal microscopy.

2. Materials (Principles of Techniques)

More than a decade ago, new optical sectioning techniques were described for fluorescence microscopy. The invention and development of the confocal optical microscope originated from the work of J. G. White, W. B. Amos, and M. Fordham in the late 1980s (6). Key elements in confocal laser scanning fluorescence microscopy are to direct, focus, and scan a laser beam over a specimen and to collect fluorescent light emitted only from the immediate vicinity of the focal plane. This was achieved by using a fully variable confocal aperture (pinhole) and a novel form of an all-reflective scanning system. Use of a pinhole in front of an internal detector helps to eliminate out-of-focus fluorescence.

The newest innovation in fluorescence microscopy is multi-photon microscopy, in which fluorescence excitation is strictly confined to the optical section by the process of two- or three-photon absorption. The first serious theories, and laboratory tests for this new technology were carried out by W. Denk, J. H. Strickler, and W. W. Webb at Cornell University in 1990 (7). Two-photon microscopy involves the illumination of a sample with light of a wavelength approx twice that of the absorption peak of the particular fluorophore being used. Thus, two-photon excitation involves simultaneous absorption of two photons of 1/2 energy (double λ), and this happens only at the focal plane. For example, indo-1, which has an absorption peak (excitation wavelength) of approx 360 nm, is excited at 720 nm using two-photon microscopy. Importantly, no excitation of the fluorophore above or below the focal plane occurs at this wavelength (720 nm) and thus no bleaching of the fluorophore will occur in the bulk of the sample. However, if a high-powered pulsed laser source (**Fig. 1**) is used with a peak power of >2 kW contained in pulses shorter than a picosecond (so that the mean power levels are moderate and do not damage the specimen), two-photon events will occur at the point of focus. During the picosecond pulse, photon density becomes sufficiently high, that two photons are absorbed simultaneously by the fluorophore. In terms of the energy necessary for excitation of the fluorophore, the absorption of two photons of a long wavelength is equivalent to the absorption of one photon of short wavelength, and thus can lead to fluorescence excitation. Thus, in a two-photon fluorescence system one has the ideal situation in which fluorescence excitation only occurs in the focal region. This new approach in fluorescence microscopy offers a number of important advantages, particularly when studying living cells. Since fluorescence excitation occurs only in the focal region, every single-fluores-

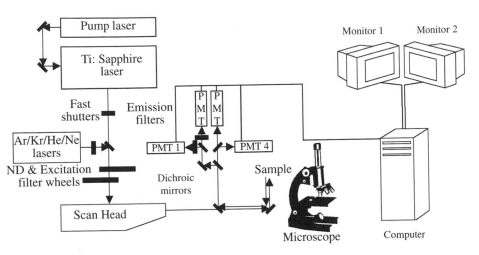

Fig. 1. Schematic drawing of the multi-photon imaging system. (*See* text for details.)

cence photon carries spatial information. Therefore, three-dimensional (3D)-imaging is possible solely by excitation, and there is no need for the expensive confocal pinhole. In addition, with two-photon fluorescence imaging, because there is no out-of-focus fluorescence, there is also no out-of-focus bleaching. Although bleaching can be higher in the focal plane with two-photon microscopy (for example, because of the high photon density), bleaching is restricted to the focal region. All these features of two-photon microscopy result in reduced photo damage of living specimens. Also, longer time periods of continuous tissue scanning is possible which provides for real-time imaging. For certain applications, UV dyes, such as indo-1 can be excited with red, near infrared, and infrared light. Longer wavelengths allow for deeper penetration into tissues, and avoid the deleterious effects of conventional ultraviolet illumination on living specimens. Also, no expensive UV optical components are required. Taken together, all these principles, features, and advantages of two-photon fluorescence microscopy allow for ultra-high quality of deep optical sectioning of living tissue samples.

3. Methods

3.1. Methods of Isolation and Microperfusion of Various Nephron Segments

Detailed methods of dissection and microperfusion of isolated renal tubule segments are described in previous publications (*8–10*) and in Chapter 31. Methods of microdissection and perfusion of an afferent arteriole (AA) with

MD have been described in detail *(11)*. Briefly, a superficial AA with its glomerulus and associated tubular segment (consisting of the cortical thick ascending limb, cTAL, the MD, and distal convoluted tubule) was microdissected using free-hand techniques from the kidneys of New Zealand white rabbits (1.0–1.5 kg) fed standard rabbit chow (Purina, St. Louis, MO), and transferred to a temperature-regulated chamber mounted on an inverted microscope. In order to prevent intracellular accumulation of NaCl prior to the experiment, the dissection solution was an isosmotic, low NaCl containing Ringer's solution consisting of (in mM): 25 NaCl, 120 N-methyl-D-glucamine (NMDG) cyclamate, 5 KCl, 1 $MgSO_4$, 1.6 Na_2HPO_4, 0.4 NaH_2PO_4, 1.5 $CaCl_2$, 5 D-glucose, and 10 N'-2-hydroxyethyl-piperazine-N'-2-ethanesulfonic acid (HEPES). The control tubular perfusate was identical to the dissection Ringer solution and the perfusion rate was maintained at about 10 nl/min. The bath (150 mM NaCl-containing Ringer solution) was identical to the arteriolar perfusate and was continuously aerated with 100% O_2, and exchanged at a rate of 1 mL/min. The preparation was kept in the low (NaCl) dissection solution, and temperature was maintained at 8°C until cannulation of both the arteriole and tubule was completed, and then gradually raised to 37°C for the remainder of the experiment. In our experience, this maneuver greatly improved the responsiveness of the preparations *(9)*. A 30-min equilibration period was allowed before taking any measurements.

3.2. Fluorescence Microscopy

Confocal and two-photon fluorescence microscopy of the isolated tubule preparations were carried out using a Leica confocal system (**Fig. 1**) that consists of Ar/Kr/He/Ne lasers (for conventional confocal microscopy) parallel with a photo-diode pump laser (Verdi, 5 W) and a mode-locked titanium:sapphire laser (Mira, both from Coherent Laser Group, Santa Clara, CA, for multiphoton microscopy). We used the Mira Ti:sapphire laser, because it is fully tunable between 690 and 1000 nm and provides the flexibility of using different fluorophores—e.g., in our studies indo-1, which is excited at 720 nm. When building a multiphoton system for applications that require the 690–1000 tunable range, another alternative for the two-photon laser source that we have also used *(4)*, is a Millennia series all-solid state pump laser (5–10 W) with the Tsunami mode-locked Ti:sapphire laser, both from Spectra Physics.

Tissue preparations were transferred to a thermoregulated chamber on a Leica DM IRBE (Leica, Germany) inverted microscope and visualized using a X63 oil-immersion lens. When studying tissue-cell morphology (**Figs. 2–4**), a fluorescent membrane-staining dye 1-(4-trimethylammoniumphenyl)-6-phenyl-1, 3,5-hexatriene *p*-toluenesulfonate (TMA-DPH, Molecular Probes, Eugene, OR) was used. Using a final concentration of 5 µM from a stock solution dissolved in

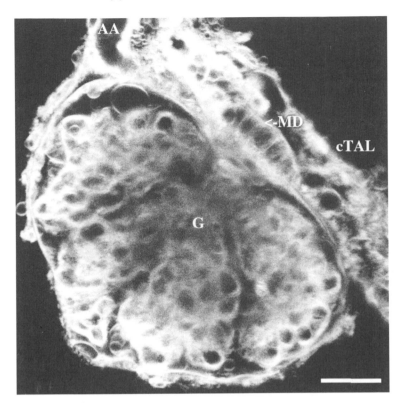

Fig. 2. Visualization of the isolated simultaneously perfused afferent arteriole (AA)-attached glomerulus (G) and cortical thick ascending limb (cTAL) containing the macula densa (MD) *in situ* with two-photon excitation fluorescence microscopy. Tissue was stained with TMA-DPH. Bar = 20 µm.

N, N'-dimethylformamide, TMA-DPH was added to both the bathing solution and the tubular fluid and, in double-perfused applications, to the arteriolar perfusion solutions in order to visualize cellular structures of the preparation. TMA-DPH is a lipid marker cationic linear polyene that acts as a surface anchor and readily incorporates in the plasma membrane of living cells (*12*). TMA-DPH is virtually nonfluorescent in water (fluorescent excitation wavelength is 755 nm with two-photon system and emission peak is 430 nm), and binds in proportion to the available membrane surface. Its fluorescence intensity is therefore sensitive to physiological processes that cause a net change in membrane-surface area, making it an excellent probe for monitoring events such as changes in cell volume. Staining of cell membranes by TMA-DPH is very rapid (1–2 min), and the duration of plasma-membrane surface staining before internalization into

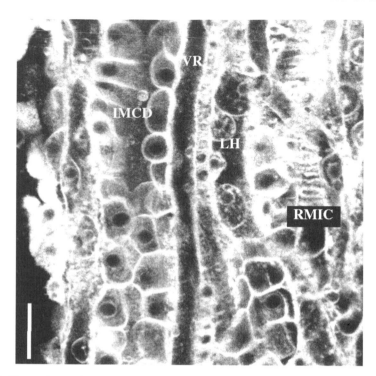

Fig. 3. Two-photon image of various tubular and vascular structures in the medulla. Inner medullary collecting duct (IMCD), vasa recta (VR), loop of Henle (LH), and renal medullary interstitial cells (RMIC). Tissue was stained with TMA-DPH. Bar = 20 μm.

the cytoplasm is quite prolonged (1–2 h). These characteristics of TMA-DPH make it a very useful tool for visualization of both overall morphology and individual cells of our preparation, as demonstrated in **Figs. 2–4**.

Another application and fluorophore that we used was indo-1 for calcium imaging **(Fig. 5)**. Indo-1 (Molecular Probes, Eugene, OR) is a ratiometric Ca^{2+} indicator, which is the preferred dye, instead of fura-2, in systems (such as two-

Fig. 4. *(opposite page)* Comparison of two-photon **(A)** and single-photon **(B)** excitation confocal imaging. The two techniques were used at the same Z section of the same isolated perfused cortical thick ascending limb (cTAL) containing the macula densa (MD) and attached glomerulus (G). two-photon and confocal measurements were obtained within 1 min of each other. Tissue was stained with TMA-DPH. Bar = 20 μm.

Fig. 5. *(opposite page)* Ca^{2+}-image of the perfused cortical thick ascending limb (cTAL) containing the macula densa (MD) with the attached glomerulus. Tissue was loaded with Indo-1 from both the tubular lumen and bathing solution. Bar = 20 μm.

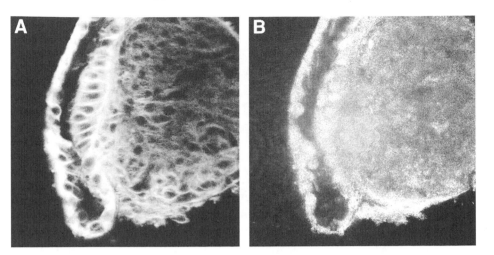

Fig. 4.

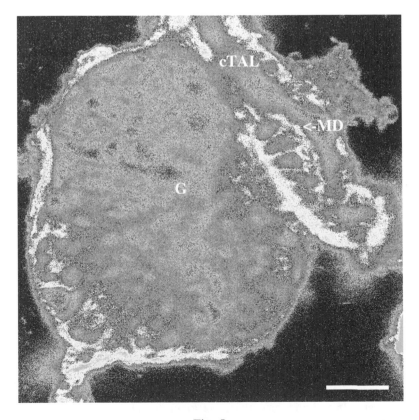

Fig. 5.

photon microscopy), where it is more practical to use a single laser for excitation (720 nm with a two-photon system) and monitor two emission wavelengths (453 and 405 nm). Indo-1 undergoes a large shift in peak emission wavelength at 405 nm upon binding Ca^{2+}, whereas the signal monitored at 453 nm does not change with Ca^{2+} binding. Indo-1 does not require special quartz optics for microscopy and may be less subject to compartmentalization than fura-2. We used the acetoxymethyl (AM) ester form of indo-1, which can passively diffuse across cell membranes. Once inside the cell, AM esters are cleaved by intracellular esterases to yield the cell-impermeant fluorescent indicator indo-1; no invasive loading techniques are required. In order to obtain absolute $[Ca^{2+}]i$, indo-1 must be calibrated, and this can be done easily with the "Physiology" function of the Leica TCS software. A 405 ± 17 nm bandpass filter was used to select the indo-1 emissions that increase with increasing Ca^{2+} concentrations prior to detection by a PMT (channel 2). A 453 ± 2 nm band pass filter was used to select isosbestic emission of indo-1, which is independent of Ca^{2+} concentration, before it was detected at a second PMT (channel 1). Fluorescent intensities at both wavelengths were background subtracted, and the ratio of indo-1 fluorescence (405 nm/453 nm) was converted into absolute Ca^{2+} values with the Leica TCS software.

Images were collected in time (xyt) or z-series (xyz), depending on the purpose of study, with the Leica TCS NT imaging software. The most frequently used xyt application had a cycle time of 10 sec, and 30 cycles were collected in each series. However, much faster data acquisition is possible.

4. Notes

1. TMA-DPH is a very useful fluorescent marker for imaging tissue-cell structure and morphology. Loading requires only a few minutes, and excitation and emission spectra have several maximums, making it a very easy-to-use fluorophore.

    Caution: TMA-DPH cannot pass through tight junctions, and it is very sensitive to light. Thus, it is highly recommended to turn off the room lights after opening the stock solution and throughout the experiments. Also, the image quality is improved if TMA-DPH is continuously present in the perfusate/bath. Do not remove it, but maintain the same concentration of TMA-DPH when switching between various perfusate/bath solutions.

2. Indo-1 was selected for calcium imaging because it is a ratiometric dye. Indo-1 is excited with a single wavelength (720 nm) light, and the 405 nm/453 nm emission ratios are calculated. The emission ratio is independent of changes in cell volume—a major technical issue in fluorescence microscopy that occurs, for example, in macula densa cells, which swell during increases in tubular [NaCl]. Thus, using Indo-1 and the emission ratio, in two-photon applications, is a great solution for a technical problem that exists for many research laboratories.

3. To date, tuning of the wide-range Ti:sapphire lasers in two-photon applications takes time. In our experience, e.g., switching from TMA-DPH experiments (755 nm excitation) to indo-1, e.g., calcium measurements (720 nm excitation) requires manual tuning of the laser, which takes at least 5 min. Consequently, if one needs simultaneous use of two fluorochromes, or sequential scanning with two photons, it may require two separate laser sources.

4. Although two-photon microscopy is ideal for deep tissue sectioning, a major limitation is the ability to distribute fluorophores throughout the tissue. Most fluorophores, including very lipophylic ones, do not penetrate very far into tissues. This is one advantage of the perfused JGA, because fluorophores can be delivered deep into the glomerulus (via the arterioles) or into the tubules or to the surface structures (bath).

5. An important issue that one must consider when planning to perform multi-photon imaging is cost. To date, the price for a two-photon system only, without additional visible lasers—including only the pump and Ti:Sapphire lasers, beam conditioning units, and various optical elements, microscope, photomultipliers, computer and software—is in the $500,000 range. This same system with additional Ar/Kr/He/Ne visible lasers and an upgraded system is about $850,000. Try to think in terms of core facilities.

6. Interpretation:

   Two-photon excitation fluorescence microscopy, in our experience, has three important advantages over confocal fluorescence imaging methods. i) First, two-photon images, in case of the highly photon-scattering kidney tissue, have far superior image quality compared to one-photon confocal imaging, as exemplified in **Fig. 4**. Various tubular and vascular structures in both the renal cortex *(4)* (**Fig. 2**) and medulla (**Fig. 3**) can be visualized in striking detail. In some experiments (**Fig. 3**), a small portion of the papillary tubular rays was dissected and the medulla visualized. The highly complex structure of the inner medulla can be visualized on the individual cell level. ii) Also, the time period of either continuous scanning or xyt time-series data collection is significantly prolonged with two-photon imaging before causing any damage to the living tissue. Reactivity of the isolated perfused tubules was well-preserved for the duration of our experiments. A 5-min-long xyt time-series experiment (e.g., in **ref. 4**) with continuous scanning can be repeated, and identical findings reproduced from the same preparation 3–4 times. iii) Another important advantage of two-photon microscopy, in our experience, is the deep optical sectioning ability. When z-sectioning through an entire glomerulus (**Fig. 4**), two-photon microscopy provides superior images for every section throughout the entire 100-μm scan. Doing the same scan with conventional one-photon excitation confocal microscopy, after the initial 20 μm, fluorescence intensity is significantly reduced, and image quality is very poor.

   In summary, multi-photon excitation imaging is a powerful new optical sectioning technique for fluorescence microscopy. This technique offers considerable advantages over confocal imaging for in vivo applications and applications that require the maximum information from images of deep optical sections.

Acknowledgments

We thank the High Resolution Imaging Facility, directed by Dr. Kent Keyser, at the University of Alabama at Birmingham for giving us access to the multi-photon/confocal site. Albert Tousson and Mark Bolding provided outstanding technical assistance. This work has been supported by grants from the National Institute of Health (DK-32032) and the American Heart Association (AHA SDG 0230074N).

References

1. Schnermann, J. and Briggs, J. (1985) Function of the juxtaglomerular apparatus: local control of glomerular hemodynamics, in *The Kidney* (Seldin, D. W. and Giebisch, G., eds.), Raven, New York, pp. 669–697.
2. Phillips, C. L., Arend, L. J., Filson, A. J., Kojetin, D. J., Clendenon, J. L., Fang, S., and Dunn, K. W. (2001) Three-dimensional imaging of embryonic mouse kidney by two-photon microscopy. *Am. J. Pathol.* **158,** 49–55.
3. Nitschke, R., Henger, A., Ricken, S., Muller, V., Kottgen, M., Bek, M., et al. (2001) Acetylcholine increases the free intracellular calcium concentration in podocytes in intact rat glomeruli via muscarinic M(5) receptors. *J. Am. Soc. Nephrol.* **12,** 678–687.
4. Peti-Peterdi, J., Morishima, S., Bell, P. D., and Okada, Y. (2002) Two-photon excitation fluorescence imaging of the living juxtaglomerular apparatus. *Am. J. Physiol. Renal Physiol.* DOI, 10.1152/ajprenal.00356.2001.
5. Yoder, E. J. and Kleinfeld, D. (2002) Cortical imaging through the intact mouse skull using two-photon excitation laser scanning microscopy. *Microsc. Res. Tech.* **56,** 304–305.
6. White, J. G., Amos, W. B., and Fordham, M. (1987) An evaluation of confocal versus conventional imaging of biological structures by fluorescence light microscopy. *J. Cell Biol.* **105,** 41–48
7. Denk, W., Strickler, J., and Webb, W. W. (1990) Two-photon laser scanning fluorescence microscopy. *Science* **248,** 73–76.
8. Burg, M. B. (1983) Perfusion of isolated renal tubules. *Yale J. Biol. Med.* **45,** 321–326.
9. Peti-Peterdi, J. and Bell, P. D. (1999) Cytosolic [Ca^{2+}] signaling pathway in macula densa cells. *Am. J. Physiol. Renal Physiol.* **277,** F472–F476.
10. Peti-Peterdi, J., Chambrey, R., Bebok, Z., Biemesderfer, D., St. John, P. L., Abrahamson, D. R., et al. (2000) Macula densa Na:H exchange activities mediated by apical NHE2 and basolateral NHE4 isoforms. *Am. J. Physiol. Renal Physiol.* **278,** F452–F463.
11. Ito, S. and Carretero, O. A. (1990) An in vitro approach to the study of macula densa-mediated glomerular hemodynamics. *Kidney Int.* **38,** 1206–1210.
12. Cupers, P., Veithen, A., Kiss, A., Baudhuin, P., and Courtoy, P. J. (1994) Clathrin polymerization is not required for bulk-phase endocytosis in rat fetal fibroblasts. *J. Cell Biol.* **127,** 725–735.

9

Atomic Force Microscopy in Renal Physiology

Robert M. Henderson

1. Fundamentals of Atomic Force Microscopy

The atomic force microscope (AFM) (**Fig. 1**) is one of a family of "scanning-probe" microscopes. It was developed by Binnig, Quate, and Gerber in 1986 *(1)* from the scanning tunneling microscope (STM), which was invented by Binnig and Rohrer in the first half of the 1980s *(2)*. The STM produces images of surfaces of relatively highly electrically conductive specimens, and has primarily been used in the physical sciences. The AFM extends the technique of STM to nonconductive as well as conductive specimens, making it suitable for biological applications. AFM obtains information by transduction of a signal produced as a sharp probe moves across perturbations on a surface. The probe is typically pyramid-shaped, and is made from silicon nitride (Si_3N_4). It is mounted on a gold-coated, highly reflective, sprung cantilever. The probe is drawn back and forth in a raster pattern across a sample (prepared on a suitably flat substrate). This arrangement is shown in **Fig. 2A**. The figure shows the sample, suitably prepared and placed upon a piezoelectric scanner. The probe makes contact with the surface of the sample. The scanner can move in three dimensions, and is under electronic control via a computer. This control is such that the probe and sample can be positioned relative to each other in either the x or y raster dimensions or in the vertical z dimension very accurately, even down to the Angstrom level. A low-powered laser is focused onto the gold-coated cantilever and is reflected onto a series of photodiode detector elements. As a result, when the sample is moved back and forth, and the probe encounters an obstacle and the cantilever is deflected, thus changing the reflected angle of the laser and affecting the signal detected by the photodiodes. The photodiodes' signals are fed into a computer that can construct a three-dimensional (3D) image from the information received and can also feedback information and instructions to the piezoelectric drives. Thus, the AFM, in

From: *Methods in Molecular Medicine, vol. 86: Renal Disease: Techniques and Protocols*
Edited by: M. S. Goligorsky © Humana Press Inc., Totowa, NJ

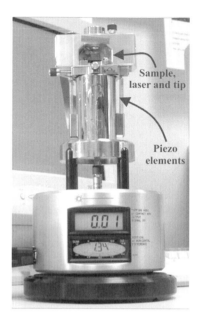

Fig. 1. A photograph of an atomic force microscope. The instrument is shown in front of a computer monitor for scale, and it is approx 28 cm in height.

contrast to optical and electron microscopes, produces an image that is not compromised by the limitations of the wavelengths of the various types of electromagnetic radiation. The resolution is very high—less than 1 nm with some biological specimens—and thus AFM makes possible the production of images of biological macromolecules under near-physiological conditions, and allows real-time imaging of dynamic interactions between macromolecules. Some microscopes, as shown in **Fig. 2B**, are designed to be used with biological specimens (*3*). Here, the probe is mounted on the bottom of the piezo assembly, which is itself moved across the sample that remains static. The laser is focused through an optical element that runs through the piezo assembly. This means that the sample can be simultaneously observed using an inverted optical microscope and the AFM. In its bare essentials, the technique of AFM is very simple—it works like a rather sophisticated miniature gramophone,—but its successful application has been dependent upon the development of a number of technological features.

The first is related to the types of probes used. Although for most purposes a tip with a conventional pyramidal profile produces good images, various types of other probes with tips of different aspect ratios can be produced. This is

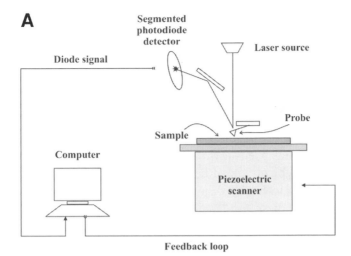

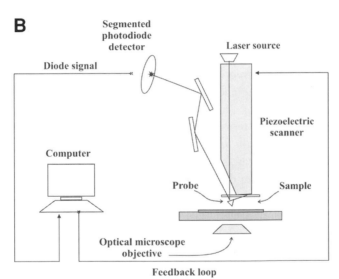

Fig. 2. Schematic diagrams of two models of AFMs. (**A**) shows the more conventional type, as illustrated in **Fig. 1**. (**B**) shows a configuration designed to be placed down directly onto samples, which might be on the stage of an optical microscope.

important because if the tip is broader than the features being imaged, then distortion of the image will take place. Under certain circumstances, it is important to use probes that have a sharper profile, effectively tapering at a sufficiently acute angle at the tip so that they are able to penetrate small crevices in the sample. If they are unable to do so, fine details of the structure will be lost. Probes are commercially available that have been sharpened or that have sharply tapering columns of Si_3N_4 deposited at their ends to improve resolution, but great interest exists in the use of Si_3N_4 probes that have had carbon "nanotubes" attached to their tips (4). These nanotubes are up to 1 nm long and thin (1–5 nm in diameter at the tip), and should prove useful in optimizing the production of images because of their ability to gain access to small recesses in surfaces without exerting large forces. Studies are continuing in the development and application of nanotubes for AFM of biological macromolecules (5–6), but progress has been slow.

The cantilevers typically must have very low spring constants (sometimes less than 0.1 pN nm^{-1}). Numbers like this are rather difficult concepts to appreciate, but effectively these spring constants are close to or lower than the intermolecular forces that produce attraction between biological molecules. This means that as the probe moves across a sample it will—ideally—be deflected vertically by features it may encounter without the danger of the cantilever being so stiff that it sweeps away all obstacles in its path. In addition, the force applied as the tip scans can be reduced by fine adjustment of the microscope at the start of an experiment. This is achieved by means of a "force curve" (**Fig. 3**). To construct the force curve, the probe is held stationary (in the horizontal directions) on the substrate and is oscillated vertically. As the probe and substrate make contact (during the downward-moving "approaching" phase), the cantilever bearing the probe is deflected, and this deflection is registered by the photodiode array. As the probe and substrate are drawn apart (during the "withdrawal" phase) the cantilever is again deflected, returning to its original position, but is often further deflected as a result of the probe maintaining contact with the substrate—a result of the molecular adhesion forces between probe and substrate. By examination and by adjustment of the force curve, the instrument can be optimized in such a way that excessive vertical forces are not applied to the sample. Too much force would "squash" the sample, and too little usually causes the probe to be displaced as it scans—effectively jumping off the surface like a car moving too rapidly along a bumpy road. Adhesive forces between probe and substrate are reduced considerably if imaging is conducted under fluid, which is in any case useful for much biological imaging. Increasingly, the force curve is being used to study the degree of attraction between probe and substrate, and can thus be used to distinguish different areas of the same sample if they have differing physical characteristics. This feature is exploited using the technique known as "force-volume" imaging. Here, force curves are generated at a number of points along each raster line, and an image is built up that effectively produces a map of probe-substrate interactions across the surface of a sample at regular intervals, which is displayed together with the conventional topographical AFM image.

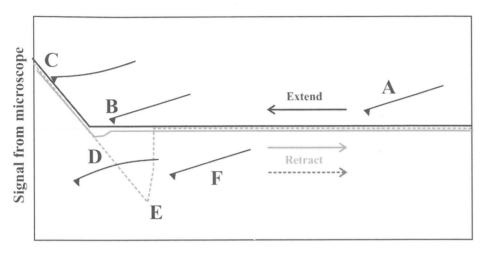

Fig. 3. Examples of force curves contrasting the situation with a sample in air with one under fluid. The probe is held stationary over the substrate and then oscillated up and down ("extended" and "retracted"). At point **A** the probe is not in contact with any substrate and thus no deflection is registered. At **B** the probe meets the substrate, and at **C** it is advanced further downward onto the substrate, and the cantilever bearing the probe is deflected. This is shown in the "y" axis of the curve, which illustrates the signal registered by the computer. The piezo drivers then begin to withdraw the probe upwards ("retract"). Because the probe and substrate are physically attracted, they maintain contact **D**, even when the probe has been withdrawn before the point where it originally made contact with the substrate. At point **E**, the probe loses contact with the substrate and jumps back to its original position **F**. The important point concerning the force curve is that the degree of attraction between the probe and substrate must be minimized. The measure of this attraction is given broadly by the size and shape of the triangle lying below the dotted line in the two diagrams. Forces are minimized when recordings are made under fluid, which is demonstrated by the solid gray line. In air, the force of attraction between probe and sample is much greater, as shown by the dotted gray line.

If the tip and sample interact and that interaction can be measured using the force curve, then it should be possible to functionalize the AFM tip—essentially, to coat it with some substance and look at the force of interaction of that substance with the specimen being investigated. Early work with the AFM focused on the interaction of streptavidin and biotin *(7)*, with one-half of the streptavidin-biotin ligand-receptor pair used to coat an AFM tip, and the other half of the pair attached to the substrate. These studies have highlighted the potential of the AFM for measurements of interactions between a large number of biologically important molecules and to allow identification of sites on biological surfaces *(8)*.

The use of cantilevers with low spring constants has proven valuable in producing data for physical, non biological specimens. However, biological materials bring with them their own problems in the application of AFM, and only with the regular and persistent technical developments that have been introduced to atomic force microscopy has high-resolution imaging been made possible. The first problem to be overcome involves the force applied by the probe, which affects the images obtained by conventional AFM on biological specimens (which are relatively soft compared with physical specimens). As the probe is drawn across the surface of the sample, it applies lateral force and thus can distort the image produced. As described here, if the force applied is too high, the sample can be damaged or even pushed around the substrate by the probe, which behaves like a small snow-plough. If the applied force is too low, then the probe can bounce off the sample as it moves over topographical features. These limitations can be overcome by setting the tip to oscillate at a high frequency (around 300 kHz and 12 kHz in air and fluid, respectively), a mode of recording known as "tapping mode" (rather than the more conventional "contact mode" described here). The reflected signal from the cantilever detected by the photodiodes then describes a sine wave, with an amplitude that is altered as the probe moves over any physical feature on the surface. This technique is illustrated in **Fig. 4**. The tapping-mode technique results in much lower lateral (and apparently vertical) forces being applied to the sample, and produces concomitantly clearer images with less scope for distortion of samples. Even with the use of tapping mode, the adhesive forces between a dry sample and the probe can be such that distorted images can result, and the ability to make tapping-mode recordings under fluid *(9)* is a useful technique to minimize adhesive forces and distortion of images or samples. These features make possible the production of high-resolution images of biological macromolecules under near-physiological conditions, and allow real-time imaging at such high resolution of dynamic interactions between macromolecules. A further development of tapping mode is "phase imaging" *(10)*. In what might now be called "classical" tapping mode recording, the cantilever is oscillated at high frequencies. If the cantilever is oscillating freely in air, then the waveform signal detected by the photodiodes should be exactly in phase with the signal driving the piezoelectric element that produces the oscillation. However, if the probe comes into contact with some substrate and there is any attractive force between the probe and substrate, this will tend to cause the tip to be held back in contact with the substrate—briefly "sticking" to it, and so the photodiode signal will move out of phase with the piezoelectric driver's waveform. This phase lag can be detected by the controlling computer and used to construct an image for the AFM that gives a measure of adhesive forces between the probe and substrate. The technique is useful because it provides

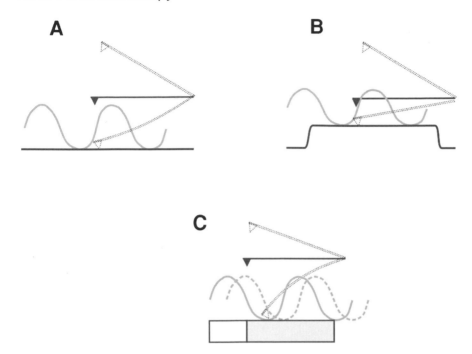

Fig. 4. Illustrating the principle of "tapping mode" **A** and **B** and "phase imaging" **C**. In tapping mode, the probe is set oscillating, describing a sine wave "**A**". The amplitude of the oscillation is altered when the probe meets any perturbation on the substrate **B**, and the change in amplitude is used to produce an image. In phase imaging, tapping mode is also used, but the behavior of the probe in comparison to that predicted by the signal produced by the computer driving it is monitored. In **C**, the tip is physically attracted to the gray area of the substrate, and thus there is a lag between the expected oscillation (solid gray sine wave) and that observed (dotted gray sine wave). This phase difference is recorded, and gives a measure of the degree of attraction between probe and substrate.

information on probe-substrate interactions that do not always need to be reflected in apparent changes in topographical features of the sample.

2. AFM Techniques Used in Renal Research

Even before the introduction of the AFM, researchers had made tentative steps in examining biological specimens using STM *(2)*. The more sympathetic nature of the interaction of the AFM with biological materials meant that very soon after its introduction, work began to be published in which cells and macromolecules were imaged. By early 1993, the technique had been adopted by renal and epithelial physiologists. Initial experiments were on intact cells, but during recent years AFM has become more sophisticated, and scientists have become more skilled in the preparation and manipulation of biological specimens for the microscope. Today, experiments are performed on intact cells, isolated organelles, isolated membranes, purified molecules, and artificial lipid membranes. Broadly speaking, the success in obtaining images of biological specimens with AFM depends upon techniques of sample preparation and upon physical aspects of the microscope (e.g., tip dimensions, force applied, rate of scan, and scan size). Rather than describe the very wide range of experiments and their results, this chapter focuses on several preparations that have been studied by various groups around the world, and identifies the technical difficulties posed and the way in which these difficulties have been addressed by the authors. The papers examined all contain extensive technical descriptions of the details of the experiments. There are a number of detailed reviews, with varying degrees of technical description, concerning AFM and the kidney (for example, *see* **ref. *10–14***), and a good, comprehensive account of AFM in biology is to be found in **ref. *15***.

2.1. Intact Cells

In 1993 and 1994, several groups published work on AFM of Madin-Darby canine kidney (MDCK) cells. MDCK cells form a good starting point for AFM of intact cells because they are relatively well-characterized physiologically, and represent a stable cell line. Later experiments broadened to include A6 toad kidney cells and CV-1 African green monkey cells (all reviewed in **ref. *11***). Intact cells are perhaps the simplest form of preparation to use for the study of renal physiology by scanning-probe microscopy. They are easy to prepare, and possess in their plasma membranes numerous transport proteins of a dimension amenable to imaging by AFM. The cells can be grown on a glass or plastic substrate and simply transferred to the microscope for imaging alive under fluid (and the type of microscope shown in **Fig. 2B** is designed for this type of experiment), or fixed and dehydrated so that they can be studied dry. Experiments on cells in vivo afford the possibility of examining dynamic events in the cell. For example, in early work by Oberleithner et al., the migration across the substrate of MDCK cells that had been transformed by alkaline stress was observed *(16)*. The AFM was able to reveal invaginations appearing in real time in the lamellipodia of the cells as they moved forward.

The major disadvantage of using intact cells for AFM is really the fact that they are intact cells. Although very impressive images can be obtained, high scanning forces (in the nanonewton range) have proven to be necessary when imaging intact cells. This means that it is difficult to produce fine detail of membrane proteins—the probe distorts the membrane and associated structures as it moves back and forth, and the high forces can even result in structures lying below the cell membrane becoming visible *(17)*. This may be an advantage in some cases, providing the ability to "see inside" intact cells, yet it may obscure other membrane structures. The plasma membrane of intact cells is a crowded and complex structure, and identification of specific proteins is difficult without some sort of marker. It is possible to improve images by enzymatic treatment of the cell membrane to remove the glycocalix (although the use of enzymes should be discouraged because of potential nonspecific damage to membrane features), and it is possible to label proteins of interest with antibodies conjugated to colloidal gold. This has been done with some success in experiments to localize epithelial sodium channels in A6 cells *(18)*. The problem posed by this approach is that the quality of the image of the membrane structure under study can be compromised by the antibodies used to identify it, and by the gold particle. However, this technique can be used for gross localization of proteins and the patterns of their location can be revealed. This can be helpful in the identification of unlabeled proteins.

2.2. Isolated Cell Membranes

Rather than using intact cells, pieces of cell membrane can be isolated and attached to a suitable substrate for subsequent imaging. This is useful because the substrate (usually glass or mica, the latter being "atomically flat") provides a robust surface to support the membrane, improving resolution of the image and thus making imaging much easier. It is necessary to physically treat the surface of the substrate in order to encourage the membrane to adhere. Both the membrane and the mica or glass have net negative charges, and thus without treatment, it is difficult to neutralize or reverse the charge of the substrate adhesion. The simplest treatment is to coat the glass or mica with poly-L-lysine *(19)*, but silanes and detergents may also be used *(20,21)*. An example of the potential for using the AFM to study isolated membranes and to produce information complementary to that obtained by other techniques is seen in the work of Lärmer et al. *(19)*, who performed patch-clamp experiments on MDCK cells, then excised the patch, attached it to poly-L-lysine-coated mica, and imaged it using AFM. The apical plasma-membrane surface of the MDCK cells showed a complex structure with multiple protruding particles that could be identified as membrane proteins. The technique is described fully in **ref. *19***, where the authors comment that "the resolution could be increased considerably... as compared to experiments on intact cells, where plasma membrane proteins were hardly detectable." Incidentally, Lärmer et al. took advantage of the technique of making a calculation of the mol wt of proteins imaged by AFM by using the microscope to measure the dimensions of the imaged particles. After obtaining these dimensions (diameter and height), the molecular volume of the proteins can be calculated by treating the imaged particle as a segment of a sphere and using the equation:

$$V_m = (h/6)\,(3r^2 + h^2)$$

In this equation V_m is the molecular volume, and h and r are the height and the radius of the particle, respectively. The molecular volume of the protein can also be calculated (V_c) using the following equation:

$$V_c = (M_0/N_0)\,(V_1 + dV_2)$$

Here, M_0 is the mol wt, N_0 is Avogadro's number, and V_1 and V_2 are the partial specific volumes of the individual protein (0.74 cm^3 g^{-1} and 1 cm^3 g^{-1} water, respectively). d is the extent of protein hydration (0.4 mol H$_2$O/mol protein) (21). There is remarkable correspondence between the measured volume and the calculated volume for a large array of proteins, and this molecular volume measurement has proved a useful method for distinguishing individual protein species in AFM experiments.

A further development of the technique of membrane isolation came in 2000. Images were produced of the isolated plasma membrane of *Xenopus laevis* oocytes using AFM. Details of the membrane preparation technique are given in Schillers et al. (22). *Xenopus* oocytes are ideal for expression of numerous proteins, so using this technique it should be possible to express non-native membrane proteins in oocytes and then study them using AFM. This has been achieved with the cystic fibrosis transmembrane-conductance regulator ion-channel (CFTR) that was expressed in oocytes, with clusters of the channels identified using AFM (23).

Although they represent an advance compared to intact cells, there are disadvantages with isolated membrane preparations. As with intact cells, the architecture of the preparation is complex. Although membrane proteins are evident in these membrane preparations, so are any other structures, notably cytoskeletal elements. There is always a requirement to find some way, either directly or indirectly, to identify the structures of interest from among the large number present. The preparation of the membranes is not necessarily complicated, but requires some skill and practice.

2.3. Isolated Membrane Proteins

The description provided here should make it clear that the native environment is not an ideal medium for study of single molecules or molecular complexes in membranes using AFM. The logical step is to use molecular biological techniques to purify proteins, or the use of recombinant proteins. This approach has been taken in studies of the renal potassium channel ROMK1 (24). Using a fusion protein of glutathione S-transferase (GST) with the renal

K$^+$ channel, the authors identified dimeric particles of appropriate size. The authors suggested that the dimer reflected the normal conformation of GST. The experiments were performed with the protein immobilized on mica, either dry or in an aqueous solution. However, the great difficulty is that simply immobilizing renal-membrane proteins (or other membrane proteins) on mica or some other substrate does not usually produce images of very great detail. The reason for this is that membrane proteins are hydrophobic, by nature, and the environment provided in aqueous solution (or dry, which is something of a misleading description here, as AFM samples examined at room temperature in a normal laboratory tend to gather a coat of water that may only be monomolecular in depth, but is discernible by the microscope) on mica does not reflect the proteins' native environment. The proteins usually arrange themselves in a globular configuration. The other consideration is that membrane proteins are difficult to produce in large quantities, and are quite difficult to purify. The use of isolated membrane proteins is thus of limited value. The prospects are more propitious for soluble proteins, but immobilization on mica can compromise their structural integrity, and limits the usefulness of the approach.

2.4. Coating (Functionalization) of Tips

The Introduction to this chapter mentions the study of the interaction of streptavidin and biotin that involved coating an AFM tip with one-half of the streptavidin-biotin ligand-receptor pair, with the other half of the pair attached to the substrate *(7)*. There is hope that studies of this type will prove to have been a prelude for measurements of interactions between other biologically important molecules. The facility to measure the force of interaction between molecules, one of them attached to the AFM tip, can be extended to force volume imaging to produce a map of interaction across the surface of a cell. Thus, the pattern of receptor expression across a cell might be mapped by attaching the appropriate ligand to the tip. This type of force-volume experiment has not thus far been a feature of renal physiology, but there is potential. For example, polysaccharides have been mapped on the surface of the yeast *Saccharomyces cerevisiae* using this technique. Tips were functionalized with concanavalin A, and the authors measured the binding force between concanavalin A and mannan polymers on the yeast-cell surface. A more sophisticated functionalization was used by Schneider et al. *(25)* who identified areas of ATP release on the plasma-membrane surface of lung epithelial cells. Here, the tips were coated with ATPase S1. As the tip passed over the cell surface, the ATPase hydrolyzed ATP on the cell membrane, which produced a disturbance in the normal scanning process of the cantilever. This appeared as a feature in the image produced. The authors point out that this was "an example of modifying the scanning probe substrate to measure simultaneously high-resolution topography and a biologically important molecule in the surface microenvironment of living cells."

The application of ligands, receptors, and other molecules to AFM tips is complicated. The techniques for coating can be crude (often simply dipping the tip into an appropriate solution), and this compromises the shape of the tip and gives no information about how many molecules of the coating agent are attached to it. Furthermore, the binding and unbinding of ligand-receptor pairs on tip and substrate will be a dynamic process unless it is covalent, and the likelihood of binding will be dependent upon the affinity between the two molecules of the pair. Beyond this, it is necessary for the ligands (or other molecules) to attract each other strongly enough to allow a change in force to be registered during the scan, but they must not attract each other so strongly that the tip is interrupted in its progress over the substrate, or that undue distortion of the sample takes place.

2.5. Artificial Lipid Membranes: Reconstitution of Proteins

It is difficult to identify and study membrane proteins in the native environment, and it is difficult to isolate such proteins and examine them in isolation. The best prospect for examining the structure and behavior of membrane proteins lies in producing purified proteins and then reconstituting them into suitable artificial lipid environment—reflecting the structure of the native plasma membrane. Such experiments are in their early stages, but physical scientists have extensively studied Langmuir-Blodgett films (see ref. 26). Partly derived from this work, artificial bilayers have been produced by spreading lipids onto mica substrate, and these have been manipulated by the AFM (27). In recent elegant experiments, lipid mixtures were made to mimic the membrane composition of the renal brush border, and imaged on mica supports (28). This work was closely followed by a study in which the proportion of cholesterol in an artificial phosphatidylcholine/sphingomyelin membrane was varied (sphingolipids are believed to be important in the development of membrane microdomains or "rafts" and rafts in turn play a significant role in the distribution and location of certain membrane proteins [29]). The results indicated that cholesterol was not crucial for the integrity of raft microdomains in this model membrane (30).

Since it is usually difficult to produce large quantities of eukaryotic membrane proteins, progress in the reconstitution of purified proteins into artificial membranes remains frustratingly slow, but there is cause for optimism as knowledge of microdomains and artificial reconstitution of microdomains develops. The closest the AFM has come to producing high-resolution images of renal membrane proteins in their native form is with the water channel aquaporin 1 (AQP1) (31). AQP1 is expressed in the nephron and in high concentrations in erythrocyte-cell membranes, from which it can be purified in sufficiently large quantities to produce two-dimensional (2D) crystals in the presence of phospholipids. The images (AFM and electron microscopic) are not of the protein directly, but are striking, and a notable achievement nevertheless. They show metal-shadowed, freeze-dried crystals of AQP1 that reveal a tetramer, with an internal central pore.

References

1. Binnig, G., Quate, C. F., and Gerber, C. (1986) Atomic force microscope. *Phys. Rev. Lett.* **56,** 930–933.
2. Baró, A. M., Miranda, R., Alamán, J., García, N., Binnig, G., Rohrer, H., et al. (1985) Determination of surface topography of biological specimens at high resolution by scanning tunnelling microscopy. *Nature* **315,** 253–254.
3. Hansma, P. K., Drake, B., Grigg, D., Prater, C. B., Yashar, F., Gurley, G., et al. (1994) A new, optical-lever based atomic-force microscope. *Journal of Applied Physics* **76,** 796–799.
4. Dai, H. J., Hafner, J. H., Rinzler, A. G., Colbert, D. T., and Smalley, R. E. (1996) Nanotubes as nanoprobes in scanning probe microscopy. *Nature* **384,** 147–150.
5. Hafner, J. H., Cheung, C., Woolley, A. T., and Lieber, C. M. (2001) Structural and functional imaging with carbon nanotube AFM probes. *Prog. Biophys. Mol. Biol.* **77,** 73–110.
6. Umemura, K., Komatsu, J., Uchihashi, T., Choi, N., Ikawa, S., Nishinaka, T., et al. (2001) Atomic force microscopy of RecA-DNA complexes using a carbon nanotube tip. *Biochem. Biophys. Res. Commun.* **281,** 390–395.
7. Florin, E.-L., Moy, V. T., and Gaub, H. E. (1994) Adhesion forces between individual ligand-receptor pairs. *Science* **264,** 415–417.
8. Hinterdorfer, P., Baumgartner, W., Gruber, H. J., Schilcher, K., and Schindler, H. (1996) Detection and localization of individual antibody-antigen recognition events by atomic force microscopy. *Proc. Natl. Acad. Sci. USA* **93,** 3477–3481.
9. Proksch, R., Lal, R., Hansma, P. K., Morse, D., and Stucky, G. (1996) Imaging the internal and external pore structure of membranes in fluid: TappingMode scanning ion conductance microscopy. *Biophys. J.* **71,** 2155–2157.
10. Lesniewska, E., Giocondi, M. C., Vié, V., Finot, E., Goudonnet, J. P., and Le Grimellec, C. (1998) Atomic force microscopy of renal cells: Limits and prospects. *Kidney Int.* **Suppl. 65,** S42–S48.
11. Henderson, R. M. and Oberleithner, H. (2000) Pushing, pulling, dragging and vibrating renal epithelia using atomic force microscopy. *Am. J. Physiol. Renal Physiol.* **278,** F689–F701.
12. Oberleithner, H., Geibel, J., Guggino, W., Henderson, R. M., Hunter, M., Schneider, S. W., et al. (1997) Life on biomembranes viewed with the atomic force microscope. *Wien. Klin. Wochenschr.* **109,** 419–423.
13. Oberleithner, H., Schneider, S., Larmer, J., and Henderson, R. M. (1996) Viewing the renal epithelium with the atomic force microscope. *Kidney Blood Press. Res.* **19,** 142–147.

14. Oberleithner, H., Brinckmann, E., Giebisch, G., and Geibel, J. (1995) Visualising life on biomembranes by atomic force microscopy. *Kidney Int.* **48,** 795–801.

15. Morris, V. J., Kirby, A. R., and Gunning, A. P. (2000) *Atomic Force Microscopy for Biologists.* Imperial College Press, London.

16. Oberleithner, H., Giebisch, G., and Geibel, J. (1993) Imaging the lamellipodium of migrating epithelial cells in vivo by atomic force microscopy. *Pfluegers Arch.* **425,** 506–510.

17. Hoh, J. H. and Schoenenberger, C. A. (1994) Surface morphology and mechanical properties of MDCK monolayers by atomic force microscopy. *J. Cell Sci.* **107(Pt. 5),** 1105–1114.

18. Smith, P. R., Bradford, A. L., Schneider, S., Benos, D. J., and Geibel, J. P. (1997) Localization of amiloride-sensitive sodium channels in A6 cells by atomic force microscopy. *Am. J. Physiol.* **272,** C1295–C1298.

19. Lärmer, J., Schneider, S. W., Danker, T., Schwab, A., and Oberleithner, H. (1997) Imaging excised apical plasma membrane patches of MDCK cells in physiological conditions with atomic force microscopy. *Pfluegers Arch.* **434,** 254–260.

20. Butt, H. J., Downing, K. H., and Hansma, P. K. (1990) Imaging the membrane protein bacteriorhodopsin with the atomic force microscope. *Biophys. J.* **58,** 1473–1480.

21. Schneider, S. W., Lärmer, J., Henderson, R. M., and Oberleithner, H. (1998) Molecular weights of individual proteins correlate with molecular volumes measured by atomic force microscopy. *Pfluegers Arch.* **435,** 362–367.

22. Schillers, H., Danker, T., Schnittler, H. J., Lang, F., and Oberleithner, H. (2000). Plasma membrane plasticity of Xenopus laevis oocyte imaged with atomic force microscopy. *Cell Physiol. Biochem.* **10,** 99–107.

23. Schillers, H., Danker, T., Madeja, M., and Oberleithner, H. (2001) Plasma membrane protein clusters appear in CFTR-expressing Xenopus laevis oocytes after cAMP stimulation. *J. Membr. Biol.* **180,** 205–212.

24. Henderson, R. M., Schneider, S., Li, Q., Hornby, D., White, S. J., and Oberleithner, H. (1996) Imaging ROMK1 inwardly-rectifying ATP-sensitive K+ channel using atomic force microscopy. *Proc. Natl. Acad. Sci. USA* **93,** 8756–8760.

25. Schneider, S. W., Egan, M. E., Jena, B. P., Guggino, W. B., Oberleithner, H., and Geibel, J. P. (1999) Continuous detection of extracellular ATP on living cells by using atomic force microscopy. *Proc. Natl. Acad. Sci. USA* **96,** 12,180–12,185.

26. Bourdieu, L., Ronsin, O., and Chatenay, D. (1993) Molecular positional order in Langmuir-Blodgett films by atomic force microscopy. *Science* **259,** 798–801.

27. Beckmann, M., Nollert, P., and Kolb, H. A. (1998) Manipulation and molecular resolution of a phosphatidylcholine-supported planar bilayer by atomic force microscopy. *J. Membr. Biol.* **161,** 227–233.

28. Milhiet, P. E., Domec, C., Giocondi, M. C., Van, M., Heitz, F., and Le Grimellec, C. (2001) Domain formation in models of the renal brush border membrane outer leaflet. *Biophys. J.* **81,** 547–555.

29. Brown, D. A. and London, E. (2000) Structure and function of sphingolipid- and cholesterol-rich membrane rafts. *J. Biol. Chem.* **275,** 17,221–17,224.
30. Milhiet, P. E., Giocondi, M. C., and Le Grimellec, C. (2002) Cholesterol is not crucial for the existence of microdomains in kidney brush-border membrane models. *J. Biol. Chem.* **277,** 875–878.
31. Walz, T., Tittmann, P., Fuchs, K. H., Müller, D. J., Smith, B. L., Agre, P., et al. (1996) Surface topographies at subnanometer-resolution reveal asymmetry and sidedness of aquaporin-1. *J. Mol. Biol.* **264,** 907–918.

10

Freeze-Fracture Analysis
of Renal-Epithelial Tight Junctions

Hiroyuki Sasaki

1. Introduction

The freeze-fracture replica method was designed in the 1950s as a technique for analysis of fine structure of biological membranes. This method was furthered along with development and establishment of the fracture devices and cryotechniques in the 1970s.

In this method, the specimen is frozen, fractured, and replicated with platinum and carbon under the high vacuum. It is generally assumed that the fracture passes along the midline of the biological membrane through the hydrophobic phospholipid interior. Both fracture faces display various integral membrane proteins as two-dimensional (2D) arrangement of small particles. When water in the samples is sublimed (etched) under the high vacuum after the fracture, the fine structures directly under the fracture plane can buoy up. This is a deep-etching replica method. In this method, subliming intracellular ice exposes the fine structures under the fracture faces. Then the metals are evaporated, and the replica films are made.

The junctional complex of simple epithelial cells is located at the most apical part of the lateral membrane and consists of three distinct components: tight junctions, adherens junctions, and desmosomes. On ultra-thin section electron micrographs, tight junctions appear as a series of apparent fusions ("kissing points") involving the outer leaflets of the plasma membranes of adjacent cells. At kissing points of tight junctions, the intercellular space is completely obliterated, whereas in adherens junctions and desmosomes, the opposing membranes are 15–20 nm apart. In simple epithelial cellular sheets, adherens junctions and desmosomes mechanically link adjacent cells, whereas tight junctions are responsible for intercellular sealing.

The tight junctions between epithelial cells of the proximal tubules are manifested as a strand protuberance in the protoplasmic fracture face (P face,

From: *Methods in Molecular Medicine, vol. 86: Renal Disease: Techniques and Protocols*
Edited by: M. S. Goligorsky © Humana Press Inc., Totowa, NJ

cell membrane side where it faces the cytoplasm) of the freeze-fracture replica method. It is observed as a groove corresponding to the protuberance in the extracellular fracture face (E face, as a membrane facing the intercellular space). In the renal proximal tubules, tight junctions are less prominent, and adherence junctions predominate *(1)*. The opposite is seen in distal tubules and collecting ducts. The tight junctions between epithelial cells of the human proximal tubules are of roughly single strand *(2)*. In the rat and the rabbit proximal tubules, one or two tight-junction strands are observed *(3)*. The tight junctions of the human tubules have 2–4 strands in the thin segments, 1–5 in the pars recta, and 2–6 in the pars convoluta *(2)*. Adherence junctions are located below tight junctions, and both form a continuous belt between the epithelial cells. Desmosomes are seen under the adherence junctions, although there are few desmosomes between the epithelial cells of the mammalian proximal tubules *(4,5)*.

The ellipsoidal intramembrane particles with twice the length of usual spherical particles are found in the P face of the intercalated cells (dark cells) of the collecting duct. It is believed that this characteristic ellipsoidal particle relates to the reabsorption of potassium, since the number of these particles increases because of potassium deficiency *(6,7)*. These characteristic particles are rare in the basolateral membrane of the intercalated cells.

2. Materials

1. Kidney: Biopsy, autopsy or nephrectomy samples of human or laboratory animals.
2. Phosphate buffer stock solution: 0.2 M phosphate buffer and pH 7.3. This buffer is prepared by mixing two stock solutions: 0.2 M sodium phosphate solution (27.6 g $NaH_2PO_4 \cdot H_2O$ is dissolved in distilled water, 1000 mL) and 0.2 M sodium phosphate solution (35.6 g $Na_2HPO_4 \cdot 2H_2O$ is dissolved in distilled water, 1000 mL) followed by pH adjustment. This solution can be stored for several weeks at 4°C. However, this solution gradually becomes contaminated and precipitates may appear during storage.
3. Phosphate buffer: 0.1 M and pH 7.2. Phosphate-buffer preservation liquid (*see* **Subheading 2., step 2**) is diluted twofold with H_2O.
4. Fixative: 2% (v/v) glutaraldehyde in 0.1 M phosphate buffer, pH 7.4. This is prepared by mixing 8 mL of 25% glutaraldehyde liquid, 50 mL of phosphate-buffer stock solution (*see* **Subheading 2., step 2**), and 42 mL of H_2O. This solution can be stored for approx 1 mo at 4°C.
5. Cryoprotectant A: 15% (v/v) glycerol in phosphate buffer.
6. Cryoprotectant B: 30% (v/v) glycerol in phosphate buffer.
7. The coolants: Propane or ethane is used. The cylinder container made of the metal or the heat-resistant glass (cup) is cooled by the liquid nitrogen. Next, it is liquefied by injecting the gas (propane or ethane) from the gas cylinder in the con-

tainer. The propane and the ethane do not freeze for about 5 min after it liquefies because their melting points are near the liquid nitrogen temperature. Meanwhile, the specimen freezing is completed. It is necessary to liquefy the gas and freeze the samples in the draft for prevention of dangerous flammable and/or toxic gases.

8. Tissue solvent: Household bleach is used.
9. Tissue solvent for immunolabeling method: 2.5% sodium dodecyl sulfate (SDS), 10 mM Tris-HCl buffer, 30 mM sucrose, and pH 8.3. This solvent is prepared from 20% (W/V) SDS and 1 M Tris-HCl buffer (pH 8.3), with addition of sucrose at the final concentration of 30 mM, and can be stored at room temperature for approx 6 mo.
10. Bovine serum albumin (BSA)-phosphate buffer. 10% (W/V) BSA is dissolved in phosphate buffer. This solution should be made as required.
11. Primary antibody: The antibody stock solution is diluted to the optimal concentration with the phosphate buffer including BSA.
12. Secondary antibody: the 5–20-nm gold-labeled antibodies diluted to the optimal concentration with the phosphate buffer, including BSA.
13. Grid for electron microscopic observation: 150–300 meshes grids for electron microscopy. The grids that contain collodion or formvar membrane are used if necessary.

3. Methods

3.1. Fixation of the Kidney

1. The biopsy, or removed human kidneys are finely cut to about 1-mm cubes, and immersed in fixative (*see* **Subheading 2., step 4**).
2. Kidneys of the laboratory animals are similarly immersed in fixative (*see* **Subheading 2., step 4**). Alternatively, fixative (*see* **Subheading 2., step 4**) is perfused through the left ventricle or large blood vessel, and the whole body is fixed, or the fixative is perfused through the renal artery, and only the kidney is fixed.
3. The fixed kidney is cut in small pieces that are suitable for the specimen carrier of the freeze-fracture device with the razor blade on boards such as vinyl chloride and carbowaxes, and then immersed in the fixative (*see* **Subheading 2., step 4** and **Note 1**). It is easy to specify uriniferous tubules at the electron microscopic observation when the kidney is divided into the renal cortex and renal medulla. The glomerulus, the convoluted part of the proximal tubule, the straight part of proximal tubule, the straight part of the distal tubule, the convoluted part of the distal tubule, and the cortical collecting duct are seen in the renal cortex. The Henle's thick and thin limbs, the straight part of the distal tubule, and the collecting duct are observed in the medulla.

3.2. Freezing Method for Tissues

The cells generally contain 70–80% water, and all cellular functions are conducted in this environment. Therefore, when the fine structures are observed by the freeze-fracture replica method, the samples should be near the normal water content. For this, the ideal method is a rapid-freezing method, yet the execution of this technique is considerably difficult. Therefore, an understanding of the behavior of intracellular water during sample freezing is necessary.

The basis of the rapid-freezing method is to prevent ice-crystal formation. The reason for this is that volume expansion during crystallization of water produces the distortion of the cellar fine structures. In general, it is believed that the ice crystals of 10 nm or less do not introduce a fatal problem for the ultrastructural observation of the biological samples. This freezing state of the water is known as the vitrification or the amorphous ice. To obtain the state of vitrification, the cooling rate of 10^{-4}/sec or more is needed. Utilization of cryoprotectants such as glycerol, dimethyl sulfoxide (DMSO), ethylene glycol, sucrose, polyvinyl pyrolidone, or dextran enables to freeze without formation of ice crystals. This is because of cryoprotectant's permeation into the cells, an increase in the intracellular solute concentration, and a decrease in the amount of water. However, it is necessary to chemically fix the cell by the aldehyde before cryoprotection, since these cryoprotectants at effective concentrations injure the living cell (*see* **Note 2**).

The freezing methods developed thus far have been classified into the following four methods:

1. Plunge-freezing method
2. Metal contact-freezing method
3. Spray-freezing method
4. High-pressure freezing method

The plunge-freezing method is a method that involves immersing the sample in coolant directly and freezing. The metal contact-freezing method is a method that involves slamming the specimen against the surface of a precooled metallic block with high thermal conductivity and freezing. The spray-freezing method is a method that freezes by spraying coolant directly to the sample. The high pressure-freezing method freezes by spraying liquid nitrogen pressurized to 2100 bar on the sample.

3.2.1. Plunge Freezing Method

In this method, the plunge speed into the coolant of the samples should be fast. The coolant with a small temperature difference between the melting point and the boiling point evaporates around the samples, since the coolant is warmed by the sample. This evaporation gas surrounds the sample, disturbs the heat exchange between the sample and the coolant, and decreases the cooling rate dramatically. Therefore, selecting a coolant with a large temperature difference is important in this method. The liquid nitrogen, liquid propane, and liquid ethane are used in this method.

1. Fixed samples are washed with phosphate buffer (*see* **Subheading 2., steps 3, 4**).
2. For cryoprotection, samples are then immersed in the cryoprotectant A (*see* **Subheading 2, step 5**) for 1–2 h.
3. Samples are then immersed in the cryoprotectant B (*see* **Subheading 2., step 6**) overnight. When the samples are immersed to the cryoprotectant such as glycerin for a long time, the cell and/or tissue shrinks. It is necessary to appreciate this, since the possibility of artifacts is present (*see* **Note 2**).
4. Samples are put on the specimen carrier of the freeze-fracture device (*see* **Note 3**). At this time, an excess cryoprotectant, which adheres to the sample, is absorbed by the filter paper.
5. Samples on the carriers are quickly plunged into a coolant (*see* **Subheading 2., step 7**).
6. The frozen samples can be preserved in the liquid nitrogen.

3.2.2. High-Pressure Freezing Method

The high-pressure freezing method is based on the depression of the melting point of water under the high-pressure state, thus preventing ice-crystal formation. As a result, the range of the vitrification broadens considerably by the high-pressure freezing compared to the metal contact-freezing and the plunge-freezing methods *(8–10)*.

The metal contact-freezing method has been used as a rapid-freezing method of the cells and tissues in the freeze-fracture replica method, especially the deep-etching replica method and the freeze-fracture replica immunolabeling method. However, it is necessary to fracture at the depth of 10–20 μm, the regions that are well frozen. Therefore, proteins available for observation are limited by this depth. In addition, the risks of observing artificial products because of a subtle defect in freezing are present. The depth of the vitrification region in the high-pressure freezing method seems to become an advantage, which opens many possibilities in the deep-etching replica method and the freeze-fracture replica immunolabeling method.

The high-pressure freezing devices, that are commercially available are two models of High-Pressure Freezing Machine (HPM-010) (BalTec Co.) and EM-PACT High-Pressure Freezer (Leica Co.). The author uses BalTec HPM-010 for the high-pressure freezing and BalTec BAF-060 for the freeze-fracture (the advantage is that the specimen carriers used for freezing can be brought into the fracture device of this company).

1. The high-pressure freezing device is turned on, and the interior of the device is cooled by the liquid nitrogen.
2. Removed tissues are finely cut to the size suited for the specimen carrier of the freezing machine under the stereoscopic microscope. Samples are put in phosphate-buffered saline (PBS) and cooled on ice.

3. Samples are put on the specimen carrier and set on the holder (*see* **Notes 3** and **4**).
4. To make a sample sandwich, a similar specimen carrier is placed on the specimen (*see* **Note 4**), and the carrier holder fixes the sandwich.
5. The sandwich in the carrier holder is placed in the object head of high-pressure freezing device.
6. The liquid nitrogen is quickly jetted in the high-pressure freezing device, and the sample is frozen rapidly.
7. The carrier holder is pulled out from the high-pressure freezing device after the freezing, and its tips with the frozen sample are quickly plunged into the liquid nitrogen.
8. The sample sandwich is removed from carrier holder in the liquid nitrogen.
9. Since the sample protrudes on the carrier when the other side of the sandwich is removed in the liquid nitrogen, it is loaded directly into the freeze-fracture device, and is ready for fracturing. The frozen samples can be preserved in the liquid nitrogen.

3.3. Freeze-Fracture Replica Method

Although the details of handling and the operation are different for each fracture device, the BALTEC BAF060 Freeze-Fracture System is described here because the basic operational steps are almost invariant.

1. The cold stage and the knife of the fracture device are cooled by the liquid nitrogen before freeze-fracture.
2. The platinum-carbon and the carbon as the evaporation source are installed in the device, the platinum-carbon is set to 45°, and the carbon is set to 90° of coating angles, respectively.
3. It is necessary to always carry out a trial coating of the platinum-carbon and the carbon prior to a freeze-fracture process in order to check that the evaporation device functions correctly.
4. The specimen table is cooled to liquid nitrogen temperature in a liquid nitrogen Dewar vessel.
5. Frozen samples on the specimen carriers are inserted in the specimen table.
6. The specimen table is loaded to the cold stage of the fracture device using a manipulator.
7. The manipulator is withdrawn from the device.
8. Wait for approx 15 min until the stage and the samples come to a preset temperature of −100°C.
9. To obtain the fracture surface, the vertical motion of the knife is adjusted to the lever of the samples.
10. The knife is rotated, and the sample fractures momentarily.
11. The platinum is coated on the fracture surface of the sample by heating the platinum-carbon. Coating thickness is adjusted to approx 2 nm. The coating stops automatically when it reaches the preset film thickness, since it synchronizes with the film-thickness measuring device in BAF060.

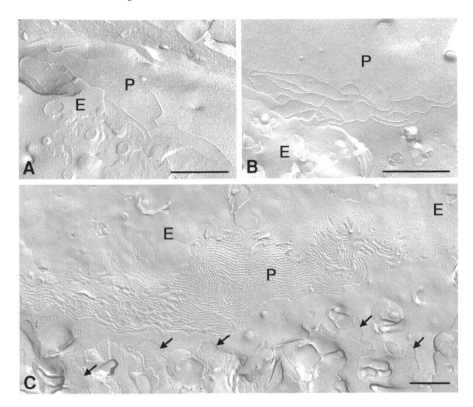

Fig. 1. Freeze-fracture replica image of mouse kidney. **(A)** Proximal tubule; **(B)** Distal tubule; **(C)** Collecting duct; P, protoplasmic fracture face; E, extracellular fracture face. Arrows: ellipsoidal intramembranous particles on the cell membrane of the collecting duct. Bar: 0.5 μm.

12. The carbon is coated by heating the carbon at approx 20 nm of the thickness.
13. The manipulator is inserted into the device, and the specimen table is taken out from the device.
14. The specimen carriers with coated samples are removed from the specimen table.
15. The samples are carefully taken out of the specimen carriers under the stereo-scopic microscope.
16. The samples are carefully floated on the surface of the household bleach.
17. When the tissues dissolve completely from the replica films (from 1 h to over-night, *see* **Note 5**), the replica films are removed and floated on the distilled water carefully for washing. Washing with distilled water is repeated 3 or 4 times.
18. The replica films are picked up on the grids with formvar film and dried in air.
19. The replica films are observed with the transmission electron microscope.

The results of such experiments are shown in **Fig. 1.**

3.4. Deep-Etching Replica Method

Rapidly frozen cells and tissues are fractured in the freeze-fracture device, the temperature of cold stage is raised at once to the sublimating point of ice, and the intercellular ice is sublimed (etching). Next, the fracture surface is coated with the platinum while rotating at the low-angle degree, and the replica is made (*see* **Note 6**). Although the etching conditions may differ in the deep-etching replica method depending on the ultimate vacuum of the freeze-fracture device used and the accuracy of control of the cold-stage temperature, the condition in the freeze-fracture device (BalTec Co. and BAF060) that we are using now is described here.

1. The frozen samples are freeze-fractured according to **Subheading 3. 3., steps 1–10**.
2. After samples are fractured, the knife in the fracture device is placed on the surface of the fractured samples.
3. The temperature of cold stage is warmed up to –100°C.
4. When the stage temperature rises to the preset temperature, samples are left for 10 min, and then are etched.
5. The coating angle of the platinum-carbon is set at 15° during **step 4**.
6. When the etching terminates, the platinum-carbon is coated with the thickness of 1–2 nm while rotating the samples.
7. The carbon coating angle is set at 90°, and the carbon is coated with the thickness of 2–5 nm while rotating the samples.
8. The rotation of the sample stage is stopped, and the specimen table is taken out with the manipulator.
9. To make the replica films, the samples are processed according to **Subheading 3.3., steps 14–19**.

The result of such an experiment is shown in **Fig. 2.**

3.5. Freeze-Fracture Replica Immunolabeling Method

Various membrane proteins preserved by the freeze-fracture replica method are detected as intramembrane particles of an almost uniform size on the replica films. Thus, there were difficulties in identification and the functional analysis of individual particles. To overcome this problem, Fujimoto designed the method of immunocytochemical reactions on the freeze-fracture replica membrane—the freeze-fracture replica immunolabeling method. Identification and 2D distributions of membrane proteins can be analyzed by this method on the replica films (*11,12*).

Although the metal contact-freezing method, which uses liquid helium, was used in an original method for the freezing of the samples, the author applies the high-pressure freezing method to the freeze-fracture replica immunolabeling method, with excellent results (*13–15*).

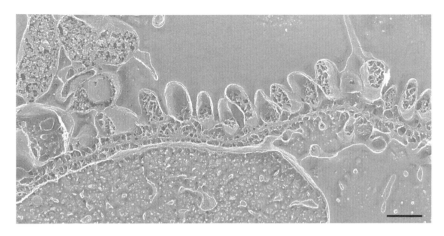

Fig. 2. Deep-etching replica image of mouse kidney. The foot processes and slit membranes of the podocytes in the renal glomerulus are observed. Bar: 0.5 μm.

The details of the actual manipulations and the techniques of the freeze-fracture replica immunolabeling method have been previously reported *(11,12)*. In the freeze-fracture replica immunolabeling method, the cells and tissues are dissolved by the sodium dodecyl sulfate (SDS) solution from the replica. Immunocytochemical reactions occur with the membrane antigen on the replica films, and identification and the localization of the proteins of interest are analyzed on the replica membrane.

1. The freeze-fracture replica immunolabeling method basically uses unfixed and rapidly frozen samples (*see* **Subheading 3.2.2.**).
2. The samples on specimen carriers are loaded into the freeze-fracture device.
3. In the freeze-fracture device, the portions of the sample, that are protruding from the carriers, are fractured.
4. The platinum-carbon is coated to the fracture surface at a thickness of 2 nm unidirectionally at 45° of the coating angle.
5. The carbon is coated to the fracture surface at a thickness of 20 nm while rotating the sample at 90° of the coating angle.
6. The coated samples are taken out of the device, and the samples are collected in phosphate-buffered saline (PBS).
7. The coated samples are immersed in the tissue solvent (*see* **Subheading 2., step 9**), and are solubilized while stirring (*see* **Note 7**).
8. The replica films are then washed in the BSA-phosphate buffer (*see* **Subheading 2., step 10**) for 10 min. Washing with BSA-phosphate buffer is repeated 3 or 4 times.
9. According to a conventional colloidal gold immunolabeling technique, the primary antibody and the secondary antibody are utilized against the replica membranes.

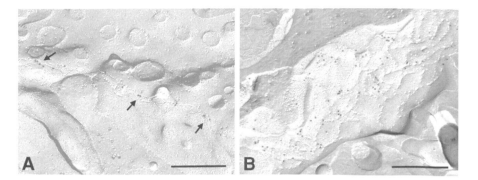

Fig. 3. Detection of tight junction (TJ) constituent proteins of cultured Madin-Darby Canine Kidney I cells. **(A)** Localization of Claudine-1. Claudin-1 (15 nm colloidal gold) was precisely localized at tight-junction strands. **(B)** Localization of Junctional Adhesion Molecules. Junctional Adhesion Molecules (20 nm colloidal gold, arrows) are adjacent to the tight junction strands. Bar: 0.5 μm.

10. The labeled replica films are washed with distilled water several times.
11. The replica films are collected on the grid for the electron microscopy observation.

The electron microscopic images of the replica films processed by this method are the same as images of a usual freeze-fracture replica method, and the localizations of gold particles is observed on the replica images **(Fig. 3)**.

4. Notes

1. In the immersion-fixation method, the operation and its time until tissues are removed and placed in the fixative greatly influences the final electron microscopic images. It is especially important to avoid the physical damage of the sample when removing and cutting it. Moreover, it is necessary to perform operations of tissue removal, cutting in pieces, and fixation in as short a time as possible to minimize postmortem changes.

   However, the conditions for perfusion-fixation differ depending on the animal species and the tissue. The important factors are the chemical composition, concentration, osmotic pressure, pH, temperature, and perfusion pressure of a fixative.

2. In a chemical fixation and cryoprotection used in of freeze-fracture replica method, artificial products (artifacts) of the structural changes, the transport and outflow of the constituents may become a problem. Moreover, since a certain time is necessary for the immobilization and the infiltration of the fixative, it is difficult to preserve early chemical changes, that have occurred in vivo.

3. In order to improve the adhesiveness of the specimens on the carrier platelets, they must be cleaned prior to their usage.

4. Although the specimen carriers of various shapes are prepared according to need, the author uses a dome-shaped gold carriers and cylinder-shaped gold carriers.

The dome-shaped carriers are treated with lecithin (1,2-dipalmitoyl-sn-glycero-3- phosphocholine monohydrate) before freezing. It is easier for a dome-shaped carrier to come off by this treatment after the freezing.

5. The time needed to solubilize the cell components is different for different samples, yet in this case, the cultured cells, the free cells, and the soft tissues are solubilized for 12–24 h at room temperature. The duration of solubilization depends on the amount of the connective-tissue components. It is difficult to dissolve samples that are rich in connective tissues.

6. In the deep-etching replica method, because of the necessity to freeze them without cryoprotectants that are not sublimed easily, the rapid freezing of the cells and tissues *in situ* has been proposed. By instantaneously freezing the samples, the rapid-freezing method was designed as a method of preserving the conditions similar to a native tissue.

7. It is difficult to dissolve samples that are rich in connective tissues completely. For this purpose, tissues or replica samples are processed by collagenase before the rapid freezing or SDS treatment, thus improving the results *(13)*. However, antigens to be detected are decomposed with the protease products, and since the epitopes may be lost for immunolabeling, the trial-and-error experiments testing the concentration and digestion time with collagenase treatment are required.

During solubilization of the replica samples, if the SDS solution is warmed (as in pretreatment of sodium dodecyl sulfate polyacrylamide gel electrophoresis [SDS-PAGE]), the time required for solubilization will be dramatically shortened. Actually, the SDS solution is processed for several minutes by the heat block warmed at 50–95°C. Since the temperature and time may vary depending on the type of the cells or tissues, the proteins to be detected or the primary antibody used, conditions should be optimized.

References

1. Farquhar, M. G. and Palade, G. E. (1963) Junctional complexes in various epithelia. *J. Cell. Biol.* **17,** 375–413.
2. Kuhn, K. and Peale, E. (1975) Functional complexes of the tubular cells in the human kidney as revealed with freeze-fracture. *Cell Tissue Res.* **160,** 193–205.
3. Roesinger, B., Schiller, A., and Taugner, R. (1978) A freeze-fracture study of tight junctions in the pars convoluta and pars recta of the renal proximal tubule. *Cell Tissue Res.* **186,** 121–133.
4. Tisher, C. C. (1986) Anatomy of the kidney, in *The Kidney* (Brenner, B. M. and Rector, F. C. eds.), W. B. Saunders Co., Philadelphia, PA, vol. 1, pp. 3–60.
5. Silverblatt, F. J. and Bulger, R. E. (1970) Gap junction occurs in vertebrate renal proximal tubule cells. *J. Cell. Biol.* **47,** 513–515.
6. Stetson, D. L., Wade, J. B., and Giebisch, G. (1980) Morphologic alterations in the rat medullary collecting duct following potassium depletion. *Kidney Int.* **17,** 45–56.
7. Orci, L., Humbert, F., Brown, D., and Perrelet, S. (1981) Membrane ultrastructure in urinary tubules. *Int. Rev. Cytol.* **73,** 183–242.

8. Moor, H. (1987) Theory and practice of high pressure freezing, in *Cryotechniques in Biological Electron Microscopy* (Steinbrecht, R. A. and Zierold, K., eds.), Springer-Verlag, Berlin, vol. 1, pp. 3–60.

9. Studer, D., Michel, M., and Muller, M. (1989) High pressure freezing comes of age. *Scanning Microsc.* **S3,** 253–269.

10. McDonald, K. (1999) High-pressure freezing for preservation of high resolution fine structure and antigenicity for immunolabeling, in *Methods in Molecular Biology, Vol. 117: Electron Microscopy Methods and Protocols* (Hajibagheri, N., ed.), Humana Press, Totowa, NJ, pp. 77–97.

11. Fujimoto, K. (1995) Freeze-fracture replica electron microscopy combined with SDS digestion for cytochemical labeling of integral membrane proteins. Application to the immunogold labeling of intercellular junctional complexes. *J. Cell. Sci.* **108,** 3443–3449.

12. Fujimoto, K. (1997) SDS-digested freeze-fracture replica labeling electron microscopy to study the two-dimensional distribution of integral membrane proteins and phospholipids in biomembranes: practical procedure, interpretation and application. *Histochem. Cell Biol.* **107,** 87–96.

13. Morita, K., Sasaki, H., Fujimoto, K., Furuse, M., and Tsukita, S. (1999) Claudin-11/OSP-based tight junctions of myelin sheaths in brain and Sertoli cells in testis. *J. Cell. Biol.* **145,** 579–588.

14. Morita, K., Sasaki, H., Furuse, M., and Tsukita, S. (1999) Endothelial claudin: claudin-5/TMVCF constitutes tight junction strands in endothelial cells. *J. Cell. Biol.* **147,** 185–194.

15. Itoh, M., Sasaki, H., Furuse, M., Ozaki, H., Kita, T., and Tsukita, S. (2001) Junctional adhesion molecule (JAM) binds to PAR-3: a possible mechanism for the recruitment of PAR-3 to tight junctions. *J. Cell. Biol.* **154,** 491–497.

III

STUDIES OF RENAL DEVELOPMENT

11

Organ Culture of Intact Metanephric Kidneys

Simon J. M. Welham and Adrian S. Woolf

1. Introduction

This chapter describes the methodology for culture of the metanephros, the direct precursor of the adult mammalian kidney (1). The metanephros initially has two tissue compartments (**Fig. 1A,B**): i) the ureteric bud epithelium, a branch of the mesonephric (Wolffian) duct, which itself branches recurrently to form the renal collecting ducts; and ii) the renal mesenchyme, a caudal section of intermediate mesoderm, which undergoes an epithelial transformation via comma and S-shaped bodies to form nephron components including glomerular and proximal tubule epithelia (**Fig. 1C**). The metanephric mesenchyme also differentiates into interstitial cells and at least some renal capillaries. The ureteric bud also forms the urothelium of the renal pelvis and the ureter. The junction of the bud and the mesonephric duct becomes incorporated into the cloaca, forming the urinary bladder trigone. The remainder of the bladder epithelium is derived from endoderm, and both the ureter and bladder become enveloped in mesodermal-derived smooth muscle.

The human metanephros appears at 5 wk of gestation, and lies in close proximity to the mesonephros, which is programmed to involute, and the gonadal ridge (1). The first layer of glomeruli form by 9 wk. Branching and nephron formation continue in the outer rim of the kidney, the nephrogenic cortex, until 34 wk, whereas further maturation, in the form of growth and differentiation, continues postnatally. Recent studies suggest that about two-thirds of nephrons are generated in the last third of human gestation, and that the range of nephrons found in healthy human kidneys is rather large, approx $0.5–1.1 \times 10^6$ (2). When the finely tuned processes, including branching and nephron formation, go wrong, malformations occur such as agenesis (absent kidney), dysplasia (incomplete differentiation, often with cysts) and hypoplasia (too few nephrons). Lower-urinary-tract malformations such as vesicoureteric reflux, duplex ureters, and posterior urethral valves can accompany renal dysplasia and hypoplasia (2).

From: *Methods in Molecular Medicine, vol. 86: Renal Disease: Techniques and Protocols*
Edited by: M. S. Goligorsky © Humana Press Inc., Totowa, NJ

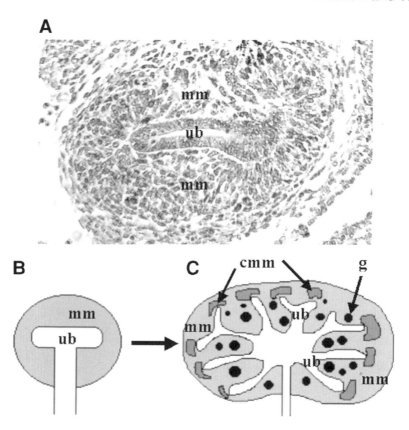

Fig. 1. Differentiation of the metanephric kidney. (**A**) Histology of a rat metanephric kidney *in situ* at d 12.5 of gestation (the equivalent stage in mouse is 11 d of gestation). This is called the "utereric bud" stage. Note that the ureteric bud (ub) has branched once and is surrounded by condensing metanephric mesenchyme (mm). There are no glomeruli present at this stage. (**B**) This frame represents the ureteric bud stage diagrammatically. (**C**) This frame depicts a metanephric kidney after about 4 d of development, when the ureteric bud has branched recurrently. In the outer part of the organ, the ureteric bud branch tips are surrounded by condensed metanephric mesenchyme (cmm), and the first glomeruli (g) have appeared.

Mechanisms of normal and abnormal kidney development have been studied in several ways. For example, development can be modulated in vivo by maternal dietary manipulation *(3)*, surgical obstruction of urinary flow *(4)*, and generation of mice that either overexpress or fail to express defined genes *(2)*. Furthermore, cell lineages can be studied after microtransplantation of metanephroi into the cortex of neonatal mice *(5)*, and primary cultures and cell lines can be generated from cell lines from normal metanephroi *(6,7)* and renal malformations *(8)*. Although each of these techniques has its unique advantages, only organ culture provides an opportunity to study the way in which the embryonic kidney develops as an integrated unit in a tightly controlled ex vivo setting. The method has generally been used to study murine organogenesis, although the techniques are applicable to other species, including humans *(9)*.

The technique for culturing the early metanephric kidney is fairly straightforward, and should provide few problems. Metanephric kidneys are dissected from embryos during the first few days after initiation of the organ, which occurs on embryonic d 11 in mice and d 12.5 in rats **(Fig. 1A)**. They are explanted onto Millipore filters and fed with either serum-containing or defined media (e.g., DMEM-F12 supplemented with insulin, transferrin, and selenium) *(10,11)*. In this manner, organs can be maintained in a viable state for up to 1 wk, with the formation of nephron (e.g., glomerular, proximal tubule, and loop of Henle) epithelia from mesenchyme and at the same time, the ureteric bud branches into the collecting-duct system. When explants are cultured in a normoxic atmosphere, few if any capillaries form; in contrast, hypoxic culture favors the formation of some capillaries that derive from renal mesenchyme *(12,13)*.

Metanephric differentiation in organ culture can be manipulated by addition of growth factors *(6,7,14,15)* and other soluble molecules, including adhesion proteins *(16)* and vitamins *(17)*. Conversely, antisera can be used to block the bioactivity of growth factors *(6,7)* and adhesion molecules *(16)*, and anti-sense oligonucleotides *(18)* have been used to downregulate expression of nephrogenic transcription factors. The latter technique has been regarded as controversial because of poor penetration of oligonucleotides into cells and lack of specificity of effects. In any experiment, the contralateral kidney may be used as the control, thereby minimizing variation within experiments.

Several methods may be used to examine experimental outcomes with metanephric kidneys cultured in vitro, such as direct observation through an inverted or confocal microscope, histology, immunohistochemistry, *in-situ* hybridization, and cell sorting. In addition, time-lapse video microscopy may be employed to examine the rate of change of size and structure of the organs. Organ culture also allows examination of secreted molecules such as growth factors through analysis of the conditioned media *(19,20)*.

There are some limitations to the usefulness of metanephric organ culture. These include the fact that after prolonged culture, cells in the center of the organ, which are relatively distant from nutrients in the culture medium, undergo necrosis. This is more of a problem if larger explants are used from larger stages of gestation. In addition, the medulla does not form as a discrete region—and, of course, glomeruli that do form, do not filter any blood.

However, as long as these restrictions are kept in mind, metanephric organ culture may be valuable in the study of kidney development.

2. Materials

Reagents can be obtained from Sigma Chemical Company (Poole, Dorset, UK), unless otherwise specified.

1. Binocular dissecting microscope (Zeiss, Oberkochen, Germany).
2. 1-mL syringes (Merck, Poole, UK).
3. 25-gauge needles (Merck).
4. Leibovitz L15 medium (Gibco, Invitrogen, Paisley, UK). Store at 4°C.
5. 6-well multicell dishes (Marathon, London, UK).
6. Millicell-CM culture-dish filter inserts (0.4 µm; Millipore, Merck).
7. Dulbecco's Modified Eagle's Medium(DMEM)-F12 (Gibco, Invitrogen). Store at 4°C.
8. Insulin. Store at 4°C.
9. Transferrin. Store at 4°C.
10. Selenium. Store at 4°C.
11. Penicillin/streptomycin. Store at <0°C.
12. Fetal calf serum (FCS). Store at <0°C.
13. Incubator (Heraeus Instruments).

3. Methods
3.1 Dissection of Embryonic Kidneys

1. This protocol is based on starting with the metanephric kidney on the first day of its inception, when it is the "ureteric bud" stage. In other words, the ureteric bud has penetrated the renal mesenchyme and may have branched up to one time. In mice, this corresponds to embryonic d 11 (with the day of the vaginal plug designated as embryonic d 0); in rats, the corresponding stage occurs about 36 h later. The equivalent human stage would be 5–6 wk after conception. Refer to **Fig. 2** for a pictorial guide to isolation of the metanephric kidney.
2. Pregnant mice are sacrificed, and the uterus is immediately removed from the mother and stored in Leibovitz L15 medium on ice prior to removal of embryos.
3. The uterus is cut and embryos are removed using watchmaker's forceps. Care should be taken to avoid damaging the hindquarters of the freshly exposed embryo.
4. The embryos are dissected in ice-cold Leibovitz L15 medium using a pair of 1-mL syringes with 25-gauge needles under a binocular dissecting microscope. **Figure 2** demonstrates how the fetus should be dissected. The first cut removes the hindquarters from the torso; this should be just above the level of the hindlimbs. Next, gently remove the dorsal-most rim of tissue comprised of the neural tube and skin. Once this is removed, turn the remaining tissue so that the ventral (front) surface of the embryonic hindquarters is downwards. Two translucent oval structures are visualized medial to the hindlimbs; these are the metanephric kidneys.

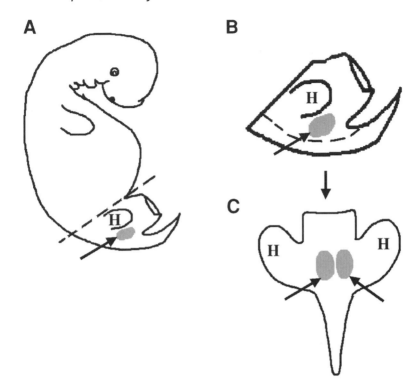

Fig. 2. Dissection of the metanephric kidney. (**A**) This frame depicts the whole embryo (rat d 12.5 or mouse d 11.0) seen from the right side. The dotted line represents the line below which the hindquarters should be removed. The arrow marks the metanephric kidney. H represents hindlimb. (**B**) This frame shows the separated hindquarters, and the dotted line highlights where to cut in order to remove the tissue (spinal cord) dorsal to the metanephroi. (**C**) This frame depicts the fully dissected hindquarters from a dorsal aspect. The metanephric kidneys are indicated by arrows.

5. The metanephric kidneys are carefully dissected out from loosely adherent connective tissue. Place kidneys either individually or in groups (depending on your statistical requirements; *see* **Notes**) on Millicell-CM filter inserts.
6. Transfer each platform into a well of a 6-well culture plate containing 1 mL DMEM-F12 supplemented with insulin (5 μg/mL), transferrin (5 μg/mL) selenium (2.8 μM), penicillin (100 U/mL), and streptomycin (100 μg/mL), amphotericin (0.25 μg/mL), and any additional compounds that your experimental protocol requires (e.g., antibodies or growth factors). Finally, place the top of the tissue-culture plate on the base.
7. Incubate at 37°C, in an atmosphere of air/5% CO_2 and 100% humidity. If all the wells are not being used in any one experiment, each unused well should receive 1 mL of medium to maintain humidity in the tissue-culture plate.

8. Medium should be changed either daily or every two days. Metanephric kidneys can be maintained for several days in this condition.

9. For examination of antibody staining (e.g., PAX2 or WT1 transcription factors as markers of induced mesenchyme, or E-cadherin and laminin as markers of epithelia) in whole-mount preparation using a confocal microscope, the following protocol may be followed. Fix metanephroi with 4% paraformaldehyde in phosphate-buffered saline (PBS), for 15–30 min. Wash in PBS (3 × 10 min). Permeabilize tissues in ice-cold methanol at −20°C for 10 min. Incubate in 10% vol/vol FCS, 1% weight/vol bovine serum albumin (BSA) in PBS for 1 h at room temperature to block nonspecific binding. Incubate organs with the relevant primary antibody in PBS containing 10% BSA overnight at 4°C. Wash in PBS (3 × 10 min). Incubate organs with the appropriate, fluorescent (e.g., fluorescein isothiocyanate [FITC])-labeled, secondary antibody at an appropriate concentration in PBS containing 10% BSA overnight at 4°C. Wash in PBS (3× 10 min). Counterstain with propidium iodide (100 µg/mL, containing RNase A) for the visualization of nuclei, if required. Create a small reservoir on a microscope slide by cutting a hole in a piece of sticky tape and sticking it to the slide. Place the organ in the reservoir, mount in Citifluor™ (Citifluor Ltd., UK), and cover with a cover slip. The stained organ may now be visualized with a confocal microscope.

10. For examination of the cultured organs using conventional histology, the following protocol may be followed. Fix organs in 4% paraformaldehyde in PBS. Dehydrate tissues by transferring them through ethanols (once in 30%, 50%, 70%, 90%, and twice in 100% ethanol) for 2 min each, and place the samples in Histoclear for 2 min, 2×. Place samples in paraffin wax at 65°C, for 10 min, replacing the wax 3×. Embed tissues in paraffin wax poured into molds, and allow to set. Sections may now be cut from the wax blocks. Dewax the sections by reversing the dehydration step described here, finishing with the slides being placed in water for 5 min. Permeabilize tissue by placing in citric acid (pH 6.0) and microwave at full power for 1–5 min (alternative methods of permeabilization include use of proteinase K, trypsin, or protease incubated at 37°C for 10–30 min). Wash in PBS, then quench endogenous peroxidase by incubating slides in 3% hydrogen peroxide made up in methanol for 30 min. Wash in PBS, then incubate slides with an appropriate primary antibody, as previously described.

4. Notes

1. When dissecting out the metanephric kidneys, the mesonephric kidney may be encountered. It is larger than the metanephros and has an elongated shape. Near the mesonephros are the round gonads, which are relatively undifferentiated at this stage. Neither structure should be mistaken for the metanephros, with its unique, centrally inserted ureteric bud.

2. When explanted, metanephric kidneys are oval structures, approx 200 µm long. In culture, they tend to flatten on the filters, forming a disc-like structure. This is more pronounced when defined, serum-free media is used.

3. As growth proceeds, the areas that become distant from contact with the medium, and the atmosphere will begin to die by necrosis because of lack of oxygen. This should be considered when designing experiments, particularly if levels of apoptosis are being examined.

4. It is often preferable to culture metanephroi in a defined, serum-free medium, as it removes possible confounding (known and unknown) factors that are present within serum. Alternatively, if the experiments do not demand a defined medium, DMEM-F12 can simply be supplemented with 5% FCS and antibiotics.

5. It may be helpful to consider the statistics to be used for analysis prior to culture. If individual metanephric kidneys are used to represent an *n* of 1, then they should be cultured individually. For large numbers of metanephroi, then several may be cultured on the same filter, and their results used within a multilevel statistical model *(3)*. This will take account of intra-dish variation and avoid problems of pseudoreplication. If rigid control of the *n* number is not required for statistical analysis, then several organs can be cultured in the same dish, thus saving money and time.

6. Flow cytometry may be a useful method for examining the outcome of experiments using metanephric organ culture. Cell populations may be isolated and examined by cell sorting via fluorescently labeled antibodies. Simple flow-cytometric analyses can provide useful information, such as cell number and cell size *(15)*.

7. Isolated metanephric mesenchyme can be cultured, after induction with embryonic spinal cord. The methodology is beyond the remit of this chapter, but readers can refer to other publications *(16,21)*.

Acknowledgments

We thank the Kidney Research Aid Fund and the National Kidney Research Fund (R16/1/2001) for grant support.

References

1. Risdon, R. A. and Woolf, A. S. (1998) Development of the kidney, in *Heptinstall's Pathology of the Kidney*, 5th ed. (Jennette, J. C., Olson, J. L., Schwartz, M. M., and Silva, F. G., eds.), Lippincott-Raven, Philadelphia New York, pp. 67–84.

2. Woolf, A. S. and Winyard, P. J. D. (2002) Molecular mechanisms of human embryogenesis: developmental pathogenesis of renal tract malformations. *Pediatr. Dev. Pathol.* **5,** 108–129.

3. Welham, S. J. M., Wade, A., and Woolf, A. S. (2002) Protein restriction in pregnancy is associated with increased apoptosis of mesenchymal cells at the start of rat metanephrogenesis. *Kidney Int.* **61,** 1231–1242.

4. Yang, S. P., Woolf, A. S., Quinn, F., and Winyard, P. J. D. (2001) Deregulation of renal transforming growth factor-$\beta 1$ after experimental short-term ureteric obstruction in fetal sheep. *Am. J. Pathol.* **159,** 109–117.

5. Loughna, S., Hardman, P., Landels, E., Jussila, L., Alitalo, K., and Woolf, A. S. (1997) A molecular and genetic analysis of renal glomerular capillary development. *Angiogenesis* **1,** 84–101.

6. Woolf, A. S., Kolatsi-Joannou, M., Hardman, P., Andermarcher, E., Moorby, C., Fine, L.G., et al. (1995) Roles of hepatocyte growth factor/scatter factor and the met receptor in the early development of the metanephros. *J. Cell Biol.* **128,** 171–184.

7. Towers, P. R., Woolf A. S., and Hardman P. (1998) Glial cell line-derived neurotrophic factor stimulates ureteric bud outgrowth and enhances survival of ureteric bud cells in vitro. *Exp. Nephrol.* **6,** 337–351.

8. Yang, S. P., Woolf, A. S., Yuan, H. T., Scott, R. J., Risdon, R. A., O'Hare, M. J., et al. (2000) Potential biological role of transforming growth factor β1 in human congenital kidney malformations. *Am. J. Pathol.* **157,** 1633–1647.

9. Matsell, D. G. and Bennett, T. (1998) Evaluation of metanephric maturation in a human fetal kidney explant model. *In Vitro Cell Dev. Biol.* **34,** 138–148.

10. Avner, E. D., Piesco, N. P., Sweeney, W. E., Studnicki, F. M., Fetterman, G., and Ellis, D. (1984) Hydrocortisone-induced cystic metanephric maldevelopment in serum-free organ culture. *Lab. Invest.* **50,** 208–218.

11. Avner, E. D., Sweeney, W. E., Piesco, N. P., and Ellis, D. (1985) Growth factor requirements of organogenesis in serum-free metanephric organ culture. *In Vitro Cell. Dev. Biol.* **21,** 297–304.

12. Tuffro-McReddie, A., Norwood, V. F., Aylor, K. W., Botkin, S. J., Carey, R. M., and Gomez, R. A. (1997) Oxygen regulates vascular endothelial growth factor-mediated vasculogenesis and tubulogenesis. *Dev. Biol.* **183,** 139–149.

13. Loughna, S., Yuan, H. T., and Woolf, A. S. (1998) Effects of oxygen on vascular patterning in Tie1/LacZ metanephric kidneys in vitro. *Biochem. Biophys. Res. Commun.* **247,** 361–366.

14. Kolatsi-Joannou, M., Li, X. Z., Suda, T., Yuan, H. T., and Woolf, A. S. (2001) Expression and potential role of angiopoietins and Tie-2 in early development of the mouse metanephros. *Dev. Dyn.* **222,** 120–126.

15. Cale, C. M., Klein, N. J., Morgan, G., and Woolf, A. S. (1998) Tumor necrosis factor-α inhibits epithelial differentiation and morphogenesis in the mouse metanephric kidney in vitro. *Int. J. Dev. Biol.* **42,** 663–674.

16. Bullock, S. L., Johnson, T. M., Bao, Q., Hughes, R. C., Winyard, P. J., and Woolf, A. S. (2001) Galectin-3 modulates ureteric bud branching in organ culture of the developing mouse kidney. *J. Am. Soc. Nephrol.* **12,** 515–523.

17. Vilar, J., Gilbert,T., Moreau, E., and Merlet-Benichou, C. (1996) Metanephros organogenesis is highly stimulated by vitamin A derivatives in organ culture. *Kidney Int.* **49,** 1478–1487.

18. Rothenpieler, U. W. and Dressler G. R. (1993) Pax-2 is required for mesenchyme-to-epithelium conversion during kidney development. *Development* **119,** 711–720.

19. Rogers, S. A., Ryan, G., and Hammerman, M. R. (1991) Insulin-like growth factors I and II are produced in the metanephros and are required for growth and development in vitro. *J. Cell Biol.* **113,** 1447–1453.

20. Santos, O. F., Barros, E. J., Yang, X. M., Matsumoto, K., Nakamura, T., Park, M. M., et al. (1994) Involvement of hepatocyte growth factor in kidney development. *Dev. Biol.* **163,** 525–529.

21. Leimeister, C., Bach, A., Woolf, A. S., and Gessler, M. (1999) Screen for genes regulated during early kidney morphogenesis. *Dev. Genet.* **24,** 273–283.

12

The Ureteric Bud

*Tissue-Culture Approaches
to Branching Morphogenesis and Inductive Signaling*

Alan O. Perantoni

1. Introduction

As demonstrated in the development of many parenchymal tissues, the metanephros is the product of an epithelial-mesenchymal interaction involving the proliferation, invasion, and branching morphogenesis of an epithelium into a juxtaposed stromal component that creates an appropriate growth environment for the epithelium and helps determine its structural patterning *(1)*. However, unlike the majority of such tissues, metanephric development depends upon an epithelium and mesenchyme that both originate from mesoderm, and a characteristic mesenchymal-epithelial conversion that provides the hallmark event of this process. The metanephros itself is derived from reciprocal interactions between an epithelial outgrowth of the mesonephric/Wolffian duct—i.e., the ureteric bud, and the surrounding metanephric mesenchyme, which comprises the caudal aspect of the nephrogenic cord/urogenital tract. The ureteric bud regulates morphogenesis of the mesenchyme both directly through elaboration of inductive factors that determine specification of the mesenchymal component and indirectly through the production of a defined number of branch termini, each of which induces a single nephron. As the progenitor population for the collecting duct, it provides the stimulus in the form of soluble patterning molecules and extracellular matrix (ECM) components for induction, differentiation, and recruitment of cells from the metanephric mesenchyme, generating interstitial stroma as well as the podocytes of the glomeruli and the epithelia of the proximal/distal tubules and the loop of Henle. Furthermore, the extent of ureteric-bud branching is a direct determinant of the number of nephrons derived in the adult organ and is now believed to predispose individuals to certain nephropathies based upon a genetic deficiency in glomerular numbers *(2)*.

From: *Methods in Molecular Medicine, vol. 86: Renal Disease: Techniques and Protocols*
Edited by: M. S. Goligorsky © Humana Press Inc., Totowa, NJ

Therefore, the availability of model systems for the study of the activities of the ureteric bud can help delineate the regulatory events in formation of both the nephron and the collecting-duct network. To this end, explant and cell-culture models have been established from isolated ureteric buds of primitive rudiments and used for an examination of the process of bud arborization as well as the factors that modulate it. Furthermore, they have allowed for the purification and identification of inductive signaling factors required for condensation and epithelialization of the metanephric mesenchyme.

This chapter describes reagents and techniques required for isolation and culture of primary ureteric bud tissues along with approaches for continuous propagation of these cells in the production of a non-tumorigenic established cell line. In addition, it presents specific approaches to address questions on development of the bud/collecting duct and events associated with this process—namely, survival, growth, and branching morphogenesis.

2. Materials

1. Properly staged rat (13.5 or 14.5 d post-coitum [dpc]) or mouse (11.5 or 12.5 dpc) embryos.
2. Sterile phosphate-buffered saline (PBS) with and without calcium and magnesium.
3. No. 11 and no. 15 surgical blades with scalpels.
4. Dissecting stereo microscope (minimum 10–25×) with substage illumination.
5. 1% trypsin solution in PBS lacking calcium and magnesium with 500 µg/µL DNase.
6. Soybean trypsin inhibitor (2.5 mg/mL) in culture medium.
7. 50:50 Dulbecco's minimum essential medium (DMEM): Ham's F12 with L-glutamine (2 mM) and gentamicin (50 µg/mL).
8. Stock solutions of the following: sodium selenite (1000X stock: 5×10^{-5} M in DMEM/F12), hydrocortisone (1000X stock: 5×10^{-5} M in 95% ethanol), insulin (100X stock: 500 µg/mL in 0.006 N HCl), prostaglandin E1 (1000X stock: 25 µg/mL in 95% ethanol), iron-saturated transferrin (1000X stock: 5 mg/mL in DMEM/F12), and triiodothyronine (1000X stock: 1×10^{-6} M in dimethyl sulfoxide (DMSO).
9. Growth supplements such as fetal bovine serum (FBS) (final concentration not to exceed 2% in basal medium), recombinant transforming growth factor (TGF)-α or epidermal growth factor (EGF) (1000X stock: 10 µg/mL in DMEM:F12 with 0.1% bovine serum albumin [BSA]), recombinant fibroblast growth factor-7 (KGF) or fibroblast growth factor-1 (FGF-1, 200–1000X stock: 10–50 µg/mL in DMEM:F12 with 0.1% BSA), and recombinant hepatocyte growth factor (HGF, 5 µg/mL in PBS with 0.1% BSA).
10. Gelled collagen prepared from commercially available bovine skin type I collagen (0.1% solution in 0.1 N in acetic acid) mixed with 10× F12 and 10× sodium bicarbonate (11.76 mg/mL) to neutralize the acidified collagen, allowing it to crosslink.
11. Collagenase (0.1 U/mL) mixed with dispase (0.8 U/mL).

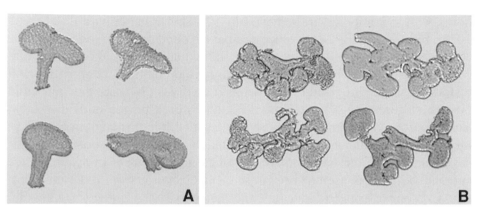

Fig. 1. Isolated ureteric buds from **(A)** 13.5-dpc and **(B)** 14.5-dpc rat metanephroi. Considerable branching has occurred over this 24-h period, significantly increasing the difficulty of bud dissection from the metanephros.

3. Methods

3.1. Isolation of Metanephroi

Although this section describes techniques developed principally for the rat ureteric bud, these approaches have been equally effective with mouse buds, allowing us to successfully establish cultures and bud lines from both rat and mouse embryos.

The techniques and original studies involving isolation of metanephroi were pioneered by Grobstein in the early 1950s and have changed little since that time *(3)*. For accurate staging of embryos, breeding pairs are caged together only overnight, and the presence of a plug in the morning is designated as d 0.5. For this purpose, metanephrogenesis begins at 12.5-dpc in the rat and 10.5-dpc in the mouse (*see* **Note 1**). We isolate metanephroi for study from 13.5- or 14.5-dpc rat and 11.5- or 12.5-dpc mouse embryos. At these early stages in organogenesis, the bud has just initiated its arborization in the mesenchyme. As shown **(Fig. 1A)**, the earlier buds isolated from 13.5-dpc rat embryos have undergone only secondary branching, yielding a T-shaped structure, and the mesenchymal component at this time reveals no obvious gross morphogenesis, such as tubule formation or even condensation. Within 24 h, however, extensive branching has occurred **(Fig. 1B)**, and signs of induction are evident as condensations around bud ampullae.

To isolate metanephroi, timed-pregnant females are euthanized, and the abdominal area is soaked with 70% ethanol to sterilize the surgical field. The abdominal area is then opened with scissors and forceps, and the intact uterine horns with the embryos are removed to 100-mm tissue culture dishes with 10 mL PBS, washed 1–2× to reduce numbers of contaminating red blood cells, and then placed on ice. The embryos are individually removed from their placental sacks, taking care not to pull them by the umbilical cord, which will distort or tear the urogenital tissues. Intact embryos *(3–4)* are then placed in 60-mm culture dishes with 1 mL PBS and stored on ice until dissected. Embryos should not be left for more than about 1 h in this condition to minimize tissue degradation (*see* **Note 2**). Isolation of the metanephroi and physical separation of the buds requires practice and patience. In acquiring the surgical skills, it is useful to begin with metanephroi from older embryos, e.g., 14.5-dpc or even 15.5-dpc rats, and then move to an earlier stage in order to recognize tissue position (prior to body elongation, the metanephroi are located in the caudal extremity between the hindlimbs and tail) and appreciate its friable nature (at 13.5 dpc, simple tissue teasing will tear the rudiment). Access to the metanephroi is most readily attained by first cutting through the embryo just under the liver rudiment (noted externally by its red-blood-cell production) and then teasing apart the lower abdominal ectoderm to open the surgical field. Once located underneath the mass of forming intestines, the urogenital tract—which includes the mesonephros—can be rolled off of the spinal cord with the embryo positioned on its side using a no. 15 surgical blade. Upon removal, the surrounding urogenital tissue is separated from the metanephroi with no. 11 and no. 15 blades. Alternatively, some prefer the use of small gauge needles for these dissections, but either way, sharp dissecting instruments are essential. Once the metanephroi have been excised, they are collected in PBS at 4°C until separated. Storage in PBS for more than 1–2 h is not recommended, as gradual tissue degradation increases the difficulty of bud-mesenchyme separations.

3.2. Bud Isolations

Following successful removal of intact metanephroi, buds are dissociated from mesenchymes with trypsin/DNase solution in PBS. The DNase substantially reduces the "stickiness" of the mesenchymes and buds during surgical manipulation. After a 5–min incubation in these enzymes, buds can be readily removed from the metanephroi using scalpels equipped with no. 11 surgical blades. Once separated, they are transferred into culture medium containing soybean trypsin inhibitor until explanted to matrix-coated filters or culture dishes for propagation.

As demonstrated in **Fig. 1**, it is possible to cleanly separate the bud from the mesenchyme at both 13.5-dpc and 14.5-dpc stages. Although the metanephroi at the earlier stage are considerably smaller and more difficult to remove intact from the embryo, isolation of the bud is significantly easier at this stage because branching is limited. Once branching occurs, the separations require considerably more surgical manipulation to tease out the mesenchyme surrounding the bud without also damaging the bud.

Isolated buds from either age can be effectively cultured. A consideration that may enter into the decision regarding bud age is the segment to be studied. It is apparent that bud ampullae are phenotypically distinct from the shafts of the dividing ducts, based upon expression patterns of molecular markers. For example, *ret*, the receptor for glial-derived neurotrophic factor (GDNF) *(4)*, and secreted patterning molecule *wnt11 (5)* are most prominent at the tips of the bud, and *wnt7b (6)*, patterning molecule *sonic hedgehog (6)*, and cell-adhesion molecule *Ksp-cadherin (7)* are found in the shafts. Thus, it may be useful to surgically select for one population over another prior to cultivation if one aspect is more desirable.

3.3. Cell-Culture Medium

Appropriate selection of components for the culture medium is critical for the continuous propagation of bud cells. For this purpose, numerous growth and survival factors, such as peptide growth factors, steroids, eicosanoids, and a variety of hormones, have been evaluated in the ultimate optimization of growth conditions *(8,9)*. These studies have revealed that high levels of FBS (greater than 2%) are perhaps the most detrimental component to bud growth *(9)*. With such treatments, the bud cells become elongated (fibroblast-like) and enlarged, cease proliferation, and eventually die. Lower concentrations (1–2%), however, are required for continuous bud-cell proliferation, at least initially in the absence of a matrix. For bud-cell propagation, we use DMEM/F12 supplemented with selenium, hydrocortisone, insulin, prostaglandin E1, iron-saturated transferrin, and triiodothyronine. In addition to the basal components listed here, inclusion of a growth factor/cytokine is also required to stimulate expansion of the cultured buds. For this, TGF-α, (5–10 ng/mL) or epidermal growth factor (EGF; 10–20 ng/mL) are effective. Alternatively or in addition to an EGF family member, 1–2% FBS facilitates bud-cell propagation. In the absence of either a growth factor or FBS, buds may attach to and spread on a substratum, but little proliferation occurs. All stock components are stored at –20°C, and are stable for more than 6 mo under these conditions. However, once diluted in culture medium, they are considerably less stable, so complete medium with supplements is not used beyond 2 wk (*see* **Note 3**). Furthermore, growth factors such as TGF-α are added directly to culture media at the time of cellular exposure to ensure biological potency.

All of the components mentioned here have been described as enhancers of renal epithelial-cell propagation, but not necessarily collecting duct epithelia. However, in cell-growth studies in which single components were deleted *(9)*, only the individual loss of selenium severely impaired bud-cell survival, but the loss of transferrin, hydrocortisone, insulin, or an EGF family member resulted in a significant reduction in growth and deletion of others had no apparent impact upon bud growth.

3.4. Explant Culture of Isolated Buds

It is considerably more effective to culture buds intact rather than subject them to the rigors of dissociation. Individual or small clumps of cells dissociated from isolated buds show poor survivability, presumably because of the lengthy trypsin digestions required for single-cell dispersion of these tightly cohesive epithelia or alternatively to the loss of cross-feeding. For this reason, 13.5-dpc rat buds are generally cultured without further manipulation, but the larger 14.5-dpc buds can be reduced in size simply through mechanical fragmentation.

The type of substratum applied to bud cultures can dramatically impact the attachment, survival, and outgrowth of bud cells. We have found gelled type I collagen to provide the most effective matrix for bud attachment and growth. However, this significantly complicates cell passaging, which then requires collagenase/dispase treatment. Inactivation of these enzymes only occurs with dilution and replating on the matrix following extensive washing after cell dissociation. Alternatively, buds can attach, albeit over several days, to uncoated tissue-culture plastic or plastic coated with a thin or dried layer of a matrix component such as type I collagen. Thinly coated plates are commercially available. To produce a pad of gelled collagen, a commercial preparation of bovine skin type I collagen is mixed with 10X F12 and 10X sodium bicarbonate, allowing the collagen to gel. Once mixed, the collagen solution solidifies as the temperature is raised from 4°C to room temperature or 37°C. If this occurs too rapidly, gas bubbles trapped in the gel will distort it. Culture medium is added after collagen has gelled, which takes approx 45 min (*see* **Note 4**).

A consideration for the ultimate culture of any cell type is development of a culture milieu that will select for the growth of a cell population of interest and against any possible contaminating population(s)—e.g., in this case, metanephric mesenchyme (MM). Fortunately, the factors in the basal medium with the described supplements are not inductive or growth-promoting for MM, and therefore the few remaining cells of MM attached to the buds following isolation have little potential for survival. On collagen, the few cells of MM can be observed to invade the gelled matrix; however, these cells show little ability to proliferate or become established in competition with the bud cells.

When they grow on plastic, primary bud cells retain a cuboidal epithelial morphology (**Fig. 2A**) and continue to expand in the presence of an EGF family member *(8)*. With the addition of 1–2% serum, this growth is sustained,

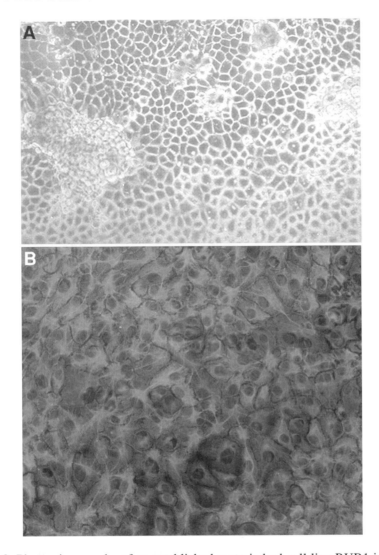

Fig. 2. Photomicrographs of an established ureteric bud-cell line RUB1 in bright-field (**A**) and analyzed for cytokeratin expression (**B**). The cells are morphologically epithelial, showing a cobblestone appearance, dome-like cystic structures typical of secreting cells, and uniform cytokeratin expression.

allowing cells to be dissociated and passaged. We have now successfully propagated bud cells for more than 50 passages without an apparent crisis. These cells continue to express characteristics of epithelia, including the synthesis of intermediate filaments typical of epithelia, such as cytokeratins (**Fig. 2B**), formation of tight junctions and desmosomes, and dome/cyst formation in

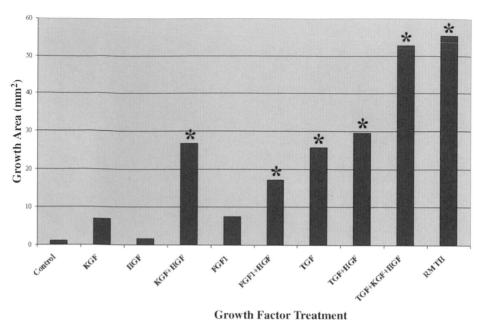

Growth Factor Treatment

Fig. 3. Regulation of growth in primary cultures of ureteric bud cells cultivated on a collagen substratum. Growth factors (HGF, 50 ng/mL; FGF1, 50 ng/mL; KGF, 50 ng/mL; and TGF-α, 10 ng/mL) function synergistically in stimulating proliferation and expansion of the bud cells. * indicates statistical significance with $p < 0.01$.

confluent culture. They also retain their ability to elaborate inductive signaling factors for MM, a topic that is described later in this chapter.

Various cytokines/growth factors differentially affect proliferation of freshly isolated buds that are explanted onto a gelled type I collagen matrix. Individual factors stimulate only limited growth, but certain combinations of factors significantly enhance proliferation (**Fig. 3**). Individually, keratinocyte growth factor (KGF or FGF7) and HGF cause no significant stimulation, yet, together they function synergistically to increase growth rates. TGF-α (10 ng/mL) treatment with KGF (50 ng/mL) and HGF (50 ng/mL) further enhance growth to a level comparable to that of a renal mesenchymal tumor homogenate (RMTH). The RMT is a perinatally induced rat tumor of renal stroma that resembles the congenital mesoblastic nephroma, and is often observed to have ductular cystic hyperplasia. The effect of the homogenate suggests that it may be a useful renewable source and model system for mitogens of the ureteric bud. HGF also complements the effects of other FGF family members, such as FGF1, yet TGF-α, by itself stimulates growth.

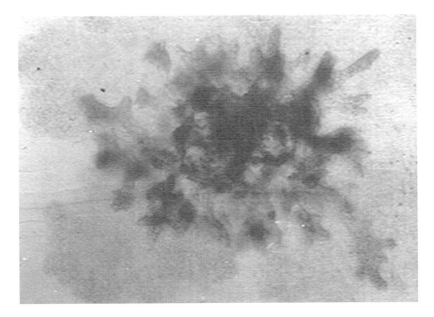

Fig. 4. A primary rat ureteric bud suspended in a collagen matrix. Extensive branching morphogenesis occurs in this explant treated with HGF (50 ng/mL), KGF (50 ng/mL), and TGF-α (10 ng/mL).

3.5. Primary Buds in a Matrix Suspension

In addition to the ability to explant and grow buds on gelled collagen, it is also possible to suspend isolated intact tissue directly in a matrix to study branching morphogenesis. For this purpose, we have submerged 13.5-dpc rat buds in gelled type I collagen as prepared previously, and have found that they can branch independently of the MM *(9)* (*see* **Note 5**). Although branching is neither as extensive nor rapid as in vivo, tertiary arborization is evident (**Fig. 4**), suggesting that the program for patterning/branching is at least partially inherent in the buds themselves, and that soluble factors secreted by the mesenchyme may primarily provide survival and growth-enhancement functions during bud morphogenesis. Of the various factors examined other than those already described, higher concentrations of FBS (5%) or TGF-β1 are both potent inhibitors of bud growth. A number of factors have been implicated by others in branching morphogenesis using a variety of approaches, including transgenic and knockout studies as well as in vitro analyses. For example, Wnt-2b (formerly Wnt-13) supports bud growth and branching when expressed by NIH-3T3 cells in cocultivation experiments *(10)*. Branching is also severely restricted in double knock-outs for the retinoic acid receptors Rara and Rarb2 *(11)*.

Subsequent to our own studies, Qiao et al. *(12)* used a 50:50 blend of type I collagen with Matrigel as a matrix into which buds could be suspended for studies of branching morphogenesis. The matrix was placed in the upper well of a Transwell tissue culture insert, which contained a polycarbonate filter with a 3-µm pore size. In their system, concentrated conditioned medium from a cell line derived from MM in combination with 10% FBS and a mixture of growth factors were added. The factors included GDNF, which is required for branching of the bud in vivo, EGF, insulin-like growth factor (IGF), FGF2, and HGF. When either the growth factors or the conditioned medium are deleted, bud survival, growth, and branching are severely inhibited. These effects are dependent upon the source of conditioned medium, requiring cells from MM. However, of the growth factors, only GDNF can facilitate extensive growth and branching in combination with conditioned medium. In addition, cocultivation of isolated buds retrieved from matrix cultures and freshly prepared 13.5-dpc rat MMs results in nephron induction within the MM, demonstrating the functional retention of bud inductive activity despite their explantation.

Application of this system to an examination of a variety of growth factors expressed in the developing metanephros has proven somewhat fruitful in analyzing branch patterns *(13)*. In the presence of FGF1 and FGF10, branch stalks become elongated in a similar manner as occurs in vivo, and branches develop clearly defined ampullae. For FGF2 and FGF7, however, the stalks are more "globular and less ordered." FGF7 is considerably more potent in inducing growth and branching than other family members. A similar approach may be useful for delineating the factors that modulate patterning in efforts to repair or regenerate diseased tissues.

3.6. Matrix Suspension of Cells from Established Lines

Another approach used in studying branching morphogenesis involves the Madin-Darby canine kidney (MDCK) epithelial-cell line. This line expresses many characteristics of collecting duct cells. When dissociated and suspended in a three-dimensional (3D) gelled collagen matrix, cells from this line form cystic structures unless incubated with HGF *(14)*. For this, confluent cultures of MDCK cells are trypsinized and suspended at 4×10^4 cells/mL in type I collagen, which is prepared as previously described except for replacement of F12 with F11 medium. The suspension is aliquoted into 4-well Nunclon plates at 300 µL/well. Under these conditions, the cells invade the matrix, generating a complex network of branched duct-like structures. Despite attempts to reproduce these studies with our bud-cell lines, our efforts to induce a comparable network of structures have been unsuccessful. Our RUB1 cell line is capable, once dissociated, of forming spherical cysts in the presence of EGF when suspended in gelled type I collagen but without any apparent potential for branching morphogenesis despite the inclusion of HGF. This may simply reflect the nature of the buds themselves as we have apparently selected for the stalk portion of the bud.

3.7. Ureteric Bud Cells as a Source of Inductive Factors for MM

As previously mentioned, the ureteric bud elaborates and secretes factors that direct morphogenesis of metanephric mesenchyme, including mesenchymal-epithelial conversion. In this regard, we recently reported the identity of several of these factors and their ability to induce morphogenesis *(15)*. To accomplish this, we exploited the capacity of these cells to grow in the absence of serum, once it was established that concentrated medium from flasks of these cells potentiated tubulogenesis *(6)*. The established rat ureteric-bud-cell line RUB1 was expanded into 10–12 tissue-culture flasks (162 cm^2). Basal medium, as described with TGFα but in the absence of any serum, was collected and concentrated 10-to-1 using a Filtron mini-ultraset (8-*Kd* cut-off) and then 5-to-1 by microfiltration in a Filtron MacroSep unit (8–10 *Kd* cutoff). Subsequent chromatographic separations were dependent upon the nature of the unknown factor (*see* **ref.** *15*), but our approach generally included anion- or cation-exchange chromatography, hydrophobic interaction chromatography, or heparin-affinity chromatography, which is especially effective because the inductive cytokines are heparin-binding but the vast majority of cellular proteins are not. Using this approach, we implicated FGF- (FGF2), IL-6- (leukemia inhibitory factor), and TGF-β- (TGF-β2, activin A and B, and growth/differentiation factor-11) family members in this complex morphogenetic process. Because of its complexity, it would have been extremely difficult to accomplish this initially through genetic studies, but by using the original inductive cell, even with its multiplicity of factors, it was possible to individually fractionate and subsequently demonstrate complementation of factors in this critical morphogenetic pathway. As methods of protein fractionation become automated with direct input into mass spectrometers, such an approach will eventually prove rapid and comprehensive, yet will lack the labor-intensive nature of our own studies.

Further examination of factors expressed by the bud cells using reverse transcriptase-polymerase chain reaction (RT-PCR) techniques have implicated additional factors. In addition to FGF2, FGF1 and FGF9 are produced by the rat bud-cell line RUB1 (**Fig. 5**). Of course, this does not identify the biological target of ligand signaling, i.e., the bud itself in autocrine stimulation or MM, but evaluation of the influence of these factors on morphogenesis in the individual progenitor populations can readily address this issue.

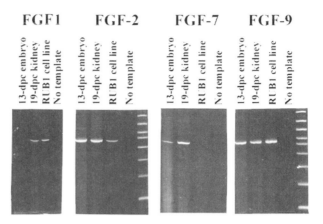

Fig. 5. Expression of FGF family members by the rat ureteric bud-cell line RUB1. RUB1 is shown to express multiple forms of FGF family members by RT-PCR, a finding that is consistent with known expression patterns for the ureteric bud.

4. Notes

1. To limit the variability of developmental stage, it is critical that breeders only be mated for a minimum period, not to exceed overnight. Commercial breeders may use up to a 24-h breeding period, which can significantly impact these studies.
2. From the time of euthanasia to the end of the surgery, the tissues are continuously degrading, so it is imperative to work through the process until the buds are in their final culture milieu. Since an average litter contains six embryos, one person should probably euthanize only three animals at a time to minimize the problem of tissue degradation.
3. Because of problems with protein denaturation and inactivation of growth factors as a result of freeze-thawing, individual aliquots of growth supplements in aqueous solutions should be frozen in small enough quantities that only one freeze-thaw cycle is applied.
4. Since glass and plastic surfaces bind a variety of proteins, including growth factors, it is useful to reconstitute biologically active proteins in 0.1% BSA and if necessary, to sterilize such reagents with low protein-binding filters, storing them in polypropylene plastics to minimize loss.
5. When suspending buds/cells in a matrix, it is useful to mix the growth supplements in the collagen as well, so permeability is not an issue. Many of these factors bind to collagen, and may be sequestered as a result.

5. Conclusions

Culture of the ureteric bud as a primary explant on a gelled collagen matrix or suspended within a matrix has provided an effective model for the study and identification of regulatory factors that are responsible for the differentiation and patterning of this epithelial progenitor from the metanephros. Furthermore, through expansion in culture, ureteric bud-cell lines have functioned as a renewable source of inductive signaling factors for the specification and morphogenesis of the mesenchymal progenitor cells. Although isolation of the buds initially requires some practice, dissections eventually come with ease, and culture conditions are sufficiently defined to allow successful explantation and propagation of normal bud cells without the need for viral immortalization. Since some congenital nephropathies may involve a failure of the bud to undergo appropriate branching and subsequent nephronic induction, the use of the models described here could contribute significantly to our understanding of the regulation of this critical morphogenetic process.

References

1. Saxén, L. (1987) *Organogenesis of the Kidney.* Cambridge University Press, New York, NY, pp. 1–173.
2. Mackenzie, H., Lawler, E. L., and Brenner, B. M. (1996) Congenital oligonephropathy: the fetal flaw in essential hypertension. *Kidney Int.* **49**, Suppl. 55, S30–S34.
3. Grobstein, C. (1953) Morphogenetic interaction between embryonic mouse tissues separated by a membrane filter. *Nature* **172**, 859–871.
4. Pachnis, V., Mankoo, B., and Costantini, F. (1993) Expression of the c-ret proto-oncogene during mouse embryogenesis. *Development* **119**, 1005–1017.
5. Kispert, A., Vainio, S., Shen, L., Rowitch, D. H., and McMahon, A. P. (1996) Proteoglycans are required for maintenance of Wnt-11 expression in the ureter tips. *Development* **122**, 3627–3637.
6. Karavanova, I. D., Dove, L. F., Resau, J. H., and Perantoni, A. O. (1996) Conditioned medium from a rat ureteric bud cell line in combination with bFGF induces complete differentiation of isolated metanephric mesenchyme. *Development* **122**, 4159–5167.
7. Thomson, R. B. and Aronson, P. S. (1999) Immunolocalization of Ksp-cadherin in the adult and developing rabbit kidney. *Am. J. Physiol.* **277**, F146–F156.
8. Perantoni, A. O., Kan, F. W. K., Dove, L. F., and Reed, C. D. (1985) Selective growth in culture of fetal rat renal collecting duct anlagen. *Lab. Investig.* **53**, 589–596.
9. Perantoni, A. O., Williams, C. L., and Lewellyn, A. L. (1991) Growth and branching morphogenesis of rat collecting duct anlagen in the absence of metanephrogenic mesenchyme. *Differentiation* **48**, 107–113.
10. Lin, Y., Liu, A., Zhang, S., Ruusunen, T., Kreidberg, J. A., Peltoketo, H., et al. (2001) Induction of ureter branching as a response to Wnt-2b signaling during early kidney organogenesis. *Dev. Dyn.* **222**, 26–39.
11. Batourina, E., Gim, S., Bello, N., Shy, M., Clagett-Dame, M., Srinivas, S., et al. (2001) Vitamin A control epithelial/mesenchymal interactions through Ret expression. *Nat. Genet.* **27**, 74–78.

12. Qiao, J., Sakurai, H., and Nigam, S. K. (1999) Branching morphogenesis independent of mesenchymal-epithelial contact in the developing kidney. *Proc. Natl. Acad. Sci. USA* **96,** 7330–7335.

13. Qiao, J., Bush, K. T., Steer, D. L., Stuart, R. O., Sakurai, H., Wachsman, W., et al. (2001) Multiple fibroblast growth factors support growth of the ureteric bud but have different effects on branching morphogenesis. *Mech. Dev.* **109,** 123–135.

14. Montesano, R., Matsumoto, K., Nakamura, T., and Orci, L. (1991) Identification of a fibroblast-derived morphogen as hepatocyte growth factor. *Cell* **67,** 901–908.

15. Plisov, S. Y., Yoshino, K., Dove, L. F., Higinbotham, K. G., Rubin, J. S., and Perantoni, A. O. (2001) TGFβ2, LIF and FGF2 cooperate to induce nephrogenesis. *Development* **128,** 1045–1057.

13

Studies of Cell Lineage in the Developing Kidney

Maria Luisa S. Sequeira Lopez and R. Ariel Gomez

1. Introduction

The development of the definitive (metanephric) kidney in mammals depends on the reciprocal inductive interactions between two mesoderm-derived structures: the metanephric mesenchyme (MM) and the epithelial ureteric bud. The ureteric bud secretes factors that induce the mesenchyme to condensate, proliferate, and convert to an epithelium, resulting in the formation of an epithelial vesicle that matures into a glomerulus. The induced mesenchyme in turn sends signals to the ureteric bud, causing its division and growth. When the ureteric bud has branched once, the MM already possesses precursor cells with the ability to differentiate into epithelial, vascular, interstitial, and mesangial cells *(1–3)*. As a result of these processes, the ureteric bud generates the collecting and the pelvic and ureteric epithelia, whereas the MM gives rise to glomeruli, vessels, and proximal tubules.

The introduction of a replication-defective retrovirus carrying a reporter gene into individual cells of the MM revealed that the MM contains cells that can generate all the epithelial regions of the nephron *(4)*. However, with this method it is difficult to control the cellular site of injection, making interpretation of results ambiguous.

Generation of transgenic mice, with cell-specific promoters driving a fluorescent reporter gene such as the *Hoxb 7*, which is expressed in the ureteric bud, allowed the visualization, in an organ-culture model, of the pattern of growth and branching of the ureteric bud *(5)*. These mice can be used to track the fate of cells derived from the primitive ureter.

Transplantation studies of the MM between genetically labeled and wild-type mice demonstrated that all vascular elements (endothelial cells, smooth-muscle cells, and renin-producing cells) differentiate within the MM *(1,3)*.

Much of our knowledge of the lineage of kidney cells comes from studies performed in multiple laboratories. Considering that the developed kidney

From: *Methods in Molecular Medicine, vol. 86: Renal Disease: Techniques and Protocols*
Edited by: M. S. Goligorsky © Humana Press Inc., Totowa, NJ

possesses more than 30 differentiated cell types, innumerable questions must still be answered. It is important to identify the signals and mechanisms that regulate the expression of genes that control the differentiation and fate of renal cells. This fundamental knowledge is instrumental to acquiring a deeper understanding of the cellular and molecular basis of kidney development. Therefore, multiple analyses between "related" cell types at different time-points during development are still required. For instance, to study the lineage relationship between two related cell types, a first and simple approach is the comparison of cell-specific protein expression throughout development by double immunohistochemistry. For example, before the renal vasculature is assembled, renin-expressing cells develop within the MM, which do not contain smooth-muscle-cell proteins (such as α-smooth-muscle actin [α-SMA]). However, when cells assemble into the vasculature, they begin expressing α-SMA as a later event in their differentiation pathway *(1)*. Although it has been suggested for many years that renin cells were derived from smooth-muscle cells *(6)* because they contain myofilaments in the adult animal, we now know that the acquisition of smooth-muscle proteins occurs later in the differentiation pathway, and renin cells probably give rise to smooth-muscle cells.

Multiple transgenic lines of mice expressing reporter genes are currently available, either commercially or from independent investigators (e.g., *Tie 2 Lac-Z [7]*, *Tie 2 GFP [8]*, *Flk Lac Z [9]*, *Ren1d GFP [10]*, *Tie 2 Cre [11]*, *Hoxb 7 GFP [5]*, or *β-globin Lac Z [12]*). Kidneys from mice expressing Lac-Z driven by cell-specific promoters can be subjected to the X-Gal reaction to visualize the β-galactosidase expression, and further double-immunostained to evaluate the co-expression or lack of co-expression of several markers on the same tissue section at a specific time frame.

Another method available to study the lineage of kidney cells is to determine the mRNA expression of two markers on a single kidney embryonic cell. The cell in question can be identified by morphology (renin cells are large granulated cells) or by the fluorescence expression in embryonic kidneys from transgenic mice *(5,8,10)*.

An elegant but laborious way of labeling cells and its descendants is by generating a transgenic mouse by homologous recombination that expresses the cre recombinase gene driven by the promoter of a gene expressed in a specific cell type. Then, by crossing the Cre-mouse with a reporter mouse—for example, the ROSA 26 reporter *(13)*—in which the Lac-Z gene is prevented from ubiquitous expression by the presence of a stop codon, which in turn is flanked by lox P sites. Once the cell-specific promoter is activated, cre recombinase is expressed, and it excises the stop codon region via recombination using the lox P sites. From then on, that cell and all its descendents will express β-galactosidase. In addition to the ROSA 26 reporter mouse, there are other reporter mice available *(14,15)*.

Regular transgenic mice generated by the pronuclear injection of DNA could be valuable tools for lineage studies. However, their major disadvantages are that i) they require a thorough characterization of the promoter, in itself time-consuming, ii) there is no control over the number of copies of the integrated transgene, and iii) random integration makes the transgene expression susceptible to the local chromosomal environment. One way to overcome this problem is to combine the promoter of the gene of interest with an intron fragment containing an already identified enhancer for that gene *(7)*.

However, for these reasons, we strongly recommend lineage studies to label the candidate genes by targeted insertion of a selectable marker into the embryonic stem-cell genome using homologous recombination. Although more laborious, it guarantees regulation of the gene within the native locus of the gene in question, thus avoiding the uncertainty of bona fide specific expression.

This chapter describes the materials and methods required to identify protein and transgene expression on tissue sections and mRNA expression in single embryonic cells.

All the transgenesis techniques are described in *Methods in Molecular Biology*, Volume 180.

2. Materials

2.1. Double and Triple Labeling Studies by Immuno/Histochemical Techniques

2.1.1. Animals

1. Wild-type mice.
2. Transgenic mice expressing Lac-Z driven by cell-specific promoters (e.g., *Flk-1*, *Tie2*, or β-*globin*).

2.1.2. X-Gal Reaction

1. Phosphate-buffered saline (PBS).
2. Buffered formalin 10%.
3. Lac-Z wash: 0.1 M phosphate buffer pH 7.4 containing 2 mM MgCl$_2$, 0.01% sodium deoxycholate, and 0.02% tergitol NP-40.
4. Staining solution: Lac-Z wash, 5 mM potassium ferricyanide, 5 mM potassium ferrocyanide, and 1 mg/mL 5-bromo-4-chloro-3-indolyl-B-D-galactopyranoside (X-gal, Gold Bio Technology, Inc., cat. # X4281C) in dimethylformamide.

2.1.3. Paraffin Embedding and Tissue Sectioning

1. Ethanol (70%, 95%, and 100%).
2. Xylene.

3. Paraffin wax (Surgipath, cat. # EM-400).
4. Glass slides (charged).
5. HistoEmbedder.
6. Microtome.
7. Slide warmer.

2.1.4. Double Immunostaining

1. Primary antibodies (monoclonal or polyclonal).
2. Vectastain ABC kits (Vector Lab, Burlingame, CA) appropriate for the antibodies to test.
3. SIGMA FAST DAB peroxidase substrate tablet set (Sigma, cat. # D 4168) (*see* **Note 1**).
4. Vector VIP substrate kit for peroxidase (Vector, cat. # SK-4600) (*see* **Note 1**). Prepare as follows:
   a. 5 mL of PBS + 3 drops of reagent 1 and mix well.
   b. Add 3 drops of reagent 2 and mix well.
   c. Add 3 drops of reagent 3 and mix well.
   d. Add 3 drops of hydrogen peroxide solution and mix well.
5. Ethanol (100%, 95% and 70%).
6. Xylene.
7. Methanol.
8. 30% hydrogen peroxide.
9. Antigen retrieval solution:
   a. Solution A: Citric acid · H_2O 1.02 g in 50 mL of distilled water.
   b. Solution B: Sodium citrate · $2H_2O$ 1.47 g in 50 mL of distilled water.
   c. Mix 4.5 mL of Solution A + 20.5 mL of Solution B + 200 mL of distilled water. Adjust pH to 6.0 with 1 N NaOH, then add distilled water to a total vol of 250 mL.
10. Nuclear fast red (Vector, cat. # H-3403).
11. Humidity chamber.
12. Mounting medium such as Permount (Fisher Scientific, cat. # SP15–100) or Cytoseal XYL (Richard-Allan Scientific, cat. # 8312-4).
13. Cover slips.

2.2. Cell Aspiration and Single-Cell Reverse Transcriptase-Polymerase Chain Reaction (RT-PCR) from Embryonic Kidneys

2.2.1. Organ Explant Culture

1. Organ-tissue culture plastic dishes, 60 × 15 mm style with center well (Falcon, cat. # 3037).
2. Sterile fine forceps and surgical blades.
3. Membrane filters, 25 mm, 0.8 μm (Gelman Sciences, cat. # 64677).

4. Cell-culture inserts, 6-well format, 3.0 μm pore size (Falcon, cat. # 3091).
5. Sterile tissue-culture water (Sigma).
6. Medium: serum-free organ-culture medium Dulbecco's Modified Eagle's Medium (DMEM):F12 (Gibco, cat.# 430-2500EG) with 10 m*M* HEPES (Sigma, cat. # H9136), 1.1 mg/mL NaHCO3, penicillin 50 U/mL, Nystatin 50 U/mL, ITS (insulin/transferrin/selenite, Sigma, cat. # I1884) 5 ug/mL I and T, 2.8 nm S, PGE1 25 ng/mL, T3 (Triiodothyronine, Sigma, cat. # T5516) 32 pg/mL.

2.2.2. Dissection of Embryonic Kidneys

1. Sterile gloves, mask.
2. Fine forceps and small scissors (always sterile).
3. Dissection microscope: with magnification range from ×7–40 with a black background stage and cold light source.
4. Culture plates: 35-mm plastic tissue-culture dishes, sterile.
5. Medium (*see* **Subheading 2.2.1**).

2.2.3. Cell Aspiration

1. Inverted microscope (e.g., Nikon Diaphot 300).
2. Micromanipulator (Nikon Narishige) attached to a PLI-100 Pico -Injector (Medical System Corporation, Greenvale, NY).
3. Nitrogen gas tank with a manometer.
4. Borosilicate capillary micropipets, ~ 4.5–10-cm length with tip diameter 5–15 μm (*see* **Note 2**).
5. Lysis buffer: 2.5% Triton X-100, 5 m*M* dithiothreitol (DTT), 1.2 U/μL RNasin in RNase-DNase-free water.
6. 0.6-μL microfuge tubes.
7. Microloaders (Eppendorf, Hamburg, Germany, cat. # 5242 956.003).
8. Culture plates: 35-mm plastic tissue-culture dishes sterile.
9. Medium (*see* **Subheading 2.2.1.**).
10. Liquid nitrogen.

2.2.4. Single-Cell RT-PCR

2.2.4.1. REVERSE TRANSCRIPTION REACTION

1. Moloney murine leukemia virus (MMLV) reverse transcriptase (Promega Corporation, Madison, Wisconsin).
2. RT buffer (5×): Contains 2.5% Triton X-100, 5 m*M* DTT, 1.2 U/μL RNasin. To prepare 100 μL, combine the following: 25 μL of 10% Triton X-100, 10 μL of 50 m*M* DTT, 3 μL of RNasin (40 U/μL) and 62 μL of RNase-DNase-free water.
3. 2.5 m*M* dNTP mix (prepared by mixing equal vol of 100 m*M* dATP, dCTP, dGTP, and dTTP) (Promega Corporation).
4. Oligo (dT) (Promega Corporation).
5. 0.5-mL microcentrifuge tubes.

2.2.4.2. PCR AMPLIFICATION

1. *Taq* DNA polymerase (5 U/μL) (Promega Corporation).
2. Thermophilic DNA polymerase 10X buffer, magnesium free: 500 mM KCl, 100 mM Tris-HCl (pH 9.0 at 25°C), and 1% Triton X-100.
3. 25 mM MgCl$_2$.
4. 2.5 mM dNTP mix (*see* **Subheading 2.2.4.1.**).
5. Outer primers and inner (nested) primers should be designed for each marker to be detected.
6. 0.5 mL thin-walled reaction tubes with flat caps.
7. Automated thermal cycler.
8. Bulk reaction mix: for each 50-μL reaction, combine the following:

2.2.4.3. AGAROSE GEL ELECTROPHORESIS OF DNA

1. Tris-acetate (TAE) buffer 1X: 40 mM Tris-acetate, 1 mM ethylenediamine-tetraacetic acid (EDTA).
2. Electrophoresis-grade agarose.
3. Loading buffer type III: 0.25% bromophenol blue, 0.25% xylene cyanol FF, 30% glycerol in water.
4. Ethidium bromide: 10 mg/mL solution (Amresco, cat. # X328).
5. DNA mol wt markers.
6. Horizontal gel electrophoresis apparatus.
7. Gel-casting platform.
8. Gel combs.
9. DC power supply.

3. Methods

3.1. Double and Triple Labeling Studies by Immuno/Histochemical Techniques

3.1.1. Kidney Isolation

1. Mice are anesthetized and kidneys are harvested through an abdominal incision, then decapsulated and sectioned in 2-mm slices.
2. Kidney slices are rinsed in PBS.

3.1.2. X-Gal Reaction

1. Fix kidney slices in buffered formalin 10% for 15 min (*see* **Note 3**).
2. Wash in Lac-Z wash 3× 15 min each.
3. Place the tissues in staining solution overnight in the dark in an incubator at 37°C.
4. Wash in PBS 3× 15 min each.
5. Postfix in buffered formalin 10% at 4°C overnight.
6. Place in ethanol 70% until embedded in paraffin.

3.1.3. Paraffin Embedding and Tissue Sectioning

1. The tissue can be processed with an automated tissue-processing machine or manually through graded ethanols and xylenes.
2. After processing, the tissue is embedded in paraffin blocks.
3. Cut 5-µ tissue sections with a microtome.
4. Mount on charged glass slides.
5. Leave slides on a slide warmer at 37°C, overnight.

3.1.4. Double Immunostaining

1. Deparafinize and rehydrate tissue section by putting slides through:
   a. Xylene: 3 washes, 5 min each.
   b. 100% ethanol: 2 washes, 3 min each.
   c. 95% ethanol: 2 washes, 3 min each.
   d. 70% ethanol: 1 wash, 2 min.
   e. PBS: 5 min.
2. 3% peroxide in methanol (make fresh) 30 min.
3. PBS: 2 washes, 10 min each.
4. Prepare humidity chamber. Apply blocking serum for 20 min.
5. Remove as much of blocking serum as possible (with pipet or blotting paper). Apply primary antibody at appropriate dilution overnight in the cold room or 90 min at room temperature.
6. PBS: 2 washes, 10 min each.
7. Apply appropriate biotinylated antibody for 30 min.
8. PBS: 2 washes, 5 min each.
9. Apply ABC solution for 45 min. During this step, the DAB solution can be prepared. **Caution**: The DAB tablets should be handled with care, using gloves and under the hood because it is a suspected carcinogen (*see* **Note 1**).
10. PBS: 2 washes, 5 min each.
11. Apply DAB solution let stand ~10 sec or until the tissue turns slightly brown (*see* **Note 1**).
12. Running water, 2 min.
13. Microwave in Antigen Retrieval Solution: 1 min on P.50 with a 2-min time lapse between each min for 3×. After each minute of microwaving, replenish the evaporated antigen-retrieval solution with distilled water at room temperature.
14. Allow to cool to room temperature for 30 min.
15. PBS in cold room or on ice for 30 min.
16. Repeat from **steps 4–10** with the second primary antibody to test.
17. Apply and cover VIC Purple solution for no more than 3 min or until light purple (*see* **Note 1**).
18. Running water, 2 min.
19. Counterstain with Nuclear Fast Red for 2 min (*see* **Note 4**).
20. Running water for 2 min.

21. Dehydrate by:
    a. 95% Ethanol: 2 washes—1 dip each.
    b. 100% Ethanol: 3 washes—1 dip each.
    c. Xylene: 3 washes—1 dip each.
22. Apply one drop of mounting medium and then put the cover slip on.

3.2. Cell Aspiration and Single-Cell RT-PCR from Embryonic Kidneys

3.2.1. Organ Culture Dishes Setup

1. The organ culture dishes have a central compartment. To this, 1.5 mL of organ culture medium is added.
2. Over the medium, a membrane filter is placed, which immediately soaks up the medium.
3. Over the membrane filter, the membrane from the cell-culture insert is placed. The cell-culture inserts come as a cup, at the bottom of which the membrane is present. Using a sterile surgical blade, the membrane is cut along the edge all around. Then with a sterile forceps, the membrane is carefully placed over the membrane filter.
4. Around the central compartment there is a moat. Add 2 mL of tissue culture water to this moat. This creates a humidity chamber and prevents drying up of kidneys.

3.2.2. Dissection of Embryonic Kidneys

1. To obtain embryonic kidneys for the analysis of single cells, adult male mice are mated with females in the late afternoon. Females are checked for the presence of a vaginal plug the following morning, considering that moment as embryonic d 0 (E0).
2. Pregnant females (at E11) are anesthetized, the uterus is opened and the embryo covered by its membranes is removed and placed into a 35-mm tissue-culture dish containing organ-culture medium.
3. Using a dissection microscope (×7 magnification) and fine forceps, remove the membranes, carefully tearing them open.
4. With one forceps, hold the embryo below the armpits, and with a small scissors cut off the anterior half of the embryo. Then make a cut along the ventral midline of the posterior. Half hold the embryo down with one forceps, and with another forceps scoop out entrails. The genital ridges are then visible. Insert tip of forceps closed below the genital ridges and dorsal aorta, then allow the forceps to open very gently to separate the aorto-gonado-meso/metanephric area and transfer it to a new dish with fresh medium.
5. Next, the gonads and aorta are carefully removed, and the embryonic kidneys are transferred to the organ-culture dish and placed over the membrane.
6. The culture dishes with the embryonic kidneys are placed in a 37°C, 5% CO_2 incubator until the cell picker is adjusted.

3.2.3. Cell Aspirations

3.2.3.1. PIPET PREPARATION

1. The pipets are backfilled with 2 µL of RNA lysis buffer using the microloader tips.

3.2.3.2. PICO-INJECTOR ADJUSTMENT

1. Turn on nitrogen flow.
2. Turn on Pico-Injector (stylus) movement control box. Ensure fine-tuning dials for depth are turned so that no horizontal lines are seen on the stick (*see* **Note 5**).
3. Attach pipet to the piper holder (*see* **Note 6**).
4. Check pressures on each channel (pipet must be installed on picker).
   a. P clear (pressure used to evacuate the pipet content completely).
      i. Target 105 psi. If needed adjustment, adjust fine-tuning black knob on nitrogen gas tank.
   b. P inject (pressure used to evacuate the cell or inject into a cell).
      i. Target 4.2–4.5 psi. Adjust with P inject knob on pressure-control console.
   c. P balance (pressure applied through pipet to keep liquid from coming into pipet when neither suction or injection is desired).
      i. Target = 0.9 psi. Adjust with P balance knob on pressure-control console.

3.2.3.3. ASPIRATION

1. The filter with the kidney is removed from the culture dish and transferred to a 35-mm tissue-culture dish.
2. 100–200 µL of organ culture medium is added over the kidneys and under the membrane (*see* **Note 7**).
3. The pipet (already backfilled with 2 µL of lysis buffer) is filled with medium up to about 1.5-cm length of the pipet using the "Fill" button.
4. Focus on cells. Position the pipet so the tip is just below the surface of medium.
5. Move the pipet roughly into focus with the joystick, fine-tune with dials.
6. Identify the candidate cell. Position the pipet beside the cell.
7. Hit the Fill button on the console to pick the cell.
8. Disconnect the stylus from the holder.
9. The tip of the pipet containing the cell is immediately broken off into a 0.6 µL microfuge tube containing 8 µL of lysis buffer, and is snap frozen in liquid nitrogen.
10. The tubes are transferred to a –80 freezer for further processing (*see* **Note 8**).

3.2.4. Single-Cell RT-PCR

3.2.4.1. REVERSE TRANSCRIPTION REACTION

1. 1 µL (0.5 µg) oligo (dT) is added to the cell aspirate.
2. The solution is heated 5 min at 65°C and chilled on ice to anneal the primer.
3. The RT reaction is performed in a 20-µL final vol: contains 11 µL of cell lysate + oligo (dT), 4 µL of 5X RT buffer (final concentration = 1X), 2 µL of 2.5 mM dNTP (final concentration = 0.25 m*M*), 2 µL (400 U) of MMLV RT, and 1 µL water.

4. Reactions are incubated at 23°C for 10 min, 42°C for 60 min, 94°C for 10 min, and then soaked at 4°C.
5. RT reactions are stored at –20°C until use.

3.2.4.2. PCR Amplification

1. Prepare for the first PCR the reaction mix containing 1X PCR buffer, 0.1 m*M* dNTPs, and 1.5 U of *Taq* DNA Polymerase plus the appropriate concentration of outer primers and $MgCl_2$ for the marker in question (*see* **Note 9**). The total vol for each reaction is 50 µL. Add the mix to a microfuge tube.
2. Add template cDNA (*see* **Note 10**).
3. Pulse-spin the tubes and transfer to PCR thermal cycler.
4. Adjust the cycling parameters to the outer primers of the marker in question. Perform 40 cycles.
5. For the second PCR reaction, prepare the PCR mix containing 1X PCR buffer, 0.1 m*M* dNTPs, and 1.5 U of *Taq* DNA Polymerase plus the appropriate concentration of inner (nested) primers and $MgCl_2$ for the marker in question (*see* **Note 9**). The total vol for each reaction is also 50 µL. Add 30 µL of the mix to a microfuge tube.
6. Add 20 µL of the first PCR reaction as the template.
7. Pulse-spin the tubes and transfer to PCR thermal cycler.
8. Adjust the cycling parameters to the inner (nested) primers of the marker in question. Perform 40 cycles.

3.2.4.3. Agarose Gel Electrophoresis

1. The 1% agarose gel in 1X TAE buffer is prepared in advance: 1 g of electrophoresis-quality agarose is added to 100 mL of 1X TAE buffer and heated until dissolved. Then 10 µL of ethidium bromide is added. Once cooled, the solution is poured into a gel cast, and a comb is applied. The gel is allowed to solidify for approx 1 h before the edges and comb are removed.
2. The cast gel is placed in a horizontal gel electrophoresis apparatus and covered with 1X TAE buffer to approx 2 mm above the surface of the gel.
3. Equal aliquots of DNA in small volumes of loading buffer are added to the wells. One well is for loading buffer containing DNA markers. The DNA is electrophoresed at constant voltage (1–5 V/cm of gel) until the bromophenol blue dye has migrated a distance sufficient for separation of the DNA fragments.
4. The DNA can be visualized by placing the gel on a UV light source, and the gel can be photographed.

4. Notes

1. The peroxidase substrates recommended for double-immunostaining and in combination with the X-Gal reaction are the DAB (brown color) and the Vector VIP (purple color). These colors can be easily distinguished from each other, and also from the blue product obtained by the histochemical reaction for β-galactosidase. With the first antibody to test, the peroxidase substrate used should be the DAB

because it will resist the Antigen retrieval step (microwaving in the antigen retrieval solution), whereas if the Vector VIP is used first, the color will be bleached during this step. Vector VIP should be prepared immediately before use. The color-developing step should be closely monitored, too much time of exposure to the peroxidase substrate can cause background. To avoid background, SIGMA FAST tablets can be diluted in 2 mL of distilled water instead of in 1 mL.

2. The success of microaspirations depends mostly on the performance of the pipets used. Pipets can be made in the lab with a pipet puller the day before the experiment. The pipet puller can be horizontal (Sutter Instrument, Inc.) or vertical (David Kopf Instrument). The tip diameter should be from 5–15 μm, but smaller diameters are recommended to aspirate the cell content and larger diameters to aspirate the whole cell. The pipets can also be purchased. The World Precision Instrument Company can configure the pipets as needed (borosilicate, long shank, required tip diameter), and they can also autoclave them.

3. Fixation time should be reduced to 10 min in newborn and late-gestation kidneys and to 5 min in early embryonic kidneys. Fixation time that is too long will kill the β-galactosidase, preventing the X-gal reaction from occurring.

4. The counterstaining step with Nuclear Fast Red can be avoided if the antigens to test are widely expressed, but if the antigens have low expression, the counterstaining can help to identify morphological structures.

5. This is the highest point for fine depth control, and allows you to maneuver the full range down once crude depth has been set.

6. Ensure that rubber gasket is in place in holder, or the pipet will be blown out with air flow.

7. The kidney should never be immersed in medium, as this can interfere with visualization of the cells during aspirations.

8. RT reaction on samples should be done on the day of isolation. If samples are stored at –80°C for more than 24 h, they usually turn negative for any cell marker. RT reaction is performed directly in the aspirated cell sample without previously extracting the RNA.

9. The concentration of primers usually varies from 0.25–0.5 μM, and the concentration of $MgCl_2$ from 0.5–2.1 mM.

10. 2–20 μL of the RT reaction are used as template in the first PCR reaction, depending on the abundance of the mRNA to be detected.

Acknowledgments

We thank Daniel R. Chernavvsky for critically reading the manuscript and for his advice on the single-cell section. Dr. Sequeira Lopez is a Howard Hughes Medical Institute Physician Postdoctoral Fellow.

References

1. Sequeira Lopez, M. L., Pentz, E. S., Robert, B., Abrahamson, D. R., and Gomez, R. A. (2001) Embryonic origin and lineage of juxtaglomerular cells. *Am. J. Physiol. Renal Physiol.* **281,** 345–356.

2. Robert, B., St John, P. L., Hyink, D. P., and Abrahamson, D. R. (1996) Evidence that embryonic kidney cells expressing flk-1 are intrinsic, vasculogenic angioblasts. *Am. J. Physiol.* **271,** F744–F753.
3. Hyink, D. P., Tucker, D. C., St John, P. L., Leardkamolkarn, V., Accavitti, M. A., Abrass, C. K., et al. (1997) Endogenous origin of glomerular endothelial and mesangial cells in grafts of embryonic kidneys. *Am. J. Physiol.* **270,** F886–F899.
4. Herzlinger, D., Koseki, C., Mikawa, T., and al-Awqati, Q. (1992) Metanephric mesenchyme contains multipotent stem cells whose fate is restricted after induction. *Development* **114,** 565–572.
5. Srinivas, S., Goldberg, M. R., Watanabe, T., D'Agati, V., al-Awqati, Q., and Costantini, F. (1999) Expression of green fluorescent protein in the ureteric bud of transgenic mice: a new tool for the analysis of ureteric bud morphogenesis. *Dev. Genet.* **24,** 241–251.
6. Taugner, R. and Hackenthal, E. (1989) The juxtaglomerular apparatus: structure and function. Springer Verlag, Heidelberg, pp. 1–3.
7. Schlaeger, T. M., Bartunkova, S., Lawitts, J. A., Teichmann, G., Risau, W., Deutsch, U., et al. (1997) Uniform vascular-endothelial-cell-specific gene expression in both embryonic and adult transgenic mice. *Proc. Natl. Acad. Sci. USA* **94,** 3058–3063.
8. Motoike, T., Loughna, S., Perens, E., Roman, B. L., Liao, W., Chau, T. C., et al. (2000) Universal GFP reporter for the study of vascular development. *Genesis* **28,** 75–81.
9. Shalaby, F., Rossant, J., Yamaguchi, T. P., Gertsenstein, M., Wu, X. F., Breitman, M. L., et al. (1995) Failure of blood-island formation and vasculogenesis in Flk-1-deficient mice. *Nature* **376,** 62–66.
10. Pentz, E. S., Lopez, M. L., Kim, H. S., Carretero, O., Smithies, O., and Gomez, R. A. (2001) Ren1d and Ren2 cooperate to preserve homeostasis: evidence from mice expressing GFP in place of Ren1d. *Physiol. Genomics* **6,** 45–55.
11. Kisanuki, Y. Y., Hammer, R. E., Miyazaki, J., Williams, S. C., Richardson, J. A., and Yanagisawa, M. (2001) Tie2-Cre transgenic mice: a new model for endothelial cell-lineage analysis in vivo. *Dev. Biol.* **230,** 230–242.
12. Guy, L. G., Kothary, R., DeRepentigny, Y., Delvoye, N., Ellis, J., and Wall, L. (1996) The beta-globin locus control region enhances transcription of but does not confer position-independent expression onto the lacZ gene in transgenic mice. *EMBO J.* **15,** 3713–3721.
13. Soriano, P. (1999) Generalized lacZ expression with the ROSA26 Cre reporter strain. *Nat. Genet.* **21,** 70–71.
14. Lobe, C. G., Koop, K. E., Kreppner, W., Lomeli, H., Gertsenstein, M., and Nagy, A. (1999) Z/AP, a double reporter for cre-mediated recombination. *Dev. Biol.* **208,** 281–292.
15. Novak, A., Guo, C., Yang, W., Nagy, A., and Lobe, C. G. (2000) Z/EG, a double reporter mouse line that expresses enhanced green fluorescent protein upon Cre-mediated excision. *Genesis* **28,** 147–155.

14

Transient Transfection Assays
for Analysis of Signal Transduction in Renal Cells

Robin L. Maser, Brenda S. Magenheimer,
Christopher A. Zien, and James P. Calvet

1. Introduction

Functional analysis of plasma-membrane receptors often involves the ectopic expression of receptor constructs in cultured cell lines followed by assay of the activation of cytosolic or nuclear signaling targets *(1)*. Although in the simplest cases full-length receptors are expressed and subsequently activated by ligand binding, this is not always feasible or desirable. For example, it may not be possible to clone and/or express the full-length receptor. There are also cases in which the ligand is unknown. It may also be desirable to examine the function of only a portion of the receptor, or to put a receptor under the control of an unrelated ligand. In these cases, the development of assays for receptor function can involve the cloning of fusion constructs that express membrane-targeted chimeric-receptor proteins.

In studies of the function of polycystin-1, we *(2)* and others *(3–6)* have found that fusion constructs expressing the C-terminal cytosolic tail of the polycystin-1 protein signal to downstream targets in a constitutively active fashion, making it possible to study receptor function using relatively small chimeric proteins. This chapter examines the construction of fusion-protein expression plasmids, and describes the methods used for transient transfection of cultured renal cells and for determining the expression of the transfected constructs by Western blotting. Activation of signaling targets by transfected fusion proteins usually requires cotransfection of the protein targets or promoter-reporter constructs, and the further dissection of signaling pathways can involve the cotransfection of additional wild-type or dominant-negative constructs. The introduction of multiple expression constructs can

From: *Methods in Molecular Medicine, vol. 86: Renal Disease: Techniques and Protocols*
Edited by: M. S. Goligorsky © Humana Press Inc., Totowa, NJ

be problematic, and must be done with an awareness of what each of the DNA constructs and/or the proteins expressed from these constructs is doing to the expression of the others. This chapter also describes assays used to monitor the function of the polycystin-1 fusion proteins, including the use of reporter assays for c-Jun N-terminal kinase (JNK) and AP-1, and immune-complex in vitro kinase assays for JNK.

1.1. Expression Vectors

The type of expression vector used for fusion-protein production is an important consideration. Some of the factors to consider when choosing a vector are: the origins of replication (both bacterial and eukaryotic); the selection markers (both bacterial and eukaryotic); and the eukaryotic promoter.

It is important to consider the type of bacterial origin of replication (ori), since vectors with a pUC-derived ori (pcDNA3 series; Invitrogen, Carlsbad, CA), as opposed to a ColE1 ori (pcDNA1.1/Amp; Invitrogen), result in very high plasmid DNA yields (>100 µg DNA per 40–50 mL Midi prep) from bacteria grown in rich broth, thus requiring less time for DNA isolation. Eukaryotic cells carrying the SV40 large T-antigen (e.g., HEK293T cells) efficiently replicate expression vectors with an SV40 origin of replication, resulting in high plasmid copy number and fusion-protein production. This feature can have both advantages and disadvantages. Although very high levels of fusion-protein expression can be achieved (especially when expression is driven by a strong promoter), replication of the vector can also result in very high DNA copy numbers, leading to competition for transcription factors (*see* **Subheading 3.2.**).

With newer expression vectors, the bacterial selection marker is usually ampicillin- or kanamycin-resistance, which can be used in most generic bacterial strains. It is important to consider that some of the older vectors (e.g., pCDM series) with more difficult selection systems such as supF/kanamycin require dual-plating schemes and special bacterial strains. For transient transfections, a eukaryotic selection marker (e.g., neomycin-resistance) is not necessary. However, if one decides at a later date to generate cell lines that stably express the fusion protein, it can be convenient to have this selection marker present in your construct. The most common eukaryotic promoter used in expression vectors is cytomegalovirus (CMV). Other promoters include SV40, RSV, and thymidine kinase (TK). These promoters have different activity levels in different cell lines. One can determine which promoters have weaker or stronger activity in a cell line of interest by testing them with the various promoter-Renilla luciferase or β-galactosidase-reporter vectors that are available. For example, in HEK293T cells, promoter strength increases in the following sequence: TK< SV40< CMV< RSV.

1.2. Fusion-Protein Construction

Membrane-targeted fusion proteins should have a signal sequence at the N-terminus, followed by a protein region that is normally extracellular, such as the ectodomain of a cell-surface receptor. It is also helpful to have a convenient epitope on the extracellular side, such as the heavy-chain constant (CH) regions of human IgG for which there are commercially available antibodies. This region also directly binds Protein A. Otherwise, it may be helpful to add one of the commonly used epitope tags, such as Myc, HA, and 6x His *(7)*. The fusion protein also requires the appropriate number of transmembrane domains (an odd number) for proper inside-out polarity. These can be supplied from exogenous sources, such as from the CD7 protein. The cytosolic side of the fusion-protein contains the receptor sequences of interest.

For our studies of polycystin-1 signaling, we have utilized two types of membrane-directed fusion protein constructs *(2)*. The first, utilizing the sIg.7 cassette *(3)*, includes the signal sequence of the CD5 protein, the CH2 and CH3 domains of human IgG, and the transmembrane domain of the CD7 protein cloned in-frame with the C-terminal 222 amino acid residues of murine polycystin-1 (sIg.7-LT222). The second type utilizes the endogenous transmembrane domains of polycystin-1, and consists of the CD5 signal peptide and the IgG domains cloned in-frame with the C-terminal 1,283 residues of polycystin-1 (sIg-11TM). For fusion-protein controls, we have developed a sIg.7 protein lacking polycystin-1 sequences and a sIg-11TMstop that contains an in-frame translation termination codon following the first transmembrane domain in sIg-11TM. Use of a fusion-protein control with an in-frame stop codon allows you to transfect cells with equal DNA amounts for the fusion protein and control protein constructs. This will achieve equal numbers of DNA molecules (moles) for the two constructs, and thus will provide equal numbers of promoters in the transfected cells. In some systems, it seems to be important to balance the promoter numbers so as to not unduly affect the expression of cotransfected reporter constructs by competition for transcription factors (*see* **Subheading 3.2.**). Alternatively, empty expression vector can serve as the control for your fusion protein.

1.3. Transient Transfection

A number of cell types are easy to maintain in culture, and provide high transfection efficiency. We have carried out most of our studies with HEK293T cells (American Type Culture Collection) because of their rapid growth, high transfection efficiency, and high fusion-protein expression when using vectors containing SV40 origins of replication. The following is our calcium-phosphate transfection protocol, which is based on that of Chen and Okayama *(8)*.

Detailed methods for luciferase assays and for kinase assays are provided in separate sections (**Subheadings 3.2.** and **3.4.**, respectively).

2. Materials

2.1. Transient Transfection

2.1.1. Supplies for Transient Transfection

1. Good-quality flasks and plates.
2. Sterile 1.5-mL Eppendorf tubes.
3. Sterile 15-mL and 50-mL screw-cap conical tubes.

2.1.2. Constructs

1. Appropriate chimeric fusion-protein constructs (*see* **Subheading 2.2.3.**).
2. Appropriate promoter-luciferase reporter construct (*see* **Subheading 2.2.3.**), or signaling target construct (*see* **Subheading 2.2.3.**).

2.1.3. Solutions and Reagents

1. Dulbecco's Modified Eagle's Medium (DMEM)-complete (4.5 g/L glucose) + penicillin (500 U/L)-streptomycin (0.5 mg/L) (P/S) + 10% heat-inactivated fetal bovine serum (FBS) (for maintaining cells and for transfection).
2. DMEM (4.5 g/L glucose) without P/S and FBS (for JNK and AP-1 studies).
3. Sterile phosphate-buffered saline (PBS).
4. 1x Trypsin/Tris/ethylenediaminetetraacetic acid (EDTA) in PBS (diluted from 10X stock; Sigma).
5. $2\ M\ CaCl_2$.
6. 2X HEPES buffered saline: 42 mM HEPES, 274 mM NaCl, 10 mM KCl, 1.8 mM Na_2HPO_4, pH 7.1.
7. Sterile, filtered H_2O (to dilute DNA).

2.2. Promoter-Reporter Assays

2.2.1. Supplies for Promoter-Reporter Assay

1. Luminometer (*see* **Note 4**).
2. Luminometer tubes.

2.2.2. Supplies for Western Blot Analysis

1. Mini-Protean II gel electrophoresis/transfer system (BioRad).
2. Immobilon P (PVDF membrane) (Millipore).

2.2.3. Constructs

1. sIg.7 (control) or sIg.7-LT222 (polycystin-1 tail) at 3 μg/225 μL transfection mix.
2. AP-1 *cis*-reporting construct (Stratagene) at 1 μg/225 μL transfection mix.
3. c-Jun Trans-Reporting System (Stratagene):
   a. GAL4 c-Jun at 50 ng/225 μL transfection mix.
   b. GAL4 Luc at 1 μg/225 μL transfection mix.

4. Renilla luciferase (Promega) at 5 ng/225 μL transfection mix.
5. pBluescript (Stratagene) (used to fill to 7 μg/225 μL transfection mix).

2.2.4. Solutions and Reagents

2.2.4.1. FOR PROMOTER-REPORTER ASSAY

1. PBS.
2. Dual-Luciferase Reporter Assay System (Promega):
   a. Passive lysis buffer.
   b. Luciferase assay buffer.
   c. Stop & Glo reagent.

2.2.4.2. FOR WESTERN BLOT ANALYSIS

1. SDS sample loading buffer ($1x = 62$ mM Tris, pH 6.8, 2% sodium dodecyl sulfate (SDS), 100 mM DTT, 10% glycerol, 0.05 mg bromophenol blue).
2. PVDF transfer buffer (25 mM Tris, 192 mM glycine, 0.1% SDS, 20% methanol).
3. TBST (10 mM Tris, pH 7.5, 150 mM NaCl, 0.1% Tween-20).
4. Anti-human IgG-alkaline phosphatase (AP) conjugated antibody (Jackson ImmunoResearch).
5. Chemi buffer (0.1 M diethanolamine, pH 9.5, 1 mM MgCl$_2$) and/or AP developing buffer (100 mM NaCl, 5 mM MgCl$_2$, 100 mM Tris, pH 9.5).
6. CDP-Star (Amersham) and/or BCIP and NBT (Sigma).

2.3. Immune Kinase Assay

2.3.1. Supplies for Immune Kinase Assay

1. Gel dryer.
2. Phosphorimager.

2.3.2. Supplies for Western Blot Analysis

1. Mini-Protean II gel electrophoresis/transfer system (BioRad).
2. Immobilon P (PVDF membrane) (Millipore).

2.3.3. Constructs

1. sIg.7 (control) or sIg.7-LT222 (polycystin-1 tail) (*see* **Subheading 2.2.3.**).
2. HA-tagged wild-type Jun-N terminal kinase (JNK) construct.
3. pBluescript (Stratagene).

2.3.4. Immune Kinase Assay

2.3.4.1. FOR IMMUNE KINASE ASSAY

1. PBS.
2. JNK lysis buffer: 20 mM Tris-HCl, pH 7.4, 137 mM NaCl, 25 mM β-glycerophosphate, 2 mM EDTA, 1 mM Na$_3$VO$_4$, 2 mM sodium pyrophosphate, 1% Triton X-100, 10% glycerol, 5 μg/mL leupeptin, 5 μg/mL aprotinin, 2 mM benzamidine, 0.5 mM DTT, and 1 mM PMSF.

3. JNK kinase buffer: 25 mM Hepes, pH 7.4, 25 mM β-glycerophosphate, 25 mM MgCl$_2$, 0.1 mM Na$_3$VO$_4$, and 0.5 mM DTT.
4. BCA protein assay kit (Pierce).
5. Protein A/G Sepharose beads (Santa Cruz Biotechnology).
6. Anti-HA (F-7) antibody (Santa Cruz Biotechnology).
7. γ^{32}P-ATP (6,000 Ci/mmol) (Perkin-Elmer) and cold ATP.
8. GST c-Jun (1–79) fusion protein (Stratagene).

2.3.4.2. WESTERN BLOT ANALYSIS

1. SDS sample loading buffer (1X): 62 mM Tris-HCl, pH 6.8, 2% SDS, 100 mM DTT, 10% glycerol, 0.05 mg bromophenol blue.
2. PVDF transfer buffer: 25 mM Tris, 192 mM glycine, 0.1% SDS, 20% methanol.
3. TBST: 10 mM Tris-HCl, pH 7.5, 150 mM NaCl, 0.1% Tween-20.
4. Anti-human IgG-alkaline phosphatase (AP) conjugated antibody (Jackson ImmunoResearch).
5. Anti-JNK1 (C-17) antibody (Santa Cruz Biotechnology).
6. Goat anti-rabbit IgG-AP conjugated (Sigma).
7. Gel staining solution (40% methanol, 10% acetic acid, and 0.1% Coomassie Brilliant Blue R-250).
8. Chemi buffer: 0.1 M diethanolamine, pH 9.5, 1 mM MgCl$_2$ and/or AP developing buffer (100 mM NaCl, 5 mM MgCl$_2$, 100 mM Tris-HCl, pH 9.5).
9. CDP-Star (Amersham) and/or BCIP and NBT (Sigma).

3. Methods

3.1. Transient Transfection

Day 1: Feed cells: Cells are maintained in T75 flasks. Feed cells 1 d before passaging on d 2. Culture should be about 50% confluent at this time.

Day 2: Passage cells: Remove medium, rinse cells once with 5 mL PBS, rinse with 2 mL trypsin solution per T75 flask, add 1 mL trypsin solution per T75, and leave at room temperature for ~2–4 min. Add 10 mL DMEM-complete to cells and transfer to 50-mL screw cap tube. Count cells on hemocytometer, spin down cells, and resuspend in medium at 1.5 × 10^6 cells per mL (*see* **Note 1**). To 6-well plate containing 0.8 mL medium per well, add 0.5 mL of cells per well and rock plate to evenly disperse cells (*see* **Note 2**).

Day 3: Transfect cells: Prepare DNA mixes (7–12 μg DNA/225 μL total vol for 3 wells; 14–24 μg DNA/450 μL total vol for 6 wells; *see* **Subheading 3.2.** and **Note 3**) in 1.5 mL tubes. To 225 μL DNA mix, add 30 μL 2 M CaCl$_2$. To 15-mL screw cap tubes, add 250 μL 2X HEPES buffered saline (for 3 wells). Bubble HEPES buffered saline with air, and at the same time add DNA/CaCl$_2$ mix dropwise with Pasteur pipet. Continue bubbling for ~5 sec longer. Place tubes on ice for >10 min. Add 150 μL of DNA precipitates per well dropwise. Rock plate gently after addition to each well. Check for precipitate formation with a microscope before placing cells back in incubator. Allow transfection to proceed at 37°C for 4 h. Aspirate medium and replace with 2 mL of medium required for the specific experiment (e.g., DMEM without P/S and FBS for JNK and AP-1 studies).

Day 4: Harvest cells: Following transfection, the cells are harvested and lysed either for luciferase assays (*see* **Subheading 3.2.**) or for kinase assays (*see* **Subheading 3.4.**) and for Western blot analysis (*see* **Subheadings 3.3.** and **3.4.**).

3.2. Promoter-Reporter Assays

One convenient method to assay the activation of signaling pathways is to make use of commercially available promoter-reporter constructs as signaling end points. Alternatively, one can make use of any promoter (or promoter region) cloned upstream of a suitable reporter.

Stratagene has a collection of *cis-* and *trans-*reporting systems for assaying a number of signaling pathways. The *cis-*reporting system, which is used to measure the activation of a signaling pathway, consists of a number of tandem enhancer sequences upstream of a TATA box and a green fluorescent protein (GFP) or luciferase reporter. The *trans-*system is used to measure the activation of a specific transcription factor. It consists of two constructs: one expressing the GAL4 DNA-binding domain fused to the activation domain of a transcription factor, and the other containing GAL4-binding elements, TATA box, and reporter. In our studies of polycystin signaling, we have utilized a 7x AP-1 *Cis*-Reporting System and a c-Jun *Trans*-Reporting System (Stratagene).

1. Transfect as described in **Subheading 3.1.**, considering the total amount of DNA being transfected (*see* **Note 5**), the relative amounts of each of the DNAs (**Note 6**), and the numbers of competing promoters (**Note 7**). For these experiments, we plate 7.5×10^5 HEK293T cells per well of a 6-well plate.
2. To harvest cells, aspirate medium, wash cells twice with cold PBS (not sterile), add 250 µL per well of lysis buffer (1× Passive Lysis Buffer for Dual-Luciferase assay) and rock for 10 min. Scrape cells off wells, transfer each to a 1.5-mL tube and freeze on dry ice. Tubes can be stored at –80°C or assayed immediately. Thaw samples in cool water. Vortex and pipet 20 µL into tubes for the luminometer and refreeze sample for Western analysis (*see* **Subheading 3.3.**).
3. For each 20-µL aliquot of lysate, add 50 µL of Luciferase assay buffer, pipet up and down twice, place in the luminometer, and read firefly luciferase for 10 sec. Remove the sample tube from the luminometer, add 50 µL of Stop & Glo Reagent to the sample and vortex, place in the luminometer, and read Renilla luciferase for 10 sec (**Note 4**).
4. Analysis of data: Each experiment should include an untransfected (cells only) control. To evaluate whether the control construct (e.g., sIg.7) has intrinsic activity, compare it with a mock-transfected control. Import the luciferase data into a

spreadsheet program, and plot data as relative luciferase units (RLUs) (firefly luciferase activity/Renilla luciferase activity). Renilla luciferase is included as an internal transfection control to measure variations between triplicates, and between different experimental conditions. Variations in the internal control must be noted when drug/agonist/inhibitor treatments are performed or when several DNA constructs are transfected. If the internal control changes with a particular treatment or with a certain DNA construct, it may be the result of an effect by that treatment or by the expression of that DNA construct on the expression of Renilla luciferase. In these cases, it may not be appropriate to express the data as RLUs. Instead, the internal control can be used to normalize the triplicate wells to each other by: i) averaging the Renilla values for the three wells, ii) dividing the Renilla values for each well into the average to generate a normalized Renilla value, and iii) multiplying the firefly luciferase values for each well by the normalized Renilla value. In this case, the average normalized firefly luciferase activity is plotted for each condition (*see* **Note 8**).

3.3. Western Blot Analysis

It is important to do Western blots following each transfection to verify the uniform expression of the fusion-protein construct and any other cotransfected constructs from sample to sample (*see* **Note 9**).

1. Thaw cell lysates quickly in room temperature water and place on ice (*see* **Note 10**). To an aliquot of the lysate (*see* **Note 11**), add an appropriate amount of 2X or 5X SDS sample loading buffer (to 1X final), and boil for 3 min (*see* **Note 12**).
2. Electrophorese lysates in a 10% polyacrylamide/SDS minigel at 100V through the stacking gel and at 200 V through the resolving gel.
3. Equilibrate gel and PVDF membrane in transfer buffer for 30–60 min. Transfer gel to PVDF membrane in ice-cold transfer buffer at 20V overnight at 4°C in a coldbox or cold room. Alternatively, the gel can be transferred at 100 V for 1 h at 4°C packed in ice.
4. Block PVDF membrane in TBST + 5% nonfat dry milk for 1 h. Incubate blot with 1:10,000 dilution of anti-human IgG-AP antibody (*see* **Note 13**) in TBST/milk for 1 h with agitation (on rotating or rocking platform). Wash blot 3–4 times for 10 min each in an excess of TBST.
5. For chemiluminescent development, equilibrate blot in Chemi buffer for 2 × 5 min. Place blot on plastic sheet and cover with CDP-Star substrate for 5 min. Let excess CDP-Star run off the blot, place blot between two sheets of plastic, and squeegee excess substrate off blot (*see* **Note 14**). Expose blots to blue X-ray film (X-Omat Blue; Kodak) in dark room, and develop film. A 1-min exposure is usually a good starting point, and can be used to determine the appropriate exposure.
6. Alternatively, for color (chromagenic) development of the blot, equilibrate blot in AP developing buffer for 2 × 5 min. Add substrates, BCIP (5-bromo-4-chloro-3-indolyl phosphate) and NBT (nitroblue tetrazolium) to AP buffer and add to blot. Let color develop until dark purple bands appear (anywhere from 30 sec to

overnight). Stop color development by washing blot in water for a few minutes. Let blot air-dry, but protect from light since purple product can fade with light.

3.4. Immune Complex Kinase Assays

To determine whether a signaling pathway has been activated by a transfected fusion construct, the activation of intermediates in the signaling cascade can be assayed. In our studies with polycystin-1, we have examined the activation of c-Jun N-terminal kinase (JNK). Although the following assay has been optimized for the in vitro analysis of JNK, this general procedure can be used to determine the activity of a variety of kinases.

1. Transfect as described above (**Subheading 3.1.**), considering the total amount of DNA being transfected (*see* **Note 5**), the relative amounts of each of the DNAs (*see* **Note 6**), and the numbers of competing promoters (*see* **Note 7**). For these experiments, we plate 1.5×10^6 HEK293T cells per T25 flask. Cells are transfected with the desired DNAs (2.0 µg each per flask) and pBluescript as filler DNA up to a total of 7–12 µg per flask. 450 µL of DNA precipitates per flask is added, rocked to mix, and incubated at 37°C for 4 h (although this time can be lengthened if desired). The medium is aspirated and replaced with 4 mL DMEM without P/S and FBS, and the flasks are incubated at 37°C for 12–24 h.

2. To harvest cells, put flasks on ice, aspirate medium, wash cells twice with 2 mL cold PBS. Add 0.5 mL cold JNK lysis buffer, scrape cells, and transfer to chilled 1.5-mL tubes. Vortex tubes at 4°C for 30 sec, leave on ice 20 min. Vortex tubes again for 30 sec and centrifuge at 16,000*g* for 10 min at 4°C. Transfer supernatant to clean tubes and determine protein concentration using Pierce BCA protein assay kit. This supernatant will be used for both immunoprecipitation and Western blotting.

3. For immunoprecipitation, add 50 µL Protein A/G Sepharose beads per sample to a 1.5-mL tube, and pulse (a few sec) centrifuge to pellet beads. Remove liquid and wash beads twice with 0.5 mL lysis buffer (without the protease inhibitors), and once with lysis buffer with protease inhibitors. Add 0.5 mL JNK lysis buffer and 0.4 mg per sample anti-HA antibody.

4. Rotate the beads with antibody at 4°C for 45 min (although this time can be lengthened if desired). Pulse-centrifuge beads, remove liquid, add 110 µL (100 µL + 10 µL extra) JNK lysis buffer per sample, resuspend beads by inverting tube several times, and aliquot 100 µL into each 1.5-mL tube containing 200–500 mg total sample protein in a final vol of 500 µL (*see* **Note 15**).

5. Rotate the tubes at 4°C for 2–3 h. In cold room, pulse-centrifuge beads, remove liquid, wash beads 3× with 600 µL lysis buffer and twice with 600 µL JNK kinase buffer. After removing most of the liquid from the final wash, pulse-centrifuge the tubes again to get all remaining liquid to the bottom. Remove remaining liquid and place tubes on ice.

6. For the in vitro kinase assay, add to each sample of beads a 31-µL master mix containing 32 µ*M* cold ATP (1 µL), 8 µg GST c-Jun substrate (3 µL), and 5 µCi

γ-^{32} P-ATP (1 μL) in 26 μL JNK kinase buffer. Pipet solution up and down rapidly 10 times and incubate at 30°C for 5 min. Stop reaction by adding 31 μL 2X SDS sample buffer and place tubes on dry ice until all samples are completed.

7. Boil tubes 5 min, pulse-centrifuge tubes to pellet beads, and load 20–25 μL per lane on a 10% polyacrylamide/SDS minigel. Run gel at 150 V until all tracking dye runs out of gel. Stain gel for 30–60 min in 40% methanol, 10% acetic acid and 0.1% Coomassie brilliant blue R-250. Destain gel with 40% methanol and 10% acetic acid, changing the destain solution 3–4× (*see* **Note 16**). Dry the gel on filter paper and determine kinase activity using a phosphorimager (*see* **Note 17**).

8. Western blot analysis. It is important to do Western blots following each transfection to verify the uniform expression of the fusion protein construct and any other cotransfected constructs (*see* **Subheading 3.3.** for the general method; specific differences are listed below; **Note 9**).

   a. To equal amounts of protein (from crude cell lysate) add an equivalent vol of 2X SDS sample loading buffer and boil for 5 min.

   b. Add anti-JNK1 antibody (1:500 in fresh TBST/milk) and incubate for at least 1 h.

   c. Add secondary antibody (goat anti-rabbit IgG-AP) at a dilution of 1:20,000 in TBST + 5% nonfat dry milk. Incubate for 30 min.

   d. Incubate the membrane with CDP-Star for 5 min (*see* **Note 14**), and expose to x-ray film to identify the endogenous JNK (lower band) and HA-JNK (upper band) (*see* **Note 18**).

4. Notes

1. The optimal plating-cell number is determined by plating various numbers of cells (e.g., 0.1 to 1×10^6 cells per well) onto 6-well plates, transfecting with 1 μg of a GFP expression construct (Invitrogen) plus filler DNA, and looking for the plating-cell number that has the highest percentage of cells appearing green under fluorescence microscopy.

2. Cells can also be plated in T25 flasks (*see* **Subheading 3.4.**) at 1.5×10^6 cells per flask.

3. One of the most critical aspects of successful transfection-based experiments is the quality of the transfected DNA. Previously, only CsCl gradient-purified DNA was used in transfections, but now a number of vendors offer DNA isolation kits that yield transfectable DNA (e.g., Qiagen, GibcoBRL, BioRad), and there are different recommendations from different laboratories. We have been most successful with the BioRad Quantum Midi prep system (the Maxi prep system, produced more DNA, yet had a noticeable genomic DNA contamination). Be sure to follow the manufacturer's recommendations for culture volumes and optimal growth of bacteria (e.g., flask-to-liquid ratios of 5–10; inoculating from a single, freshly streaked colony; and <16 h growth time). One clear indication of a "bad" DNA preparation is when the Renilla luciferase activity drastically drops.

4. Single-tube luminometers are significantly more sensitive than plate-type luminometers.

5. To determine the optimal amount of total DNA, keep the amount of luciferase reporter constant and add increasing amounts of filler DNA (a vector without a eukaryotic promoter, such as pBluescript). Harvest the transfections and carry out the luciferase readings. The conditions with the highest luciferase readings will indicate the optimal total DNA amount.

6. Another consideration is the relative amount of each of the multiple DNA constructs within the transfection mix. The most important DNA construct should be at the highest concentration followed by amounts of DNA constructs in order of their importance. This will ensure that every cell that receives the luciferase reporter will also receive the other constructs.

7. One must be aware of the possibility of having too many copies (or unequal numbers of copies) of promoters, thus swamping out the available transcription factors or setting up competition for transcription factors. This becomes particularly important when attempting to transfect and express multiple proteins. Maximal levels of a promoter can be simply determined by transfecting increasing amounts of a fusion-protein construct and assaying levels of fusion-protein expression by Westerns, and noting when fusion-protein expression levels off. Competition between two promoters can be assayed in a similar fashion by using two protein-expression constructs with different promoters.

8. To be on the safe side, the firefly luciferase and Renilla luciferase values should be at least 10× higher than those of untransfected (cells only) or mock-transfected control cells.

9. Cotransfection of two expression constructs will sometimes result in one affecting the level of expression of the other, compared to a control sample that does not express a protein. This could lead to misinterpretation of the data, suggesting an experimental effect by one protein when it is actually caused by an increase or decrease in the other. These problems can be easily detected by Western blotting.

10. For most analyses, fusion-protein expression can be assayed directly from the Passive Lysis Buffer cell lysate. Addition of protease inhibitors (e.g., 1 m*M* PMSF, 1 μg/mL aprotinin and leupeptin) to the lysis buffer is not necessary (but should not affect luciferase activity measurements) if lysates are kept briefly on ice and refrozen in dry ice for storage at –70°C. Western blots are performed after the cell lysate has undergone at least one freeze-thaw cycle.

11. Volumes of cell lysates to be compared for fusion-protein production are determined based on the method used to report luciferase activity. If RLUs are used, one can calculate an average Renilla for the entire experiment and use the formula: average Renilla/sample Renilla × standard lysate volume. In deciding the amount of the standard lysate volume to use, keep in mind the total volume that the gel wells can hold and allow for addition of loading dye. If the average normalized firefly luciferase is used (*see* **Subheading 3.2.**), then one simply substitutes the average Renilla for each triplicate sample in the equation listed here. It is preferable to check at least two samples (or all three if space permits) from each experimental condition when determining relative fusion-protein expression levels.

12. If fusion protein tends to aggregate upon boiling (sometimes giving higher molecular weight bands or a smear in the Western analysis) or if fusion protein stays in the pellet (giving low yields of fusion protein), one can further extract the Passive Lysis Buffer cell lysates with a 1/6.25 vol of the following detergent mix: 6.25% Triton X-100, 3.1% Na deoxycholate (DOC), and 0.6% SDS (for a final concentration in lysate of 1% Triton, 0.5% DOC, 0.1% SDS). The detergent mix is added to each aliquot of cell lysate, vortexed, incubated on ice for 1 min, and spun 3 min at 16,000g in a 4°C microfuge (in coldbox or cold room) to pellet nuclei. The supernatant is removed and denatured by the addition of SDS sample loading buffer and heating at 37°C for 15 min. If chromosomal DNA interferes with sample loading, the samples can be vigorously vortexed immediately after boiling to shear the chromosomal DNA.

13. Fusion proteins containing the human IgG CH2-CH3 domains can be directly detected with an anti-human IgG-AP antibody using chemiluminescent or chromagenic assays, with no need for a secondary antibody. If other proteins have been cotransfected, additional gels should be run and assayed with primary and secondary antibodies (*see* **Subheading 3.4.**).

14. CDP-Star is very sensitive to the presence of scratches on the PVDF membrane caused by tweezers. Therefore, to avoid lines and scratches in the exposure, be very careful with the tweezers, touching only the edges of the blots.

15. The amount of protein used for immunoprecipitation will depend on the type of cells and the level of expression of the tagged enzyme. To aliquot beads, use pipet tips with the ends cut to avoid clogging the tip with beads. Also, resuspend beads before each sample is taken, since beads tend to settle rapidly.

16. Staining the gel will allow you to determine whether the protein samples were loaded equally. Destaining helps remove unincorporated radioactivity from the gel, and will lower background.

17. It is sometimes a good idea, but not necessary, to also carry out autoradiography.

18. Although the endogenous JNK band serves as a control for equal protein loading, it is important to check HA-JNK abundance, for uneven expression may affect interpretation of the kinase activity results.

References

1. Dohlman, H. G., Thorner, J., Caron, M. G., and Lefkowitz, R. J. (1991) Model systems for the study of seven-transmembrane-segment receptors. *Annu. Rev. Biochem.* **60**, 653–688.
2. Parnell, S. C., Magenheimer, B. S., Maser, R. L., Zien, C. A., Frischauf, A. M., and Calvet, J. P. (2002) Polycystin-1 Activation of c-Jun N-terminal kinase and AP-1 is mediated by heterotrimeric G proteins. *J. Biol. Chem.* **277**, 19,566–19,572.
3. Arnould, T., Kim, E., Tsiokas, L., Jochimsen, F., Gruning, W., Chang, J. D., et al. (1998) The polycystic kidney disease 1 gene product mediates protein kinase C alpha-dependent and c-Jun N-terminal kinase-dependent activation of the transcription factor AP-1. *J. Biol. Chem.* **273**, 6013–6018.

4. Kim, E., Arnould, T., Sellin, L. K., Benzing, T., Fan, M. J., Gruning, W., et al. (1999) The polycystic kidney disease 1 gene product modulates Wnt signaling. *J Biol. Chem.* **274,** 4947–4953.

5. Delmas, P., Nomura, H., Li, X., Lakkis, M., Luo, Y., Segal, Y., et al. (2002) Constitutive activation of G-proteins by polycystin-1 is antagonized by polycystin-2. *J. Biol. Chem.* **277,** 11,276–11,283.

6. Nickel, C., Benzing, T., Sellin, L., Gerke, P., Karihaloo, A., Liu, Z. X., et al. (2002) The polycystin-1 C-terminal fragment triggers branching morphogenesis and migration of tubular kidney epithelial cells. *J. Clin. Investig.* **109,** 481–489.

7. Koller, K. J., Whitehorn, E. A., Tate, E., Ries, T., Aguilar, B., Chernov-Rogan, T., et al. (1997) A generic method for the production of cell lines expressing high levels of 7-transmembrane receptors. *Anal. Biochem.* **250,** 51–60.

8. Chen, C. and Okayama, H. (1987) High-efficiency transformation of mammalian cells by plasmid DNA. *Mol. Cell. Biol.* **7,** 2745–2752.

IV

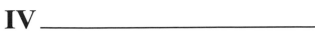

APPROACHES TO STUDY MOLECULAR MECHANISMS OF DISEASE

15

The Study of Gene Polymorphisms

How Complex Is Complex Genetic Disease?

Sylvia Bähring, Atakan Aydin, and Friedrich C. Luft

1. Introduction

1.1. Basic Definitions

What is a polymorphism? Strictly speaking, a polymorphism is the occurrence in a population of two or more genetically determined forms in such frequencies that the rarest of them could not be maintained by mutation alone. For our purposes, we are examining polymorphic DNA, so that the polymorphic information content is the amount of variation at a particular site in the DNA. When dealing with complex genetic diseases, particularly for mapping, we often rely on satellite DNA. Satellite DNA is a class of DNA sequences, that separates out on density-gradient centrifugation as a shoulder or "satellite" to the main peak of DNA. Satellite DNA corresponds to 10–15% of the DNA in the human genome consisting of tandemly repeated DNA sequences. Minisatellites (also termed variable numbers of tandem repeats, or VNTR) have repeat units 6–24 basepairs in length, and microsatellites have repeat units of only 1–4 basepairs in length. We rely on microsatellites. Microsatellite DNA consists of polymorphic variation in DNA sequences caused by VNTR of the dinucleotide CA, tri- or tetranucleotides. Microsatellites are generally less than 300 basepairs long. Fortunately for us, there are thousands of microsatellites scattered all along the genome. Every person on earth has microsatellites at precisely the same location as all other persons. However, the microsatellites vary (are polymorph) in terms of their length. A hypothetical example is shown in **Fig. 1**. The microsatellite is named D12S310, and is located on the short arm of chromosome 12. There are six variants that differ in their length. Every individual will have two of these variants, one on each copy of chromosome 12. The

From: *Methods in Molecular Medicine, vol. 86: Renal Disease: Techniques and Protocols*
Edited by: M. S. Goligorsky © Humana Press Inc., Totowa, NJ

Chromosome 12p Marker D12S310

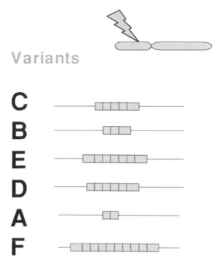

Fig. 1. A hypothetical example of a microsatellite marker is shown. D12S310 actually exists. Let us assume this microsatellite consists of six variants. They differ in terms of their length. CA tandem repeats are a common marker pattern. Each person on earth carries two of these markers on one or the other of their chromosomes 12. The variants can be amplified by the polymerase chain reaction and separated by means of electrophoresis. The longer variants travel more slowly in the gel than the shorter variants.

variants can be amplified with the polymerase chain reaction (PCR) and then separated by electrophoresis.

1.2. Gene Mapping

Now that we have dealt with these definitions, we can address the problem of mapping genes. Monogenic disease mapping is generally done by recruiting a large family or several families that harbor the disease. We conduct the search for microsatellite variants that are always inherited with the disease. The process of gene mapping relies on "linkage." Linkage is strictly defined as two loci situated close together on the same chromosome, the alleles of which are usually transmitted together in meiosis in gamete formation. The reasoning is that if the disease gene and the microsatellite marker variant are sufficiently close to one another, they will be inherited together without a recombination occurring in between. When we find such microsatellites, we assume that they are located close to the gene of interest. A statistical method is used to give us inference into how close they are located—namely the logarithm of the odds

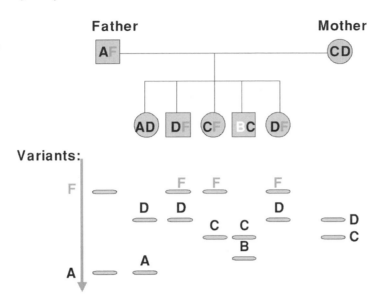

Fig. 2. A hypothetical family consisting of parents and their five children. Let us assume that the father harbors a disease gene located on the short arm of chromosome 12, directly next to the longest (F) variant of D12S310. On his other chromosome 12, he has the shortest variant (A) of D12S310. The mother has two different variants of D12S310. Each parent transmits one of the markers to each of the children. Can you pick out the child that cannot belong to the father?

ratio or LOD score. The LOD score describes the relative likelihood of two loci being linked. The score is a logarithm. In genetics, when the LOD score is >3, even the most bored and skeptical geneticists gradually develop interest.

A family tree is shown in **Fig. 2**. Let us assume that the father (square) has an autosomal-dominant disease. The mother (circle) is normal. The family has five children. Let us also assume the disease gene sits directly next to marker D12S310 on the short arm of chromosome 12. The father has two variants of D12S310: a long variant next to the disease gene, and on his other chromosome 12, he has a very short variant. The mother also has two variants of D12S310: one is a bit shorter than the long variant of the father, and the other is a bit longer than the short variant of the father. Each parent can transmit one of the variants to each of the children. Clearly, the children who inherit the long variant of D12S310 from the father will be affected by the disease. The electrophoresis gel runs from top to bottom. The short variants travel faster through the gel than the long variants. Can you select the children who are bound to be affected? Can you pick out the child who cannot belong to the father?

Microsatellites are favorite tools in forensic medicine because they enable "ownership" to be established as well as inheritance. O. J. Simpson was a lucky exception. The jurors evidently failed to appreciate this method of detection.

1.3. Sibpairs

To use linkage in complex genetics, we generally rely on affected sibling pairs (sibpairs). For instance, if both siblings have hypertension, we would assume that they both carry genetic variants, wherever they may be, that contribute to the hypertensive trait (phenotype). We gather as many affected sibling pairs as possible (identical-by-trait) and amplify microsatellites across the genome. The closer they are together (denser), the greater are our chances of finding linkage; however, the larger our grant must be to afford the analysis. Microsatellites are amplified from genomic DNA with the PCR and then fluorescent probes are used for genotyping. In our analysis, we look for spots along the genome, where many or hopefully most of our sibling pairs share marker variants. For a problem such as hypertension, 1000 or more sibling pairs would be necessary for a reasonable linkage analysis. Those performed to date have occasionally yielded LOD scores of >3. However, the scans seldom are in accord, and no new gene for essential hypertension has been found in man on the basis of a linkage analysis. Unfortunately, the same is true for almost all other complex genetic diseases. Do not despair, there may be other approaches.

To give our affected sibpair linkage analysis a bit more pep and power, we might try an identity-by-descent linkage analysis. We would still gather siblings, but would now need DNA from their parents. The parental DNA tells us where the allelic variants are coming from. This information is vitally important because it has a great influence on the informative nature of the alleles. Comparative details are given in **Fig. 3**. If we consider the mother to possess variants AB, and the father to possess CD, then we would expect 25% of the children to share both alleles in common, 25% no alleles in common, and 50% one of the alleles in common. Deviation from the expectation can be analyzed statistically. However, if we have no DNA from Mom and Dad, we are unable to determine what the distribution likelihood will be in the children and how many more pairs are necessary. Unfortunately, for conditions such as hypertension, the parents are already dead and their DNA is unavailable. This state of affairs complicates the problem.

We have used linkage analyses in analyzing dizygotic (DZ) twin pairs and their parents. The subjects are young, and therefore their parents were able to allow us access to DNA. Since blood pressure is a continuous variable and since the definition of hypertension changes relatively frequently, our analysis views blood pressure as continuous or quantitative, rather than a qualitative trait. Recruiting DZ twins has the distinct advantage of minimizing environmental

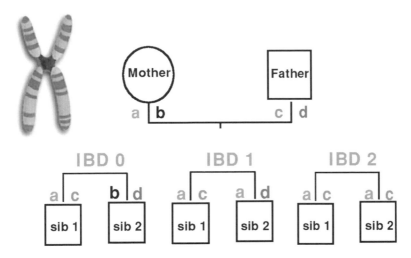

Fig. 3. Sib-pair linkage analysis can be either identical-by-state or identical-by-descent. If DNA is available from the parents, an identity-by-descent analysis is possible. By chance, if the parents both have different marker alleles, we would expect one-fourth of the offspring to share no alleles in common, one-half to share one allele in common, and one-fourth to share both alleles in common. Deviation from this expected statistic, increased sharing of marker alleles, may indicate the presence of linkage.

effects on the phenotype. However, DZ twins are rare and we do not have 1000 pairs. Thus, it is unlikely that we would achieve a LOD score of >3, although there are some exceptions. For instance, we mapped a locus on chromosome 3 as related to the phenomenon of DZ twinning, and achieved a LOD score considerably greater than three (*1*). Finally, if we examine gene loci of genes that have already been declared as candidates on the basis of other criteria, the LOD scores are not as stringent as they would be if we were operating blindly.

1.4. Association

Pundits point out that "getting there is half the fun." In terms of complex disease genetics, "getting there,"—that is, answering the "Where is it?" question—isn't any fun at all. Again, no gene has ever been discovered for essential hypertension on the basis of a linkage analysis. We could stop the discussion at this point if it were not for the "candidate gene" approach. Physiologists, pathologists, pharmacologists, physicians, and surgeons have been working on essential hypertension and other complex genetic conditions for decades. Thus, information on basic mechanisms is readily available. Examples include the renin-angiotensin-aldosterone system, the respective receptors, signaling molecules, and effectors, and the sympathetic nervous system and all its ramifications, as well as many hormones, transmitters, enzymes, and other mechanisms. There are hundreds of candidate genes. These candidate genes are polymorphic—they are filled with polymorphisms, such as microsatellites and other forms of repeats. In addition, the candidate genes contain single-nucleotide polymorphisms, or SNPs.

The single-nucleotide DNA-sequence variations or SNPs occur every 1/500 to 1/2000 basepairs. Some SNPs may result in amino acid substitutions that may influence gene-product function. However, most do not. Simple arithmetic tells us that if the genome is 3 billion basepairs long, we can expect 3 million SNPs. With SNPs and other polymorphisms, we can have a field day with candidate genes. An example is the insertion/deletion polymorphism in the angiotensin-converting enzyme (ACE) gene. Over a thousand papers have been written on this topic, but please do not go out and read them all. Here, we use genetic association rather than linkage. Presumably, we already know where we are—the ACE gene, for example. We gather patients with our favorite disease, such as hypertension, myocardial infarction, stroke, or intractable pruritis. We gather a group of people without this condition. We then genotype everyone for the ACE gene insertion/deletion polymorphisms. The polymorphism in the ACE gene is not a SNP. Instead, the polymorphism is a so-called ALU repeat in intron 16 of the gene. An ALU repeat is a short, repeated DNA sequence that appears to have homology with transposable elements in other organisms. The repeat is amplified by the PCR and the product separated on a gel. We then look to see if either of the variants turn up more frequently among the "haves" (those associated with the trait), compared to the "have-nots." With this method, investigators determined that the D polymorphism in the ACE gene is associated with risk of myocardial infarction, as well as numerous other things. An example of the approach is shown in **Fig. 4**. Association is defined as the occurrence of a particular allele in a group of patients more often than can be accounted for by chance. The chi square statistic helps us here. However, Doctors Hardy and Weinberg predicted a problem with allelic distribution at the beginning of the last century, long before microsatellites or SNPs were discovered. The learned gentlemen pointed out that for a society to be genetically stable, it must be in Hardy-Weinberg equilibrium, which means the maintenance of allele frequencies in a population with random mating and absence of selection. The Hardy-Weinberg equilibrium implies that the relative proportion of the different genotypes remain constant from one generation to the next. Please do not ask your subjects if they are mating randomly! Instead, a simple binomial equation in population genetics can be used to determine the frequency of the different genotypes from one of the phenotypes. In any event, the first question to be posed of any association study is "were the groups in Hardy-Weinberg equilibrium?" If not, put your money in a different bank.

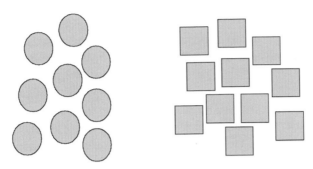

"Top-down" association study or "bottom-up" association study

Fig. 4. Association studies are case-control. If the circles are the cases and squares are the controls, a particular variant of a candidate gene (ACE deletion polymorphism, for example) may occur more frequently in the cases than in the controls. Alternatively, we can recruit persons carrying the variant (homozygosity for the ACE D allele, for example) and persons not carrying the variant (homozygosity for the ACE I allele, for example). We could then measure the blood pressure of both groups to determine whether or not higher blood pressures are "associated" with the D allele.

Association studies also have other problems. We must assume that the "cases" and "controls" are matched, perhaps in terms of genetic background, race, gender, income tax group, or whatever. We must also be certain that the cases indeed have the "disease" and the controls do not. In the case of hypertension, this problem is not trivial. As indicated previously, the definition changes frequently, is arbitrary, and highly age-dependent. Thus, your normotensive control may be a case tomorrow, and you have little means of ruling the possibility out. As pointed out in a scholarly editorial recently, genetic-association studies are a risky business *(2)*. The risks include undermining public confidence if the results are first published or cannot be replicated—or worse, are then refuted and must be retracted. Thus, a confirmation cohort—a second association study, if you will—is necessary. The studies should have large sample sizes and small P values, and they should report associations that make biological sense. The alleles should affect the gene product in a meaningful way. Ideally, the association should be observed both in family-based and population-based studies. Few association studies will meet all these criteria. Unfortunately, many published association studies meet none of the criteria. Thousands of association studies have been done to elucidate hypertension and other complex genetic conditions. Clearly, the association strategy is absolutely necessary if we are to approach complex genetics at all. However, the studies must be done properly.

1.5. Linkage Dysequilibrium Mapping

Investigators have worked very hard to improve the association approach and to make it more informative. Spielman et al. *(3)* were highly successful in our view. They recognized that as a means for identifying genes for complex diseases, both the association and the affected-sib-pairs linkage approaches have limitations. They pointed out that population association between a disease and a genetic marker can arise as an artifact of population structure, even in the absence of linkage. However, linkage studies with modest numbers of affected sib pairs may fail to detect linkage, especially if there is linkage heterogeneity. Spielman et al. *(3)* developed an alternative method to test for linkage with a genetic marker when population association has been found. They used data from families with at least one affected child, and then evaluated the transmission of the associated marker allele from a heterozygous parent to an affected offspring, as shown in **Fig. 5**. In their paper, they described the statistical basis for this "transmission test for linkage disequilibrium"—or, as they called it, the "TDT." They then showed the relationship of this test to tests of cosegregation that were based on the proportion of haplotypes or genes identical by descent in affected sibs. They concluded that their analysis applies to the study of disease associations when genetic markers are closely linked to candidate genes. When a disease is found to be associated with such a marker, the TDT may detect linkage, even when haplotype-sharing tests, such as identity-by-descent linkage tests, do not. What Spielman and associates did was to combine the linkage and association approaches, termed "linkage dysequilibrium" mapping.

The TDT test requires DNA from parents, but what if the parents are deceased? Spielman and Ewens have developed a way to avoid this problem *(4)*. They developed a method known as the "sib TDT," which overcomes the problem of deceased parents by use of marker data from unaffected sibs instead of from parents. Thus, they were able to apply of the principle of the TDT to sibships without parental data. They then showed how all the data may be used jointly in one overall TDT-type procedure that tests for linkage in the presence of association. Their extensions of the TDT are valuable for the study of diseases of late onset, such as hypertension.

Can we use SNPs for mapping? Recently, Horikawa et al. showed that the gene (CAPN10) for the protein calpain-10 is associated with type 2 diabetes mellitus *(5)*. Their study was a cloning effort that followed a linkage analysis performed in Mexican-American subjects from Starr County, Texas *(6)*. The linkage study localized a susceptibility gene to the region of closely spaced microsatellites on chromosome 2. The investigators selected a 1.7-Mb region defined by the 1-LOD support interval to focus their search. The area contained seven known genes and 15 expressed sequence tags. The investigators

Trios permit parental control studies

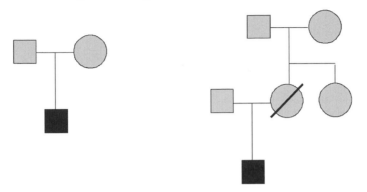

Fig. 5. Trios permit parental control studies. Ideally, the index patient and both parents are recruited. However, if one parent is missing, the genotype of that parent may be deduced (exhumed) by genotyping close relatives. Alternatively, other analyses can be done.

examined 21 SNPs to detect an association between type 2 diabetes mellitus and multi-locus haplotypes at three consecutive SNPs, an example of linkage disequilibrium mapping. The haplotype frequency led to the discovery of additional SNPs in the region, some of which were associated with diabetes. They then sequenced a 66-kb interval in 10 diabetic persons, which revealed three genes, including calpain (CAPN)10 and 179 polymorphisms. A complex statistical approach was used to implicate a single SNP in CAPN10, namely an intronic G/A polymorphism. The G allele was associated with a risk for diabetes. Altshuler et al. referred to the result as "guilt by association," emphasizing the association approach in the analysis *(7)*. The work was difficult and tedious; the authors spent four years doing the study.

1.6. Haplotypes

When single SNPs do not help, haplotypes may be better. The term "haplotype" was conventionally used to refer to the particular alleles present at the four genes of the HLA complex on chromosome 6. However, today we use the term to describe DNA-sequence variants—SNPs for example—on a particular chromosome adjacent to or closely flanking a locus of interest. Thus, we can expand our region by considering more than merely a single point. We have already introduced the term "haplotype sharing" when we introduced the TDT test. Haplotypes can be used in association studies, and may be more informative than single SNPs. We recently had the opportunity to test this notion *(8)*.

2. Materials

2.1. Microsatellite Mapping

1. Primers for amplification of microsatellite markers.
2. DNA sequencer.

2.2. SNP Genotyping

1. Fluorescent probes with the TaqMan system.
2. Specific primers for minisequencing.
3. Fluorescently labeled ddNTPs.

3. Methods

3.1. Microsatellite Mapping

Mapping of disease-associated genes relies on microsatellites. Because dinucleotide repeats are prone to replication slippage during PCR, tri- and tetranucleotide repeats usually provide clearer results. Fluorescent-labeled PCR primers can be used with every specific target DNA to amplify specific loci. As explained earlier, the closer the marker is to the gene, the lesser the probability that it is separated from the gene by recombination processes during the first meiotic cell division. Primers must be ordered or constructed to amplify the microsatellite markers. The amplified marker products from each individual are loaded onto the DNA sequencer. The sequencer has an electrophoresis capillary or gel, which permits separation of the marker products and automated reading. The PCR marker products are separated according to their lengths. The software precisely calculates the varying lengths of the amplification products of the PCR as shown in **Fig. 6**. To map a gene in question in either families or in sib-pair models, we will need about 350 microsatellites spread across all 22 pairs of autosomes.

3.2. SNP Genotyping

With the sequencing of the entire human genome, SNPs have gained in significance. An industrial consortium is committed to identifying >300,000 SNPs in the human genome (*9*). Gene mapping with SNP analysis has been shown to be feasible, and multiple SNP analyses in single genes or gene series are becoming commonplace (*10*). To master such complex genotyping needs, new technologies such as Maldi-Tof, biochips, novel enzymes, and fluorophores are being developed (*11,12*). However, investigators are currently faced with conventional technologies. A widely used method for detection of an interesting region on the DNA and to discriminate SNPs is the PCR. We frequently employ one of three PCR-based methods for SNP classification, namely allelic discrimination using fluorescent probes with the TaqMan system (5' nuclease

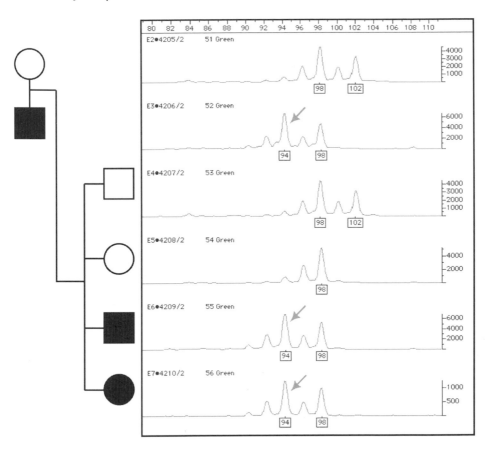

Fig. 6. Separation and automated calculation of the different allele length of a microsatellite marker is shown. The red arrow shows the paternal allele that cosegregates with the disease.

reaction), minisequencing with specific primers and fluorescence-marked ddNTPs and a capillary sequencer, and an oligonucleotide ligation assay (OLA), relying on a conventional gel sequencer. We have described a comparison of these techniques in detail elsewhere *(13)*. The principles behind the three assays are shown in **Fig. 7**.

For the 5' nuclease reaction with the TaqMan, fluorescent probes are used that consist of an oligonucleotide labeled with both a fluorescent reporter dye and a quencher dye. Both probes have the quencher dye TAMRA, yet, each has its own specific reporter dye. Doing the PCR one-reporter oligonucleotide probe, labeled with TET, hybridizes with the wild-type allele. The other probe,

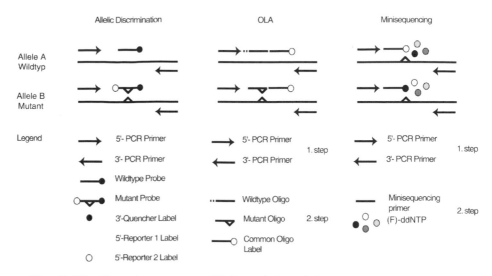

Fig. 7. The 5' nuclease assay, OLA, and the minisequencing reaction. In the 5' nuclease assay (allelic discrimination), probes are used to classify the mutation. Together with the two PCR primers flanking a polymorphism, two additional allele-specific probes are used, spanning the SNP. Both probes are marked with a quencher fluorescence molecule (TAMRA) at the 3'-end. A different reporter fluorescence molecule (TET or FAM) resides at the 5'-end. During the PCR reaction, the probes hybridize and are completely degraded by the 5' nuclease activity of Taq polymerase. For the OLA, a PCR product is used that contains the SNP. To distinguish the sequence variations, two allele-specific oligonucleotides of different length and a third—the labeled common oligonucleotide—are hybridized to one strand of the PCR product. At the 5' end of the common oligonucleotide, one of the allele-specific oligonucleotides is ligated by the thermostable DNA ligase. For the minisequencing reaction, a PCR product distinguishes the sequence variations. A detection primer anneals to the nucleic acid sequence at the 3' end of the nucleotide position of the mutation. ddNTPs labeled with four different fluorescent dyes serve for the detection of the product and terminate the reaction.

labeled with FAM, hybridizes with the mutant allele. The TaqMan instrument reads and records each individual sample and determines which alleles are present. Homozygous allele A, homozygous allele B, and heterozygous individuals were clearly separated.

For the minisequencing reaction (*14*), a PCR product is used to distinguish the sequence variations. After the PCR amplification, the PCR product is in solution along with primers (oligonucleotides), dNTPs, enzyme, and buffer components. To avoid participation in the subsequent minisequencing reaction, PCR primers and unincorporated dNTPs must be removed. Subsequently, a detection primer is needed that anneals to the nucleic acid sequence immediately at the 3' end of the nucleotide position of the polymorphism-position. Dideoxynucleotide triphosphates (ddNTPs) labeled with four different fluorescent dyes serve for the detection of the product. The ddNTPs terminate the reaction. If a homozygous for allele A or B is present, only one signal from the labeled ddNTP is obtained. In case of heterozygosity, two signals from the ddNTP are obtained.

For the OLA, a PCR product is used that contains the SNP. To distinguish the sequence variations, three different oligonucleotides are used. Two allele-specific oligonucleotides of different length and a third common oligonucleotide are hybridized to one strand of the PCR product *(15,16)*. At the 5' end of the common oligonucleotide, one of the allele-specific oligonucleotides is ligated by the thermostable DNA ligase. Linear amplification of product is achieved by *Thermus aquaticus* ligase. This sets up a competitive hybridization-ligation process between the two allelic oligonucleotides and the common oligonucleotide at each locus. Since the common oligonucleotide is labeled with a fluorescent dye, its defined electrophoretic mobility and fluorescent color can identify each ligation product. If homozygosity for allele A or B is present, one of the allele-specific forward primers hybridizes with the common oligonucleotide. In the case of heterozygosity, both allele-specific oligonucleotide hybridize with the common oligonucleotide.

The 5'-nuclease assay incorporates ease of design and the commercial availability of analysis software, which provides for rapid data analysis. The reaction run is simple and fast. Contrary to OLA, the allelic discrimination offers no high multiplex ability. However, by the use of modified oligonucleotides and different dyes such as FAM, TET, VIC, and NED, a higher multiplex ability can be achieved. Contrary to allelic discrimination, the minisequencing reaction requires more steps. Specifically, together with two PCR primers that flank a polymorphism, a PCR reaction must be done (*see* **Note 1**). The minisequencing reaction is universal, and does not require a fluorescent marked oligonucleotide. Therefore, the flexibility is high. The minisequencing reaction with varying length of primers is also suitable for analyzing more than one SNP at a time *(13)*. The OLA is suitable when many samples must be run or in which multiple SNP must be detected simultaneously. OLA takes the most time for optimization; however, once it is running, it is the least expensive method. In the OLA and minisequencing reactions, the products are separated and detected by the gel or capillary system. In the allelic analysis, the fluorescent signal for the allelic discrimination is measured directly in PCR reaction tubes. For the all SNP genotyping experiments, we include two controls that contain no template DNA (*see* **Note 2**).

4. Notes

1. This problem represents a bottleneck because more work steps are needed in the minisequencing technique. But an advantage, compared to allelic discrimination and to oligonucleotide ligation assay, is that all four variable nucleotides are identified during the same reaction.
2. Both negative controls show no signal in every reaction. The control method (gold standard) we employed to compare the three methods described here direct sequencing of the SNPs. We routinely apply direct sequencing when the results of the three methods are not in agreement.

References

1. Busjahn, A., Knoblauch, H., Faulhaber, H. D., Aydin, A., Uhlmann, R., Tuomilehto, J., et al. (2000) A region on chromosome 3 is linked to dizygotic twinning. *Nat. Genet.* **26**, 398–399.
2. [Anonymous] (1999) Freely associating. *Nat. Genet.* **22**, 1–2.
3. Spielman, R. S., McGinnis, R. E., and Ewens, W. J. (1993) Transmission test for linkage disequilibrium: the insulin gene region and insulin-dependent diabetes mellitus (IDDM). *Am. J. Hum. Genet.* **52**, 506–516.
4. Spielman, R. S. and Ewens, W. J. (1998) A sibship test for linkage in the presence of association: the sib transmission/disequilibrium test. *Am. J. Hum. Genet.* **62**, 450–458.
5. Horikawa, Y., Oda, N., Cox, N. J., Li, X., Orho-Melander, M., Hara, M., et al. (2000) Genetic variation in the gene encoding calpain-10 is associated with type 2 diabetes mellitus. *Nat. Genet.* **26**, 163–175.
6. Hanis, C. L., Boerwinkle, E., Chakraborty, R., Ellsworth, D. L., Concannon, P., Stirling, B., et al. (1996) A genome-wide search for human non-insulin-dependent (type 2) diabetes genes reveals a major susceptibility locus on chromosome 2. *Nat. Genet.* **13**, 161–166.
7. Altshuler, D., Daly, M., and Kruglyak, L. (2000) Guilt by association. *Nat. Genet.* **26**, 135–137.
8. Knoblauch, H., Bauerfeind, A., Krahenbuhl, C., Daury, A., Rohde, K., Bejanin, S., et al. (2002) Common haplotypes in five genes influence genetic variance of LDL and HDL cholesterol in the general population. *Hum. Mol. Genet.* **11**, 1477–1485.
9. Roses, A. D. (2000) Pharmacogenetics and future drug development and delivery. *Lancet* **355**, 1358–1361.
10. Martin, E. R., Gilbert, J. R., Lai, E. H., Riley, J., Rogala, A. R., Slotterbeck, B. D., et al. (2000) Analysis of association at single nucleotide polymorphisms in the APOE region. *Genomics* **63**, 7–12.
11. Lipshutz, R. J., Fodor, S. P., Gingeras, T. R., and Lockhart, D. J. (1999) High density synthetic oligonucleotide arrays. *Nat. Genet.* **21**, 20–24.
12. Ross, P., Hall, L., Smirnov, I., and Haff, L. (1998) High level multiplex genotyping by MALDI-TOF mass spectrometry. *Nat. Biotechnol.* **16**, 1347–1351.

13. Aydin, A., Baron, H., Bahring, S., Schuster, H., and Luft, F. C. (2001) Efficient and cost-effective single nucleotide polymorphism detection with different fluorescent applications. *Biotechniques* **4,** 920–928.

14. Syvanen, A. C. (1999) From gels to chips: "minisequencing" primer extension for analysis of point mutations and single nucleotide polymorphisms. *Hum. Mutat.* **13,** 1–10.

15. Barany, F. (1991) Genetic disease detection and DNA amplification using cloned thermostable ligase. *Proc. Natl. Acad. Sci. USA* **88,** 189–193.

16. Baron, H., Fung, S., Aydin, A., Bahring, S., Luft, F. C., and Schuster, H. (1996) Oligonucleotide ligation assay (OLA) for the diagnosis of familial hypercholesterolemia. *Nat. Biotechnol.* **14,** 1279–1282.

16

Laser-Capture Microdissection

Laura Barisoni and Robert A. Star

1. Introduction

The kidney is an anatomically complex organ with exceptional cellular heterogeneity. Our understanding of renal physiology has been advanced by studies of hand-dissected individual tubules (microdissection). Glomeruli or renal tubules are dissected away from surrounding structures, and subjected to microassays for enzymatic activity and receptor function, in vitro microperfusion for transport rates, and single-tubule reverse transcriptase-polymerase chain reaction (RT-PCR) *(1)*. Thus, microdissection methods have allowed assay of activity and mRNA and protein expression in single-nephron segments in normal or uninjured kidneys. Renal disease may be global, but more typically involves selective injury to the glomerulus, portions of the nephron, interstitium, or blood vessels. Less is known about renal pathophysiology and the nephron-specific response to injury. For example, how do different portions of the nephron interact during renal injury? Why are some renal diseases focal? How do individual glomeruli react in focal semental glomerulosclerosis (FSGS)? Does the interaction tend to propagate or to defend against further injury? Microdissection techniques have not been widely used to study renal injury because microdissection is often limited by tissue necrosis or fibrosis. In addition, the time required for microdissection often exceeds the time-course of rapid and transient changes in a cellular response such as certain metabolic intermediates or early-response genes. Instead, these questions are usually approached using immunohistochemistry or *in situ* hybridization. However, this depends upon the availability of specific antibodies that function in tissue sections, or optimization of complicated hybridization conditions. Also, genes must be studied one at a time, and, there is little specific information about human injury because of limited tissue availability.

Increasingly, the identification of disease mechanisms, markers, or therapeutics has benefited from newer genomic and proteomics techniques. These

From: *Methods in Molecular Medicine, vol. 86: Renal Disease: Techniques and Protocols*
Edited by: M. S. Goligorsky © Humana Press Inc., Totowa, NJ

techniques can be performed using the whole organ, but the biologically important cell type is often in the minority. This problem of obtaining a pure population of defined tissue cuts across many scientific disciplines. Several microdissection methods have been developed that allow structures to be isolated from stained tissue sections. Cells can be mechanically separated by a sharp pipet, needle, or blade *(2)*. However, this requires patience, manual dexterity, and correct orientation of tissue planes. The drawbacks of these manual methods have been overcome recently with the advent of laser-capture microdissection (LCM) by Lance Liotta's laboratory at that National Institute of Health (NIH) *(3–5)*, and laser catapult microdissection *(29)*. LCM was developed by oncology researchers to identify differences between a tumor and its adjacent stroma, early events in tumorigenesis, and to examine changes in the metastatic front *(6)*. LCM is especially useful for isolating structures from injured or fibrotic tissue, since manual dissection under these conditions is impossible *(7)*. It is now possible to obtain information from a single glomerulus, or single cross-section of a tubule. The use of LCM for single-cell analysis is described at the end of the chapter.

2. Principles of Technique

LCM allows a precise one-step isolation from tissue sections of single glomeruli, single tubules, small group of cells, or large single cells of interest *(3,4)*. This technique is based on the selective adherence of visually targeted cells or fragments of tissue to a thermoplastic membrane that is activated by a high-energy infrared laser pulse. The LCM system available from Arcturis is composed of an inverted microscope, with the slide holder located between the lens and a laser beam. The microscope is attached to a computer through which the laser is controlled and the images can be archived. A vacuum system in the base of the slide holder immobilizes the slide during the capturing. An optically clear cap containing a 6-mm-diameter sticky thermoplastic polymer membrane (capture film) is inserted into a mechanical transport arm (**Fig. 1**). One side of the cap faces the laser beam, and the side with the attached thermoplastic membrane faces the slide.

The cap is placed on the desired area of the tissue section, and the group of cells to study are visually selected. The stage is moved until the guide laser spot overlays the cells of interest. When the laser is pulsed at higher energy, the thermoplastic capture film made from ethylene vinyl acetate melts onto the tissue at the selected site, then solidifies (**Fig. 1**). The cells are thermally fused to the capture film. After sufficient numbers of spots are fused, the film is lifted away from the section (**Figs. 1** and **2**). Since the adhesive forces between the membrane and the tissue are stronger than those between the tissue and the glass slide, the targeted cells are detached from the tissue section. The cap

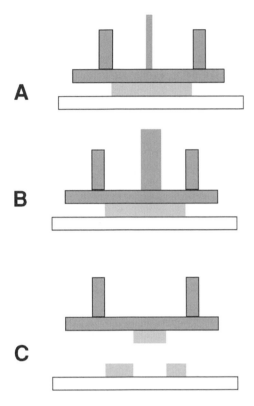

Fig. 1. Diagram of Laser-capture microdissection. (**A**) The cap (dark gray) is placed on the desired area of the tissue section (light gray), and the stage is moved until the guide laser spot (red) overlays the cells of interest. (**B**) When the laser is pulsed at higher energy (red), the thermoplastic capture film melts onto the tissue at the selected site then solidifies. (**C**) After sufficient numbers of spots are fused, the film is lifted away from the section.

is placed into a PCR tube containing the solution required for isolation of DNA, RNA, proteins, or enzymes. The cells are lysed, and desired material is purified and analyzed for DNA, RNA, or proteins. This one-step transfer method overcomes many of the problems of traditional microdissection techniques. The diameter of the laser beam is 7.5, 15, or 30 μm. Depending on dissection conditions, the diameter of melted plastic may be larger because the melting plastic flows into the surrounding area. In theory, this can be controlled by refocusing the beam and adjusting the laser energy. However, in our experience, the transferred spot is approximately twice the diameter of the laser beam.

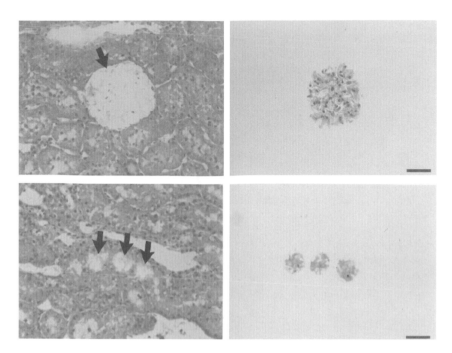

Fig. 2. LCM capture of glomerulus and proximal straight tubule. Two micron sections of freshly frozen tissue were fixed in 70% ethanol, and stained with H&E. Left panels show histologic section after transfer and right panel shows recovery of renal glomerulus (top, 70-μm spot size) and proximal straight tubules (bottom, 35-μm spot size) on transfer film. Arrow indicates the transferred area. Bar = 50 μm; × 200. Modified and used with permission from *Kidney Int.* (2000), **57**, 323.

3. Methods

3.1. LCM on Frozen Kidney Sections

Studies by Emmert-Buck et al. *(4)* showed that LCM could capture a single glomerulus on the transfer film. Kohda et al. measured gene expression in the glomerulus and portions of the nephron *(7)* (**Fig. 2**). Several groups have optimized fixation and staining methods for renal LCM *(4,7–11)*. Tissue sections must be clean, flat, and dry to optimally adhere to the transfer film. All new LCM laboratories discover that the sections must be completely dehydrated, or the capture film will not adhere to the desired cells. Work must be carried out rapidly to prevent RNA degradation. **Table 1** shows general methods that are applicable to LCM. Several groups have found that RNA recovery from kidney sections is best when LCM is performed on frozen sections that are fixed with acetone, ethanol, or methanol, then lightly stained with Hema-

Table 1
General Methods

1. All solutions (ice-cold acetone, diethyl pyrocarbonate [DEPC]-treated water or PBS, ethanol, xylene, etc.) are prepared freshly each day under RNAse free conditions. Place 50 mL of each solution in 50 mL plastic conical test tubes (Falcon) or glass staining jars and arrange in a row. All solutions are at room temperature unless noted. All containers must be autoclaved.
2. The cryostat blade, glass slides and other tools used for the cutting should be cleaned with ethanol and RNase Away, or autoclaved.
3. After cutting and storing sections at –80°C, sections are processed rapidly one at a time because RNases degrade tissue RNA rapidly.
4. Rapid washing steps (< 20 sec) are performed by repeatedly dipping the slide up and down once per sec.
5. Longer incubations (> 20 sec) are performed by dipping the slide up and down once per sec for 5–10 times, then letting sit in the solution for the remaining time.
6. Slides are air dried for 2 min at room temperature. Correctly dried slides will be dark. Do not use a hair dryer to speed up the process; the quality and quantity of RNA will be worse, even when no additional heading is applied.

toxylin under RNase-free conditions *(7,10)*. The optimized protocol, with comments, follows.

3.1.2. Preservation Method

Traditionally, tissue is snap-frozen at –80°C, then embedded in OCT (frozen tissue-embedding medium). Parlato recently described a new method of sucrose preservation that preserves morphology and permits extraction of intact RNA *(12)*. Tissue is washed with diethyl pyrocarbonate (DEPC)-treated phosphate-buffered saline (PBS), then incubated at 4°C for 4–12 h in 30% sucrose in PBS. The tissue is then rinsed in PBS and embedded in OCT and snap-frozen. This method has not been utilized on kidney tissue, but shows great promise.

3.1.3. Cutting

Two to four μm frozen cryosections are cut under sterile conditions in a RNAase-free environment. The cryostat blade, glass slides and other tools have to be cleaned with 100% ethanol and RNase Away or autoclaved. If immunostaining is not necessary, noncoated glass slides can be used to reduce adhesiveness of the sections to the glass. Gloves should be changed after completing every sample.

Table 2
Rapid Hematoxylin and Eosin Staining

1. Prepare sections as in **Table 1**, store at −80°C, and process one at a time.
2. Fix section with 70% ethanol for 2 min at room temp.
3. Wash twice in two successive tubes of DEPC-treated water for 5 sec each.
4. Stain rapidly with hematoxylin stain (CS 401-1D, Fisher Scientific) for 30 sec.
5. Immerse in the hematoxylin solution for 1 min.
6. Wash twice in two successive tubes of DEPC-treated water for 10 sec.
7. Dehydrate sides through an ethanol gradient (70, 100, and 100% ethanol) for 1 min each.
8. Counterstain with alcoholic eosin Y solution (HT110-1-16; Sigma Chemical Co., St. Louis, MO) for 30 sec.
9. Wash 3× with three successive tubes of 100% ethanol for 1 min each.
10. Wash twice in two successive tubes of xylene for 1–2 min each.
11. Air dry.

3.1.4. Fixation and Storage

Unfixed sections can be immediately stored at −80°C. Fixation methods that do not alter the three-dimensional (3D) structure of proteins (e.g., acetone, methanol, or ethanol) preserved RNA the best, and yielded the best tissue architecture in the kidney cortex and outer medulla (*7*). Stronger crosslinking fixatives such as formalin and paraformaldehyde greatly inhibited dissolution of the tissue in GTC and degraded RNA. The former can be overcome by adding proteinase K to the isolation buffer (*13*).

3.1.5. Staining

Sections can be left and used unstained if the purpose of the microdissection is simply to select glomeruli over tubules. Goldsworthy and colleagues and Kohda and colleagues found that RNA survived hematoxylin & eosin (H&E) staining but was degraded considerably by PAS staining (*7,10*), similar to that proposed in the original description of the LCM technique (*4,14*). **Table 2** shows the optimized H&E staining protocol (*7*), and similar protocols have been used by Tanji and Parlato (*12*). Eosin should be avoided if protein assays will be performed.

3.1.6. RNA Extraction and Reverse Transcription

A microdissected fragment of tissue, adherent to the cap, can be transferred to a sterile 1.5-mL microcentrifuge tube and lysed in 200 mL of RNA lysis buffer. We and others use a standard GTC method because it was believed to be superior to many of the commercially available kits (**Table 3**) (*7,11*). RNA

Table 3
RNA Isolation and RT/PCR

1. Incubate transfer film with 200 µL of 4 *M* guanidine thiocyanate, 25 m*M* Na$_3$ citrate, 0.5% sarcosyl, and 0.72% β-mercaptoethanol for 10 min at room temperature. We found that the tissue did not completely dissolve at 4°C; however, incubation at room temperature worked much better.
2. Add 160 µL water-saturated phenol (bottom layer).
3. Add 40 µL chloroform.
4. Vortex vigorously.
5. Put on wet ice for 15 min.
6. Centrifuge samples at 16,000*g* for 30 min at 4°C.
7. Remove supernatant to a new 500 µL test tube.
8. Add 200 µL of the chloroform and vortex sample for 30 sec.
9. Centrifuge samples at 16,000*g* for 30 min at 4°C.
10. Remove supernatant to a new 500 µL test tube.
11. Add 1 mL of ice-cold isopropanol and invert tube 10×.
12. Freeze for 1 h at –80°C
13. Centrifuge at 16,000*g* for 40 min at 4°C
14. Wash samples with ice cold 70 % ethanol, then ice cold 100% ethanol.
15. Air dry samples.

can be purified by phenol and chloroform extractions followed by precipitation with an equal volume of isopropanol in the presence of 0.1 vol of 3 mol/L sodium acetate (pH 4.0), and 1 µL of 10 mg/mL of carrier glycogen at –20°C. The RNA pellet can be washed once in 70% ethanol, dried, and resuspended in 10 mL of RNase-free water. Alternatively, RNA isolation kits from PicoPure or Arcturus are stated to allow RNA recovery from LCM samples containing 10 cells. An alternative method to analyze mRNA without RNA isolation *(15)*, although we have not tried this method.

3.1.7. Sensitivity

Liotta's laboratory has shown that LCM/PCR can isolate DNA and mRNA from small numbers of 60 µm laser spots and can be optimized to potentially target single cells *(4,14,16,17)*. A cylinder-based LCM instrument that employs a novel convex geometry of the transfer film can detect hepatitis B virus in single hepatocytes *(18)*. Kohda found that LCM/RT-PCR detected mRNA for podoplanin in 2% of a single glomerulus, rat basic amino acid transporter in 6% of a single cross-section of proximal straight tubule, and renin in 8 proximal convoluted tubule cross-sections *(7)*. LCM/RT-PCR could isolate pure populations of proximal convoluted tubules, proximal straight tubules, and thick ascending limbs from renal histologic sections, although we could not isolate pure collecting ducts. LCM/RT-PCR localized ischemia-reperfusion induced induction of KC/interleukin-8 primarily to the medullary thick ascending limb, and detected TGF-β mRNA in glomeruli of a patient with membranous glomerulonephropathy. Tanji and colleagues found that mRNA for WT-1 could be detected in as few as five glomeruli, and the tubule-specific gene aminopeptidase N could be detected in as few as five microdissected tubule cross-sections, with no cross-contamination from surrounding tubulds *(11)*.

3.1.8. Immunohistochemistry-Enhanced LCM

Many papers have used LCM to isolate cells based upon morphologic (cell size) or histologic staining characteristics. For example, differentiation of cancer vs normal cells or small vs large neurons is easily performed on lightly stained sections *(19)*. However, many cells cannot be differentiated by histologic criteria. Differentiation of cells in mixed populations of tumors, or structurally heterogenous organs such as the kidney, is often difficult in paraffin sections, and may be impossible in frozen sections. Identification of injured nephron segments was difficult even in hematoxylin-stained sections *(7)*. If more sophisticated selection of the tissue elements is necessary, sections can be stained by a rapid immunohistochemistry technique before LCM. This allows isolation of cells based upon their expression of function-related proteins or specific immunophenotype *(9)*. Frozen sections are rapidly immunostained, then subjected to LCM, RNA extraction, and PCR. The total aqueous time is shortened to 8–10 min; 4–5 min of antibody exposure and 4–5 min of color development. Although immunohistochemistry staining protocols were optimized to reduce the time of aqueous incubation and thus lessen mRNA degradation, 99% of the mRNA for beta-actin was lost *(7,13)*. RNA loss occurred even in the absence of antibody, suggesting that endogenous RNases were not inhibited sufficiently during the aqueous-phase incubations. Thus, this method works well for analysis of DNA, but not for RNA analysis.

To surmount the RNA loss, several groups have developed intervening LCM *(16)*, or navigated LCM, whereby desired cell populations are defined on IH- or IF- stained sections, then the adjacent serial section is lightly stained with H&E, and used for LCM *(20)*. These methods might be useful to identify individual glomeruli, but are unlikely to be useful for tubular studies because of the difficulty in following a single tubule from section to section.

3.1.9. Immunofluorescent-Enhanced LCM

Targeting of specific cells may be difficult using routine morphologic stains. Immunohistochemistry can identify cells with specific antigens; however, exposure to aqueous solutions destroys 99% of the mRNA. Murakami et al. developed a rapid immunofluorescence LCM (IF-LCM) procedure that allows

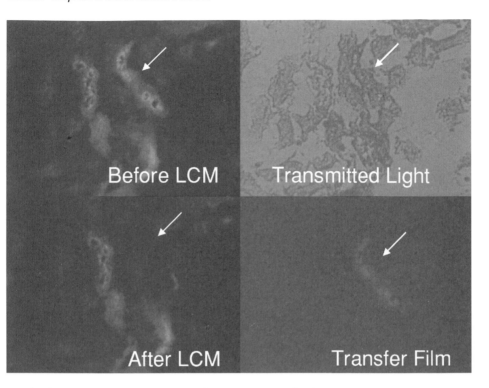

Fig. 3. LCM capture of immunofluorescently stained mouse kidney. A 2 μm section of freshly frozen mouse kidney tissue was fixed in 100% acetone, and rapidly immunostained with anti-THP (*see* **Subheading 3**). Top left and right panels show the immunofluorescent and transmitted light image before transfer, respectively. Bottom left panel shows the fluorescent image of the tissue section after dissection. Bottom right panel shows a fluorescent image of the thick ascending limb recovered on the transfer film. Arrow indicates the transferred area. Modified and used with permission from *Kidney Int.* (2000), **58**, 1349.

targeted analysis of gene expression in specific cells from frozen sections without mRNA loss *(21)* (**Fig. 3**). Immunofluorescence methods offer several advantages over immunohistochemical methods. First, immunofluorescence methods are more sensitive, and thus can detect lower concentrations of antigens. Second, immunofluorescence methods do not require additional enzymatic reactions for visualization. Since immunofluorescent labeling could be performed more rapidly, there was less time for RNA degradation. This technique requires few adaptations on the conventional LCM microscope. A low-light video camera is added to the side port of the microscope. Since the low-light level video camera is sensitive to the laser light, 1–2 heat filters must be added inside the camera extension tube to shield the image intensifier from

Table 4
Immunofluorescent LCM

1. Set up freshly prepared solutions.
2. Incubate high concentrations of primary antibody (1:20 dilution; 20-fold greater than routine immunohistochemistry), secondary antibody (1:7 dilution; 100/7 = 14-fold greater than routine IH), and RNase inhibitor (400 U/mL; N251A, Promega, Madison, WI) for 10 min at room temperature, and store at 4°C in the dark until use (*see* **steps 8–9**). Each section will require 10 µL of solution.
3. Cut freshly frozen tissue sections, store at –80°C as above. Process one slide at a time.
4. Fix section for 2 min with cold acetone.
5. Hydrate section for 5 sec DEPC-treated PBS (pH 7.6). Repeat using a second container of DEPC-treated PBS.
6. Dry section by snapping 2× and wiping with Kimwipe.
7. Warm the premixed primary and secondary antibody solution to room temp for approx 10 min before use.
8. Incubate section with 10 µL of the premixed primary and secondary antibody for 1 min. The solution is dropped onto the section, and the section is gently rocked for 1 min.
9. Rapidly wash the section in two successive tubes of DEPC-treated PBS (5 sec each).
10. Dehydrate slide in two successive vials of 100% ethanol, 1 min each.
11. Dehydrate slide in 100% Xylane for 1–2 min.
12. Air-dry slides for 2 min at room temperature.
13. View slides with a FITC filter cube and low-light level video microscopy.
14. Perform LCM; keep dissections less than 30 min after staining to prevent the degradation of RNA.
15. As a control, incubate sections with a different primary antibody (anti human alpha-smooth muscle actin; M085, DAKO, Carpintera, CA) or with only the secondary antibody.

the laser. The protocol is shown in **Table 4**. After rapid fixation and rehydration, sections are incubated for 1' at room temperature, with a solution made of primary antibody, ALEXA-linked secondary antibody at high concentration (1:7), and RNase inhibitor, which has been prepared 10' before and kept in the dark. Sections are then rinsed with DEPC-treated water, twice × 5' and rehydrated in 100% alcohol, twice × 1' *(21)*.

3.2. LCM on Paraffin-Embedded Tissue

Adaptation of LCM for use on paraffin-fixed tissue allows the use of LCM on archived human pathology slides that are uniformly available, instead of needing special flash-frozen specimens. LCM can be used to isolate DNA from single glomeruli or tubule cross-sections *(11)*, or establish molecular micro-heterogeneity in complex neoplasms *(22)*. RNA analysis is more difficult because formalin degrades RNA, crosslinks proteins that shear RNA during tissue processing, and covalently modifies RNA by addition of mono-methylol groups *(23)*. mRNA can be detected using RT-PCR with moderate-sized amplicons (400–500 basepairs); however, the levels are only 1% of frozen sections *(7)*. Recently, Specht et al. found quantitative recovery of small amplicons (60–122 bp) from formalin-fixed paraffin-embedded material *(13)*, and this result has been confirmed by another group *(24,25)*. The recovery was excellent, compared to frozen sections, even with as few as 50–100 cells. Evidently, the small amplicons gets around the formalin-induced crosslinking problems. Tissue samples were fixed in formalin for 20 h, cells isolated by laser-assisted microdissection, and mRNA extracted with proteinase K digestion and organic extraction *(23)*. Use of a novel RNase inhibitor increased cDNA yields, increased dissection time, and allowed gene detection by quantitative Taqman analysis from 1% of a single glomerulus *(25)*. Alternatively, the use of 70% ethanol as a fixative allows for superior recovery of both proteins and nucleic acids *(26)*. 70% ethanol functions as a coagulative fixative, but does not crosslink sulfhydryl groups of proteins or cause RNA damage. Histology is well retained, and this fixative is easily implemented because it is the second step in standard processing protocols.

3.2.1. Cutting

Formalin-fixed and paraffin-embedded sections are cut at 5–8 μm on a microtome with disposable blades in an RNase-free environment.

3.2.2. Deparaffinization

Sections are deparaffinized in two changes of xylene for 10 min each. Failure to properly deparaffinize the section will impede microdissection.

3.2.3. Staining

Generally, no staining is necessary to discriminate between glomeruli and tubules. If a more sophisticated discrimination is necessary (e.g., proximal vs distal tubules), a light hematoxylin staining can be performed. Sections are rehydrated with an ethanol scale at 2 min each step and are stained with hematoxylin alone for 15–30 sec, or followed by eosin for 45 sec, rinsed in RNase-free water for 30 sec and dehydrated in 100% ethanol for 1 min. If the kidney parenchyma is not injured, the H&E staining could be enough to discriminate between proximal and distal tubules. However, under conditions such as tubulo-interstitial damage of any origin, tubules may lose their morphologic characteristic features, and additional staining may be necessary. Unfortunately, antigen retrieval with enzymes or microwaving, typically used with formalin-fixed tissue, cannot be used because of RNA destruction. Although we have not tested this theory, we suspect that antibodies can be used if they are sufficiently "robust," do not need antigen retrieval techniques or microwaving, and are detected by immunofluorescent methods. It should be possible to use fluorescent-labeled lectins to discriminate among different segments of tubules.

3.2.4. RNA Extraction and Reverse Transcription

Processing is similar to frozen tissue samples, except that a proteinase K step is required *(23)*.

3.3. Variations of LCM

Fend has reviewed some of the newer alternatives to LCM, including laser-pressure catapulting and laser-manipulated microdissection *(27)*. Laser-manipulated microdissection can detect mRNA from single cells *(28)*, and has been applied to the kidney *(29)*. A 6 μm kidney section is placed on a metallic or polyethylene membrane. The desired structures are traced with a very fine laser. When the outline is completed, the desired structure falls (or is pushed up) into a collection tray for further analysis. Nagawasa used this to isolate glomeruli in a Thy1.1 glomerulonephritis model, and found upregulation of TGF-β mRNA expression by real-time PCR *(29)*. This technique may be quite useful for structures that are hard to isolate by LCM, and might allow improved targeting, since it is easier to define the desired area. However, the technique requires more operator concentration and takes longer.

3.4. Conclusion

This decade has witnessed the development of genomics and proteomics that may allow an understanding of biological networks of interacting genes and proteins at a scale not envisioned at the beginning of the decade. The development of laser-assisted microdissection techniques, coupled with sensitive detection methods, allow the measurement of mRNA, and soon, protein expression of a single cell. We have found these techniques to be extremely helpful in pinpointing expression of newly discovered genes in the kidney. However, extreme care must be taken to ensure the that microdissected cells are taken from the correct tubule segment.

4. Notes

1. The advantages of this method are its speed, precision, versatility for analysis of DNA, RNA, and proteins. LCM has been applied to a wide range of tissue preparations. The morphology of the captured tissue is well-preserved, as well as the

Table 5
Analysis of LCM Samples

	Detection # spots	Single gene	Many genes	References
DNA	1	LOH		*3*
	1	Gene mutations		*22*
mRNA	1	RT-PCR		*3,4*
	few	qRT-PCR		*10,20,23,30*
	1000+		cDNA libraries	*19,31,32*
	1000+		cDNA microarrays	*19,30,33*
Protein	250–2000	Western blotting		*8,34–36*
	50	ELISA		*37*
	7,000–30,000		2D gels	*8,33,34,36*
	25–500		SELDI/TOF	*17,37*
	2000+		Protein arrays	*38*
	2000+		Antibody arrays	*17*

morphology of the remaining tissue, allowing multiple sampling from the same slide. Since the resolution of unstained sections is generally poor, rapid staining protocols and immunofluorescent-enhanced LCM have been developed that preserve RNA. Although LCM is considered a fast technique, the amount of time required to carry out microdissection is still considerable, especially for genomic and proteomic applications.

2. The LCM process, like any sensitive technique, has a number of technical and methodological hazards. Reagents must be fresh, especially xylenes, alcohols, and stains. RNases may contaminate all reagents, and are found in the tissue sections. The LCM microscope and surrounding area must be kept clean, and work must proceed rapidly to prevent RNA degradation. Tissue sections must be clean, flat, and completely dehydrated to adhere to the transfer film. Care must be taken to remove any nondesired tissue elements that nonspecifically adhere to the capture membrane, especially when working at the single-cell level. This is especially true when isolating tubule segments, since the molten plastic easily flows past the tubule basement membrane if the spot size is too large *(22)*. Finally, the targeted cells must be clearly differentiated from the surrounding area. This last requirement is especially true when targeting kidney tubules.

3. LCM-dissected material can serve as the input material for a wide range of assays, including many assays described in other chapters of this book. These range from analysis of DNA mutations to gene expression, proteomics, and even single cells (**Table 5**). We will highlight some of the uses of LCM, but because of space, are unable to review all the published papers.

   a. One of the first uses of LCM was to measure loss of heterozygosity (LOH) in tumors *(3,4)*. More recently, Fend et al used LCM to examine the molecular micro-heterogeneity of complex neoplasms *(22)*. They sequenced heavy-chain gene rearrangements to find that low-grade B-cell lymphomas with two distinct cell populations come from two different clones. LCM-captured cells can also be analyzed for genetic anomalies by fluorescence *in situ* hybridization (FISH) *(39)*. LCM samples have also been used to measure cell-cycle parameters and provide ploidy analysis, even on paraffin-embedded archived cancer specimens *(39)*. Samples from a single glomerulus or tubule cross section are sufficient for DNA analysis *(11)*.

b. As discussed here, mRNA analysis is more difficult. LCM-derived RNA can be used to measure mRNA abundance of single genes by RT-PCR quantitative PCR *(10,20,23,30,32)*, or generate expression libraries, perform subtractive hybridization cloning, or screen high-density cDNA arrays *(4,19,30)*. Differential gene profiling of normal and diseased tissue can provide clues to the pathogenesis of disease, if the two populations are accurately selected. Regulation of the identified genes can be validated using quantitative RT-PCR, immunohistochemistry, or tissue arrays *(30,40)*. The first use of LCM to detect changes in large numbers of genes was by Luo et al. who analyzed the gene-expression profile of small and large neurons in the dorsal-root ganglion *(19)*. RNA was isolated from small (< 25 μm) and large (>40 μm) neurons (5000 spots per sample), subjected to two rounds of linear T7-based RNA amplification, tagged with ^{33}P, and hybridized to custom-spotted microarrays containing 477 target cDNAs. They found dramatically different gene patterns in the two cell types. Sgroi performed a similar study to monitor gene expression in LCM-purified normal, invasive, and metastatic breast cancer cells (10,000 cells per group) from a single patient using high-density cDNA arrays *(30)*. They found 90 genes that had two-fold changes in expression. Some of the changes were verified by real-time PCR and tissue microarrays. Studies by Hooper and colleagues used a hybrid model; they analyzed global changes in gene expression in the intestine before and after colonization of germ-free mice with *Bacteriodes thetaiotaomicron*. They then used LCM to localize the resulting changes in gene expression *(41)*. Because of the major changes seen with bacterial colonization, they only needed to dissect small numbers of cells from the tissue compartments to confirm and localize the array results. Finally, Sugiyama et al. compared the RNA expression profile of RNA extracted from cancer cells obtained by LCM with that of RNA from the bulk cancer tissue *(42)*. They found no correlation between the expression levels of the two samples; with notable enrichment in immune-system proteins in the bulk tissue (from the surrounding stroma), and enrichment of transcription factors (? targets for chemotherapy) in the LCM-procured cancer cells. This study demonstrates the need for microdissection for the profiling of clinical tumor specimens.

These studies are extremely difficult because of the large number of laser spots needed (generally 500–2000 spots) that must be rapidly procured, and the technically demanding amplification procedure. The T7 amplification procedure used in most studies is extremely tricky and tedious. Whereas several commercial amplification kits are on the market, the sensitivity and linearity of these kits should be carefully scrutinized.

c. More recently, LCM is being used to measure protein expression and protein-expression patterns in tissue from human cancers, primarily in the field of oncology. LCM offers the ability to examine changes in protein composition of human cancers, not cell lines, and detect differences between protein and protein activity in normal, premalignant, and malignant tissue, and the surrounding stroma. The problems with cell lines are illustrated by the findings of Ornstein et al.—that there was only 20% overlap in protein profile between cultured cancer-cell lines and malignant tissue captured by LCM *(18)*.

Known proteins can be measured by enzyme-linked immunosorbent assay (ELISA) or Western blotting. Prostate specific antigen levels have been measured in LCM-isolated prostate cancer tissue. Simone et al. report special extraction buffers that have been developed for secreted and membrane-bound proteins. As few as five cells are needed in this very sensitive sandwich immunoassay *(43)*, allowing quantitation of protein levels in pure populations of cells. An exciting but technically challenging development is the use of LCM samples to construct protein microarrays *(38)*, and the analysis of LCM-procured samples by antibody array *(17)*. LCM-derived material can be spotted onto protein arrays, and immunoblotted with activation state-specific phosphorylation antibodies to describe the activation state of different tissue compartments within tumors *(38)*. LCM-derived material could also be placed in liquid protein arrays *(44)*, allowing preparation of up to 800 identical arrays for testing using conventional immunohistochemical techniques.

LCM has also been used to detect new potential biomarkers using one- and two-dimensional (2D) polyacrylamide gel electrophoresis (PAGE) followed by mass spectrometry *(8,14,18,34,35,45)*. The microdissection process apparently does not alter protein migration or mass spectrometry identification *(8,34)*. Nearly identical 2D profiles have been found in microdissected normal vs malignant renal cancer *(8)* or from normal vs adjacent esophageal cancer *(34)*. However, selective enrichment has been detected. For example, analysis of LCM-dissected normal esophageal squamous epithelium or cancer (50,000 cells each) revealed that 17 of 675 2D gel spots showed tumor-specific alterations *(34)*. Ten spots were uniquely present in the tumor and 7 in normal tissue. High-sensitivity mass spectrometry was used to identify two of the differentially expressed genes as cytokeratin 1 and adenexin 1 *(34)*, which was confirmed using Western blotting and immunohistochemistry of samples obtained in a longitudinal study *(36)*. Whereas the initial 2D gels required 40–50,000 cells (7000 laser shots), the western blotting "only" required 2500–6500 cells *(33–36)*. Craven et al. recently extended their testing of different tissue preparation methods on the recovery of proximal tubule proteins *(14)*. They found acceptable protein recovery using routine H&E staining, although omission of eosin improved the isoelectric focusing resolution. They also report an exciting rapid staining protocol using ethanol-fixed tissue that allows visualization of proximal tubules with preservation of protein recovery. It is hoped that this technique can be adapted to other antibodies that localize to rarer tissue compartments (distal convoluted tubules, thick ascending limb, collecting ducts) or individual cells (intercalated cells). Taken together, the studies indicate that LCM can be used to search for novel genes in clinically important environments. However, these studies require extensive dissection (13 h to 4 d of dissection *[8,14]*) for each sample.

LCM-purified samples can be subjected to surface-enhanced laser desorption/ionization mass spectrometry (SELDI-TOF) followed by heuristic cluster analysis *(17,37)*. Since the SELDI-TOF method is extremely sensitive, it can be naturally coupled with LCM samples. This would allow the development of disease-specific fingerprint patterns that could differentiate normal from cancer, as has been recently reported for using proteomic patterns in serum to identify ovarian cancer *(46)*. However, the identity of the specific peaks is extremely difficult to determine *(17)*.

4. The minimum laser-spot size of 7.5 µm is probably too large to capture single small cells in the kidney; however, it has been used to isolate larger single cells from B-cell lymphomas, and foam cells from atherosclerotic lesions *(22)*. Alternatively, one can add a lens above the capture membrane to reduce the spot size by approx 50% *(7)*, use specially designed caps that include a 10-µ spacer to reduce contact area, or perform LCM on cytospin material *(13,47)*. None of these methods appears to be sufficiently robust for single podocytes or inflammatory cells in the kidney. However, Arcturus has developed a new LCM microscope (PixCell IIe) that has a narrower laser beam and superior image quality, and is said to be capable of transferring smaller spot sizes. It is not presently known if this new instrument can be used for single-cell capture in the kidney. With any of these techniques, it is critical to eliminate the dissection of fragments from other nearby cells.

References

1. Moriyama, T., Murphy, H. R., Martin, B. M., and Garcia-Perez, A. (1990) Detection of specific mRNAs in single nephron segments by use of the polymerase chain reaction. *Am. J. Physiol.* **258,** F1470–F1474.
2. Whetsell, L., Maw, G., Nadon, N., Ringer, D. P., and Schaefer, F. V. (1992) Polymerase chain reaction microanalysis of tumors from stained histological slides. *Oncogene* **7,** 2355–2361.
3. Bonner, R. F., Emmert-Buck, M., Cole, K., Pohida, T., Chuaqui, R., Goldstein, S., et al. (1997) Laser capture microdissection: molecular analysis of tissue. *Science* **278,** 1481–1483.
4. Emmert-Buck, M. R., Bonner, R. F., Smith, P. D., Chuaqui, R. F., Zhuang, Z., Goldstein, S. R., et al. (1996) Laser capture microdissection. *Science* **274,** 998–1001.

5. Simone, N. L., Bonner, R. F., Gillespie, J. W., Emmert-Buck, M. R., and Liotta, L. A. (1998) Laser-capture microdissection: opening the microscopic frontier to molecular analysis. *Trends Genet.* **14**, 272–276.

6. Liotta, L. A. and Kohn, E. C. (2001) The microenvironment of the tumour-host interface. *Nature* **411**, 375–379.

7. Kohda, Y., Murakami, H., Moe, O. W., and Star, R. A. (2000) Analysis of segmental renal gene expression by laser capture microdissection. *Kidney Int.* **57**, 321–331.

8. Banks, R. E., Dunn, M. J., Forbes, M. A., Stanley, A., Pappin, D., Naven, T., et al. (1999) The potential use of laser capture microdissection to selectively obtain distinct populations of cells for proteomic analysis—Preliminary findings. *Electrophoresis* **20**, 689–700.

9. Fend, F., Emmert-Buck, M. R., Chuaqui, R., Cole, K., Lee, J., Liotta, L. A., et al. (1999) Laser capture microdissection of immunostained frozen sections for mRNA analysis. *Am. J. Pathol.* **154**, 61–66.

10. Goldsworthy, S. M., Stockton, P. S., Trempus, C. S., Foley, J. F., and Maronpot, R. R. (1999) Effects of fixation on RNA extraction and amplification from laser capture microdissected tissue. *Mol. Carcinog.* **25**, 86–91.

11. Tanji, N., Ross, M. D., Cara, A., Markowitz, G. S., Klotman, P. E., and D'agati, V. D. (2001) Effect of tissue processing on the ability to recover nucleic acid from specific renal tissue compartments by laser capture microdissection. *Exp. Nephrol.* **9**, 229–234.

12. Parlato, R., Rosica, A., Cuccurullo, V., Mansi, L., Macchia, P., Owens, J. D., et al. (2002) A preservation method that allows recovery of intact RNA from tissues dissected by laser capture microdissection. *Anal. Biochem.* **300**, 139–145.

13. Jin, L., Thompson, C. A., Qian, X., Kuecker, S. J., Kulig, E., and Lloyd, R. V. (1999) Analysis of anterior pituitary hormone mRNA expression in immunophenotypically characterized single cells after laser capture microdissection. *Lab. Investig.* **79**, 511–512.

14. Craven, R. A., Totty, N., Harnden, P., Selby, P. J., and Banks, R. E. (2002) Laser capture microdissection and two-dimensional polyacrylamide gel electrophoresis: evaluation of tissue preparation and sample limitations. *Am. J. Pathol.* **160**, 815–822.

15. To, M. D., Done, S. J., Redston, M., and Andrulis, I. L. (1998) Analysis of mRNA from microdissected frozen tissue sections without RNA isolation. *Am. J. Pathol.* **153**, 47–51.

16. Darling, T. N., Yee, C., Bauer, J. W., Hintner, H., and Yancey, K. B. (1999) Revertant mosaicism: partial correction of a germ-line mutation in COL17A1 by a frame-restoring mutation. *J. Clin. Investig.* **103**, 1371–1377.

17. Knezevic, V., Leethanakul, C., Bichsel, V. E., Worth, J. M., Prabhu, V. V., Gutkind, J. S. , et al. (2001) Proteomic profiling of the cancer microenvironment by antibody arrays. *Proteomics* **1**, 1271–1278.

18. Craven, R. A. and Banks, R. E. (2001) Laser capture microdissection and proteomics: possibilities and limitation. *Proteomics* **1**, 1200–1204.

19. Luo, L., Salunga, R. C., Guo, H., Bittner, A., Joy, K. C., Galindo, J. E., et al. (1999) Gene expression profiles of laser-captured adjacent neuronal subtypes. *Nat. Med.* **5**, 117–122.

20. Wong, M. H., Saam, J. R., Stappenbeck, T. S., Rexer, C. H., and Gordon, J. I. (2000) Genetic mosaic analysis based on Cre recombinase and navigated laser capture microdissection. *Proc. Natl. Acad. Sci. USA* **97**, 12,601–12,606.

21. Murakami, H., Liotta, L., and Star, R. A. (2000) IF-LCM: laser capture microdissection of immunofluorescently defined cells for mRNA analysis rapid communication. *Kidney Int.* **58**, 1346–1353.

22. Fend, F., Quintanilla-Martinez, L., Kumar, S., Beaty, M. W., Blum, L., Sorbara, L., et al. (1999) Composite low grade B-cell lymphomas with two immunophenotypically distinct cell populations are true biclonal lymphomas- A molecular analysis using laser capture microdissection. *Am. J. Pathol.* **154**, 1857–1866.

23. Specht, K., Richter, T., Muller, U., Walch, A., Werner, M., and Hofler, H. (2001) Quantitative gene expression analysis in microdissected archival formalin-fixed and paraffin-embedded tumor tissue. *Am. J. Pathol.* **158**, 419–429.

24. Cohen, C. D., Frach, K., Schlondorff, D., and Kretzler, M. (2001) Quantitative gene expression analysis in renal biopsies: a novel protocol for multicenter applications. *J. Am. Soc. Neph.* **12**, 674A. (abstract)

25. Cohen, C. D., Grone, H. J., Grone, E., Nelson, P. J., Schlondorff, D., and Kretzler, M. (2001) Laser microdissection and gene expression analysis on formaldehyde-fixed tissue: IP-10 and RANTES in renal allograft rejection. *J. Am. Soc. Neph.* **12**, 674A. (abstract)

26. Gillespie, J. W., Best, C. J., Bichsel, V. E., Cole, K. A., Greenhut, S. F., Hewitt, S. M., et al. (2002) Evaluation of non-formalin tissue fixation for molecular profiling studies. *Am. J. Pathol.* **160**, 449–457.

27. Fend, F. and Raffeld, M. (2000) Laser capture microdissection in pathology. *J. Clin. Pathol.* **53**, 666–672.

28. Bernsen, M. R., Dijkman, H. B., de Vries, E., Figdor, C. G., Ruiter, D. J., Adema, G. J., et al. (1998) Identification of multiple mRNA and DNA sequences from small tissue samples isolated by laser-assisted microdissection. *Lab. Investig.* **78**, 1267–1273.

29. Nagasawa, Y., Takenaka, M., Matsuoka, Y., Imai, E., and Hori, M. (2000) Quantitation of mRNA expression in glomeruli using laser-manipulated microdissection and laser pressure catapulting. *Kidney Int.* **57**, 717–723.

30. Sgroi, D. C., Teng, S., Robinson, G., LeVangie, R., Hudson, J. R., Jr., and Elkahloun, A. G. (1999) In vivo gene expression profile analysis of human breast cancer progression. *Cancer Res.* **59**, 5656–5661.

31. Krizman, D. B., Chuaqui, R. F., Meltzer, P. S., Trent, J. M., Duray, P. H., Linehan, W. M., et al. (1996) Construction of a representative cDNA library from prostatic intraepithelial neoplasia. *Cancer Res.* **56**, 5380–5383.

32. Emmert-Buck, M. R., Strausberg, R. L., Krizman, D. B., Bonaldo, M. F., Bonner, R. F., Bostwick, D. G., et al. (2000) Molecular profiling of clinical tissue specimens: feasibility and applications. *Am. J. Pathol.* **156**, 1109–1115.

33. Ahram, M., Best, C. J., Flaig, M. J., Gillespie, J. W., Leiva, I. M., Chuaqui, R. F., et al. (2002) Proteomic analysis of human prostate cancer. *Mol. Carcinog.* **33**, 9–15.

34. Emmert-Buck, M. R., Gillespie, J. W., Paweletz, C. P., Ornstein, D. K., Basrur, V., Appella, E., et al. (2000) An approach to proteomic analysis of human tumors. *Mol. Carcinog.* **27,** 158–165.
35. Ornstein, D. K., Englert, C., Gillespie, J. W., Paweletz, C. P., Linehan, W. M., Emmert-Buck, M. R., et al. (2000) Characterization of intracellular prostate-specific antigen from laser capture microdissected benign and malignant prostatic epithelium. *Clin. Cancer Res.* **6,** 353–356.
36. Paweletz, C. P., Ornstein, D. K., Roth, M. J., Bichsel, V. E., Gillespie, J. W., Calvert, V. S., et al. (2000) Loss of annexin 1 correlates with early onset of tumorigenesis in esophageal and prostate carcinoma. *Cancer Res.* **60,** 6293–6297.
37. Paweletz, C. P., Liotta, L. A., and Petricoin, E. F., III (2001) New technologies for biomarker analysis of prostate cancer progression: Laser capture microdissection and tissue proteomics. *Urology* **57,** 160–163.
38. Paweletz, C. P., Charboneau, L., Bichsel, V. E., Simone, N. L., Chen, T., Gillespie, J. W., et al. (2001) Reverse phase protein microarrays which capture disease progression show activation of pro-survival pathways at the cancer invasion front. *Oncogene* **20,** 1981–1989.
39. DiFrancesco, L. M., Murthy, S. K., Luider, J., and Demetrick, D. J. (2000) Laser capture microdissection-guided fluorescence in situ hybridization and flow cytometric cell cycle analysis of purified nuclei from paraffin sections. *Mod. Pathol.* **13,** 705–711.
40. Moch, H., Schraml, P., Bubendorf, L., Mirlacher, M., Kononen, J., Gasser, T., et al. (1999) High-throughput tissue microarray analysis to evaluate genes uncovered by cDNA microarray screening in renal cell carcinoma. *Am. J. Pathol.* **154,** 981–986.
41. Hooper, L. V., Wong, M. H., Thelin, A., Hansson, L., Falk, P. G., and Gordon, J. I. (2001) Molecular analysis of commensal host-microbial relationships in the intestine. *Science* **291,** 881–884.
42. Sugiyama, Y., Sugiyama, K., Hirai, Y., Akiyama, F., and Hasumi, K. (2002) Microdissection is essential for gene expression profiling of clinically resected cancer tissues. *Am. J. Clin. Pathol.* **117,** 109–116.
43. Simone, N. L., Remaley, A. T., Charboneau, L., Petricoin, E. F., III, Glickman, J. W., Emmert-Buck, M. R., et al. (2000) Sensitive immunoassay of tissue cell proteins procured by laser capture microdissection. *Am. J. Pathol.* **156,** 445–452.
44. Miyaji, T., Hewitt, S. M., Liotta, L., and Star, R. A. (2002) Liquid protein arrays. *Proteomics* **2,** 1489–1493.
45. Ornstein, D. K., Gillespie, J. W., Paweletz, C. P., Duray, P. H., Herring, J., Vocke, C. D., et al. (2000) Proteomic analysis of laser capture microdissected human prostate cancer and in vitro prostate cell lines [In Process Citation]. *Electrophoresis* **21,** 2235–2242.
46. Petricoin, E. F., Ardekani, A. M., Hitt, B. A., Levine, P. J., Fusaro, V. A., Steinberg, S. M., et al. (2002) Use of proteomic patterns in serum to identify ovarian cancer. *Lancet* **359,** 572–577.
47. Maitra, A., Wistuba, I. I., Virmani, A. K., Sakaguchi, M., Park, I., Stucky, A., et al. (1999) Enrichment of epithelial cells for molecular studies. *Nat. Med.* **5,** 459–463.

17

Serial Analysis of Gene Expression

M. Ashraf El-Meanawy, Shrinath Barathan, Patrick S. Hayden, Sudha K. Iyengar, Jeffrey R. Schelling, and John R. Sedor

1. Introduction

Molecular medical research has traditionally required hypothesis-driven strategies, often focusing on identification of linear signaling pathways that mediate disease pathogenesis. This approach does not identify novel pathways, or genes that act together to produce pathology or a disease-permissive milieu. To generate new hypotheses that require no *a priori* assumptions about disease pathogenesis, gene-expression profiles of normal and diseased tissues or cell types can be compared. Although determining protein-expression patterns would be preferable, necessary methodologies are not readily available, and protein diversity generated by post-translation modifications adds technical complexities to this strategy. On the other hand, techniques for the study of RNA-expression patterns are available, and represent a reasonable "data mining" alternative. Complex relationships between multiple molecules that regulate disease pathogenesis should be identified, at least in part, by analyzing transcript profiles generated from normal and diseased states. Differential display (1,2), subtractive hybridization (3), and subtraction libraries (4) are semi-quantitative, comparative tools that have been utilized previously. However, molecular pathway discovery has been revolutionized by development of high-throughput, quantitative techniques, including serial analysis of gene expression (SAGE) and hybridization array (5,6). Because both of these methods generate transcript libraries or transcriptomes, which catalog thousands of simultaneously expressed genes, a small laboratory can comprehensively determine differential gene-expression profiles within months.

The SAGE technique was initially developed in Kenneth Kinzler's laboratory at Johns Hopkins University (5). SAGE is a reverse transcriptase-polymerase chain reaction (RT-PCR)-based technique that produces a quantitative

From: *Methods in Molecular Medicine, vol. 86: Renal Disease: Techniques and Protocols*
Edited by: M. S. Goligorsky © Humana Press Inc., Totowa, NJ

compilation of gene-specific, 9–13-basepair, cDNA sequence tags that represent mRNA species in a particular pool of mRNAs. The relative abundance of these tags in the SAGE expression library reflects the relative abundance of the corresponding mRNA in the total mRNA population. This technique has several key principles. First, it is quantitative. The 9–13 basepair cDNA sequence tags, derived from 3'-ends of mRNAs, are counted, providing a digital characterization of a transcriptome in contrast to the fluorescent dye ratios or spot intensities (analog output) provided by hybridization array. Second, tags are sufficiently unique to map to specific genes, although ambiguity in tag-to-gene mapping has increased as numbers of known gene sequences increase (*see* **Subheading 4.**). Third, individual tags are ligated together to form longer cDNA concatemers (typically 0.7–1.5 kb in length). Concatemer sequence, containing many gene tags, can quickly be determined in a single sequencing reaction. Use of an automated sequencer allows high-throughput sequencing of many concatemers, enabling individual tag sequences to be identified, counted, and catalogued into libraries. Fourth, SAGE uses PCR amplification in a manner that avoids the introduction of distortion. SAGE therefore simultaneously quantifies expression of a large number of genes, measured in different experimental samples or in tissues corresponding to different clinical phenotypes, which can then be analyzed using classical statistical approaches, hidden Markov models, and/or Bayesian probabilities. Finally, SAGE libraries contain tags of both known and unknown genes, whereas arrays contain only previously identified cDNAs/Ests. For this reason, SAGE may be a preferable strategy for identification of new genes. However, either approach represents a powerful strategy to obtain global snapshots of gene-expression patterns, which can better define basic pathways that regulate cell function and provide insights into disease pathogenesis by simultaneously determining the net consequences of gene-gene and gene-environment interactions on the expression of thousands of genes.

1.1. Overview of SAGE Protocol

SAGE requires the isolation of 9–13 cDNA fragments (tags) from the 3' end of mRNA, which are ligated together to form concatemers for high-throughput sequencing and computerized identification and counting of individual gene tags. Although SAGE uses basic molecular biological techniques that are commonly practiced in most laboratories, the protocol involves many steps, and understanding its general strategies prior to processing samples will increase the likelihood of success. **Figure 1** is a schematic overview of SAGE. Briefly, polyadenylated RNA (A+) is isolated (**step 1**) and used to synthesize 3' biotinylated cDNA (**step 2**). The cDNA is then digested by a restriction enzyme with a 4-nucleotide recognition sequence (anchoring enzyme), thus

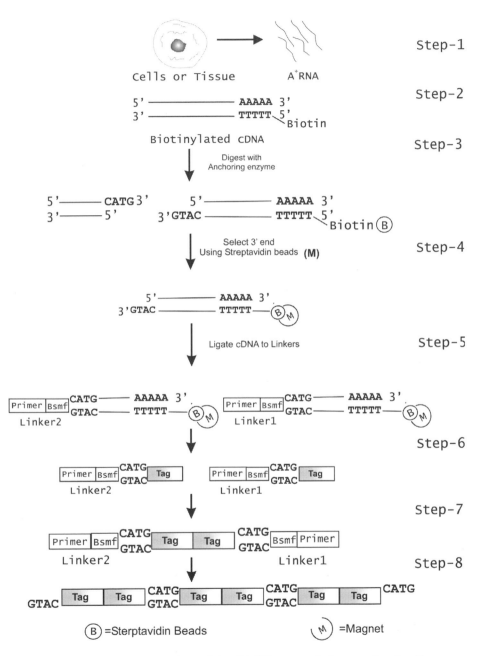

Fig. 1. Schematic overview of the SAGE protocol. *See* text for details.

allowing cleavage on average every 256 (4^4) bp (**step 3**). The resulting 3' ends of the cDNAs are captured and isolated from the rest of the cDNA fragments using streptavidin-coated magnetic beads (**step 4**). The pool of bead-bound, 3'-cDNA ends is divided in half, and each half is ligated to a different, DNA linker, containing an anchoring enzyme sequence overhang (linker 1 and linker 2) (**step 5**). In addition to the anchoring enzyme overhang, the linkers contain a PCR primer template and a class II-S (shift) endonuclease recognition site (tagging enzyme), such as *BsmF*-I. Digestion with the tagging enzyme cleaves DNA 10–14 nucleotides downstream from the recognition site, releasing cDNA-linker sequence from the beads (**step 6**). The cDNA-linker pools (A and B) are mixed and ligated using T4DNA ligase, resulting in linker-cDNA tag-cDNA tag-linker (linker-ditag-linker) molecules (**step 7**). The ligation products are then PCR-amplified and digested with anchoring enzyme, releasing ditags from linkers. After gel purification, ditags are concatenated (**step 8**), and concatemers are subcloned and sequenced. Concatemer sequences are analyzed with software programs that are available in the public domain, and tag sequences are extracted to produce a tag library. Tools for mapping tags to specific genes and library analysis are discussed in detail in the data analysis section (**Subheading 3.2.**).

2. Materials

1. Poly-adenylated RNA isolation reagents or kits: e.g., Qiagen product, combination of RNeasy (total RNA) and Oligotex (mRNA extraction) (Qiagen, Valencia, CA).
2. Streptavidin magnetic beads M-280 (Dynal Biotech, Oslo, Norway).
3. Superscript cDNA synthesis system (Invitrogen, Carlsbad, CA).
4. Restriction endonucleases: *Nla*-III, *BsmF*-I, *Sph*-I, and modifying enzymes T4DNA polymerase and T4DNA ligase (high and low concentration) (New England Biolabs, Beverly, MA).
5. Glycogen, molecular-biology grade (Roche Molecular Biochemicals, Indianapolis, IN).
6. *Taq* Platinum DNA polymerase (Invitrogen).
7. pZero Cloning system (Invitrogen).
8. Electromax (electrocompetent) DH10B *Escherichia coli* bacteria (Invitrogen).
9. DMSO (Sigma, St. Louis, MO).
10. Phenol/chloroform/isoamyl alcohol 25:24:1 (v:v:v) and chloroform/isoamyl alcohol (v:v) (Invitrogen).
11. Pre-casted Tris-borate/ethylenediaminetetraacetic acid (EDTA) (TBE) 8% and 12% acrylamide gels (Invitrogen).
12. 10X polymerase chain reaction (PCR) Buffer: 166 mM (NH$_4$)$_2$SO$_4$, 670 mM Tris-HCl, pH 8.8, 67 mM MgCl$_2$,100 mM β-mercaptoethanol.
13. LoTE: 3 mM Tris-HCl, 0.2 mM EDTA, pH 7.5.
14. 2X bind and wash buffer (B&W): 10 mM Tris-HCl (pH 7.5), 1 mM EDTA, 2.0 M NaCl.

15. Oligonucleotides (polyacrylamide gel electrophoresis [PAGE] purified) (Integrated DNA Technologies, Coralville, IA).
16. Magnet and magnetic tube holder (Dynal Biotech), either single or multi-slot (for pulling-down the magnetic beads).
17. Sybr Green I dye.
18. Linker 1 A: 5'-TTTGGATTTGCTGGTGCAGTACAACTAGGCTTAATAGGG ACATG-3'.
19. Linker 1 B (5'-phosphorylated, 3'-amino modified C7): 5'-TCCCTATTAAGCCT AGTTGTACTGCACCAGCAAATCC-3'.
20. Linker 2 A: 5'-TTTCTGCTCGAATTCAAGCTTCTAACGATGTACGGGGAC ATG-3'.
21. Linker 2 B (5'-phosphorylated, 3'-amino modified C7): 5'-TCCCCGTACATCGT TAGAAGCTTGAATTCGAGCAG-3'.
22. Primer 1: 5'-(biotin)2-GGATTTGCTGGTGCAGTACA-3'.
23. Primer 2: 5'-(biotin)2-CTGCTCGAATTCAAGCTTCT-3'.
24. Biotinylated oligo dT: 5'-(biotin) T_{20}-3'.
25. M13 Forward (gel purification unnecessary): 5'-GTAAAACGACGGCCAGT-3'.
26. M13 Reverse (gel purification unnecessary): 5'-GGAAACAGCTATGACCATG-3'.

3. Methods

3.1. Molecular Methods

3.1.1. RNA Preparation (*Fig. 1; step 1*)

RNA is extracted from tissue or cultured cells by standard methods, and mRNA (or poly A+ RNA) is selected using commercially available kits, and is quantified by spectrophotometry. The original SAGE protocol recommended a minimum input of 5 µg poly A+ RNA for cDNA synthesis (5), which worked without difficulty in our SAGE analysis of a normal murine kidney transcriptome (7). High-quality poly A+ RNA is essential, and can be verified using agarose gel electrophoresis. Miniaturized protocols that require 500- to 5,000-fold less input RNA—e.g., from as few as 15,000–50,000 cells (8–10) have been used for SAGE analysis of small samples, such as nephron segments, glomeruli, or kidney cells isolated from biopsies, using laser-capture microdissection (LCM) (11). Alternatively, quantitative RNA amplification can be used to obtain sufficient starting material from small samples (12). These technical advances should allow expression libraries to be generated from as little as a few thousand cells.

3.1.2. Synthesis of 3' Biotinylated cDNA (*Fig. 1; step 2*)

A key aspect of SAGE is the synthesis of 3'-biotin-labeled cDNA to permit affinity separation of the 3'-cDNA ends from the rest of the molecule after anchoring enzyme restriction endonuclease digestion.

1. 5 μg A⁺ RNA is used to generate double-stranded cDNA following manufacturer recommendations, with the exception that 2.5 μg biotinylated oligo-dT is substituted for unbiotinylated oligo-dT. At least 75%–85% cDNA synthesis efficiency should be expected. We recommend including a parallel cDNA synthesis reaction, using 100 ng of input poly A⁺ RNA and including [^{32}P]α-dCTP as tracer, to evaluate the quality and efficiency of cDNA synthesis. Good quality cDNA should produce a smear ranging from a few hundred bp to 10 kbp.

2. Purify the generated cDNA by phenol-chloroform/isoamyl alcohol (phenol/chloroform) extraction. Bring the vol of the cDNA to 200 μL with LoTE. Add 200 μL of phenol-chloroform and mix by vortexing for 1 min. Spin in a microfuge for 1 min and transfer the aqueous (upper) layer to a new tube, and add 200 μL of chloroform:isoamyl alcohol. Mix by vortexing for 1 min, spin for 1 min and transfer the aqueous layer into a new microfuge tube.

3. Ethanol-precipitate by adding 1/10 vol of 3*M* sodium acetate (pH 5.2) and 2.5 vol of absolute (nucleic acid-grade) ethanol and placing the mixture on dry ice. After 10 min, precipitate the cDNA by spinning in a microfuge at 4°C. Decant the supernatant and wash the pellet with 300 μL of 70% ethanol (do not disturb pellet, and if necessary, recentrifuge the sample for 3 min at room temperature). Remove all alcohol and dry the pellet (either on the bench for 5 min or in Speed-Vac for 1 min). Resuspend the cDNA pellet in 20 μL LoTE.

3.1.3. Digestion of Biotinylated DNA with Anchoring Enzyme (**Fig. 1**; *step 3*)

1. Digest 10 μL cDNA with *Nla*III (anchoring enzyme) for 1 h at 37°C in 200 μL of the appropriate buffer (*see* manufacturer's directions). Phenol-chloroform extract the digested cDNA, as in **Subheading 3.1.2.**, ethanol-precipitate, and suspend the pellet in 20 μL LoTE.

3.1.4. Capture of 3'-Biotinylated cDNA Fragment with Streptavidin Beads (**Fig. 1**; *step 4*)

1. In two 1.5 mL microfuge tubes, wash 100 μL streptavidin-coated magnetic beads using 200 μL 1X B&W buffer. Pellet beads with the magnet and resuspend in 100 μL 1X B&W buffer.

2. Add 10 μL of the digested cDNA, 90 μL water, and 100 μL 2X B&W buffer to each tube and rotate at room temperature for 15 min.

3. Pellet the beads and wash them 3× with 200 μL 1X B&W buffer and once with 200 μL LoTE. Use a magnet to pellet the streptavidin bead-bound cDNA. In this step, the 3'-most *Nla*-III digestion fragment of the cDNA (downstream of the last *Nla*-III site) remains bound to the beads, and the rest of the cDNA fragments are washed away.

3.1.5. Ligation of Linkers to Bead-Bound cDNA (**Fig. 1**; *step 5*)

1. Linker 1 and linker 2 are generated prior by mixing equimolar amounts of linkers 1A and 1B and linkers 2A and 2B in separate microcentrifuge tubes. Heat each

mixture to 90°C for 1 min and gradually cool to room temperature for efficient annealing of the component oligonucleotides.

2. Resuspend in two tubes the streptavidin bead-bound cDNA in 25 µL of LoTE by gentle mixing, spin briefly in a microcentrifuge and add 5 µL of linker 1 or linker 2 (200 ng/µL).

3. Heat the microcentrifuge tubes at 50°C for 2 min, incubate at room temperature for 15 min, and add 8 µL of 5X T4 ligase buffer and 2 µL high-concentration (5 U/µL) T4 ligase to each microcentrifuge tube. Incubate for 2 h at 16°C with intermittent mixing.

4. After ligation, wash the beads 3× with 200 µL 1X B&W buffer and transfer the mixture to a new tube. Wash once with 200 µL 1X B&W buffer and twice with 200 µL 1X tagging enzyme buffer, and remove the supernatant.

3.1.6. Digestion with a Tagging Enzyme (*Fig. 1; step 6*)

The tagging enzyme (usually *BsmF*-I) cleaves target DNA approx 10–14 bp downstream of the recognition sequence, thus releasing short, staggered-end DNA fragments containing gene-specific cDNA sequences (tags) ligated to linkers (e.g., linker-cDNA tag hybrid sequences).

1. To each tube, add 10 µL tagging enzyme in 10X buffer, 2 µL 100X bovine serum albumin (BSA) (supplied with the tagging enzyme from New England Biolabs) and 4 units *BsmF*-I. Bring vol to 100 µL with water.

2. For *BsmF*-I, incubate at 55°C for 2 h (rather than manufacturer-suggested 65°C, to increase the efficiency and reproducibility of the reaction and to minimize temperature-induced cDNA leaching from beads) while continuously rotating in a hybridization oven.

3. Pellet the beads with a magnet and collect the supernatant, containing the linker-cDNA tag hybrid DNA. Phenol-chloroform extract the linker-cDNA tags and ethanol-precipitate using 10–20 µg glycogen as carrier. Resuspend the pellets in 10 µL LoTE.

3.1.7. Blunting the End of Released cDNA Tags

Blunt ends are created on *BsmF*-I generated linker-cDNA tags, using Klenow fragment of DNA polymerase-I.

1. To the resuspended pellets, add 10 µL 5X second-strand cDNA synthesis buffer (Invitrogen cDNA kit), 1 µL 100X BSA (Invitrogen), 2.5 µL of 10 m*M* dNTP mix, 23.5 µL water, 3 µL Klenow fragment of DNA polymerase-I, and incubate at 37°C for 30 min.

2. Phenol-chloroform extract and ethanol-precipitate the linker-cDNA tags. Resuspend each pellet in 5 µL LoTE.

3.1.8. Generation of Ditags from Linker-cDNA Constructs (*Fig. 1; step 7*)

The blunt-ended L1-cDNA tags and L2-cDNA tags are ligated to form L1-linker-ditag-L2-linker (linker-ditag-linker) PCR templates.

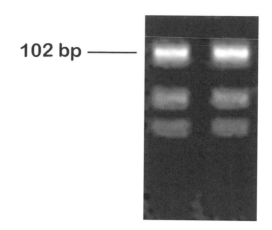

102 bp

Fig. 2. Amplification of ditags. Sybr green I-stained polyacrylamide gel demonstrating 102-bp ditag bond and less intense 90 bp linker-tag-linker and 80 bp linker-linker bands.

1. Mix L1-cDNA tags (2 µL) and L2-cDNA tags (2 µL) with 1.2 µL 5X ligase buffer and 0.8 µL T4 ligase (5 U/µL).
2. Incubate overnight at 16°C and add 14 µL water.
3. Prepare a duplicate reaction, omitting T4 ligase, as a negative control for the large-scale PCR amplification of ditags (*see* **Subheading 3.1.9.**).

3.1.9. PCR Amplification of Ditags

1. Ditags are amplified using primer 1 and primer 2. Prior to large-scale amplification, the PCR conditions are optimized. The linker-ditag-linker templates are serially diluted (1:10 through 1:200), and the different dilutions of the ligation products (0.6 mL) in a reaction buffer containing 10X PCR buffer (3.0 µL), dimethyl sulfoxide (DMSO) (1.8 µL), 10 m*M* dNTPs (4.5 µL), primer 1 (350 ng/µL) (0.6 µL), primer 2 (350 ng/µL) (0.6 µL), water (18.3 µL), and Taq Platinum polymerase (5 U/µL) (0.6 µL).
2. PCR amplification conditions: 1 cycle at 95°C for 2 min; 26–30 cycles: 94°C for 30 sec, 55°C for 1 min, 70°C for 1 min (the ligation sample prepared without T4 ligase [negative control, *see* **Subheading 3.1.8, step 3**] should be amplified for 35 cycles); and 1 cycle at 70°C for 5 min.
3. Analyze 10 µL of each PCR product by PAGE using 8% TBE acrylamide gel and staining with Sybr green I (1:10,000 dilution). The template dilution, which generates the most intensely stained 102-bp product, is used for large-scale (96 × 100 µL) PCR reactions with the same amplification parameters. Contaminating 80-bp (linker-linker dimer) and 90-bp (linker-tag-linker hybrid) bands may be seen on Sybr green I-stained gels, but both products should be less intense compared to the 102-bp linker-ditag-linker band (**Fig. 2**). Although we have not

experienced significant problems with linker-dimer contamination, several protocol modifications, which reduce linker-dimer production and increase ditag
yields, have been published *(13,14)*.

4. After large-scale PCR, pool individual PCR reactions, phenol-chloroform extract
   and ethanol-precipitate. Purify the PCR products using preparative, non-denatur-
   ing 8% TBE polyacrylamide gel electrophoresis (PAGE). We recommend that
   DNA derived from the 102-bp band be excised from the gel and electroeluted in
   0.5X TBE inside dialysis tubing (size exclusion of 6000–8000 D). Although this
   is an added step to the original protocol, we found that this procedure improves
   ditag concatenation by removing contaminating genomic DNA fragments with
   Nla-III restriction sites. After electroelution, collect the buffer from dialysis tubing, phenol-chloroform extract, ethanol-precipitate and resuspend in 100 μL
   LoTE. Quantification of DNA is useful at this point, and the yield should be
   between 10 and 20 μg.

3.1.10. Isolation of Ditags

Gel-purified, linker-ditag-linker constructs are digested with *Nla*-III, which
releases ditag cDNA (22–26 bp in length) from linkers (40 bp).

1. Mix the electroeluted PCR products (100 μL), 10X *Nla*-III 10X buffer (40 μL),
   water (216 μL), BSA 100X (4 μL), and Nla-III (10 U/μL) (40 μL). Incubate for
   1 h at 37°C and add 2X B&W (400 μL).
2. Ditags, which contain unique 9–11-bp tag sequences for two genes in 3' tail to
   3' tail orientation, are separated from linkers using streptavidin-coated magnetic
   beads, followed by 12% PAGE. Pipet 800 μL of streptavidin beads into each of
   two microcentrifuge tubes. Wash twice with 1X B&W buffer, pellet with a magnet, and then discard supernatant. Add the *Nla*-III digestion mixture (400 μL) to
   each tube, and incubate at room temperature for 15 min. Pellet with a magnet
   and collect the supernatant. Wash the beads in each tube with 200 μL 1X B&W
   buffer, collect the supernatant, and combine with the first aliquot. Place on ice,
   phenol-chloroform extract and ethanol-precipitate. Resuspend the ditag pellet in
   40 μL LoTE, run 10 μL per lane in 4 lanes on a 12% acrylamide gel in parallel
   with the 20-bp DNA marker (160 V for 2–2.5 h). Stain the gel with Sybr green I,
   excise the 24–26-bp band, and elute the DNA as follows.
3. Pierce the bottom of a 0.5-mL tube with a 21-gauge needle, add the gel fragment
   containing the 24–26 bp band, place the 0.5-mL tube in a 2.0-mL siliconized
   microcentrifuge tube, and spin in a microcentrifuge at full speed for 2 min. Discard the 0.5-mL tubes, and add 250 μL LoTE and 50 μL 7.5 *M* ammonium acetate
   to 2.0-mL tubes. Vortex the tubes and place at 37°C for 15 min. Use SpinX columns to isolate eluted DNA from gel fragments. Phenol-chloroform extract the
   DNA. Ethanol-precipitate and resuspend the DNA in LoTE (7.5 μL).

3.1.11. Ligation of Ditags to Form Concatemers (**Fig. 1; step 8**)

Ditags with *Nla*-III cohesive termini are ligated together using T4 DNA
ligase. The resulting concatemers contain the transcript signature tags in tail-

to-tail orientation punctuated by the anchoring enzyme recognition sequence (CATG in the case of *Nla*-III).

1. Mix ditags (7 µL), 5X T4 ligase buffer (2 µL), and T4 DNA ligase (5U/µL) (1 µL). Incubate at 16°C for 1–3 h. Add 2 µL 5X gel-loading dye, and heat at 65°C for 5 min. Load one well of an 8% TBE PAGE gel with the 10-µL sample and another well with 1-kb ladder. Apply direct current (130 V for 3 h). Stain with Sybr green I and excise the DNA with a size range from 700–1200 bp from the gel. Electroelute by placing the gel slice in dialysis tubing (6000-D cutoff), add 0.5X TBE buffer (500 µL), clamp the tube, and place it in TBE buffer. Apply direct current (150 V for 1 h) and collect the buffer from inside the dialysis tubing. Phenol-chloroform extract the concatemers, ethanol-precipitate, and then resuspend in LoTE (6 µL).

3.1.12. Cloning of Concatemers into pZero

The isolated concatemers are cloned into pZero vector, and the plasmid is electroporated into E. coli strain DH10B. Bacteria are plated on zeosin-containing selection medium.

1. Digest pZero (100 ng) for 30 min with *Sph* I (generates a cohesive end that is compatible with *Nla*-III termini of the concatemers). Phenol-chloroform extract and ethanol-precipitate the *Sph* I-linearized vector and resuspend in 4 µL LoTE. Mix the electroeluted concatemers (6 µL), *Sph* I-linearized pZero (1 µL), and 5X T4 ligase buffer (2 µL). Heat at 50°C for 2 min and place on ice. Add T4 DNA ligase (1 U/µL) (1 µL) and incubate overnight at 16°C. Phenol-chloroform extract, ethanol-precipitate, and resuspend the ligation reaction in LoTE (10 µL). Use 1 µL of the ligation reaction for electroporation into Electromax DH10B. After recovery, incubate at 37°C in SOC media for 30 min, plate the bacteria on zeosin-LB agar, and incubate overnight at 37°C.

3.1.13. Isolation of Recombinant Clones and Sequencing

Individual clones are analyzed for recombinants by direct PCR using M13 forward and reverse primers (appropriate recognition sites flank the multiple cloning site). PCR products are resolved by agarose gel electrophoresis, and DNA products ranging from 800–1500 bp in size are excised from the gel. We recommend gel purification of DNA fragments, rather than phenol-chloroform extraction, to remove excess primers and incomplete PCR products, which may reduce the efficiency of the sequencing reaction. Concatemers are sequenced using an automated sequencer. Approximately 25–40 tag sequences can be routinely obtained from each concatemer.

1. Mix 10X PCR buffer (2.5 µL), DMSO (1.25 µL), 10 m*M* dNTP (1.25 µL), M13 forward primer (350 ng/µL) (0.5 µL), M13 reverse primer (350 ng/µL) (0.5 µL), water (19 µL), and *Taq* Platinum polymerase (0.2 µL).

2. Use sterile pipet tips to touch individual colonies and place in PCR mix. PCR according to the following protocol: 1 cycle: 95°C for 2 min; 25 cycles: 95°C for 30 sec, 52°C for 1 min, 72°C for 1 min; and 1 cycle: 70°C for 5 min.
3. Electrophorese the total PCR reaction vol in 1% agarose gel. Cut out products 800–1500 bp in size. Use Qiaquick gel extraction kit to isolate DNA according to the manufacturer recommendations, except PCR products should be eluted in water rather than 10 mM Tris.
4. Sequence the concatemers using T7 or SP6 primers. Use of an automated, high-throughput sequencer is recommended.

3.2 Tag Identification and Library Analysis

Several analytic programs, which are freely available to the academic community, can be used to extract and catalog individual tag sequences from concatemer sequences to generate a library of expressed genes (**Table 1**). The number of times a specific tag is identified and extracted from concatemer sequence represents the relative expression level of the corresponding gene in a total population of transcripts. After the tag expression library is generated, the gene products identified by the tags must be determined, and appropriate comparisons must be made between libraries generated from various experimental conditions (**Fig. 3**).

3.2.1. Tag to Gene Mapping

In contrast to array technology, in which the identity of the cDNAs or oligonucleotides spotted on the chip is known, SAGE tags must be linked to a specific gene after extraction from concatemer sequence. Although several software programs for tag identification are available, the National Center for Biotechnology Information has developed the most comprehensive tool for tag-to-gene mapping, SAGEmap *(15)*. Tag-to-gene assignments are computationally generated using sequence data contained in the Unigene project (http://www.ncbi.nlm.nih.gov/Unigene). Unigene automatically partitions GenBank source sequences (cDNA, EST, protein) into nonredundant clusters, each of which represents a unique transcript. SAGEmap uses sequence information in each cluster to generate tags that represent a specific transcript. Tag-to-gene mappings, as well as gene-to-tag mappings, are available for human, rat, mouse, Arabidopsis thaliana, cow, and pig libraries, generated with *Nla*-III- and *Sau*3A-anchoring enzymes.

3.2.2. Statistical Analysis of SAGE Data

The optimal analysis of large, complex data sets remains controversial. A number of tools are available to investigators for analysis of SAGE libraries, both to evaluate data quality and to identify differentially expressed genes.

Table 1
Freely Available SAGE Resources for Data Management and Analysis

Resource	Capabilities	Contact
SAGE2000	Tag extraction and distribution Hidden Markov Model (Monte Carlo simulations) Library comparisons Significance calculations	http://www.sagenet.org/
SAGEmap	Tag-to-gene and gene-to-tag mappings Tag distribution Differential data analysis statistics (Bayesian) Online comparison SAGE library repository	http://www.ncbi.nlm.nih.gov/SAGE/
USAGE	Tag extraction and identification Data pooling and storage Statistical comparison and normalization SAGE experimental design	http://www.cmbi.kun.nl/usage/bin/login.cgi
eSAGE[a]	Tag extraction and identification Statistical analysis Library comparison	e-mail: ehm@umich.edu
SAGEstat[b]	Statistical test (based on binominally distribution) Libraries can be unequal in size	e-mail: j.m.ruijter@amc.uva.nl
Analysis of digital transcription profile[c]	Significance calculations	http://igs-server.cnrs-mrs.fr/~audic/significance.html

From: Schelling, J.R., et al. (2002) *Exp. Nephrol.* **10**, 82–92.
Additional resources are available at Genzyme (http://www.genzyme.com/sage/welcome.htm) and Compugen (http://www.labonweb.com/).
[a]Marguilies, E. H., et al. (2000) *Bioinformatics* **16**, 650–652.
[b]van Kampen, A. H. C, et al. (2000) *Mol. Biol. Cell* **10**, 1859–1872.
[c]Audic, S. and Claverie, J. M. (1997) *Genome Res.* **7**, 986–995.

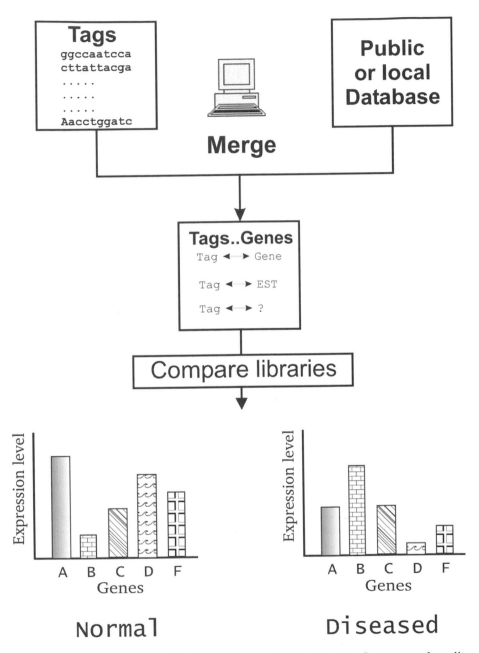

Fig. 3. Strategy for comparing SAGE-generated tag libraries from normal vs diseased samples.

These packages can also extract and count tag sequences derived from concatemer sequence, and in some instances, plan SAGE experiments based on sample size and expected tag frequencies. The statistical approaches differ, and include a variety of methodologies. The developers of SAGE used hidden Markov models and a simulation approach to determine the probability of obtaining significantly different expression levels by chance *(16,22)*. Other investigators have applied classical statistical approaches, such as using a Poisson distribution to define confidence intervals *(23)*. We have used a Bayesian approach for SAGE data analyses *(27)*, which was originally applied to expressed sequence tag (EST) data *(24)*. Alternative Bayesian methods have also been proposed and implemented in SAGEmap (*see* **refs.** in *[15]*). More recently, a comparison of different statistical methods, using simulated SAGE libraries, has suggested that the Chi-square test has the best power, and performs well for a broad range of data and probability distributions *(25)*. Consultation with bioinformatics experts will facilitate appropriate analysis of SAGE data sets.

4. Notes

Specific issues with molecular methods have been incorporated into the protocol. We have previously discussed aspects of SAGE library analysis *(27)*, and summarize our comments here.

1. Tag Uniqueness: Computer analysis originally demonstrated that a 9-bp tag had a 95% probability of being unique *(5,16)*, but our experience indicates that short tags can be ambiguous (e.g., the tag can represent different genes), or that a single gene can have different corresponding tags resulting from alternative splicing, heterogeneity in polyadenylation cleavage sites *(17)*, or population polymorphisms (e.g., when the tag is not specific). For example, almost 3% of 9600 human genes screened had at least two SAGE tags resulting from alternative polyadenylation signals *(17)*. The prevalence of ambiguous tags or tags lacking specificity is unclear, but has increased with the growth of the sequence databases. The number of genes contained in a genome also contributes to tag non-uniqueness. For 15,000 genes, a 10-bp tag has approx 95% probability of being unique, but for a genome containing 75,000 genes, the probabilities are approx 26% and 8% that a 9- and 10-bp tag, respectively, will be found in more than one gene *(18)*.

2. Gene identification: A corollary issue in tag-library analysis is reliability of tag-to-gene assignments. SAGEmap categorizes tag-to-gene mappings according to reliability, based on sequence annotation and orientation *(15)*, and allows users to download either reliable or full tag-to-gene mappings by file transfer protocol (FTP). We concur with the recommendation, proposed by Velculescu et al. *(5)*, that tag sequence most reliably maps to a unique gene if it identifies sequence most 3'-adjacent to the 3'-most tagging enzyme-recognition site (e.g., CATG if

Nla-III is used). Gene tags should preferably match a well-characterized cDNA or mRNA sequence. However, most investigators would also prefer to use the information available in the EST databases for tag-to-gene assignments. For example, the mouse RefSeq database of curated mRNA transcripts contains approx 8478 records, and the murine dbEST entries exceed 2.5 million. Tags, which match an EST with a poly-A signal or poly-A tail, have a considerable degree of reliability, especially if annotated as 3' sequences.

The possibility of sequencing error complicates use of ESTs for gene identity assignment. Since ESTs and concatemers are only single-pass sequences, and the sequencing error rate has been estimated to be between 0.7% and 1%, SAGE may rarely be complicated by incorrect tag-to-gene identification and transcript quantification. To reduce sequencing artifact, SAGE tags should be identified at least in duplicate to be considered reliable, although this strategy would discard some rare transcripts, and more than 83% of transcripts are expected to be present at levels as low as one copy per cell *(19)*. In addition, we recommend that all tags of interest be experimentally validated using other quantitative tools for RNA analysis (Northern blot, solution hybridization, or real-time RT-PCR). Since mRNA levels may not accurately predict protein abundance *(20)*, immunoblot or immunoprecipitation can confirm differential expression of a protein if appropriate antibodies are available. Finally, several modifications of SAGE have been published, that generate longer tag sequences that may result in more specific and less ambiguous tag-to-gene assignments *(14,21)*.

3. Number of tags necessary to define a transcriptome: The minimum number of tags needed to define a transcriptome is a matter of debate, which is partly predicated on the goals of the experiment, as well as the actual number of genes contained in a particular genome. Two studies have addressed this issue. First, using Monte Carlo simulations, Velculescu demonstrated that a yeast library containing 60,000 tags would provide a 97% probability that a single-copy transcript would be detected, assuming that yeast contain 15,000 mRNA molecules per cell *(22)*. The rate of rise in numbers of unique genes, identified in the yeast transcriptome, decreased after analysis of approx 40,000 tags and plateaued at 60,000 tags. A second analysis of a HeLa cell-tag library *(14)* found that, in contrast to yeast, new transcripts were identified even after sequencing 80,000 tags. This difference in the numbers of unique genes identified in yeast and HeLa transcriptomes may reflect the larger, more complex human genome and the likelihood that mammalian cells contain 300,000 transcripts. If correct, simulations predict that a 300,000-tag library would provide only a 92% likelihood of identifying a transcript expressed at three copies or greater *(16)*. Analysis of a transcriptome generated from colon-cancer cell lines demonstrated that the fraction of new transcripts identified did not approach zero until 650,000 tags were sequenced *(19)*. However, the largest fraction of new transcripts found in the total tag population decreased asymptotically, with the largest yield of new genes identified in the first 100,000 tags. Sequencing errors, as discussed here, may also contribute by generating "novel" tags without matches in the databases.

4. Reliability in identifying differentially expressed genes: A major goal of expression profiling, using both array and SAGE platforms, is to identify clusters of differentially expressed genes in two or more samples. In most reports using SAGE, differential expression has been used to identify candidate genes that regulate a disease process, and then other methods were used to confirm differential transcript abundance. However, most investigators do not comment on the numbers of differentially expressed genes, which may have resulted from inaccurate quantification or tag-to-gene mapping. Yamamoto and colleagues examined the reliability of profile comparison in a HeLa cell-tag library *(14)*. The 80,000-tag library was randomly divided in smaller transcriptomes ranging in size from 2,000–40,000 tags. No differences in relative abundance were noted for highly expressed genes in small tag libraries. In contrast, transcript quantity for genes, expressed at less robust levels, was less reliable in transcriptomes defined by smaller numbers of tags. These data indicate that comparison of transcriptomes defined by large tag libraries more reliably identifies differentially expressed genes, further underscoring the need for confirmation of differential transcript abundance with alternative methods.

5. Other considerations: Despite the tremendous strengths of SAGE as a high-throughput technique to evaluate pathobiologic mechanisms, the method has several limitations. We have already highlighted potential technical and analytical issues, but several other significant issues also deserve attention. First, the costs of concatemer sequencing can be prohibitive, particularly if a large tag library is desired. Even at $0.07/base, a 60,000-tag library would cost approx $55,000 to sequence. Establishing a contractual arrangement for "bulk" sequencing can significantly reduce costs. Personnel costs can also be substantial, because the SAGE technique requires a minimum of 2–3 mo for a dedicated researcher with significant molecular biology expertise to generate the tag libraries. Second, generation of replicate SAGE libraries for data validation is not practical, mostly because of the expense. Replication of these large data sets becomes less critical if the experimental goal is to identify a small number of differentially expressed genes, since these comparative analyses can be confirmed by less cumbersome, quantitative techniques and functionally characterized in hypothesis-driven experiments. However, if the goal is to explore expression of large clusters or pathways of genes, data validation of transcript identities using other techniques is difficult. SAGE data can be rapidly confirmed and validated if the SAGE transcriptome is used to fabricate a custom array containing gene clusters of interest and appropriate controls, an approach used to characterize breast tumor-cell lines *(26)*. Third, analytic tools for SAGE data are relatively limited, although as discussed previously, groups of computational biologists are working to establish cross-platform relational databases for storage and analysis of expression data.

Finally, SAGE transcriptomes have inherent biases. For example, in rare cases, some transcripts may lack a tagging-enzyme recognition site and will not be represented in the final library. In theory, different tagging and anchoring enzymes can be used to generate SAGE libraries from the same mRNA samples *(14)*, but this approach is not practical for most laboratories. In addition, genomic DNA sequence is known to be nonrandom because of mutations, selective pressure, and repetitive sequences, potentially resulting in the more frequent occurrence of some tag sequences, and thereby reducing the number of unique tags *(18)*.

References

1. Amson, R. B., Nemani, M., Roperch, J. P., Israeli, D., Bougueleret, L., Le Gall, I., et al. (1996) Isolation of 10 differentially expressed cDNAs in p53-induced apoptosis: activation of the vertebrate homologue of the *Drosophila* seven in absentia gene. *Proc. Natl. Acad. Sci. USA* **93,** 3953–3957.
2. Babity, J. M., Armstrong, J. N., Plumier, J. C., Currie, R. W., and Robertson, H. A. (1997) A novel seizure-induced synaptotagmin gene identified by differential display. *Proc. Natl. Acad. Sci. USA* **94(6),** 2638–2641.
3. Stevens, C. J. M., Te Kronnie, G., Samallo, J., Schipper, H., and Stroband, H. W. J. (1996) Isolation of carp cDNA clones, representing developmentally-regulated genes, using a subtractive-hybridization strategy. *Roux's Arch. Dev. Biol.* **205,** 460–467.
4. Kohda, Y., Murakami, H., Moe, O. W., and Star, R. A. (2000) Analysis of segmental renal gene expression by laser capture microdissection. *Kidney Int.* **57(1),** 321–331.
5. Velculescu ,V. E., Zhang, L., Vogelstein, B., and Kinzler, K. W. (1995) Serial analysis of gene expression. *Science* **270,** 484–487.
6. Schena, M., Shalon, D., Davis, R. W., and Brown, P. O. (1995) Quantitative monitoring of gene expression patterns with a complementary DNA microarray. *Science* **270(5235),** 467–470.
7. El-Meanawy, M. A., Schelling, J. R., Pozuelo, F., Churpek, M. M., Ficker, E. K., Iyengar, S., et al. (2000) Use of serial analysis of gene expression to generate kidney expression libraries. *Am. J. Physiol.* **279(2),** F383–F392.
8. Datson, N. A., Van der Perk-de Jong, J., Van den Berg, M. P., de Kloet, E. R., and Vreugdenhil, E. (1999) MicroSAGE: a modified procedure for serial analysis of gene expression in limited amounts of tissue. *Nucleic Acids Res.* **27(5),** 1300–1307.
9. Virlon, B., Cheval, L., Buhler, J. M., Billon, E., Doucet, A., and Elalouf, J. M. (1999) Serial microanalysis of renal transcriptomes. *Proc. Natl. Acad. Sci. USA* **96(26),** 15,286–15,291.
10. Ye, S. Q., Zhang, L. Q., Zheng, F., Virgil, D., and Kwiterovich, P. O. (2000) MiniSAGE: gene expression profiling using serial analysis of gene expression from 1 μg total RNA. *Anal. Biochem.* **287(1),** 144–152.
11. Emmert-Buck, M. R., Strausberg, R. L., Krizman, D. B., Bonaldo, M. F., Bonner, R. F., Bostwick, D. G., et al. (2000) Molecular profiling of clinical tissue specimens: feasibility and applications. *Am. J. Pathol.* **156(4),** 1109–1115.
12. Luo, L., Salunga, R. C., Guo, H., Bittner, A., Joy, K. C., Galindo, J. E., et al. (1999) Gene expression profiles of laser-captured adjacent neuronal subtypes. *Nat. Med.* **5(1),** 117–122.

13. Powell, J. (1998) Enhanced concatemer cloning—a modification to the SAGE (Serial Analysis of Gene Expression) technique. *Nucleic Acids Res.* **26(14)**, 3445–3446.

14. Yamamoto, M., Wakatsuki, T., Hada, A., and Ryo, A. (2001) Use of serial analysis of gene expression (SAGE) technology. *J. Immunol. Methods* **250(1–2)**, 45–66.

15. Lash, A. E., Tolstoshev, C. M., Wagner, L., Schuler, G. D., Strausberg, R. L., Riggins, G. J., et al. (2000) SAGEmap: A public gene expression resource. *Genome Res.* **10(7)**, 1051–1060.

16. Zhang, L., Zhou, W., Velculescu, V. E., Kern, S. E., Hruban, R. H., Hamilton, S. R., et al. (1997) Gene expression profiles in normal and cancer cells. *Science* **276(5316)**, 1268–1272.

17. Pauws, E., Van Kampen, A. H. C., Van de Graaf, S. A. R., De Vijlder, J. J. M., and Ris-Stalpers, C. (2001) Heterogeneity in polyadenylation cleavage sites in mammalian mRNA sequences: implications for SAGE analysis. *Nucleic Acids Res.* **29(8)**, 1690–1694.

18. Stollberg, J., Urschitz, J., Urban, Z., and Boyd, C. D. (2000) A quantitative evaluation of SAGE. *Genome Res.* **10(8)**, 1241–1248.

19. Velculescu, V. E., Madden, S. L., Zhang, L., Lash, A. E., Yu, J., Rago, C., et al. (1999) Analysis of human transcriptomes. *Nat. Genet.* **23(4)**, 387–388.

20. Gygi, S. P., Rochon, Y., Franza, B. R., and Aebersold, R. (1999) Correlation between protein and mRNA abundance in yeast. *Mol. Cell Biol.* **19(3)**, 1720–1730.

21. Ryo, A., Kondoh, N., Wakatsuki, T., Hada, A., Yamamoto, N., and Yamamoto, M. (2000) A modified serial analysis of gene expression that generates longer sequence tags by nonpalindromic cohesive linker ligation. *Anal. Biochem.* **277(1)**, 160–162.

22. Velculescu, V. E., Zhang, L., Zhou, W., Vogelstein, J., Basrai, M. A., Bassett, D. E., Jr., et al. (1997) Characterization of the yeast transcriptome. *Cell* **88(2)**, 243–251.

23. Madden, S. L., Galella, E. A., Zhu, J. S., Bertelsen, A. H., and Beaudry, G. A. (1997) SAGE transcript profiles for p53-dependent growth regulation. *Oncogene* **15(9)**, 1079–1085.

24. Audic, S. and Claverie, J. M. (1997) The significance of digital gene expression profiles. *Genome Res.* **7(10)**, 986–995.

25. Man, M. Z., Wang, X. N., and Wang, Y. X. (2000) Power SAGE: comparing statistical tests for SAGE experiments. *Bioinformatics* **16(11)**, 953–959.

26. Nacht, M., Ferguson, A. T., Zhang, W., Petroziello, J. M., Cook, B. P., Gao, Y. H., et al. (1999) Combining serial analysis of gene expression and array technologies to identify genes differentially expressed in breast cancer. *Cancer Res.* **59(21)**, 5464–5470.

27. Schelling, J. R., El-Meanawy, M. A., Barathan, S., Dodig, T., Iyengar, S. K., Sedor, J. R. (2002) Generation of kidney transcriptomes using serial analysis of gene expression. *Exp. Nephrol.* **10(3)**, 82–92.

18

RNA Labeling and Hybridization
of DNA Microarrays

Erwin P. Böttinger, Akiva Novetsky, and Jiri Zavadil

1. Introduction

DNA array technologies provide powerful tools for comprehensive genomic and transcriptomic exploration in renal research. Applications of DNA arrays include analysis of disease predisposition by using single-nucleotide polymorphism (SNP) microarrays (*1*), reliable detection of chromosomal deletions and amplifications using microarray-based comparative genomic hybridization (array-CGH) (*2*), and global gene-expression patterns by cDNA microarrays (*3*). A DNA microarray consists of a small membrane or glass slide containing samples of many genes arranged in a regular pattern. Genetic content for DNA arrays may consist of cDNA fragments amplified from extensive (EST) clone libraries by high-throughput polymerase chain reaction (PCR) methods. Production of cDNA arrays is error-prone because of requirements for maintenance and processing of large numbers (tens of thousands) of bacterial stock of expressed sequence tag (EST) clones. Synthetic long oligonucleotide probes (45-mer to 70-mer), designed for optimal sequence specificity and annealing temperatures, can be spotted as an alternative to cDNA fragments, and pose lesser logistic and quality-control demands during array production. Ready-to-print oligonucleotide libraries containing probes for human, mouse, or rat Unigene clusters are available from several vendors. Although precise knowledge of exon-specific probe sequences can be a distinct bioinformatics advantage for spotted oligonucleotides, it may pose a considerable problem for genes with extensive alternative splicing of exons. An alternative method, based on fabrication of gene arrays by high-density *in situ* synthesis of oligonucleotides on wafers using photolithographic masking techniques, was developed by Steve Fodor and colleagues, and provides the basis for commercially available Affymetrix's GeneChip technology (*4*). Although DNA array production,

From: *Methods in Molecular Medicine, vol. 86: Renal Disease: Techniques and Protocols*
Edited by: M. S. Goligorsky © Humana Press Inc., Totowa, NJ

sample probe preparation and hybridization, and image acquisition with dual-color laser scanners are similar for spotted cDNA and spotted oligonucleotide arrays, Affymetrix GeneChip methodology differs significantly in all aspects of experimental protocol. Each spot on DNA arrays contains one nucleic acid species (cDNA or long oligo) for examination of expression of a single transcript. Affymetrix GeneChip use so-called probe cells containing multiple short oligonucleotide sequences derived from different regions of a single target transcript. Spotted DNA arrays are typically co-hybridized with two independent samples that are labeled with different color fluorophores. Image acquisition with laser scanners allows parallel processing of two separate data sets, providing an option for inclusion of standard "reference" RNA samples in the experimental design that can be advantageous for data normalizations and direct data comparison across multiple arrays and samples. Affymetrix GeneChip methodology is limited to hybridization with single samples, and depends on the inclusion of quality-control probe sets to allow intra-array data normalization and interarray data comparability by complex statistical models. High quality of input images derived from DNA array scanning is an essential prerequisite for successful data analysis and output. Thus, robust and reproducible procedures for labeling of cDNA samples, array prehybridization, and hybridization and washing of DNA arrays are important to achieve consistently high signal intensities and low background intensities (optimal signal-to-noise ratios).

In this chapter, we describe methods for dual-color fluorescence-based DNA array experiments for massively parallel interrogation of gene-expression levels in total RNA samples derived from kidney, or cells maintained in culture media. Because the specifications of DNA arrays may vary considerably from institution to institution, it is important to emphasize that materials and methods described here have been optimized for use with poly-L-lysine-coated glass arrays containing spotted cDNA PCR fragments. **Subheadings 2** and **3** contain footnotes as indicated, describing modifications to the standard protocols to optimize performance when spotted long oligonucleotide arrays and/or different slide-coating materials are used.

2. Materials

Meticulous attention to detail of reagent storage and use are essential for successful DNA array experiments. Because of the significant cost involved in this type of experiment, we routinely test new reagents and solutions using routine bulk-stock RNA samples and test DNA arrays provided at no charge from our DNA Microarray Core Facility. This precaution helps to prevent waste of precious RNA samples and expensive DNA arrays resulting from experiments conducted with defective solutions or reagents.

2.1. Reverse Transcription and RNA Labeling

2.1.1. Direct Reverse-Transcriptase (RT) Labeling Method

1. 70–100 μg of pelleted RNA: precipitated using 7.5 M Ammonium Acetate and 95% ethanol.
2. Oligo dT/DEPC-H$_2$O mixture: 17 μL DEPC-H$_2$O + 2 μL Oligo dT (12–18) (Invitrogen) 0.5 μg/μL.
3. Low dTT dNTP mixture: 50 μL of each 100 mM dATP, dCTP, and dGTP + 20 μL of 100 mM dTTP + 830 μL DEPC-H$_2$O.
4. Labeling mix: 8 μL 5x First-strand buffer (Invitrogen) + 4 μL 0.1 M dithiothreitol (DTT) (Invitrogen) + 4 μL low dTT dNTP + 1 μL RNAse inhibitor (Invitrogen) + 2 μL Superscript II RT enzyme (Invitrogen).
5. Cy3-dUTP and Cy5-dUTP dyes (4 μL of each): available from Amersham.
6. RNase One mixture: 44.2 μL filtered ddH$_2$O + 9.8 μL RNase One buffer (Promega) + 2 μL RNase One Enzyme (Promega).
7. Microcon YM-50 columns (Amicon).

2.1.2. Reverse Transcription and Aminoallyl Coupling (Indirect) Labeling Method

1. 5-(3-Aminoallyl)-2'-deoxyuridine 5'-triphosphate (aa-dUTP) (Sigma).
2. Fluorolink Cy5 and Fluorolink Cy3 Monofunctional Dye 5-Pack available from Amersham. Each tube should be resuspended in 48 μL of dimethyl sulfoxide (DMSO), aliquoted in 4 μL aliquots, and dried in a speed vac.
3. 2–20 μg RNA precipitated using 7.5 M ammonium acetate and 95% ethanol.
4. Random primer or Oligo dT/DEPC-H$_2$O mixture: 13.4 μL DEPC-H20 + 1 μL 2 μg/μL Oligo dT (12–18) (Invitrogen) or 1 μL 2ug/ul Random Primer.
5. dNTP + aa-dUTP mixture: 10 μL each of: 100 mM dATP, 100 mM dCTP, 100 mM dGTP + 6 μL 100 mM dTTP + 4 μL 100 mM aa-dUTP + 200 μL DEPC-H$_2$O (*see* **Note 1**).
6. cDNA synthesis mixture: 6 μL 5X first-strand buffer (Invitrogen) + 3.6 μL aa-dNTP mixture + 3 μL DTT + 2 μL SuperScript II RT enzyme (Invitrogen) + 1 μL RNase inhibitor.
7. 1 N NaOH.
8. 0.5 M ethylenediaminetetraacetic acid (EDTA).
9. 1 M TRIS or HEPES pH 7.0 for neutralization.
10. Microcon YM-30 columns (Fisher).
11. 0.05 M sodium bicarbonate buffer, pH 9.0.
12. 4 M hydroxylamine (Sigma).
13. QIAquick PCR Purification Kit (Qiagen).

2.2. Prehybridization and Hybridization

1. Prehybridization solution: 3.5 mL formamide + 2 mL 20X SSPE + 0.5 mL 10% SDS + 0.5 mL 50X Denhardt's Solution + 0.2 mL salmon sperm DNA + 3.3 mL ddH$_2$O.

2. Hybridization solution: 700 μL formamide + 50 μL 20% SDS + 100 μL 50X Denhardt's solution + 400 μL 20X SSPE.

3. 20X Blocking solution: 40 μL 1 μg/μL polydA + 8 μL 10 μg/μL type V tRNA (from wheat germ) + 200 μL 1 μg/μL human/mouse Cot1 DNA. Ethanol-precipitate and resuspend in 20 μL of filtered ddH$_2$O.

4. Slide-blocking solution: Dissolve 0.56 g succinic anhydride + 36 mL N-methylpyrrilidinone. Add 4 mL of 0.2 M sodium borate pH 8.0 to the dissolved mixture and stir until the solution is clear (see **Note 2**) (required only for Poly-L-Lysine slides).

5. Slide chambers are available from Telechem International, Catalog #AHC-6.

6. Slide covers are regular cover slips, available from Fisher.

2.3. Array Wash Solutions

1. Solution 1: 1X SSC/0.1 sodium dodecyl sulfate (SDS).
2. Solution 2: 0.2X standard saline citrate (SSC)/.1% SDS.
3. Solution 3: 0.2X SSC.

3. Methods

Generation of fluorescent-labeled cDNA target samples is a critical step in procedures that use cDNA or oligonucleotide arrays spotted on glass. A number of different procedures have been developed for generation of fluorescent-labeled cDNA targets from experimental RNA samples. The two most widely used methods are the direct RT labeling method and an aminoallyl indirect labeling method. The term "direct" refers to the use of fluorescent dNTP in the RT reaction. Cy3-dUTP and Cy5-dUTP are the most widely used dye-conjugated dNTPs. Because of their different physical properties, incorporation rates of Cy3-dUTP and Cy5-dUTP often vary depending on template sequences that require application of data normalization algorithms to correct for this dye bias. Dye incorporation bias is less significant with the aminoallyl indirect method, because it relies on incorporation of aminoallyl nucleotides via first-strand cDNA synthesis followed by a coupling of the aminoallyl groups to either Cyanine 3 (Cy3) or Cyanine 5 (Cy5) fluorescent molecules. Alternative methods have been developed by the commercial sector, and include dendrimer tagging procedures and products developed by Genisphere, Hatfield, PA (5).

We recommend the direct labeling method (see **Subheading 3.2.**) in situations in which highest sensitivity for detection of low-abundance transcripts is desired, and generous amounts of total RNA (e.g., 70–100 μg) can be generated readily. Typically, a single kidney from ~ 7-d-old mice, or 2–6 dishes (100 mm) subconfluent to confluent adherent cells is sufficient to generate a single sample. The aminoallyl indirect protocol achieves sufficient sensitivity when used with as little as 5–20 μg of total RNA. Protocols for both methods are described in **Subheading 3.2.** (direct labeling) and **Subheading 3.3.** (aminoallyl indirect labeling).

3.1. RNA Extraction, Purification and Quality Measures

Most methods for extraction of total RNA from mammalian samples provide high-quality RNA suitable for DNA-array analysis. We usually extract RNA using Trizol (Invitrogen) following the manufacturer's protocol. Alternatively, RNA can also be extracted using the RNeasy Mini Kit (Qiagen) or modified LiCl extraction protocol (*6*) with equally good results. Verification of RNA purity and RNA integrity is essential. Standard methods include measurement of absorbance at 260 nm and 280 nm and denaturing formaldehyde agarose gel electrophoresis. Indicators of high-quality RNA should be A260/A280 ratio over 1.9 and intact ribosomal 28S and 18S RNA bands. However, RNA electrophoresis requires significant (µg) quantities of RNA and is not very sensitive for detection of RNA degradation. We are now using Agilent's 2100 Bioanalyzer instrumentation and LabChip nucleic acid analysis based on Calipers Lab-on-a-chip technology to quantitate RNA and verify RNA integrity. Analysis can be performed with as little as 5 ng total RNA. In general, results of LabChip RNA quality control correlate strongly with satisfactory outcome for DNA array experiments. Note that a yield of 800–1000 µg total RNA can usually be extracted from a mouse kidney weighing ~ 200 mg (4–6-wk-old mouse) after homogenization in 5 mL Trizol solution.

3.2. RNA Labeling

3.2.1. Direct RT Labeling of RNA

The protocol is a modified protocol based on an original method developed by Dr. Geoffrey Childs at the Albert Einstein cDNA Microarray Facility, which is available (http://sequence.aecom.yu.edu/bioinf/funcgenomic.html).

3.2.1.1. RNA Precipitation

1. Precipitate the RNA by adding 1/10 vol of 7.5 *M* ammonium acetate and 2.5 volumes of 95% ice-cold ethanol.
2. Store at –20°C for 30 min.
3. Spin at high speed (14,000*g*) for 20 min at room temperature, discard the supernatant, wash with 500 µL of ice-cold 75% ethanol, and spin for 10 min at high speed.
4. Discard the supernatant, wash with 95% ethanol, immediately pipet it out, and allow to air dry (*see* **Note 3**).

3.2.1.2. Probe Preparation

1. Resuspend the RNA pellet in 19 µL of the Oligo dT/DEPC-H$_2$O mixture and incubate for 4 min at 65°C.
2. Remove the resuspended RNA and place on ice for 2 min, pulse-spin, and put back on ice.
3. Add 4 µL of either Cy3-dUTP or Cy5-dUTP to the RNA sample (*see* **Note 4**).

4. Add 19 μL of the Labeling mix to each RNA sample mix and incubate at 42°C for 2 h.

3.2.1.3. PROBE CLEANING AND PREANNEALING

1. Add 56 μL of the RNase mix to each tube and incubate at 37°C for 10 min.
2. Pulse-spin to spin down any probe remaining on the walls of the tube and add 200 μL of filtered ddH$_2$O to the Cy5-cDNA and Cy3-cDNA probe tubes. Transfer the Cy5-cDNA probe to the tube with Cy3-cDNA tube.
3. Flush the YM-50 microcon columns with air (pressurized air duster) to remove any particles and pipet the mixture of Cy5-cDNA and Cy3-cDNA onto the column.
4. Cap and spin at room temperature for 10 min at ~12,500g.
5. Discard flowthrough and add 400 μL of ddH$_2$O to the column. Spin at ~12,500g for 10 min.
6. Repeat **step 5** an additional 2×.
7. The pellet should be visible along the edge of the column.
8. Invert column and place into a fresh tube, lightly vortex, and spin for 1 min at 1000g to collect the probe.
9. Probe volume (6.5 μL); add 12.5 μL of hybridization solution and 1 μL to blocking solution.
10. Centrifuge at high speed for 10 min and transfer supernatant to a clean tube.
11. Heat at 95°C for 2 min to denature the probe and immediately preanneal the probe at 50°C for 1 h.
12. Continue with **Subheading 3.3.** and/or **3.4.**

3.2.2. Aminoallyl Indirect RT Labeling of RNA

The protocol is derived from a method developed at Rosetta Inpharmatics, Kirkland, WA. Modifications from our laboratory and from The Institute of Genomics Research (TIGR, Rockville, MD) have been incorporated.

3.2.2.1. RNA PRECIPITATION

1. Precipitate the RNA by adding 1/10 vol of 7.5 M ammonium acetate and 2.5 volumes of 95% ice-cold ethanol.
2. Store at –20°C for 30 min.
3. Spin at high speed for 20 min at room temperature, discard the supernatant, wash with 500 μL of ice-cold 75% ethanol, and spin for 10 min at high speed.
4. Discard the supernatant, wash with 95% ethanol, immediately pipet it out, and allow to air dry.

3.2.2.2. REVERSE TRANSCRIPTASE REACTION AND AA-DUTP LABELING

1. Resuspend the RNA pellet in 14.4 μL of the Oligo dT/DEPC-H$_2$O mixture and incubate for 10 min at 70°C.
2. Remove the resuspended RNA and place on ice for 10 min, pulse-spin, and put back on ice.

3. Add 15.6 µL of the cDNA Synthesis Mixture to each tube of RNA and incubate for 2 h at 42°C.
4. To hydrolyze RNA, add 10 µL of 1 N NaOH and 10 µL of .5 M EDTA and incubate for 15 min at 65°C.
5. Neutralize the reaction with 25 µL 1 M Tris-HCl pH 7.4 and mix well.

3.2.2.3. REACTION PURIFICATION

1. Add 450 µL of filtered ddH$_2$O to each tube of cDNA.
2. Pipet the diluted cDNA onto the YM-30 Microcon columns.
3. Spin at ~12,400g for 8 min and dump flowthrough.
4. Add another 450 µL of filtered ddH$_2$O to the column and spin at 12,400g for 8 min.
5. Repeat **step 4** 1× more.
6. Elute by flipping the column and spinning at 1000g for 1 min. If the remaining vol is over 150 µL concentrate it again on a new microcon column.
7. Dry eluate in a speed vac.

3.2.2.4. COUPLING AA-CDNA TO CY DYE ESTER

1. Resuspend cDNA pellet in 9 µL 0.05 M sodium bicarbonate, pH 9.0, and let it sit for 10–15 min at room temperature.
2. Transfer the cDNA + bicarbonate buffer to the aliquoted tubes of Cy3 and Cy5 and let incubate in the dark at room temperature for 1 h.

3.2.2.5. QUENCHING AND REMOVAL OF UNCOUPLED DYE

1. The coupling reactions must be quenched before combining the Cy3 and Cy5 samples, so add 4.5 µL of 4 M Hydroxylamine and let the reaction incubate in the dark at room temperature for 15 min.
2. Use the Qia-Quick PCR Purification Kit to remove any unincorporated or quenched Cy dyes.
3. Combine Cy3 cDNA and Cy5 cDNA reactions.
4. Add 70 µL of filtered ddH$_2$O.
5. Add 500 µL of Buffer PB (Quiagen).
6. Pipet onto Qia-Quick column and spin at 10,000g for 1 min.
7. Discard the flowthrough, wash with 750 µL of Buffer PE (Qiagen), and spin for 1 min.
8. Repeat **step 7** 1× more.
9. Discard the flowthrough and spin again for 1 min at high speed to dry the column.
10. Transfer the column to a fresh tube.
11. Add 30 µL of Buffer EB (Qiagen), let it sit for 1 minute, and then spin at 10,000g for 1 min.
12. Repeat **step 11** with another 30 µL of Buffer EB (Qiagen).
13. Speed vac the eluate.
14. To probe volume (6.5 µL), add 12.5 µL of hybridization solution and 1 µL of blocking solution.

15. Centrifuge at high speed for 10 min and transfer supernatants to a clean tube.
16. Heat at 95°C for 2 min to denature the probe, and immediately preanneal the probe at 50°C for 1 h.

3.3. DNA Array Cleaning and Blocking of Nonspecific Binding Sites

1. Mark the slide edges with the pencil to denote the beginning and end of the array.
2. Spray the slide with air to remove any particulate.
3. Very briefly (fraction of second) vapor-moisturize the slide (array facing down) over boiling water.
4. Quickly place in Stratalinker (array facing up) at 200 mJ.
5. Remoisten over steam and heat snap on a hot plate for less than 3 sec (array facing up).
6. Soak slide for 15 min in slide blocking solution and shake intermittently (*see* **Note 5**).
7. Rinse slide in 0.1% SDS for 10–20 sec.
8. Rinse slide in ddH$_2$O for 10–20 sec.
9. Boil in filtered ddH$_2$O at 95° for 3 min.
10. Dunk twice in ice-cold ethanol.
11. Spin at 200g for 5 min to remove excess ethanol (*see* **Note 6**).

3.4. DNA Array Prehybridization, Hybridization, and Washes

3.4.1. Prehybridization

1. Spray slide with air to remove any particles.
2. Place 15 (minimum) to 20 µL of prehybridization solution on to of the array.
3. Place cover slip over array, being careful to avoid introducing any bubbles.
4. Add ddH$_2$O to the corners of the hybridization chamber to maintain humidity.
5. Place slide in hybridization chamber and incubate for 2 h in a 50°C water bath.
6. Remove cover slip and spin at 200g to dry slide.

3.4.2. Hybridization

1. Add the probe solution to the array and cover with cover slip (*see* **Notes 7** and **8**).
2. Place in hybridization chamber and add ddH$_2$O to the special ports in the bottom of the slide to maintain humidity.
3. Hybridize overnight (~16 h) in a 50°C water bath.

3.4.3. Array Washing and Preparation for Scanning

1. Place slide in slide holder filled with washing solution 1 and shake gently until cover slip falls off.
2. Place slide in washing solution 2 and shake slide for 10 min.
3. Place slide in washing solution 3 and shake slide for 10 min.
4. Dump the solution and add fresh washing solution 3 and shake for an additional 10 min.
5. Spin slide for 5 min at 200g with DNA side facing out and label facing down to dry slide.

3.5. Image Acquisition (Array Scanning)

To create a digital array image file, it is necessary to scan the array at fluorescence excitation wavelengths that are appropriate for the dyes used in RNA labeling. For example, appropriate wavelengths for Cy3 are 550 nm, and for Cy5, 635 nm. A number of different scanning instruments with varying technical specifications have been developed by several companies. Most scanners permit manual adjustment of the voltage settings of the photomultiplier tubes (PMTs) to adjust gain during a scan. Image acquisition software is usually provided by the manufacturer of a laser scanner, and should be used according to the respective user manual.

4. Notes

1. The ratio of aa-dUTP to dTTP can be adjusted if the signal is either too strong or too weak.
2. *N*-methyl-pyrrolidone reacts with plastics, so measuring must be done in a glass beaker using glass pipets.
3. After precipitation, the RNA can be stored as pellet at –20°C.
4. Cy3 and Cy5 dyes are light-sensitive. Care should be taken to minimize their exposure to light. Wrap all reaction tubes during incubations with aluminum foil.
5. All solutions that come in contact with the slide, except the *N*-methyl-pyrrolidone/Boric acid solution, must be filtered, and pH adjusted to 7.0.
6. When the slide is spun, the array must face the wall of the centrifuge to allow for the liquid to spin off the slide.
7. Glass cover slips must be used for the overnight hybridization, as plastic cover slips may warp because of the heat.
8. 0.05 µL of the probe mixture should be hybridized for every mm^2 of slide surface area covered by the cover slip.

Acknowledgment

The authors would like to thank the NIDDK and the NIDDK Biotechnology Center Consortium for support under grant U24 DK58768-01A1.

References

1. Hacia, J. G., Fan, J. B., Ryder, O., Jin, L., Edgemon, K., Ghandour, G., Mayer, R. A., et al. (1999) Determination of ancestral alleles for human single-nucleotide polymorphisms using high-density oligonucleotide arrays. *Nat. Genet.* **22,** 164–167.
2. Pollack, J. R., Perou, C. M., Alizadeh, A. A., Eisen, M. B., Pergamenschikov, A., Williams, C. F., et al. (1999) Genome-wide analysis of DNA copy-number changes using cDNA microarrays. *Nat. Genet.* **23,** 41–46.
3. Schena, M., Shalon, D., Davis, R. W., and Brown, P. O. (1995) Quantitative monitoring of gene expression patterns with a complementary DNA microarray. *Science* **270,** 467–470.

4. Fodor, S. P., Read, J. L., Pirrung, M. C., Stryer, L., Lu, A. T., and Solas, D. (1991) Light-directed, spatially addressable parallel chemical synthesis. *Science* **251,** 767–773.

5. Stears, R. L., Getts, R. C., and Gullans, S. R. (2000) A novel, sensitive detection system for high-density microarrays using dendrimer technology. *Physiol. Genomics* **3,** 93–99.

6. Auffray, C. and Rougeon, F. (1980) Purification of mouse immunoglobulin heavy-chain messenger RNAs from total myeloma tumor RNA. *Eur. J. Biochem.* **107,** 303–314.

19

Gene-Expression Analysis of Microdissected Renal Biopsies

Clemens D. Cohen and Matthias Kretzler

1. Introduction

The entire human genetic code has been deciphered, and the DNA sequence information of most laboratory animals will be in the public domain in the near future. This will enable the analysis of gene expression in clinical specimen and disease models, which will help to study disease mechanisms. Renal biopsy diagnostics in particular could be complemented by the identification of typical mRNA fingerprints in diseased organs and their correlation with the diagnosis, prognosis, and responsiveness to the different available treatments *(1)*. In this chapter, we will focus on the isolation of RNA/cDNA from microdissected renal tissue as a starting point for mRNA analysis and the quantification by real-time reverse transcriptase-polymerase chain reaction (RT-PCR). Other techniques to evaluate the expression profiles of a tissue, such as serial analysis of gene expression (SAGE) and cDNA array, are discussed in Chapters 17 and 18 of this manual.

To obtain human renal biopsy tissue for the analysis of gene expression, several technical and ethical considerations must be taken into account. First, renal biopsy is an invasive procedure with a small but significant risk for the patient. Any experimental protocol must not interfere with the diagnostic evaluation of the renal biopsy. The protocol demonstrated here allows gene-expression profiles to be generated by real-time RT-PCR from approx 10% of one biopsy core. The inherent RNA instability must be accounted for by any isolation protocol with sufficient RNase inhibition at any given step. Furthermore, the approach must be optimized for high RNA/cDNA yield and sensitivity of the analysis. The complex architecture of the kidney confounds gene-expression analysis. The sampling error inherent in any biopsy procedure can be at least partially compensated for by microdissection of the different

From: *Methods in Molecular Medicine, vol. 86: Renal Disease: Techniques and Protocols*
Edited by: M. S. Goligorsky © Humana Press Inc., Totowa, NJ

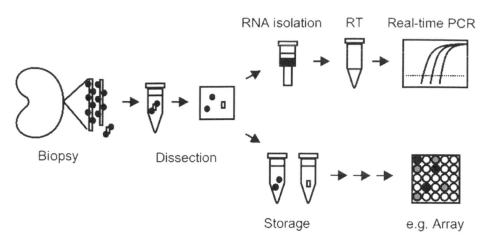

Fig. 1. Schematic view of the protocol. A section of a biopsy core is separated, stored, and microdissected. RNA may be isolated, reverse-transcribed, and analyzed by real-time PCR. Or the microdissected tissue is further stored in RNase inhibitor, and may be analyzed by additional techniques as cDNA arrays.

functional compartments—e.g., glomeruli and tubulo-interstitium. Here, a straightforward approach using manual microdissection under a stereo microscope is presented. This allows separation of the functional units in a high-throughput manner, as required in a multicenter approach, and provides maximal yield of tissue. It does not allow histological analysis and gene-expression analysis of the very same specimen. If this is essential, laser microdissection should be the preferred choice. This technique, presented in Chapter 16 even allows the investigation of mRNA expression on formalin-fixed, paraffin-embedded archival tissue *(2)*.

Finally, the protocol must be easily applicable to clinical settings, in which time is limited and the clinical staff may not be familiar with the requirements of RNA analysis. In the setting of the European Renal cDNA Bank (ERCB), the presented protocol proved to be reliable in twenty different clinical centers, which have processed several hundred renal biopsies *(3)*. A schematic overview of the tissue processing is provided in **Fig. 1**.

2. Materials

2.1. Tissue Acquisition and Storage

Specimens from routine fine-needle human kidney biopsies, open surgical biopsies, samples from a tumor-free part of a nephrectomy, or parts of a transplant nephrectomy can be used. Importantly, informed consent—according to the local ethics committee recommendations—must be obtained before separation of the specimen is done. Tissue from animal models can be handled using the same protocol. Prepare Eppendorf tubes filled with RNase inhibitor RNAlater (Ambion, Huntingdon, UK).

2.2. Manual Microdissection

A stereomicroscope, two dissection needle holders, glass dishes, or Petri dishes of two different diameters, RNase inhibitor (RNAlater, Ambion) and reaction tubes filled with RNase inhibitor and/or lysis buffer are required.

2.3. Tissue Lysis and RNA Isolation

Silica gel column-based RNA isolation techniques are preferred, e.g., RNeasy Mini Kit (Qiagen, Germany).

2.4. Reverse Transcription (RT)

RT is performed in a 45-μL volume, containing 9 μL buffer, 2 μL DTT (both Life Technologies, Germany), 0,9 μL 25 mM dNTP (Amersham Pharmacia, Germany), 1 μL RNase inhibitor (RNasin, Promega, Germany) and 0.5 μL Microcarrier (Molecular Research Center, USA), 1 μg random hexamers (2 mg/ mL stock, Roche, Germany) and 200 U RT (Superscript, Life Technologies) for 1 h at 37°C.

2.5. Real-Time Quantitative PCR

Real-time RT-PCR can be performed using anyone of the commercially available real-time RT-PCR devices. The methods reported here relate to TaqMan ABI 7700 Sequence Detection System (Applied Biosystems, Germany) using heat-activated TaqDNA polymerase (Amplitaq Gold, Applied Biosystems). After quality control of the primers and probes (*see* **Note 1**) oligonucleotide primers are mostly used at a concentration of 300 nM and of probes at nM, respectively.

3. Methods
3.1. Tissue Acquisition and Storage

The tissue must be transferred immediately after biopsy/nephrectomy into a reaction tube filled with RNase inhibitor (RNAlater, Ambion). The volume ratio of tissue:RNase inhibitor must not exceed 1:5, or RNase inhibition cannot be guaranteed. If nephrectomies or wedge biopsies are used, make sure that tissue blocks are thin enough (max. 5 mm) to be quickly permeated by fixative.

3.2. Manual Microdissection

Prepare one glass dish precooled in an ice bath—e.g., a larger dish filled with ice. Cover the bottom of the dish with RNase inhibitor (RNAlater,

Ambion). Transfer the biopsy specimen into the dish. Under a stereomicroscope, you will be able to microdissect the glomeruli with the needle holders: Fix the biopsy core with one hand, and with the other hand loosen the glomeruli sitting on the surface of the core. After separation of these, begin to comb through the specimen starting from one end and proceed to the other end (*see* **Note 2**). The glomeruli appear as cloudy balls, which are easy to separate from the tubulo-interstitium. In most cases, Bowman's capsule will not be separated with the glomeruli. Otherwise, it can be opened easily with the needles and the glomerular tuft can be separated. Routinely, effective tissue separation should be verified and documented by nephron-segment-specific gene-expression patterns such as Wilm's tumor antigen 1 (WT-1/GAPDH). The ratio should be considerably higher in glomerular specimens compared to tubulo-interstitium. In our settings, samples containing only glomerular structures give a 300-fold higher signal for WT-1—a marker for glomerular epithelial cells—than tubulo-interstitium (values depend on the given chemicals, primers, and probes) (*3*).

The microdissected tissue can be transferred immediately into lysis buffer or returned to RNase inhibitor for analysis after further storage (e.g., for cDNA microarrays).

3.3. Tissue Lysis and RNA Isolation

The tissue should be properly microdissected before transfer into lysis buffer. For cell lysis, glomeruli should be separated from the capsule and from the interstitium. The tissue must be rinsed in clear RNase inhibitor prior to transfer. This can be done in a separate dish or in an unused part of the microdissection dish. Glomeruli can be transferred with a pipet in approx 5 μL of RNase inhibitor. Tubulo-interstitium is transferred easily with the microdissection needle.

Cell lysis is performed best in the lysis buffer included in the given RNA isolation kit. Do not forget to add β-mercaptoethanol to the lysis buffer. Cell lysis is sufficient after 10 min mixture in lysis buffer (*see* **Note 3**). Additional use of shredder columns or ultrasound treatment is not needed for microdissected tissue.

3.4. Reverse Transcription

Thirty μL of eluate are obtained using the above RNA isolation protocol (*see* **Note 4**). You can add 15 μL RT chemicals given in **Subheading 2.** directly to the eluate. This mix of 45 μL is incubated at 37°C for 1 h.

After RT, the cDNA can be stored for years at –80°C or for mo at –20°C. Before use of the cDNA for RT-PCR, it is best to dilute the cDNA 1:10 with ddH$_2$O, as components of the RT may interfere with the PCR.

3.5. Real-Time Quantitative PCR

If possible, a 96-well plate setup should be used for real-time RT-PCR. With this format one can easily include positive controls and standard curves, and even analyze housekeeping genes and gene of interest in the same PCR-run. In our experience, a reaction volume of 20 μL is sufficient and very reproducible, but PCR efficiency and accuracy of the pipetting steps may vary from setting to setting. Routinely, the following cycler conditions are used: An initial hold of 2 min at 50°C activates the enzyme Amperase (included in the Master mix offered by Applied Biosystems). This digests PCR products of former PCR runs which may have contaminated your current experiment. If you prepare your own master mix, you may skip this enzyme and the given activation step, if strict contamination precautions are in place in your laboratory. This step is followed by 10 min hold at 95°C. Here, the heat-activated Taq-Polymerase (Amplitaq Gold in the case of Applied Biosystems) will be activated. Actually, not all molecules become activated, but some will be activated at later states of the PCR run, guaranteeing high PCR efficiency. Cycling conditions start with 95°C for 15 sec and 60°C for 60 sec. At the higher temperature, complementary strands separate, and at 60°C primers anneal to the cDNA strand and the polymerase is active. For real-time RT-PCR, one step for annealing and chain extension is sufficient. Routinely, 40 cycles should be performed, allowing even detection of RNA from single microdissected cells *(4)* (*see* **Notes 5** and **6**).

4. Notes

1. Tissue acquisition and storage: It is essential to keep the time from tissue acquisition to transfer into RNase inhibitor as short as possible. This is easy in animal models, but may be difficult to accomplish in clinical settings. The best method is to hand out tubes filled with a sufficient volume of RNase inhibitor to the clinician who is performing the biopsy or nephrectomy. Pre-label the tubes with a code number or, if possible, the initials of the patient and date of biopsy or nephrectomy.

   The tissue can be stored in RNase inhibitor at room temperature for hours, at 4°C for days, or without a known time limitation at –20°C. Please do not transfer the tubes to liquid nitrogen and do not store at –80°C, as it may lead to leakage of the cell membrane and loss of RNA during subsequent microdissection.

   We have determined the quality of RNA on samples stored for 6 mo in RNase inhibitor at –20°C by a microfluidic system. Tubulo-interstitial fragments were microdissected from six renal biopsies from different clinical centers, and total RNA was isolated as described here. All microdissected samples showed intact ribosomal RNA (28S/18S ratio >2). No signs of RNA degradation—as judged by the appearance of small RNA fragments, additional peaks below ribosomal bands or loss of the overall RNA signal—were detected by capillary electrophoresis *(3)*.

2. Manual microdissection: Here we describe the protocol for manual dissection giving maximal yield of RNA of nephron segments from limited starting material. Tissue harvested according to this strategy should also yield highly intact RNA if separation is performed by laser microdissection from frozen sections. For a detailed protocol, *see* Chapter 16 in this manual. For isolation of RNA from formalin fixed tissue, please refer to Cohen et al. *(2)* for details.

   Manual microdissection can be performed best with needles. We use microdissection needle holders from graphic supplies (pricker, HAFF Gmbh, Pfronten, Germany). After microdissection, the needles should be rinsed with water and dried at high heat or rinsed in sodium hydroxide.

   Some groups performed microdissection in PBS with or without vanadyl ribonucleoside complex (VRC) *(5)*. We found no significant differences in the cDNA yield with or without VRC *(3)*. The tissue appears to be softer in PBS and the microdissection of the tubulo-interstitium is easier than in RNase inhibitor. But the yield of cDNA is significantly reduced in PBS compared to microdissection in RNase inhibitor (60-fold higher yield in RNase inhibitor compared to PBS without VRC) *(3)*. If undiluted RNase inhibitor is used for microdissection, no differences in RNA yield are seen over a time period of 90 min *(3)*. A further question is, whether microdissection *per se* leads to loss of RNA compared to immediate snap-freezing and processing without microdissection. We found no difference in the yield of cDNA comparing tissue microdissected in RNase inhibitor or processed without microdissection *(3)*. Microdissection performed according to this protocol allows separation of glomerular structures without a significant loss of mRNA.

3. Tissue lysis and RNA isolation: Several lysis protocols have been reported, and most groups have used the protocol published by Peten et al. in 1992 *(5)*. We systematically compared lysis in 2% Triton-X 100 combined with freeze-thaw cycles in liquid nitrogen, lysis in β-mercaptoethanol containing lysis buffer combined with shredder columns or ultrasound treatment. The highest cDNA yield was achieved by transfer of the microdissected specimen to the β-mercaptoethanol containing lysis buffer and mix at room temperature for 10 min. Tissue fragmentation with ultrasound or shredder columns did not improve the yield *(3)*.

   Until recently, several groups avoided RNA isolation from microdissected renal specimens as Peten et al. demonstrated a higher yield of cDNA after *in situ* RT compared to standard RNA isolation followed by RT *(5)*. Eikmans et al. and our group could demonstrate that RNA isolation by the silica gel-based technique using tubulo-interstitial fragments or glomeruli gave higher cDNA yield compared to *in situ* RT *(3,6)*. In our experience, this technique produced reproducible RNA yields in several thousand RNA isolations from a minimal amount of tissue.

   In this protocol, no DNase treatment is performed, as cDNA-specific primers are available for most targets, the contamination by genomic DNA is low, and contamination of the cDNA solution by DNase may lead to the loss of template during prolonged storage. If DNase treatment is unavoidable, one may use a DNase digestion directly on the silica gel column (Qiagen, Germany). This step is easy to include into the protocol, and allows for an effective removal of the DNase after the reaction.

To test for contaminating genomic DNA, we analyzed microdissected specimens with or without RT using primers with similar amplification efficiencies on cDNA and genomic DNA. Analysis by real-time RT-PCR showed contamination by genomic DNA below 0.1% *(3)*.

4 Reverse transcription: After RNA isolation we preferably proceed immediately with the RT as cDNA is easier to store and handle than RNA.

5. Real-time PCR: The fluorescence-labeled probe is the most expensive component for real-time RT-PCR. Indirect fluorescence detection via intercalating dyes (e.g., SYBR green, Applied Biosystems) works well for many applications, but is usually not specific or sensitive enough to work with microdissected tissue. To test the primers before ordering the internal probe, we perform a PCR run under TaqMan conditions on reference cDNA (and genomic DNA). PCR products are separated on a 10% acrylamide or 2% agarose gel to evaluate PCR product length. If a product of the expected size (and no signal corresponding to the genomic DNA, if primers are cDNA-specific) is detected, the internal probe can be ordered with high rates of success. For a growing number of mRNAs, predeveloped primer and probes are available. Please contact your local nucleotide reagent supplier for the latest developments.

The complete TaqMan assay (primers and probe) should be tested for comparable amplification efficiency with the housekeeping genes assays used, if the ΔΔCt technique will be employed for quantification. For a cDNA-specific assay (e.g., primer or probe sequence spans an exon-intron boundary), no amplification signal should be obtained from 10.000 copies of genomic DNA.

Two approaches can be selected for quantification of the gene of interest: i) Quantification by a standard curve or ii) the ΔΔCt technique. Both techniques normalize the expression to a given housekeeping gene, a marker for the overall cDNA content of the specimen (e.g., β-actin, cyclophilin, GAPDH, or 18 S RNA). It is essential to normalize to several housekeepers, as regulation of these reference genes has been demonstrated in many experimental conditions and diseases.

For the first quantification technique, the generation of a template-specific standard curve is required. DNA-plasmids containing the sequence of interest are an elegant way to enable "absolute quantification" *(4)*. Using a limited dilution of known plasmid templates as a reference point, the threshold cycle of the RT-PCR and the plasmid dilution standard curve allow the calculation of the cDNA template number obtained in the amplification. If no respective plasmids are available, diluted "standard cDNA"—e.g., from a nephrectomy, can be used to generate a standard curve, allowing calculation of the cDNA concentration as relative units (e.g., dilution steps of standard cDNA).

The ΔΔCt technique is well-described in Fink et al. *(7)*. The primers of the housekeeping gene and of the gene of interest must show comparable amplification efficiencies. This can be demonstrated by analyzing serial cDNA dilutions, giving an absolute value of the slope of log input cDNA amount vs ΔCt (= Ct housekeeping gene–Ct target) of <0.1. Relative quantification can be performed using the following formula:

$$T_0/R_0 = K(1 + E)^{(Ct,R-Ct,T)}$$

$T0$ = Initial copy number of the target; $R0$: Initial copy number of reference (housekeeper) transcripts; E = Efficiency of amplification; Ct,T = Threshold cycle of target gene; Ct, R = Threshold cycle of reference (Housekeeping gene); and K = a constant that is dependent upon individual assay properties. Following this formula, the relative expression of the target, normalized to housekeeper gene expression, can be calculated by subtracting the mean Ct of a triplet for the target gene from the mean Ct for the housekeeper triplet (= ΔCt). If the amplification efficiency is 1 (documented by serial dilutions), copies of the individual target transcripts are defined as $K*2^{\Delta Ct}$ copies of housekeeper transcripts.

6. Data analysis: Gene-expression data from individual patients can be related to clinical parameters, histologic patterns, or other gene-expression profiles. Bioinformatics dealing with these issues have developed into one of the most rapidly expanding fields of biomedicine, and expert advice on this issue is strongly recommended. Handling of the information obtained from real-time RT-PCR can be done as described for DNA arrays in this book. In contrast to most gene-expression screening assays, real-time RT-PCR delivers exact quantification over several orders of magnitude and therefore high-quality numeric data. With the growing number of pre-developed real-time RT-PCR assays available for specific mRNAs and the protocol described here, quantification of defined mRNAs in microdissected nephron segments should be within the scope of most laboratories that are familiar with standard molecular biology techniques.

Concerning sample size, the unpredictable intra- and interindividual variability, together with the unknown degree of gene expression and regulation, makes an *a priori* statement of the required biopsy population very difficult. As this protocol was developed specifically for easy handling of the material by the clinician procuring the biopsies, we hope that optimal use of the limited clinical material can be achieved.

References

1. Kretzler, M., Cohen, C. D., Doran, P., Henger, A., Madden, S., Gröne, E. F., et al. (2002) Repuncturing the renal biopsy: strategies for molecular diagnosis in nephrology. *J. Am. Soc. Nephrol.* **13,** 1961–1972.
2. Cohen, C. D., Gröne, H. J., Gröne, E. F., Nelson, P. J., Schlöndorff, D., and Kretzler, M. (2002) Laser microdissection and gene expression analysis on formaldehyde-fixed archival tissue: IP-10 and RANTES in renal allograft rejection. *Kidney Int.* **61,** 125–132.
3. Cohen, C. D., Frach, K., Schlöndorff, D., and Kretzler, M. (2002) Quantitative gene expression analysis in renal biopsies: a novel protocol for a high-throughput multicenter application. *Kidney Int.* **61,** 133–140.

4. Kretzler, M., Teixeira, V. P., Unschuld, P. G., Cohen, C. D., Wanke, R., Edenhofer, I., et al. (2001) Integrin-linked kinase as a candidate downstream effector in proteinuria. *FASEB J.* **15,** 1843–1845.
5. Peten, E. P., Striker, L. J., Carome, M. A., Elliott, S. J., Yang, C. W., and Striker, G. E. (1992) The contribution of increased collagen synthesis to human glomerulosclerosis: a quantitative analysis of alpha 2IV collagen mRNA expression by competitive polymerase chain reaction. *J. Exp. Med.* **176,** 1571–1576.
6. Eikmans, M., Baelde, H. J., De Heer, E., and Bruijn, J. A. (2000) Processing renal biopsies for diagnostic mRNA quantification: improvement of RNA extraction and storage conditions. (2000) *J. Am. Soc. Nephrol.* **11,** 868–873.
7. Fink, L., Seeger, W., Ermert, L, Hanze, J., Stahl, U., Grimmiger, F., et al. (1998) Real-time quantitative RT-PCR after laser-assisted cell picking. (1998) *Nat. Med.* **4,** 1329–1333.

20

The Use of SELDI ProteinChip® Array Technology in Renal Disease Research

Eric Fung, Deb Diamond, Anja Hviid Simonsesn, and Scot R. Weinberger

1. Introduction

Proteomics approaches can be useful in identifying biomarkers of renal disease as well as in understanding biological processes specific to renal function. When combined with laser-capture microdissection (LCM), proteomics techniques can identify biomarkers that are specific to structures of the renal parenchyma such as glomeruli, proximal tubules, or distal tubules, thus increasing the specificity of markers. In addition, since proteomics can be applied to urine as well as cells of the renal parenchyma, proteomics has the potential to identify biomarkers that could be useful in non invasive clinical tests.

Proteomics itself is a generic term, and there are many methods of examining the proteome. Because the dynamic range of protein expression is so vast, all proteomics technologies consist of essentially two steps—separation followed by detection. A discussion of the merits of the respective types of proteomics technologies is beyond the scope of this chapter; which focuses upon the application of Surface-Enhanced Laser Desorption/Ionization (SELDI) ProteinChip® Array technology to the study of renal disease. ProteinChip technology, a suite of tools that includes retentate chromatography, protein identification, and multivariate analysis, allows the researcher to examine patterns of protein expression and modification. Because of its ease of use and high-throughput capabilities relative to other proteomics technologies, this approach has found a niche in efforts to dissect pathways of disease as well as to screen clinical samples for biomarkers of disease. This chapter describes the technology underlying SELDI ProteinChip analysis, and provides examples of its use in medical research, concluding with a series of protocols for the specific application of the technology to urine.

From: *Methods in Molecular Medicine, vol. 86: Renal Disease: Techniques and Protocols*
Edited by: M. S. Goligorsky © Humana Press Inc., Totowa, NJ

1.1. An Overview of SELDI and ProteinChip Array Technology

There are three widely used photo-induced ionization techniques employed for the analysis of solid-state samples by mass spectrometry: Laser Desorption/Ionization (LDI); Matrix-Assisted Laser Desorption/Ionization (MALDI), and Surface Enhanced Laser Desorption/Ionization (SELDI). Each of these techniques rely upon the energy inherent in a focused laser beam to promote the creation of gaseous ions from solid-state matter. Samples are most often presented as crystals or thin films upon a sample support that is typically referred to as a probe. LDI occurs when the sample directly absorbs energy from the laser and heats up via direct or secondary thermal changes, thus producing desorbed ions. In MALDI, thermal energy is transferred to the analyte from energy-absorbing compounds that are typically referred to as "matrix."

Analyte is first embedded as impurities within matrix crystals or thin films. Laser energy is then applied to the sample, inducing ionization and transformation from the solid to the gas state.

LDI analyses date back to the early 1960s, when LDI was mostly used to study a number of small inorganic salts *(1–3)*. Laser-based analysis of large biopolymers was first facilitated by the development of MALDI *(4–7)*. For both LDI and MALDI applications, the sample probe surface plays a passive role in the analytical scheme—the probe merely presents the sample to the mass spectrometer for analysis. Thus, crude samples must first be fractionated and desalted in order to produce a usable mass spectrometry signal. Furthermore, in the case of MALDI, biopolymer analysis is only possible when analytes are co-crystallized with a solution of matrix.

SELDI, as originally defined by Hutchens and Yip, consists of two subsets of technology: Surface-Enhanced Affinity Capture (SEAC) and Surface-Enhanced Neat Desorption (SEND) *(8)*. SEND is a process in which analytes, even those of large mol wt, may be desorbed and ionized without the need for the addition of matrix. SEND is accomplished by attachment of an energy-absorbing compound to the probe surface using the process of covalent modification or physi-adsorption *(8,9)*. Compared to SEAC, this technology is still in its germinal stages.

The SELDI application that shows the most promise to date is SEAC. In SEAC, the probe surface plays an active role in the extraction, presentation, structural modification, and/or amplification of the sample. Without question, the state of SEAC science has been most greatly advanced by researchers at Ciphergen Biosystems, Inc. (Fremont, CA), and is commercially embodied in Ciphergen's ProteinChip Array platforms.

Using ProteinChip® Array technology, sample fractionation is accomplished by retentate chromatography, and detection is accomplished by SELDI Time-of-Flight Mass Spectrometry (SELDI-TOFMS). Retentate chromatography is

Quasi-specific, Chromatographic Surfaces for General Profiling

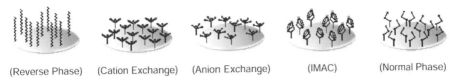

(Reverse Phase)   (Cation Exchange)   (Anion Exchange)   (IMAC)   (Normal Phase)

Preactivated Surfaces for Specific Biochemical Interaction Studies

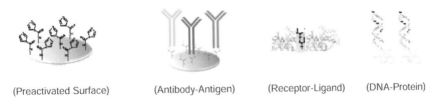

(Preactivated Surface)   (Antibody-Antigen)   (Receptor-Ligand)   (DNA-Protein)

Fig. 1. Various ProteinChip® array surfaces. Both chromatographic surfaces and preactivated surfaces are illustrated. Chromatographic surfaces are composed of reverse phase, ion exchange, immobilized metal affinity capture (IMAC), and normal-phase chemistries that function to extract proteins using quasi-specific means of affinity. Preactivated surfaces contain reactive chemical groups that are capable of forming covalent linkages with primary amines or alcohols. As such, they are used to capture specific bait molecules such as antibodies, receptors, or oligonucleotides that are often used for the study of biomolecular interactions. Figure courtesy of Ciphergen Biosystems, Inc. (Fremont, CA).

performed on ProteinChip® Arrays with varying chromatographic properties, such as anion exchange, cation exchange, metal affinity, and reverse phase (*see* **Fig. 1**). By utilizing arrays with differing surface chemistries in parallel and in series, a complex mixture of proteins, including those from cells or body fluids, can be resolved into subsets of proteins with common properties. After the arrays are washed to remove weakly bound proteins (*see* **Fig. 2**), matrix solution is added and allowed to crystallize, embedding the retained proteins within. After crystallization, features within these arrays are read in the LDI time-of-flight mass spectrometer, often simply referred to as a chip reader.

Once a peak of interest has been detected, the analyte can be enriched or purified for further analysis, which is accomplished through a combination of column and/or on-chip purification strategies. Once a protein is sufficiently purified, it is digested with proteolytic enzymes, and subsequent analysis of the peptide patterns by single mass spectrometric means can yield important identification information. Alternatively, protein mixtures upon these arrays may be studied by combining on-chip chemical (*10*) or enzymatic (*11*) pro-

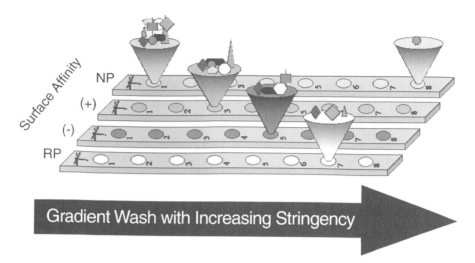

Fig. 2. Protein Profiling using retentate chromatography. Complex biological mixtures are deposited upon each feature of a number of chromatographic arrays, each with different surface affinities (NP, normal phase; RP, reverse phase; (+), anion exchange; (–), cation exchange). A gradient of wash conditions specific for each array surface is sequentially applied to remove proteins of lower binding affinity. Matrix solution is ultimately applied, and arrays are then read by SELDI-TOF MS. Figure courtesy of Ciphergen Biosystems, Inc. (Fremont, CA).

teolysis with tandem mass spectrometry to identify proteins using database-mining approaches. The platform can also be used to identify proteins purified from one-dimensional (1D) or two-dimensional (2D) gels (for an example, *see* **ref. 12**). Various applications of SELDI-TOFMS have been described in several reviews *(13–16)*, and more technical information can be found in **ref. 17**.

1.2. SELDI ProteinChip Array Technology and Medical Research

One widely used application is the study of protein modification, a strength of proteomics as compared to genomics. In fact, reliance purely on genomics information can sometimes lead to incorrect conclusions. For example, transcription array studies of *Mycobacterium tuberculosis* indicated a 4.3-fold increase in ACPm mRNA after 6-h exposure to INH, an antifungal agent known to disrupt micolic acid and cell-wall synthesis in mycobacterium and other fungi. Lysates of control and INH-treated *M. tuberculosis* cultures were examined using anion-exchange ProteinChip Arrays and SELDI-TOF MS, followed by analysis of an on-chip protein digest of a 13,217 Da protein using tandem mass spectrometry (MS/MS) *(18)*.

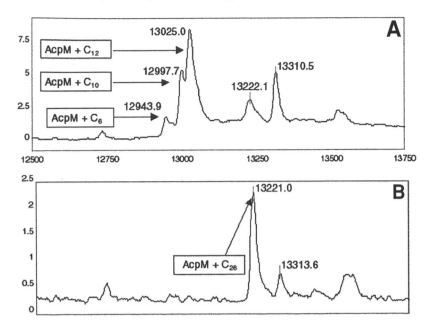

Fig. 3. Truncated forms of ACPm-fatty acid complexes. ProteinChip® Array analysis detected a variety of truncated ACPm-fatty acid complexes found within INH exposed *M. tuberculosis* lysate when compared to that of the control group. These truncated conjugates are postulated to be a direct consequence of INH exposure, indicative of disrupted cell-wall synthesis. Lysates were provided courtesy of Gary Schoolnik, Pat Brown, and Mike Wilson, Department of Infectious Diseases, Stanford University (Palo Alto, CA).

This protein, which was determined to be ACPm-conjugated with its cofactor (phosphopantetheine) and a C_{26} fatty acid, appeared to be downregulated based on ProteinChip® data, in contrast to the microarray data. However, closer examination of the ProteinChip data revealed that peaks found at 12943.9, 12997.7, and 13025.0 Da in the INH exposed lysates were in fact ACPm-phosphopantetheine conjugated with C_6, C_{10}, and C_{12} fatty acids, respectively (*see* **Fig. 3**). This finding highlights the importance of examining proteins directly.

Specific analytes can also be examined using preactivated arrays to which a bait molecule (such as an antibody or biotinylated DNA) is immobilized and a solution containing the binding partner(s) is presented to the array. This array-based immunoprecipitation or protein-binding experiment has been successfully used to study DNA-binding proteins *(19)*, receptor–ligand interactions *(20)*, and protein complexes *(21)*. Such studies can be designed to examine modification of specific proteins. For example, beta-amyloid, a protein believed to be involved in the pathogenesis of Alzheimer's disease, is proteolytically processed by several secretases, resulting in multiple cleavage products. By covalently attaching an antibody to the N-terminus of beta-amyloid to a preactivated surface ProteinChip array, these various cleavage products can be captured from a complex mixture (e.g., tissue-culture supernatant, cerebrospinal fluid [CSF], brain extracts) *(22–24)*. This strategy was used to examine the cleavage products of beta amyloid from cultured neurons isolated from mice deficient for beta secretase 1 (BACE1). Generation of the major cleavage products A1-40/42 and A11-40/42 was abolished, indicating that BACE1 is the principal beta-secretase in neurons *(25)*.

A similar approach was taken to investigate the role of beta-defensins in the oral environment, where these peptides are believed to play a role in the epithelial protective barrier function. The secretion of beta-defensins was examined in vitro and in biological fluid by immunocapture on the ProteinChip® surface using polyclonal antibodies to human beta-defensin 1 (hBD1) and human beta-defensin 2 (hBD2) *(26)*. Consistent with mRNA-expression data, hBD1 was detected in cell culture supernatants from both unstimulated and stimulated human gingival epithelial cells, and hBD2 was detected only in stimulated cells. Both peptides were also detected in gingival crevicular fluid that accumulates between gingival tissue and the tooth surface. These observations are consistent with the idea that a more general antimicrobial barrier could be achieved by secretion of beta-defensins at mucosal sites.

Clinical proteomics is intended to scan the realm of expressed proteins to identify biomarkers that can answer specific clinical questions. The most obvious are markers that can be used for diagnosis or prognosis. Another important issue that clinical proteomics promises to help resolve is the ability to predict a patient's response to a specific drug. Clinical proteomics is also useful outside of the doctor's office. For example, diagnostic markers can themselves be candidates for drug targets, and pharmaceutical companies pursue clinical proteomics to identify markers that predict the toxicity of candidate drugs.

The most straightforward approach to clinical proteomics begins with protein profiling or protein differential display studies, in which protein expression in control individuals is compared with that in patients. Physiological fluids, tissue homogenates, or cell lysates from control and disease samples are processed on the same types of array surfaces, and the arrays read under the same data collection conditions. The premise of this approach is to establish composite fingerprint profiles of both disease and non-disease states from a series of training samples, and then to use these profiles to make a diagnosis on actual unknown patient samples. Biomarker identification is not strictly required for diagnostic purposes, but is required for insight into the underlying biological process as well as to evaluate the use of the biomarker as a therapeutic target.

In general, it is expected that the markers that are specific to a given medical condition are most likely to be found in the organ or tissue—and even cellular population—afflicted. Thus, protein profiling of selected tissues or cells is often the first attempt at biomarker discovery. LCM is a powerful tool that allows researchers to examine histologic sections of tissue and specifically select the cells of interest (e.g., glomeruli, or even segments of glomeruli demonstrating evidence of focal glomerulonephritis) *(27)*. Initially, most studies used LCM to obtain samples from which mRNA could be obtained for cDNA microarray analysis. With innovative sample preparation techniques and the use of frozen sections, researchers have been able to maintain an environment that is friendly to proteins, and have thus allowed LCM to be coupled to proteomics techniques. Because of the relatively low sample requirements of ProteinChip® technology, researchers have been eager to use this technology to analyze LCM-procured samples *(28–32)*.

Although examination of tissue itself is useful for finding biomarkers, the more clinically useful biomarkers are those that are found in body fluids such as serum and urine, since these can be obtained using noninvasive techniques and are thus less stressful to the patient and less costly for the health care system. Researchers have used ProteinChip technology to perform biomarker discovery efforts in a variety of diseases, including infectious and inflammatory diseases *(33)*, neuropsychiatry *(34)*, cardiovascular disease *(15)*, and cancer *(35–40)*. A detailed discussion of these studies is not warranted here, and the focus of this chapter is on studies specifically related to renal disease.

1.3. Review of SELDI ProteinChip Array Research in Renal Disease

There is significant interest in utilizing ProteinChip technology to monitor differences in protein expression in a variety of situations that lead to renal disease. In this regard, a recently published study described the application of ProteinChip Array technology to begin investigating changes in protein expression in renal cell carcinoma (RCC) *(41)*. Extracts from normal, peripheral, and central tumor tissue were compared for differences in protein expression using reversed-phase ProteinChip Array surfaces. The protein profiles of eight well-characterized RCC cases showed up- and downregulation of specific proteins in tumor tissue. However, since the growth pattern of the tumor leads to a significant amount of heterogeneity, it is more difficult to identify unambiguous differences in protein expression in these RCC samples. This contrasts with studies using microdissected tissue samples where more homogeneous preparations allowed for more clearly defined differences in protein expression *(42)*. Although additional studies are needed to further characterize the changes in protein expression, the initial results demonstrate the utility of

ProteinChip® Array technology as a potential diagnostic and prognostic approach to the study of RCC.

In an effort to move away from invasive and labor-intensive procedures for monitoring renal and bladder disease, laboratories have turned their attention to protein biomarkers in the urine. Vlahou and colleagues described ProteinChip profiling experiments identifying biomarkers for transitional cell carcinoma (TCC) of the bladder, and demonstrated the potential of this approach to serve as a urinary TCC diagnostic test *(43)*. A total of 94 urine samples representing patients with TCC, patients with other urogenital diseases, and healthy donors were analyzed for differences in protein expression. Several differences in protein expression are described for the TCC group, and the simultaneous analysis of many protein biomarkers and protein clusters improved the sensitivity for detecting TCC. These results demonstrated the feasibility of looking for urine biomarkers associated with renal disease. A separate study described the use of ProteinChip technology to monitor changes in urine protein composition in an effort to identify markers of radiocontrast-induced renal dysfunction *(44)*. This study investigated the effect of radiocontrast medium on urinary protein composition from both an animal model and patients undergoing cardiac catheterization. In both cases, dramatic changes in urinary protein composition after injection of the radiocontrast medium were demonstrated. One of the detected differentially upregulated proteins was an 11.75-kDa peak identified as α2-microglobulin, a controversial marker of nephrotoxicity *(45–47)*.

Finally, another study describes the use of ProteinChip Array technology to monitor the interaction of serine proteases with negsin, a novel member of the serine protease inhibitor (serpin) superfamily proposed to play a role in the pathogenesis of human glomerular diseases *(48)*. A 120,163-Da peak proposed to contain a complex between negsin (46,883 Da) and plasmin (73,264 Da) was identified from a reaction mixture containing both proteins.

2. Materials

1. ProteinChip® Arrays, Immobilized Metal Affinity Capture (IMAC3)-Ni^{++}, Ion-Exchange ProteinChip® Reader, Ciphergen Bioprocessor.

3. Methods

3.1. Basic Experimental Design

The typical clinical proteomics study begins with a discovery phase, in which assay conditions are tested on a relatively small number of samples. The number of samples and types of samples are perhaps the most important parameters that determine the success of a project. We usually profile at least 30 samples in each classification group (e.g., disease vs healthy or treated vs untreated). This number of samples is usually enough to give us >90% statistical confidence in single markers with p values <0.01, and is also enough to allow us to use some forms of multivariate analysis. The samples themselves are another critical parameter. Because this sample set size is relatively small, inherent biological variability always threatens the ability to conclude that the observed differences are consequences specific to the disturbance under study. Therefore, the study must include well-chosen samples (e.g., patients of the same age group or all of a single sex), and equally important, appropriately chosen controls. Naturally, in vitro studies show less variability than do animal studies, which in turn show less variability than human studies. No matter what the source of samples, all should be handled identically, and care should be taken to minimize the number of freeze-thaw cycles.

Once the samples are procured, they can be processed directly on the arrays with minimal preparation. However, when there is adequate material (for serum, this is defined as 20 μL of vol), we typically perform some form of fractionation prior to any ProteinChip Array binding procedure. In our experience, this fractionation step significantly increases the number of peaks visualized, and therefore increases the likelihood that biomarkers will be found. For serum, we use anion-exchange fractionation, and for cells or tissues we often perform subcellular fractionation. Specific applications may make other types of fractionation worthwhile. Because urine is expected to be protein-deficient, fractionation is generally not required. In some cases in which a researcher is attempting to distinguish between two proteinuric states (e.g., different types of nephrotic syndrome), fractionation may be recommended. Following fractionation, each fraction is profiled under a series of ProteinChip Array assay conditions, which can include different permutations of array surface chemistries, choice of matrix solutions, and laser energies. Consequently, each sample in the study generates multiple spectra, and therefore generates a significant amount of data. Strategies for the analysis of the data are discussed in **ref. *13***.

3.2. ProteinChip Array Protocols for Urine Analysis

Urine samples should be immediately centrifuged at 8000*g* to sediment cellular material prior to storing supernatants frozen at −80°C until further analysis. The supernatants should subsequently be subjected to only one freeze-thaw on ice, and either centrifuged in a microfuge at ~11,200*g* for 10–15 min at 4°C or analyzed directly. The centrifugation step is intended to remove any aggregates that may form during the freeze-thaw process and subsequently interfere with analysis on the ProteinChip® Arrays. A comparison can be made of the protein-expression profiles generated in the presence and absence of the centrifugation step. It is strongly recommended that a protein assay be performed, and that all samples to be compared are applied to the ProteinChip® Arrays at the same protein concentration. Alternatively, urine protein profiles may be normalized to some other standard such as urine creatinine levels. Typical array protein profiling protocols used for urine are outlined here.

3.2.1. Profiling on a Reversed-Phase Hydrophobic ProteinChip Array Surface (Method 1)

1. Outline each ProteinChip spot with a hydrophobic (PAP) pen and allow to air dry. If using arrays whose features are already sequestered with hydrophobic boundaries, skip this step.
2. Pre-treat the spots with 5 μL acetonitrile (the same percentage that will be used for binding and wash steps).
3. Remove the acetonitrile and apply 1–5 μL of sample (0.5–1.0 μg/μL final protein concentration suspended in aqueous acetonitrile) to the surface. Typical concentrations of acetonitrile used are 0%, 10%, 30%, or 50% acetonitrile:water (v/v). Increasing acetonitrile concentration (e.g., higher stringency) results in selective enrichment of those proteins with the highest affinity for the hydrophobic surface. **Caution**: Do not allow the spots to air dry during the sample exchange.
4. Place the ProteinChip Array in a humid chamber for 20 min at room temperature to allow the sample to interact with the surface.
5. Remove the unbound proteins and other contaminants by performing 3–5 5 μL washes using the binding buffer. **Note**: An alternative method of washing can be achieved by placing the entire array into a 15-mL conical tube containing 8 mL of the desired wash buffer and rocking at room temperature for 2–5 min per wash.
6. The spots are allowed to dry, and matrix solution is then applied. For analysis of low mW proteins (<20 kDa) α-cyno-4-hydroxy-cinnanic acid (CHCA) in 50% acetonitrile and 0.5% trifluoroacetic acid is used and for high mW proteins (>20 kDa) 3–5-dimethyoxy-4-hydroxycinnamic acid (SPA) in 50% acetonitrile and 0.5% trifluoroacetic acid is used. Typically, 2–0.5 μL applications of matrix solutions are made to each spot.
7. The ProteinChip Array is then placed in the ProteinChip reader for mass analysis of the proteins captured and retained on the surface.

3.2.2. Profiling on a Reversed-Phase Hydrophobic ProteinChip Surface (Method 2)

1. Outline each ProteinChip spot with a hydrophobic (PAP) pen and allow to air dry. If arrays with features that are already sequestered with hydrophobic boundaries are used, skip this step.
2. Pretreat the spots with 5 μL acetonitrile.
3. Remove the acetonitrile and add 1–5 μL (maximum 0.5–1.0 μg total protein) urine to the spots and allow to dry. (This method allows denaturation of the proteins as the sample dries down, thus exposing hydrophobic regions that are normally present in the interior of the protein. This is meant to increase the number of proteins captured and retained on the ProteinChip surface. (The reproducibility of this method is particularly sensitive to fluctuations in protein and salt con-

centrations. Thus, if there is significant inter- and intra-sample variability, this method is not recommended.).

4. The spots are then washed with the desired buffers as described in **Subheading 3.2.1., step 5**.
5. The spots are allowed to dry, and the chip is prepared for mass analysis and analyzed as described in **Subheading 3.2.1., steps 6** and **7**.

3.2.3. Profiling on Other ProteinChip Surfaces

Although the preferred ProteinChip Array for urine profiling has routinely been the reversed-phase surface, other surfaces have been used successfully. The experimental design should take into consideration the salts present in urine and the effect of these salts on binding to a given surface. For protein-expression profiling experiments performed on a reversed-phase surface, the salt will promote hydrophobic interactions, thus facilitating binding. If a metal-affinity surface is used for profiling, the salt will minimize nonspecific interactions, thus facilitating capture of proteins that bind specifically to the chelated metal ion on the ProteinChip surface. In each of these examples, the presence of salt is not likely to present a problem during profiling unless it is sufficiently high to cause some proteins to begin precipitating. By contrast, profiling on ion-exchange ProteinChip surfaces will be compromised by the presence of salts that function as modifiers of binding to ionic surfaces. If the concentration is sufficiently high, the salts will preclude capture and detection of proteins on these surfaces. One of several methods may be considered for reducing the salt concentration in the sample prior to application on the ProteinChip surfaces. These include: dilution into desired binding buffers, dialysis against a suitable buffer (e.g., 0.1 M HEPES pH 7.0, 0.1% Tx100), and buffer exchange using a concentrator. For the latter method, we recommend trying dilution in 50 mM Tris pH 9.0 containing a final concentration of 1 M urea, 0.2% CHAPS, and subsequent concentration (Apollo high-performance concentrators from Orbital Biosciences, LLC have worked well in our experience, e.g., orbio@shore.net, www.orbio.com). With each of these methods, it is desirable to achieve a final protein concentration of ~ 0.5–1.0 µg/µL prior to profiling. In this way, small volumes of sample can be applied to the ProteinChip surface. For samples of lower protein concentration, a bioprocessor that creates a well over the ProteinChip spots may be used to apply larger volumes of sample.

3.2.4. Profiling on an Immobilized Metal Affinity Capture (IMAC3)-Ni++ ProteinChip® Surface

1. Outline each ProteinChip spot with a PAP pen and allow to air dry. If using arrays with features that are already sequestered with hydrophobic boundaries, skip this step.

2. Apply 10 μL 100 m*M* nickel sulfate to each spot and incubate in a humidity chamber for 15 min. Do not allow the solution to air dry. Repeat this step.
3. Rinse the chip under running deionized water for about 10 sec to remove the excess nickel.
4. Neutralize the array by incubating for 5 min in a humidity chamber with 10 μL sodium acetate pH 4.0.
5. Remove the sodium acetate and apply 10 μL 0.5 *M* NaCl in phosphate-buffered saline (PBS) pH 7.0 to each spot; incubate for 5 min.
6. After equilibration, remove the buffer and add 5 μL of fresh 0.5 *M* NaCl in PBS pH 7.0. Into this spike 5 μL urine and pipette up and down 3× to mix.
7. Incubate in a humid chamber at room temperature for 30 min.
8. Remove the unbound material and wash each spot with 10 μL binding buffer.
9. Wash the entire ProteinChip Array for 2 min in bulk using a 15-mL conical tube containing 8 mL binding buffer.
10. Perform a quick water rinse to remove buffer salts and allow to air dry.
11. Apply matrix solution and analyze as described previously.

3.2.5. Profiling on an Ion-Exchange ProteinChip Surface

1. Outline each spot of a Strong Anion Exchange (SAX2) or Weak Cation Exchange (WCX2) ProteinChip array with a PAP pen. If using arrays with features are already sequestered with hydrophobic boundaries, skip this step.
2. If a WCX2 chip is chosen, wash the chip in a 15-mL conical tube with 10 mL 10 m*M* hydrochloric acid on a rocker for 5 min, or perform spot washes using 5 μL per spot. Rinse the chip with 10 mL of water 3×.
3. Apply 5–10 μL binding buffer and incubate in a humidity chamber at room temperature for 5 min. Recommended starting buffers include 100 m*M* sodium acetate pH 4.0 for WCX2 and 50 m*M* Tris pH 8.0 for SAX2. **Note**: a non-ionic detergent (e.g., 0.05% TX100) is recommended to reduce nonspecific binding. If detergent is present the maximum volume loaded on the spot should not exceed 5 μL in order to avoid sample spreading. Larger volumes may be applied using a bioprocessor to contain the sample (*see* **Fig. 4**).
4. Repeat **step 3** 2×.
5. Apply 5 μL of urine in binding buffer and incubate in a humid chamber for 30 min at room temperature.
6. Perform five 5-μL washes with binding buffer followed by two 5-μL water washes. Alternatively, the chip may be washed in bulk as described in **Subheading 3.2.1.5.**
7. Add matrix solution and analyze as in **Subheading 3.2.1.6.**

3.2.6. Profiling with the Ciphergen Bioprocessor (see *Fig. 4*)

A brief description of urine-profiling experiments performed using the bioprocessor for larger sample volumes is outlined here. The arrays are placed into the bioprocessor and are then prepared as described in **Subheadings 3.2.1.–3.2.5.** with minor modifications.

For profiling on IMAC3 arrays, the spots are loaded with 50 μL of the appropriate metal solution (e.g., nickel or copper sulfate), and the wash and neutralization steps are performed with 50 μL water and sodium acetate pH 4.0, respectively. Equilibration of the arrays is accomplished using 100 μL of the appropriate binding buffer and vortexing for 5 min at room temperature. This process is repeated a second time prior to application of the sample. For screening of high-mass proteins, the samples are prepared by diluting 160 μL urine with 60 μL denaturing buffer (9 *M* urea, 2% CHAPS, 50 m*M* Tris pH 9.0) and vortexing for 30 min at 4°C. Then, 25 μL denatured urine is added to wells containing 25 μL appropriate binding buffer, and the arrays are vortexed for 30 min at room temperature. The sample is then removed and three 100-μL washes are performed with the corresponding binding buffer by vortexing for 5 min each at room temperature. The arrays are rinsed twice with water, removed from the bioprocessor, and allowed to dry. SPA is added prior to mass analysis. For screening of peptides, 1.5 mL urine is concentrated to 150 μL in an Eppendorf concentrator. Then, 10 μL of concentrated urine is added to wells containing 40 μL of appropriate binding buffer, and the arrays are vortexed for 30 min at room temperature. The sample is then removed, and washes are performed as described prior to application of CHCA for subsequent mass analysis.

4. Notes

1. When performing differential protein display experiments, it is imperative to run appropriate controls to minimize potential variability resulting from differences in sample origin, extraction, processing, and handling. As a general rule, artifactual creation of potential biomarker signals can be manifested as a direct result of differences with respect to sample origin. Under these circumstances, it is best to compare protein profiles between control and experimental groups when all samples originate from subjects of similar sex, age, and ethnicity. Of course, in many circumstances, it may be impossible to adequately stratify the sampling pool as such, and as an added insurance against artifactual biomarker detection, stratification studies among different members of the control group should be performed to evaluate protein phenotypic differences between heterogeneous members.

   Additionally, differences in sample extraction, preparation, and storage could generate anomalous results. Consequently, control and experimental group samples must be procured and handled similarly and, for long-term studies, the number of freeze-thaw cycles should be judiciously minimized.

2. It is important to realize the value of maintaining a regular policy of mass calibration for all chip readers involved during the course of a ProteinChip study. As a general rule, chip readers should be calibrated daily using a calibration mix of constant composition throughout the course of each study. Calibration mixes should be wisely chosen so that their analyte components closely mimic the target proteins under investigation with respect to physical characteristics such as

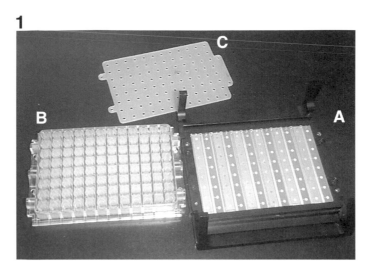

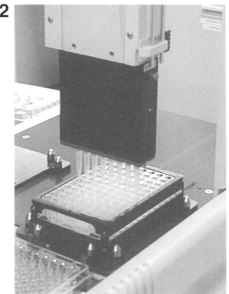

Fig. 4. Ciphergen bioprocessor unit. The Ciphergen Bioprocessor is a device that allows the juxtapositioning of up to 12 different arrays creating a 96-well or 192-well format for 8- and 16-feature arrays, respectively. Arrays are inserted into a supporting base plate (**Photo 1A**). A seal between the arrays and overlying well assembly (*see* **Photo 1B**) is created by an intervening gasket (*see* **Photo 1C**). The well assembly accepts up to 400 μL and 200 μL of solution for 96- and 192- well formats, respectively. Bioprocessor units are directly compatible with most robotic systems, for they comply with all basic microtiter-plate dimensional requirements (*see* **Photo 2**). Photo courtesy of Ciphergen Biosystems (Fremont, CA).

mol wt and post-translational modifications. Calibration runs should be performed using chip-reader settings similar to those used for each experiment, particularly mass range, applied laser energy, and time lag-focusing parameters for those devices capable of operating in time lag-focusing mode.

3. As a general rule, all control and experimental assays should be performed using the same Energy Absorbing Molecule (EAM) solution systems. Subtle differences in EAM solvent systems may potentially create differences in EAM ion profiles that may be erroneously identified as potential biomarkers. It is important to realize that these solutions are photo-sensitive, and as such, are best stored in photo-opaque containers. If refrigerated at approx 4°C, solutions should be stable for about 20 d. However, considering the ease at which EAM solutions can be prepared, researchers are encouraged to begin each new profiling experiment with freshly prepared solutions.

4. It is important to understand that the inadvertent introduction of alkali metals such as Na^+ and K^+ can create artifactual signals in both protein and EAM domains. Consequently, researchers are encouraged to guard against the accidental introduction of these ubiquitous metals. In general, all sample solutions should be prepared using plastic vessels, such as ultra-high-density polyethylene, and glass should be avoided. If glass must be used, wash all contact surfaces with acidified deionized water to remove any residual metals, that may be conjugated to the glass surface.

References

1. Isenor, N. R. (1964) High energy ions from a Q-switched laser. *Can. J. Phys.* **42,** 1413–1416.
2. Fenner, N. C. and Daly, N. R. (1966) Laser used for mass analysis. *Rev. Sci. Instrum.* **37,** 1068–1070.
3. Vastola, F. J. and Pirone, (1968) Ionization of organic solids by laser irradiation. *Advances in Mass Spectrometry* **4,** 107–111.
4. Tanaka, K., Waki, H., Ido, Y., Akita, S., Yoshida, Y., and Yoshida, T. (1987) Protein and polymer analyses up to m/z 100,000 by laser ionization time-of-flight mass spectrometry. *Proceedings of the Second Japan-China Joint Symposium on Mass Spectrometry*, Osaka, Japan.
5. Tanaka, K., Waki, H., Ido, Y., Akita, S., Yoshida, Y., and Yoshida, T. (1988) Protein and polymer analyses up to m/z 100,000 by laser ionization time-of-flight mass spectrometry. *Rapid Comm. Mass Spectrom.* **2,** 151–153.
6. Karas, M. and Hillenkamp, F. (1988) Laser Desorption Ionization of Proteins with Molecular Masses Exceeding 10,000 Daltons. *Anal. Chem.* **60,** 2299–2301.
7. Karas, M. and Hillenkamp, F. (1988) UV Laser Desorption of Ions above 10,000 Daltons. *Proceedings of the International Mass Spectrometry Conference*, Bordeaux, France.
8. Hutchens, T. W. and Yip, T-T. (1993) New desorption strategies for the mass spectrometric analysis of macromolecules. *Rapid Comm. in Mass Spectrom.* **7,** 576–580.

9. Voivodov, K., Ching, J., and Hutchens, T. W. (1996) Surface arrays of energy absorbing polymers enabling covalent attachment of biomolecules for subsequent laser-induced uncoupling/desorption. *Tetrahedron Lett.* **37,** 5669–5672.
10. Weinberger, S. R., Lin, S., Tornatore, P., King, D., and Orlando, R. (2001) Limited acid hydrolysis as a means of fragmenting proteins isolated upon ProteinChip® array surfaces. *Proteomics* **1,** 1172–1184.
11. Weinberger, S. and Merchant, M. (2000) Recent advancements in surface-enhanced laser desorption/ionization time-of-flight mass spectrometry. *Electrophoresis* **21,** 1164–1177.
12. Wang, S., Diamond, D. L., Hass, G. M., Sokoloff, R., and Vessella, R. L. (2001) Identification of prostate-specific membrane antigen (PMSA) as the target of monoclonal antibody 107-1A4 by ProteinChip® array surface-enhanced laser desorption/ionization (SELDI) technology. I. *J. Cancer* **92,** 871–876.
13. Fung, E. T. and Enderwick, C. (2002) ProteinChip clinical proteomics: computational challenges and solutions. *Biotechniques* **Suppl. 34-8,** 40–41.
14. Fung, E. T., Thulasiraman, V., Weinberger, S. R., and Dalmasso, E. A. (2001) Protein biochips for differential profiling. *Curr. Opin. Biotechnol.* **12,** 65–69.
15. Fung, E. T., Wright, G. L., Jr., and Dalmasso, E. A. (2000) Proteomic strategies for biomarker identification: progress and challenges. *Curr. Opin. Mol. Ther.* **2,** 643–650.
16. Merchant, M. and Weinberger, S. R. (2000) Recent advancements in surface-enhanced laser desorption/ionization time-of-flight mass spectrometry. *Electrophoresis* **21,** 1164–1177.
17. Weinberger, S. R., Morris, T. S., and Pawlak, M. (2000) Recent trends in protein biochip technology. *Pharmacogenomics* **1,** 395–416.
18. Chernushevich, I., Ens, W., and Standing, K. G. (1999) Orthogonal-injection TOFMS for analyzing biomolecules. *Anal. Chem.* **71,** 452A–461A.
19. Forde, C. E., Gonzales, A. D., Smessaert, J. M., Murphy, G. A., Shields, S. J., Fitch, J. P., et al. A rapid method to capture and screen for transcription factors by SELDI mass spectrometry. *Biochem. Biophys. Res. Commun.* **290,** 1328–1335.
20. Stoica, G. E., Kuo, A., Aigner, A., Sunitha, I., Souttou, B., Malerczyk, C., et al. (2001) Identification of anaplastic lymphoma kinase as a receptor for the growth factor pleiotrophin. *J. Biol. Chem.* **276,** 16,772–16,779.
21. Tassi, E., Al-Attar, A., Aigner, A., Swift, M. R., McDonnell, K., Karavanov, A., et al. (2001) Enhancement of fibroblast growth factor (FGF) activity by an FGF-binding protein. *J. Biol. Chem.* **276,** 40,247–40,253.
22. Davies, H., Lomas, L., and Austen, B. (1999) Profiling of Amyloid Peptide variants using SELDI ProteinChip® arrays. *BioTechniques* **27,** 1258–1261.
23. Austen, B., Davies, H., Stephens, D. J., Fears, E. R., and Walters, C. E. (1999) The role of cholesterol in the biosynthesis of beta-amyloid. *Neuroreport* **10,** 1699–1705.
24. Vehmas, A. K., Borchelt, D. R., Price, D. L., McCarthy, D., Wills-Karp, M., Peper, M. J., et al. (2001) beta-Amyloid peptide vaccination results in marked changes in serum and brain Abeta levels in APPswe/PS1DeltaE9 mice, as

detected by SELDI-TOF-based ProteinChip technology. *DNA Cell Biol.* **20,** 713–721.

25. Cai, H., Wang, Y., McCarthy, D., Wen, H., Borchelt, D. R., Price, D. L., et al. (2001) BACE1 is the major beta-secretase for generation of Abeta peptides by neurons. *Nat. Neurosci.* **4,** 233–234.

26. Diamond, D. L., Kimball, J. R., Krisanaprakornkit, S., Ganz, T., and Dale, B. A. (2001) Detection of beta-defensins secreted by human oral epithelial cells. *J. Immunol. Methods* **256,** 65–76.

27. Emmert-Buck, M. R., Bonner, R. F., Smith, P. D., Chuaqui, R. F., Zhuang, Z., Goldstein, S. R., et al. (1996) Laser capture microdissection. *Science* **274,** 998–1001.

28. Banks, R. E., Dunn, M. J., Forbes, M. A., Stanley, A., Pappin, D., Naven, T., et al. (1999) The potential use of laser capture microdissection to selectively obtain distinct populations of cells for proteomic analysis—preliminary findings. *Electrophoresis* **20,** 689–700.

29. Jones, M. B., Krutzsch, H., Shu, H., Zhao, Y., Liotta, L. A., Kohn, E. C., et al. (2002) Proteomic analysis and identification of new biomarkers and therapeutic targets for invasive ovarian cancer. Proteomics **2,** 76–84.

30. Verma, M., Wright, G. L., Jr., Hanash, S. M., Gopal-Srivastava, R., and Srivastava, S. (2001) Proteomic approaches within the NCI early detection research network for the discovery and identification of cancer biomarkers. *Ann. NY Acad. Sci* **945,** 103–115.

31. Wright, G. L., Jr., Cazares, L. H., Leung, S. M., Nasim, S., Adam, B. L., Yip, T. T., et al. (2000) Proteinchip surface enhanced laser desorption/ionization (SELDI) mass spectrometry: a novel protein biochip technology for detection of prostate cancer biomarkers in complex protein mixtures. *Prostate Cancer Prostatic Dis.* **2,** 264–276.

32. Wulfkuhle, J. D., McLean, K. C., Paweletz, C. P., Sgroi, D. C., Trock, B. J., Steeg, P. S., et al. (2001) New approaches to proteomic analysis of breast cancer. *Proteomics* **1,** 1205–1215.

33. Li, X., Mohan, S., Gu, W., Miyakoshi, N., Baylink, D. J. (2000) Differential protein profile in the ear-punched tissue of regeneration and non-regeneration strains of mice: a novel approach to explore the candidate genes for soft-tissue regeneration. *Biochim. Biophys. Acta.* **1524,** 102–109.

34. Johnston-Wilson, N. L., Bouton, C. M., Pevsner, J., Breen, J. J., Torrey, E. F., and Yolken, R. H. (2001) Emerging technologies for large-scale screening of human tissues and fluids in the study of severe psychiatric disease. *Int. J. Neuropsychopharmacol.* **4,** 83–92.

35. Paweletz, C. P., Gillespie, J. W., Ornstein, D. K., Simone, N. L., Brown, M. R., Cole, K. A., et al. (2000) Rapid protein display profiling of cancer progression directly from human tissue using a protein biochip. *Drug Dev. Res.* **49,** 34–42.

36. Issaq, H. J., Veenstra, T. D., Conrads, T. P., and Felschow, D. (2002) The SELDI-TOF MS approach to proteomics: protein profiling and biomarker identification. *Biochem. Biophys. Res. Commun.* **292,** 587–592.

37. Wellmann, A., Wollscheid, V., Lu, H., Ma, Z. L., Albers, P., Schutze, K., et al. (2002) Analysis of microdissected prostate tissue with ProteinChip® arrays—a way to new insights into carcinogenesis and to diagnostic tools. *Int. J. Mol. Med.* **9**, 341–347.

38. Ball, G., Mian, S., Holding, F., Allibone, R. O., Lowe, J., Ali, S., et al. (2002) An integrated approach utilizing artificial neural networks and SELDI mass spectrometry for the classification of human tumours and rapid identification of potential biomarkers. *Bioinformatics* **18**, 395–404.

39. Petricoin, E. F., Ardekani, A. M., Hitt, B. A., Levine, P. J., Fusaro, V. A., Steinberg, S. M., et al. (2002) Use of proteomic patterns in serum to identify ovarian cancer. *Lancet* **359**, 572–577.

40. Rosty, C., Christa, L., Kuzdzal, S., Baldwin, W. M., Zahurak, M. L., Carnot, F., et al. (2002) Identification of hepatocarcinoma-intestine-pancreas/pancreatitis-associated protein I as a biomarker for pancreatic ductal adenocarcinoma by protein biochip technology. *Cancer Res.* **62**, 1868–1875.

41. Von Eggeling, F., Junker, K., Fiedler, W., Wollscheid, V., Durst, M., Claussen, U., et al. (2001) Mass spectrometry meets chip technology: a new proteomic tool in cancer research. *Electrophoresis* **22**, 2898–2902.

42. von Eggeling, F., Davies, H., Lomas, L., Fiedler, W., Junker, K., Claussen, U., et al. (2000) Tissue-specific microdissection coupled with ProteinChip array technologies: applications in cancer research. *Biotechniques* **29**, 1066–1070.

43. Valhou, A., Schellhammer, P. F., Mendrinos, S., Patel, K., Kondylis, F., Gong, L., et al. (2001) Development of a novel proteomic approach for the detection of transitional cell carcinoma of the bladder in urine. *Am. J. Pathol.* **158**, 1491–1502.

44. Hampel, D. J., Sansome, C., Sha, M., Brodsky, S., Lawson, W. E., and Goligorsky, M. S. (2001) Toward proteomics in uroscopy: urinary protein profiles after radiocontrast medium administration. *J. Am. Soc. Nephrol.* **12**, 1026–1035.

45. Tataranni, G., Zavagli, G., Farinelli, R., Malacarne, F., Fiocchi, O., Nunzi, L., et al. (1992) Usefulness of the assessment of urinary enzymes and microproteins in monitoring cyclosporin nephrotoxicity. *Nephron* **60**, 314–318.

46. Lewis, L. D., Burton, L. C., Harper, P. G., and Rogers, H. J. (1992) Uroepithelial and nephrotubular toxicity in patients receiving ifosfamide/mensa: measurement of urinary N-acetyl-beta-D-glucosaminidase and beta-2-microglobulin. *Eur. J. Cancer* **28A**, 1976–1981.

47. Rashad, F. A., Vacca, C. V., Speroff, T., and Hall, P. W. (1991) Altered urinary beta 2-microglobulin excretion as an index of nephrotoxicity. *Kidney Int.* **34**, S18–S20.

48. Miyata, T., Inagi, R., Nangaku, M., Imasawa, T., Sato, M., Izuhara, Y., et al. (2002) Overexpression of the serpin negsin induces progressive mesangial cell proliferation and expansion. *Clin. Investig.* **109**, 585–593.

V

TECHNICAL MEANS
TO ASSESS FUNCTIONAL CORRELATES OF DISEASE

21

Clearance Studies in Genetically Altered Mice

William T. Noonan and John N. Lorenz

1. Introduction

Measurements of renal clearance, including the measurement of the glomerular filtration rate (GFR), renal plasma flow (RPF), and electrolyte excretion rate, form the foundation for evaluating kidney function in the intact organism. Although much of our current knowledge regarding the kidney was developed using classical in vivo clearance approaches in larger animals such as dogs and rats, new molecular approaches for producing targeted gene mutations in mice have led to a renewed interest in evaluating kidney function at the level of the whole animal. Our understanding of renal physiology and the molecular mechanisms of blood-pressure regulation and extracellular fluid (ECF) volume homeostasis by the kidney has been significantly advanced as transgenic and gene-knockout mouse models have become available. This chapter focuses on special considerations for applying clearance methods in the mouse, with the idea that adapting mouse methodologies and techniques for use in larger animals (such as the rat) is simpler than adapting large animal methods for use in the mouse. In developing and adapting techniques appropriate for the mouse, it became apparent that mice are more sensitive to stress than rats, and it was clear that the technical refinement of existing methodologies would be necessary to reliably reproduce experiments in the mouse. Over the past several years, significant advances have been made in the technologies available for evaluating renal physiology in the mouse. The following discussion is intended to introduce the inexperienced reader to the methodologies used for making clearance measurements in the mouse, and serve as a source of guidance for the seasoned investigator who may seek to adapt current techniques for use in the mouse.

1.1. Principles of Techniques

The renal clearance of a substance is defined as the volume of plasma that is completely cleared of the substance by the kidneys per unit of time. This concept

From: *Methods in Molecular Medicine, vol. 86: Renal Disease: Techniques and Protocols*
Edited by: M. S. Goligorsky © Humana Press Inc., Totowa, NJ

is extremely useful both in the experimental and clinical setting, as it provides a way of quantifying the excretory function of the kidneys. The mathematical formula for clearance is:

$$C_x = (U_x \times V)/P_x \tag{1}$$

where C_x is the clearance rate of substance x, U_x is the urine concentration of the substance, V is the urine volume per unit of time, and P_x is the plasma concentration of substance x. One important caveat is that the experimental subject must be in a steady state, and the urine and plasma concentrations of substance x must not change during the collection period.

Methods for estimating the GFR depend on the availability of a substance that is freely filtered and is not reabsorbed or secreted by the renal tubules. Therefore, the rate at which this substance is excreted ($U_x \times V$) would be equal to the rate at which it is filtered by the kidneys (GFR $\times P_x$). Thus, the GFR can be calculated as the clearance of such a substance, and the prototypical compound used in experimental settings is inulin, a fructose polymer with a mol wt of ~5,000, which meets the criteria set forth here. Since inulin is not an endogenous substance, it must be administered intravenously at a constant rate to measure the GFR in an experimental subject. As an alternative to inulin, creatinine can be used as a suitable and convenient marker for GFR, since it is endogenously produced and released into the bloodstream at a constant rate as a result of muscle metabolism. Although creatinine is freely filtered, it is secreted into the tubules to a small degree, so investigators should be aware that creatinine clearance may slightly overestimate GFR, at least in man. However, since the endogenous production of creatinine obviates the need for constant intravenous (iv) infusion, it has been proven to be an effective and convenient marker for estimating GFR, especially in a clinical setting. The effectiveness of creatinine diminishes in rats, and especially in mice, since plasma levels tend to be very low.

Clearance protocols can also be used to provide estimates of renal blood flow (RBF). The use of clearance tests to measure RPF is based on the Fick equation, in this case written as:

$$(RPF \times RA_x) - (RPF \times RV_x) = U_x \times V \tag{2}$$

which can be rearranged as:

$$RPF = (U_x \times V)/(RA_x - RV_x) \tag{3}$$

where ($U_x \times V$) is the amount of substance x excreted in the urine, and RA_x and RV_x are the concentrations of substance x in the renal artery and vein, respectively. This equation illustrates that RPF can be calculated if the amount of substance x excreted and the difference in the arterial and venous concentrations across the kidney are known. Importantly, if a substance is completely cleared from the plasma (e.g., the renal venous concentration is zero), then the previous equation reduces to a standard clearance equation:

$$RPF = (U_x \times V)/(RA_x) = C_x \tag{4}$$

Although there are no substances that are completely cleared from the kidney, there are a number of weak organic acids and bases that are avidly secreted by the proximal tubule, resulting in very low renal venous concentrations of these solutes. Since one such substance, p-aminohippuric acid (PAH), is generally about 90% cleared from the plasma, its renal clearance often used as a reasonable approximation of RPF. It should be recognized that since the extraction of PAH is less than 100%, RPF is actually underestimated with this method. If renal venous effluent can be collected, however, then the extraction ratio (RA_{PAH}/RV_{PAH}) can be used to calculate actual renal plasma flow (RPF = C_{PAH}/extraction ratio of PAH). In addition, one can calculate the renal blood flow (RBF) through the kidneys from the renal plasma flow and the hematocrit (RBF = RPF/(1-hematocrit)).

In summary, once a measurement of GFR has been made, it then becomes possible to determine whether the kidney manifests a net reabsorption or net secretion of any given substance (the word *net* is used here to indicate that some substances can undergo both reabsorption and secretion). If a particular solute has a clearance that is greater than inulin, and if the solute is freely filtered and is not synthesized by the kidney, this indicates that the solute undergoes a net secretion by the kidney. Similarly, if a solute has a clearance less than inulin and is also freely filtered, net reabsorption must predominate.

2. Materials

1. Creatinine assay reagents: prepared reagents for this assay can be obtained from Sigma-Aldrich (Catalog number 555-A). The alkaline picrate solution is a mixture of 5 vol of approx 0.6% picric acid and 1 vol of 1.0 N sodium hydroxide. The acid reagent is an unspecified mixture of sulfuric and acetic acids.
2. Dichloroacetic acid (DCA) for PAH assay: to 30 mL H_2O, add 8.29 mL of DCA (Sigma, catalog number D5,470-2), 5.7 g toluensulfonic acid (Sigma, catalog number T 3751), and 3.4 g of NaOH (Sigma, catalog number S 8045). After components are fully dissolved, bring final vol to 100 mL.
3. p-dimethylaminobenzaldehyde color reagent for PAH assay: Dissolve 1.0 g of dimethylaminobenzaldehyde (Sigma, catalog number D 2004) into 60 mL of 95% ethanol. After fully dissolved, bring final vol to 100 mL.

3. Methods
3.1. Balance Studies in Awake Animals

Successful analysis of long-term electrolyte balance has been performed in mice, using rat metabolic cages or cages designed specifically for mice that are now commercially available. In our laboratory we use a simple cage design consisting of a Plexiglas cylinder, divided into an upper chamber that houses the mouse and a lower chamber that houses a tear-drop-shaped glass ball that effectively separates feces from urine *(1)*. The use of such cages allows the determination of daily fluid and electrolyte excretion, as well as creatinine clearance. Urine is collected in a small vial under mineral oil, and since the urine output in a mouse is very small (3–5 mL/d), it is imperative that the glass collecting funnel (or in our case, a tapered ball) be rinsed thoroughly to enhance recovery of dissolved substances that have been retained on the funnel as a result of evaporation (*see* **Note 1**).

3.2. Blood Sampling from Awake Mice

Blood samples are obtained from awake mice by saphenous-vein puncture or by tail-vein cut. A detailed description of the procedure for saphenous-vein puncture in the mouse has been provided previously *(2)*. For tail-vein blood sampling, the mouse must first be warmed in order to induce blood flow to the tail; this can be accomplished using an electric heating pad or infrared light. The animal is then placed in a lucite chamber with its tail protruding from a small slit and held firmly in one hand. A small incision is made along the lateral aspect of the tail with a sharp scalpel and as a drop of blood forms, it is collected into a heparinized capillary tube. Usually up to 200 µL of blood can be readily collected by this method. The flow of blood can be halted with a cold compress.

Balance studies have been combined with the use of indwelling arterial and venous catheters to permit monitoring of blood pressure, blood sampling (with simultaneous replacement), and electrolyte infusion *(3)*. Although methods related to placement of indwelling catheters are addressed elsewhere in this volume, it is essential to recognize that the blood volume of a 30-gram mouse is quite small, typically 2–2.5 mL. Therefore, blood sampling must be kept to a minimum. A blood sample of even 200 µL represents a significant hemorrhage, and can be expected to have hemodynamic consequences. When possible, therefore, blood samples should be replaced with an equal amount of blood from a strain-matched donor mouse.

3.3. Measurement of Creatinine Clearance

To evaluate renal functional parameters in awake mice, we have used a standard picric acid-based creatinine assay to measure endogenous creatinine levels in urine and plasma (available from Sigma-Aldrich, St. Louis, MO; procedure No. 555). We use this particular assay because mouse plasma contains a large amount of non-creatinine chromagens (glucose, proteins, and acetoacetate) that add to the characteristic yellow-orange color development.

The difference between this assay and the widely used Jaffé method is the acidification of the sample that destroys the color derived from creatinine before that of the non-creatinine chromagens. Therefore, the difference in color measured at or near 500 nm before and after acidification is proportional to the creatinine concentration. Since the creatinine concentration in mouse plasma is very low (~0.25 mg/dL), relatively large sample volumes are required for this assay. We have miniaturized this assay by using half-area 96-well microplates (Costar 3696, Corning Inc., Corning, NY), so that the total reaction volume is 120 µL: 40 µL of plasma and 80 µL of alkaline picrate (*see* **Subheading 2.1.1.** for reagents). Color is allowed to develop for 8–12 min and at this time the optical density is determined on a colorimetric microplate reader at 500 nm (Bio-Tek Instruments EL 340, Winooski, VT). Then, 5 µL of acid reagent is added to the reaction mixture. A precipitate, which forms after the addition of the acid, typically dissolves after vigorous mixing. The optical density is read again after 5 min, and this second value is subtracted from the first to obtain the optical density contributed by the creatinine-picrate complex. Creatinine concentration in urine is measured in the same fashion, but the amount of non-creatinine chromagens in urine is usually negligible. Investigators should use caution in cases of renal dysfunction, such as diabetes mellitus, because some non-creatinine chromagens may be present in the urine. Other more specific methods of serum-creatinine determination include the enzymatic PAP+ assay and high-performance liquid chromatography (HPLC), which is proposed as a candidate reference method because results are similar to the definitive isotope-dilution mass spectrometry *(4)*.

3.4. Electrolyte Measurements

In our lab, we have managed to condense many of the common assays for serum and urine electrolytes so that only a few µL of sample are required. In addition, newer model ion-selective electrode-based instruments are capable of analyzing several electrolytes on small capillary samples. For example, we employ a Chiron model 348 blood gas analyzer (Medfield, MA) that can measure PO_2, PCO_2, pH, Na^+, K^+, and Cl^- (or Ca^{2+}) in only 40 µL of whole blood. In addition, using a Corning model 480 flame photometer (Medfield, MA), we measure Na^+ and K^+ in only 5 µL of plasma or urine by manually diluting the samples (1:200) using a Hamilton micro-syringe diluter (Microlab 500 Series, Reno, NV), rather than using the automatic diluter supplied with the instrument. Fecal sodium and potassium measurements can be made using the flame photometer after resuspension of the feces in 0.75 *N* nitric acid overnight. We measure plasma and urine osmolality using a Fiske One-Ten freezing-point depression osmometer (Norwood, MA), and the 15-µL sample can be largely recovered following the analysis. Finally, a Labconco model 442 digital chloridometer (Kansas City, MO) can be used to measure chloride in 10-µL samples.

3.5. Whole-Kidney Measurements in the Anesthetized Animals

Of paramount importance in any investigation of renal function in the whole animal is the monitoring and maintenance of cardiovascular function. Fortunately, the advent of genetically altered mice as models for physiological investigation has coincided with significant advancements in electronics, instrumentation, and computer technology. Micro-chip-based instrumentation has permitted the miniaturization of sensors and transducers to a size and performance level that is suitable for the mouse. In addition, computer technology and digital recording equipment, along with significant advances in data archival media, have allowed for greater accuracy, ease, and dependability in recording equipment. In general, there have been two obstacles to overcome in adapting existing methodologies for use in the mouse: the size—usually approx 30 g for an adult mouse—and the frequency-response requirements, which must faithfully monitor heart rates that can peak as high as 700 beats per min (bpm). Equipment manufacturers have responded to the particular challenges presented by an animal that weighs only 30 g. For example, transit-time flow probes (Transonics Systems, Ithaca, NY) have been miniaturized to the point that they are capable of accurately measuring flow in vessels as small as 0.25 mm in diameter, such as the renal artery (5), and further miniaturization has recently been introduced. Telemetric implants have been miniaturized so that heart rate, temperature, and blood pressure can be monitored continually in unrestrained mice for months at a time (6). Along with advancements in sensors, there have been radical improvements in data recording and analysis equipment, and there are a number of hardware/software packages on the market that greatly simplify and improve the recording of physiological signals. In our laboratory, we primarily use a PowerLab System (ADInstruments, Grand Junction, CO) that permits recording at very high sampling speeds, and has a wide array of signal recording, conditioning, and analysis options. Current technology allows for inexpensive fluid-filled catheter/transducer systems (Cobe CDX III, Argon, Athens, TX) that are properly responsive (frequency-response curves that are flat to perhaps 150 Hz), and suitable for faithful recording of blood-pressure waveforms in the mouse.

3.6. Anesthesia

Several types of anesthesia are available for use in the mouse, and the choice depends largely on the type of experiment being performed as well as the personal preference and experience of each investigator. Anesthetic regimens are of two types, injectable and inhaled, and the various compounds used in mice have been extensively reviewed *(7)*. For long non-recovery procedures, characteristic of renal clearance or micropuncture experiments, we typically use a combination of ketamine and inactin given as separate intraperitoneal (ip) injections: 2 μL/gBW of 25 mg/mL ketamine given first, followed by 2 μL/ gBW of 50 mg/mL inactin. This combination allows for quick induction and fairly prolonged action. The cardiodepressor effects are mild, as evidenced by mean arterial pressure of 80–90 mmHg and heart rates of 400–450 bpm. The advantage of using both agents in a long procedure is that the ketamine/inactin combination will initially produce a deeper anesthesia that permits relatively invasive procedures, such as kidney isolation. Then, as the shorter-acting ketamine begins to wear off, the level of anesthesia can be carefully titrated via iv supplementation and with constant monitoring of heart rate and blood pressure. It should be noted that inactin does not have the very long duration of action that is seen in the rat, and therefore must be supplemented occasionally. A tracheotomy is usually performed using a short length (2–3 cm) of PE-90 tubing to ensure airway patency, and the animal is usually allowed to breathe spontaneously without the aid of a ventilator. However, it is common to provide anesthetized mice with a stream of 100% O_2 to prevent hypoxia. It is important to note that anesthetized mice are particularly vulnerable to hypothermia and body temperature must be constantly monitored and carefully regulated. We monitor and maintain temperature with a rectal thermistor probe and a feedback-controlled, warmed surgical table (Vestavia Scientific, Birmingham, AL). Supplemental heat is often provided using a heat lamp to ensure even warming.

3.7. Surgical Procedures

Many if not most of the techniques used to evaluate renal function involve the surgical isolation and cannulation of an artery and/or vein, and the techniques used do not vary substantially from those used in larger animals. The correct tools are crucial for these procedures, and great care must be taken to prevent even slight blood loss. We have found that use of a low-power binocular dissecting microscope to be essential for procedures, and adding 0.5× objectives can increase the field of view as well as the working distance. Dissecting tools include several pairs of very fine forceps (e.g., Dumont #5, straight or angled), small dissecting scissors, and a set of Vannas scissors. For fluid-filled catheters, we have found it convenient to heat stretch very fine cannulae from large-bore, thick-walled polyethylene tubing. The resulting catheters have a relatively large internal diameter/outer diameter (ID/OD) ratio, and therefore better frequency-response characteristics than conventional PE tubing (e.g., stretched PE10) for measuring arterial blood pressure (*see* **Note 2**).

With this approach, we have been able to fashion catheters as small as 100 μm OD, and have managed to insert up to four catheters into a single femoral vein.

For actual cannulation, the vessel is carefully isolated from surrounding tissue and associated vessels using two pairs of fine forceps. We have found it useful to polish the tips of Dumont #5 forceps to remove burrs and to slightly blunt them to prevent accidental puncture of the vessel (the veins are especially delicate and can be easily torn). Once isolated, three loops of 7-0 silk suture are placed around the vessel; the distal-most ligature is tied to prevent back-flow of blood, and enough tension is placed on the proximal ligature to temporarily occlude flow. The center ligature is loosely knotted, and will be used to secure the catheter in place and prevent leakage when the proximal tie is released. Once blood flow is occluded, a short longitudinal incision is made in the vessel and the cannula is introduced. Alternatively, some investigators use a 23- or 25-gauge hypodermic needle, bent at an angle at the tip, to puncture the vessel and to use as an introducer. Once the cannula is in place, the central ligature is tightened and the tension is removed from the proximal tie; the catheter can then be advanced further and secured into place. For the collection of urine, the bladder is isolated and exteriorized via a midline incision in the lower abdomen, and a heat-flared catheter (PE 10 tubing, approx 4 cm in length) is inserted into the bladder through a small apical incision and secured with a 5-O purse-string suture. All surgical incisions are closed using cyanoacrylate adhesive, even in non-recovery procedures, in order to prevent evaporative fluid loss and tissue desiccation. The animal is then placed on its side on the temperature-regulated surgical table, and an isotonic maintenance infusion is initiated, usually at a rate of 0.1–0.2 μL/min/g body wt.

3.8. Measurement of Inulin Clearance

To evaluate glomerular filtration rate, we have successfully adapted the use of fluorescein isothiocyanate (FITC)-inulin for use in both whole-kidney and micropuncture samples (8). For whole-kidney clearance measurements, animals are infused with a 1% solution of FITC-inulin (Sigma, catalog number F 3272) at the maintenance infusion rate of 0.1–0.2 μL/min/g body wt. Following a 30–45 min equilibration period, several consecutive urine collection periods are initiated, lasting 20–30 min each, depending on urine flow rate. Typically, we collect urine through two control periods, followed by two experimental periods (e.g., volume expansion or drug treatment). Blood samples (20–30 μL) are drawn from the arterial catheter into heparinized hematocrit tubes, midway through each urine collection period, with replacement of whole donor blood. Urine is collected from the bladder catheter into preweighed microcentrifuge tubes. For the inulin assay, urine samples are prediluted 1:50 or 1:100 (again, depending on urine flow rate) with distilled water to bring the concentration of inulin into the same range as the plasma samples. Plasma or urine aliquots of 4 μL are then diluted with 196 μL of 10 mM Hepes buffer (pH 7.4), into black 96-well microplates (Costar 3792, Corning Inc., Corning, NY) using a Hamilton micro-syringe diluter. The samples are then analyzed using a microplate fluorometer with an excitation at 485 nm and emission at 538 nm. In our experience, GFR ranges between 0.8 and 1.0 mL/min/g kidney weight *(8)*, which is consistent with most of the current findings *(9,10)*. It is interesting to note that on a kidney weight basis, GFR in mice and rats are comparable, but when corrected for body wt, GFR in the mouse may be twice that in the rat, reflecting the increased kidney weight-to-body weight ratio in mice.

3.9. Measurement of PAH Clearance

The estimation of renal plasma flow using PAH has also been utilized in mice by several investigators. Spurney and colleagues used ^{3}H-PAH to measure renal plasma flow and reported values approx 2.5 mL/min/g kidney weight *(9)*. More recently, several groups have reported the use of a colorimetric assay for evaluating PAH clearance in mice infused with 2–5% PAH *(10,11)*, but the findings were limited because of sampling restrictions. These investigators reported PAH clearances ranging from 2–4.5 mL/min/g kidney weight. We have miniaturized a colorimetric assay for PAH *(12)* enabling measurement on as little as 10 μL of plasma. For these experiments, animals are prepared and treated exactly as described in **Subheadings 3.7.** and **3.8.**, except that 3% PAH (Sigma, PAH sodium salt, catalog number A 3759) is included in the maintenance infusion (0.1–0.2 μL/min/g body wt).

As with the inulin assay, urine samples are prediluted 1:50 with distilled water to achieve the same PAH concentration range as the plasma samples. Plasma and diluted urine sample are diluted 1:10 with DCA (*see* **Subheading 2.1.2.**) to precipitate proteins and to adjust pH. After centrifugation, 40-μL aliquots of the supernatant are mixed with 40 μL of p-dimethylaminobenzaldehyde color reagent (*see* **Subheading 2.1.3.**) into half-area 96-well microplates, which are read on a colorimetric microplate reader at a wavelength of 450 nm.

By cannulating the renal vein to sample renal venous effluent blood, we have found that the extraction ratio for PAH generally ranges between 0.8 and 0.9 at plasma PAH concentrations up to at least 0.08 mg/mL. These values compare favorably to those obtained in rats, which are generally reported to range between 0.6 and 0.9. It is important to note that the plasma concentration of PAH remains below 0.1 mg/mL, even at infusion rates of 6 μg/gBW/min (corresponding to an infusion of 4% PAH at a rate of 3 μL/min). Values for renal blood flow obtained from these experiments averaged approx 3 mL/min/g kidney weight.

3.10. Direct Measurement of Renal Blood Flow and Autoregulation

Direct measurements of renal blood flow (RBF) using flow probes are generally preferable to estimates using PAH clearance, and current technology utilizing transit time and/or laser-Doppler flowmetry permits such approaches. Gross and colleagues evaluated renal blood flow and pressure-natriuresis responses using a Transonics Systems 0.5-mm V-series perivascular flow probe to measure total RBF and two fiberoptic strands in conjunction with a Transonics laser-Doppler flowmeter to determine cortical and medullary flow *(5)*. To define autoregulatory and natriuretic responses in mice, these investigators used long-term changes in renal perfusion pressure, induced by ligating the celiac and mesenteric arteries and lower abdominal aorta. We and others have used an aortic clamp to transiently alter renal perfusion pressure to evaluate RBF autoregulation.

Autoregulation experimental procedures can be quite challenging because of the invasiveness of the surgical procedure and the overall length of the experiment. We and others have adopted several different maneuvers to help maintain a stable animal throughout the experimental protocol. First, the femoral artery is cannulated as described in **Subheading 3.7.**, except that the tip of the catheter is advanced approx 2 cm to a point just below the renal artery; the vein and bladder are cannulated as in **Subheading 3.7.** Mice receive an iv maintenance infusion of 150 mM NaCl containing 2.5% bovine serum albumin [BSA]/1% glucose at a rate of 0.4 (l/min/g body wt. After the animal is placed on its right side, a flank incision of approx 3 cm in length is made from back to abdomen, approx 0.5 cm caudal to the margin of the ribcage, in order to expose the abdominal wall overlying the left kidney. The muscle layer is then incised along the same line, using a small electric cautery to prevent blood loss. Wound retractors are then used to expose the kidney and the surrounding structures. The kidney is carefully dissected free from the perirenal fat, and deflected medially to expose the abdominal aorta. Using fine Dumont forceps, the celiac and mesenteric arteries, and the abdominal aorta, just above and just below the left kidney are dissected free, and 7-O silk sutures are placed loosely around them. The renal artery, which is almost always positioned dorsal to the renal vein in the mouse, is then dissected free, and two short pieces of 7-O silk are placed under the vessel to aid in placement of the artery into a 0.5-mm, V-type ultrasonic flow probe (Transonic Systems, Ithaca, NY), which is held in place with a micromanipulator. An adjustable stainless-steel clamp (Vestavia Scientific, Birmingham, AL) is placed around the aorta just above the renal artery with the aid of suture placed earlier, and it is also held in place by a micromanipulator. The final step is to tie off the superior mesenteric and celiac arteries and the aorta below the renal arteries using the silk sutures placed earlier, in order to elevate renal-perfusion pressure. The lower aortic ligature is tied around the femoral artery catheter to permit continuous recording of renal-perfusion pressure. To perform autoregulation experiments, the aortic clamp is transiently tightened for 30–60-sec periods so as to lower renal-perfusion pressure to a series of predetermined values (e.g., 120, 110, 100, 90, 80, 70, and 60 mmHg, usually in random order), and the resultant changes in renal blood flow are continuously monitored.

3.11. Micropuncture Studies

Free-flow micropuncture measurements of single-nephron clearance were reported in transgenic mice as early as 1994 *(13)*, and since then several different mutant models have been studied by analyzing samples obtained from both proximal and distal tubules *(14,15)*. Free-flow measurements have yielded a profile of nephron function that is not altogether different from that seen in the rat. Although values of single nephron GFR are lower in mice, averaging approx 12–15 nL/min as compared to 30–35 nL/min in rat, fractional reabsorption from late proximal and early distal puncture site is comparable to the rat: 40–50% and 70–80%, respectively, in normal animals. In practical terms, we have found that proximal punctures in the mouse are on the same size and flow scale as distal collections in the rat, and mouse distal collections are somewhat smaller. Pipets for making proximal tubule collections are sharpened to a tip diameter of 7–8 μm, and those for distal collections to a tip diameter of 5–6 μm. For micropuncture, preparation and kidney isolation is conducted as described in the previous section regarding placement of the renal artery flow probe, except that the aorta and mesenteric and celiac arteries are not isolated and tied. After the kidney is dissected free from the surrounding fat and fascia, and the adherent adrenal gland, it is immobilized in a small Lucite cup, which is then clamped in place (*see* **Note 3**). Space does not allow a full discussion of the methods for performing renal micropuncture; however, additional issues are addressed in Chapter 29.

We have miniaturized the technique for evaluating FITC-inulin clearance to include measurements of single nephron GFR *(8)*. Using this approach, micropuncture samples of 5 nL or greater are deposited between oil columns into a small 1-μL microcapillary tube (microcaps, Drummond Scientific, Broomall, PA). After adding 0.5–1 nL of 500 m*M* HEPES (pH = 7.4) to each sample in order to normalize pH, the microcaps are placed on the stage of an inverted microscope fluorometer (of the sort typically used for intracellular calcium measurements). Using an excitation wavelength of 480 nm and emission wavelength of 530 nm, the samples are digitally imaged and then analyzed for fluorescence intensity. This technique has the advantages of being simple to use, highly sensitive, inexpensive, and nonradioactive; furthermore, it can be performed on samples as small as 5 nL, and it does not consume the sample.

4. Notes

1. We prefer to use a spray bottle to mist small quantities of water onto the funnel to redissolve the dried urine. The resultant wash is collected in the urine collection vial, after first measuring the urine volume. We usually wash 3×.

2. Catheter fabrication for cannulating mouse vessels is challenging because of the small size requirements. In larger animals, investigators usually rely on prefabricated polyethylene micro-bore tubing, such as Intramedic PE-50 and PE-10, for the construction of catheters. However, since the available dimensions of this tubing are too large for use in the mouse, catheters are made by stretching this tubing over low heat to achieve an OD that is appropriate for mouse vessels (e.g., ~ 0.3–0.4 mm). In our experience, however, this approach results in catheters with very small-lumen diameters and less than optimal frequency-response characteristics for recording blood pressure. Therefore, we construct our catheters by heat-stretching cannulae from large-bore, thick-walled polyethylene tubing. Using this process, the tubing is placed just above a hot flame until it becomes molten and clear. It is then removed from the flame and rapidly stretched to produce a thin tapered filament, much in the same manner that fine glass capillaries can be pulled from larger glass tubes. With a little practice, this approach can be used to make catheters of almost any dimension and shape. Since the tubing retains its original wall thickness/ID ratio, the resulting catheters have relatively larger bores than similar-sized catheters fabricated from PE-10. For arterial catheters, we start with polyethylene tubing with an OD of 3/8 or even 1/2 inch and a wall thickness of 1/16 inch (9.5 or 12.7 mm × 1.6 mm; Nalgene 489 Polyethylene Tubing, product number 8010-0125, Nalge Nunc Int., Rochester, NY). To minimize the dead space for venous catheters, we use tubing with an OD of 1/4 inch and a wall thickness of 1/16 inch (6.4 mm × 1.6 mm).

3. The ureter of the mouse kidney is tightly adherent to the medial margin of the kidney, and is therefore very difficult to dissect free without bleeding. For this reason, we have modified the Lucite kidney holder by adding a second opening: the first opening is located traditionally, near the center of the holder (opposite the handle), so as to accommodate the renal vessels emerging from the hilum, and the second opening is located in one corner in order to accommodate the ureter emerging from the caudal pole of the kidney.

References

1. Meneton, P., Schultheis, P. J., Greeb, J., Nieman, M. L., Liu, L. H., Clarke, L. L., et al. (1998) Increased sensitivity to K+ deprivation in colonic H,K-ATPase-deficient mice. *J. Clin. Investig.* **101,** 536–542.

2. Hem, A., Smith, A. J., and Solberg, P. (1998) Saphenous vein puncture for blood sampling of the mouse, rat, hamster, gerbil, guinea pig, ferret and mink. *Lab. Anim.* **32,** 364–368.

3. Mattson, D. L. and Krauski, K. R. (1998) Chronic sodium balance and blood pressure response to captopril in conscious mice. *Hypertension* **32,** 923–928.

4. Rosano, T. G., Ambrose, R. T., Wu, A. H., Swift, T. A., and Yadegari, P. (1990) Candidate reference method for determining creatinine in serum: method development and interlaboratory validation. *Clin. Chem.* **36,** 1951–1955.
5. Gross, V., Lippoldt, A., and Luft, F. C. (1997) Pressure diuresis and natriuresis in DOCA-salt mice. *Kidney Int.* **52,** 1364–1368.
6. Butz, G. M. and Davisson, R. L. (2001) Long-term telemetric measurement of cardiovascular parameters in awake mice: a physiological genomics tool. *Physiol. Genomics* **5,** 89–97.
7. Rao, S. and Verkman, A. S. (2000) Analysis of organ physiology in transgenic mice. *Am. J. Physiol. Cell Physiol.* **279,** C1–C18.
8. Lorenz, J. N. and Gruenstein, E. (1999) A simple, nonradioactive method for evaluating single-nephron filtration rate using FITC-inulin. *Am. J. Physiol. Renal Physiol.* **276,** F172–F177.
9. Spurney, R. F., Fan, P. Y., Ruiz, P., Sanfilippo, F., Pisetsky, D. S., and Coffman, T. M. (1992) Thromboxane receptor blockade reduces renal injury in murine lupus nephritis. *Kidney Int.* **41,** 973–982.
10. Cervenka, L., Mitchell, K. D., Oliverio, M. I., Coffman, T. M., and Navar, L. G. (1999) Renal function in the AT1A receptor knockout mouse during normal and volume-expanded conditions. *Kidney Int.* **56,** 1855–1862.
11. Wang, D., Yoshida, H., Song, Q., Chao, L., and Chao, J. (2000) Enhanced renal function in bradykinin B(2) receptor transgenic mice. *Am. J. Physiol. Renal Physiol.* **278,** F484–F491.
12. Waugh, W. H. and Beall, P. T. (1974) Simplified measurement of p-aminohippurate and other arylamines in plasma and urine. *Kidney Int.* **5,** 429–436.
13. Sonnenberg, H., Honrath, U., Chong, C. K., Field, L. J., and Veress, A. T. (1994) Proximal tubular function in transgenic mice overexpressing atrial natriuretic factor. *Can. J. Physiol. Pharmacol.* **72,** 1168–1170.
14. Lorenz, J. N., Schultheis, P. J., Traynor, T., Shull, G. E., and Schnermann, J. (1999) Micropuncture analysis of single-nephron function in NHE3-deficient mice. *Am. J. Physiol. Renal Physiol.* **277,** F447–F453.
15. Schnermann, J., Chou, C. L., Ma, T., Traynor, T., Knepper, M. A., and Verkman, A. S. (1998) Defective proximal tubular fluid reabsorption in transgenic aquaporin-1 null mice. *Proc. Natl. Acad. Sci. USA* **95,** 9660–9664.

22

Long-Term Blood-Pressure Monitoring in Unrestrained Animals

Karen A. Griffin, Isam Abu-Amarah, and Anil K. Bidani

1. Introduction

The kidneys are not only intimately involved in the long-term regulation of blood pressure (BP), but hypertension per se leads to secondary alterations in renal function *(1–4)*. Moreover, the kidneys are a major target site for end-organ hypertensive damage. Indeed, hypertension plays a dominant role in the progression of all forms of chronic renal diseases, including diabetic nephropathy *(5–9)*. An accurate estimate of the ambient BP load is critical in defining the relationships between BP and renal damage in and between experimental models or to evaluate the impact of any therapeutic intervention on such relationships *(9)*. Additionally, the interrelationships between renal function, BP regulation, and hypertensive renal damage involve complex interactions between genetic and environmental factors that are the subject of ongoing investigations and which require rather precise and accurate characterization of the BP phenotype for valid conclusions *(10–16)*. However, BP exhibits moment-to-moment fluctuations as a result of the activity and interactions of neural, hormonal, and other components of the cardiovascular system in addition to the circadian rhythms *(17,18)*. Such BP lability is further exaggerated in hypertensive states *(17–19)*. Therefore, conventional periodic tail-cuff BP measurements, although adequate for separating relatively large differences in average BP between experimental groups, are inherently inadequate in providing an accurate assessment of the ambient BP profiles that are usually necessary to define the relationship of BP to the parameters of investigative interest *(19–22)*. The availability of radiotelemetric methods to continuously monitor BP in conscious unrestrained animals *(23,24)* has provided an extremely valuable investigative tool for such studies and has yielded important new insights into the complexity of the BP phenotype and its regulatory mechanisms *(11–14,18)* (**Fig. 1**). Radiotelemetric BP moni-

From: *Methods in Molecular Medicine, vol. 86: Renal Disease: Techniques and Protocols*
Edited by: M. S. Goligorsky © Humana Press Inc., Totowa, NJ

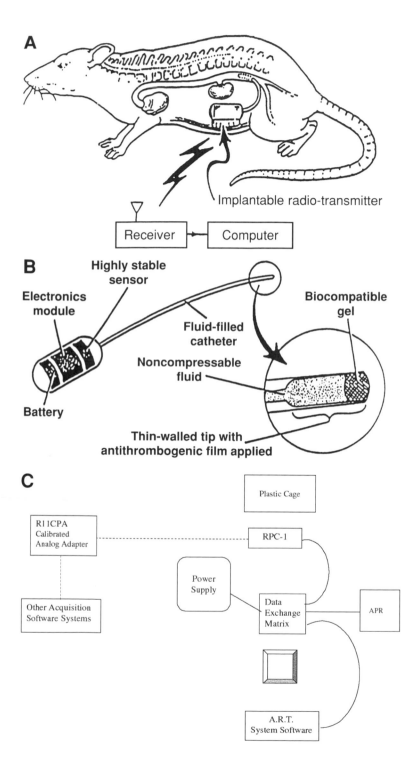

A

Implantable radio-transmitter

Receiver → Computer

B

Electronics module

Highly stable sensor

Fluid-filled catheter

Biocompatible gel

Noncompressable fluid

Battery

Thin-walled tip with antithrombogenic film applied

C

Plastic Cage

R11CPA Calibrated Analog Adapter

RPC-1

Power Supply

Data Exchange Matrix

APR

Other Acquisition Software Systems

A.R.T. System Software

Fig. 1.

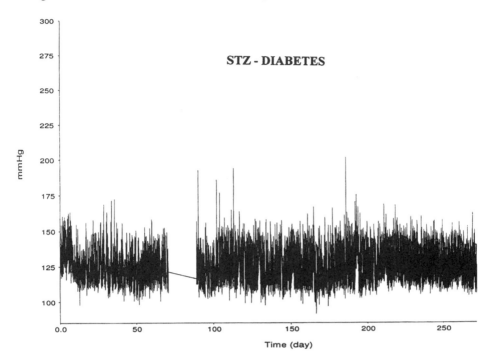

Fig. 2. Illustration of the course of systolic BP in a STZ diabetic Sprague-Dawley rat. Systolic BP was measured for 5 sec at 10-min intervals for ~300 d. The transmitter was turned off between d 75–90 and is depicted by the straight line in the graph.

toring can be successfully performed over a period of weeks and months, rendering it particularly useful for an evaluation of the chronic BP load-over-time in the investigations of hypertensive renal damage (**Fig. 2**). The superiority of such high-fidelity BP phenotyping over conventional techniques has been clearly demonstrated in a variety of experimental models investigating genetic and acquired differences in susceptibility to hypertensive renal damage and the potential role of differences in the real-time transmission of systemic BP to the renal microvasculature in the pathogenesis of such damage *(19,22,25–32)*. Very often such studies have called into question the interpretations and conclusions that had been obtained using the conventional tail-cuff BP methodology *(25–31)*.

Fig. 1. *(opposite page)* (**A**) Illustration of the TA11PA-C40 radiotransmitter in a rat aorta. The radiofrequency waves are transmitted to a receiver placed under the rat's cage and sent to the data acquisition software. (**B**) Schematic of the radiotransmitter device with insert of pressure-sensitive catheter tip containing a biocompatible gel. (**C**) Schematic of the A.R.T. radiotelemetry system setup. The dotted lines illustrate connections to other systems using the R11CPA calibrated analog adapter.

Although the radiotelemetric methodology has been available for several species—including most recently the mouse—its application has been most extensive in the rat. Therefore, the methods described here are for the rat, although the general principles are applicable to other species such as the mouse *(33,34)*. At present, Data Sciences Inc, which developed the radiotelemetric methodology for animal use, is presently the only supplier for the radiotelemetry system for these species. A detailed description of the data acquisition and analysis system software and options is beyond the scope of this text, and interested readers are strongly encouraged to contact Data Sciences, Inc.

2. Materials

2.1. Implantation of the Radiotransmitter

1. TA11PA-C40 radiotransmitter (blood pressure and physical activity).
2. Heated operating table and light source.
3. Shaver.
4. Providone solution and scrub.
5. Sodium pentobarbital.
6. One each, 14-gauge needle, 18-gauge needle.
7. 1-mL syringe and 25-gauge needle.
8. Two pairs of forceps.
9. Scissors.
10. 2% lidocaine.
11. 4-O chromic gut suture.
12. 3-O silk suture.
13. Staple gun.
14. Penicillin G.

2.2. Data Acquisition and Analysis

1. Dataquest A.R.T. system (Advanced Research Technology) 2.1 or higher.
2. Power supply.
3. R11CPA (Calibrated Pressure Analog Adapter).
4. Data Exchange Matrix.
5. RPC-1 General Purpose Receiver for Plastic Cages.
6. Computer system Minimum requirements:
   a. Pentium 133, IBM-compatible PC.
   b. 1 free half-length 16-bit ISA Bus slot.
   c. 16 megabytes of RAM.
   d. Hard drive with ~1 Gigabyte storage to install.
   e. Dataquest A.R.T. software.
   f. S.V.G.A. display adapter and monitor.
   g. CD-ROM drive.
   h. One open parallel or serial port for printer.

7. Dataquest Plug-in Card CQ2010.
8. Cables.
9. Ambient Pressure Reference.

3. Methods

3.1. Implantation of the Radiotransmitter (Femoral Artery Approach)

1. Administer sodium pentobarbital (50 mg/kg ip) and wait for adequate plane of anesthesia.
2. Shave the abdomen and inner thigh area, then disinfect.
3. Make a vertical incision along the center of the abdominal wall.
4. Make an incision along the inner thigh to expose the femoral vessels.
5. Isolate the femoral artery from the femoral vein and saphenous nerve.
6. Pass three sutures underneath the femoral artery (proximal occlusion, artery ligature, and distal occlusion).
7. Using a 14-gauge needle, pierce the abdominal wall on the femoral side to obtain access to the peritoneal cavity and leave in place.
8. Place the transmitter in the peritoneal cavity, insert the catheter tip into the needle, and advance it beyond the abdominal wall inside the needle. Carefully withdraw the needle, exposing the catheter on the femoral side of the abdominal wall.
9. Tie the distal suture to occlude the downstream portion of the femoral artery and apply tension. Lift the femoral artery by applying tension to the proximal suture to prevent bleeding and pierce the artery with a catheter introducer (bent-tip 22-gauge needle) near the distal occlusion site.
10. Very carefully, introduce the catheter into the femoral artery below the needle, using the needle tip as a guide.
11. Release enough tension on the proximal suture to allow the catheter to be advanced past the iliac vein into the aorta.
12. Tie the remaining middle suture around the femoral artery at the base of the catheter.
13. Release the proximal suture and observe for bleeding at the catheter's entry site.
14. Close the muscle layer of the abdominal incision and incorporate the suture tab affixed to the transmitter. Staple the overlying skin.
15. At the femoral site, loop the catheter subcutaneously to prevent kinking, and suture the stem of the catheter to the surrounding tissue to prevent slippage.
16. Close the femoral incision by stapling the overlying skin.
17. Penicillin G (40,000 U/kg, intramuscular) is administered at the completion of the surgery as prophylaxis against infection.

3.2. Data Acquisition and Analysis

The rats are individually housed in plastic cages placed over the radiotelemetry receiver RPC-1. The ART software provides an extensive range of options for the data acquisition and storage of the parameters of interest, and allows customization for intermittent or continuous sampling and for the selection of

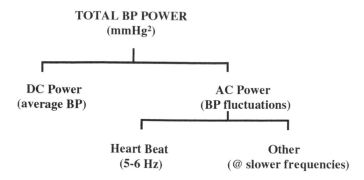

Fig. 3. The power (energy per unit time) of any given signal consists of two compo-. nents: i) that due to its average value (DC power) and ii) that resulting from its fluctuations from the average value (AC power).

sampling rates. Considerable flexibility is also available for customization of data analysis, depending upon the investigative objectives.

Blood-pressure radiotelemetry in our laboratory has primarily been used to define the relationship between ambient BP and renal damage in various experimental models. Therefore, for most of these investigations, we have chosen to sample BP continuously at 10-min intervals with a sampling duration of 10 sec for each BP sample. The average BP during 50–60 heartbeats is thus recorded as one reading, with 144 such readings obtained for each rat/day. The average BP, an average of all the readings over a 5–40-wk period depending upon the model and experimental protocol, thus provides one index of the average ambient BP load in that animal for correlation with the functional or histologic indices of renal damage. The data can additionally be analyzed for indices of BP lability, such as for diurinal rhythms (nighttime and daytime averages), daily standard deviation of the BP or for the frequency of BP readings above a certain threshold.

More recently, we have suggested that the total BP load that the kidney is potentially exposed to may be more precisely quantitated using bioengineering concepts of total BP power (energy/U time) as indicated in **Fig. 3** *(11)*. For such analysis, BP in individual animals is additionally sampled at 500 Hz for up to 24 h at designated intervals during the course of studies. Blood-pressure power spectra are then determined by applying Fast Fourier Transforms (FFT) to the obtained recordings in order to examine the differences in frequency distribution of BP power between models and/or animals for potential relationships to indices of renal injury (**Fig. 4**). We have also used BP radiotelemetry in conjunction with chronic renal arterial blood-flow probes (Transonic System) to examine the renal blood-flow response in real time to

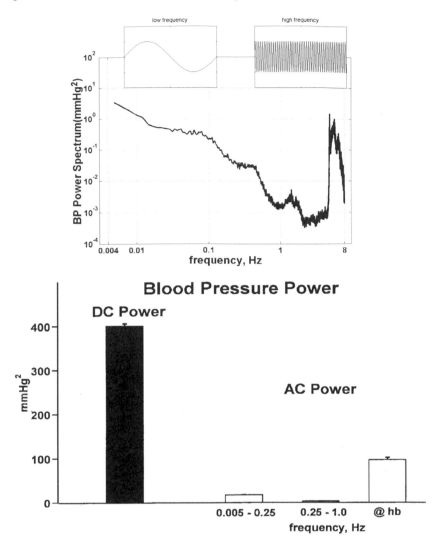

Fig. 4. Blood-pressure power spectra illustrating heartbeat frequency and frequencies less than the heartbeat in a Sprague-Dawley rat (upper panel). Relative total BP power distribution in normotensive Sprague-Dawley rats ($n = 13$) (lower panel).

BP fluctuations in conscious unrestrained rats. Because of the requirements for connecting the flow probes to flowmeters and for some animal monitoring during the recording, such data are usually only obtained for 30–60 min during a recording session. However, such sessions can be repeated several times over the course of a few weeks, and thus, provide a powerful tool to investigate the renal hemodynamic responses to spontaneous BP fluctuations in conscious animals, before and after experimental interventions. These variations in data acquisition and analysis are provided as a way to illustrate the flexibility that is available with the radiotelemetry system for adaptation to the individual investigative focus.

4. Notes

1. To prevent infection, wash the area first with Providine scrub, followed by disinfection with Providine solution. A sharp blade for shaving also helps to reduce the incidence of infection by preventing unnecessary "nicking" of the skin.
2. To reduce the incidence of ventral hernias, use the *linea alba* as a guide to make the abdominal incision.
3. Expose as much of the femoral artery as possible. This will reduce the risk of bleeding when you release the proximal suture to advance the catheter tip.
4. Irrigation of the femoral artery with 2% Lidocaine will help dilate the femoral artery and allow smooth passage of the catheter.
5. Attach a hemostat to the loose ends of the distal ligature to apply tension.
6. Bend the 14-gauge needle tip ~90° with the open side face down in the vessel to facilitate the passage of the catheter into the artery.
7. Use an interrupted suture technique to close the abdominal wall. 4-O gut chromic should be used to close the incision, with 3-O silk being used to attach the suture tab of the transmitter to the incision site.
8. Occasionally, the catheter may develop a clot. This can be detected by a decrease in BP and inspection of the waveforms (*see* **Fig. 5A,B**). When this occurs, the radiotransmitter should be replaced. This is done by removing the transmitter and tying off the femoral artery at the insertion site. A new transmitter can be placed in the femoral artery on the other side.
9. The battery lasts ~6 mo; at this time the transmitter must be returned for a complete refurbishment. If the transmitter has been used for less than that amount of time in a completed study, it can be sterilized, re-gelled, and implanted in another animal. The gel is available from Data Sciences, Inc.
10. Rinse the transmitter in water to remove blood and tissue. Direct a gentle stream of saline at the tip of the catheter to remove debris if visible. Then soak in freshly made biodetergent (Kleer-0) for 30 min. Use gauze to wipe the surface until it is clean. Thoroughly rinse the transmitter in tap water. Place the transmitter into *fresh* 2% glutaraldehyde (shelf life of 14 d after activation). The transmitter should be left in the 2% glutaraldehyde overnight. (Minimum is 4 h.) Place the transmitter into sterile saline for 15–30 min. Then place the transmitter into a second beaker of sterile saline for 15–30 min. Inspect the catheter tip and re-gel if necessary. Keep the transmitter in sterile saline until ready to use. Remove the transmitter from this beaker when ready to implant.
11. When re-gelling the catheter, the gel should be slowly infused with the dispensing tip into the catheter tip to prevent air bubbles and excess pressure. The presence of air bubbles will dampen the signal and lead to clotting/malfunction.

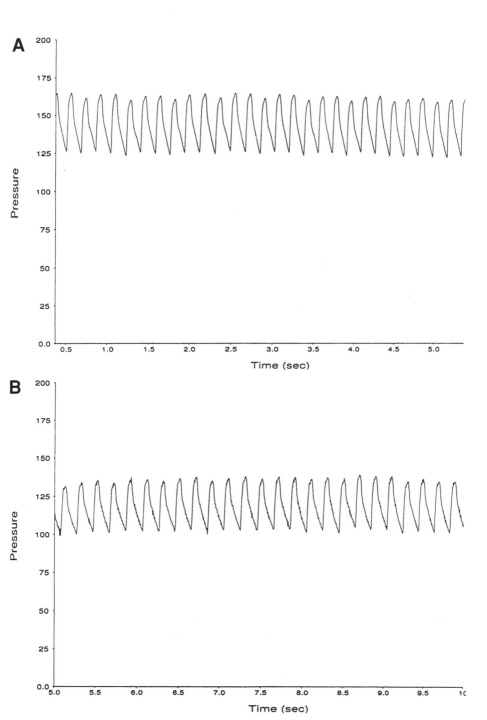

Fig. 5. **(A)** Illustration of a waveform trace over a 5-sec interval in an SHRsp rat with malfunction of the transmitter secondary to blood clot formation in the catheter tip. **(B)** Illustration of a restored normal waveform trace after replacement of the radio-transmitter in the same rat. Notice the significantly higher systolic BP compared to **Fig. 5A**.

References

1. Guyton, A. C., Hall, J. E., Coleman, T. G., et al. (1995) The dominant role of the kidneys in long-term arterial pressure regulation in normal and hypertensive states, in *Hypertension: Pathophysiology, Diagnosis, and Management, vol 1* (Laragh, J. H. and Brenner, B. M., eds.), Raven Press, New York, pp. 1311–1326.
2. Laragh, J. H. and Sealey, J. E. (1992) Renin-angiotensin-aldosterone system and the renal regulation of sodium, potassium and blood pressure homeostasis, in *Handbook of Physiology, Vol 11* (Windhager, E. E., ed.), Oxford University Press, New York, pp. 1409–1541.
3. Navar, L. G. and Majid, D. S. A. (1996) Interactions between arterial pressure and sodium excretion. *Curr. Opin. Nephrol. Hypertens.* **5,** 64–71.
4. Hayashi, K., Epstein, M., and Saruta, T. (1996) Altered myogenic responsiveness of the renal microvasculature in experimental hypertension. *J. Hypertens.* **14,** 1387–1401.
5. Neuringer, J. R. and Brenner, B. M. (1993) Hemodynamic theory of progressive renal disease: a 10-year update in brief review. *Am. J. Kidney Dis.* **22,** 98–104.
6. Klag, M. J., Whelton, P. K., et al (1996) Blood pressure and end-stage renal disease in men. *N. Engl. J. Med.* **334,** 13–18.
7. UK Prospective Diabetes Group. (1998) Tight blood pressure control and risk of macrovascular and microvascular complications in type 2 diabetes: UKPDS 38, *Br. Med. J.* **317,** 708–713.
8. Bidani, A. K., Schwartz, M. M., and Lewis, E. J. (1987) Renal autoregulation and vulnerability to hypertensive injury in remnant kidney. *Am. J. Physiol.* **252,** F1003–F1010.
9. Bidani, A. K. and Griffin, K. A. (2002) Long-term renal consequences of hypertension for normal and diseased kidneys. *Curr. Opin. Nephrol. Hypertens.* **11,** 73–80.
10. Cusi, D., Tripodi, G., Cesari, G., Robba, C., Boilini, P., Merati, G., et al. (1993) Genetics of renal damage in primary hypertension. *Am. J. Kidney Disease* **21(5),** (Suppl. 2):2–9.
11. Lemmer, B., Mattes, A., Bohm, M., Ganten, D. (1993) Circadian blood pressure variation in transgenic hypertensive rats. *Hypertension* **22,** 97–101.
12. Calhoun, D. A., Sutao, Z., Wyss, M. J., Oparil, S. (1994) Diurnal blood pressure variation and dietary salt in spontaneously hypertensive rats. *Hypertension* **24,** 1–7.
13. Churchill, P. C., Churchill, M. C., Bidani, A. K., Griffin, K. A., Picken, M., et al. (1997) Genetic susceptibility to hypertension-induced renal damage in the rat: evidence based on kidney specific genome transfer. *J. Clin. Investig.* **100,** 1373–1382.
14. Dominiczak, A. F., Clark, J. S., Jeffs, B., Anderson, N. H., Negrin, D. C., Lee, W. K., et al. (1998) Genetics of experimental hypertension. *J. Hypertens.* **16,** 1859–1869.
15. Shimamura, T., Nakajima, M., Iwasaki, T., Hayasaki, Y., Yonetani, Y., and Iwaki, K. (1999) Analysis of circadian blood pressure rhythm and target organ damage in stroke-prone spontaneously hypertensive rats. *J. Hypertens.* **17,** 211–220.

16. Freedman, B. I. and Satko, S. G. (2000) Genes and renal disease. *Curr. Opin. Nephrol. Hypertens.* **9**, 273–277.

17. Holstein-Rathlou, N. H., He, J., Wagner, A. J., and Marsh, D. J. (1995) Patterns of blood pressure variability in normotensive and hypertensive rats. *Am. J. Physiol.* **269**, R1230–R1239.

18. Persson, P. B. (1996) Modulation of cardiovascular control mechanisms and their interaction. *Physiol. Rev.* **76**, 193–244.

19. Bidani, A. K., Griffin, K. A., Picken, M., and Lansky, D. M. (1993) Continuous telemetric BP monitoring and glomerular injury in the rat remnant kidney model. *Am. J. Physiol.* **265**, F391–F398.

20. Bunag, R. D. (1983) Facts and fallacies about measuring blood pressure in rats. *Clin. Exp. Hypertens.—Theory and Practice* **A5(10)**, 1959–1681.

21. Bunag, R. D., McCubbin, J. W., and Page, I. H. (1971) Lack of correlation between direct and indirect measurements of arterial pressure in un-anesthetized rats. *Cardiovasc. Res.* **5**, 24–31.

22. Tanaka, M., Schmidlin, O., Olson, J. L., Yi, S.-L., and Morris, R. C. Jr. (2001) Chloride-sensitive renal microangiopathy in the stroke-prone spontaneously hypertensive rat. *Kidney Int.* **59**, 1066–1076.

23. Brockwqay, B. P., Mills, P. A., and Azar, S. H. (1991) A new method for continuous chronic measurement and recording of blood pressure, heart rate and activity in the rat via radio-telemetry. *Clin. Exp. Hypertens.—Theory and Practice* **A13(5)**, 885–895.

24. Bazil, M. K., Kurlan, C., and Webb, R. L. (1993) Telemetric monitoring of cardiovascular parameters in conscious spontaneously hypertensive rats. *J. Cardiovasc. Pharmacol.* **6**, 897–905.

25. Griffin, K. A., Picken, M., and Bidani, A. K. (1994) Method of renal mass reduction is a critical modulator of subsequent hypertension and glomerular injury. *J. Am. Soc. Nephrol.* **4**, 2023–2031.

26. Griffin, K. A., Picken, M., and Bidani, A. K. (1994) Radiotelemetric BP monitoring, antihypertensives and glomeruloprotection in remnant kidney model. *Kidney Int.* **46**, 1010–1018.

27. Griffin, K. A., Picken, M. M., and Bidani, A. K. (1995) Deleterious effects of calcium channel blockade on pressure transmission and glomerular injury in the rat remnant kidneys. *J. Clin. Investig.* **96**, 798–800.

28. Griffin, K. A., Picken, M. M., Bakris, G. L., and Bidani, A. K. (1999) Class differences in the effects of calcium channel blockers in the remnant kidney model. *Kidney Int.* **55**, 1849–1860.

29. Bidani, A. K., Picken, M. M., Bakris, G., and Griffin, K. A. (2000) Lack of evidence of BP independent protection by renin-angiotensin system blockade after renal ablation. *Kidney Int.* **57**, 1651–1661.

30. Griffin, K. A., Picken, M. M., Churchill, M., Churchill, P., and Bidani, A. K. (2000) Functional and structural correlates of glomerulosclerosis after renal mass reduction in the rat. *J. Am. Soc. Nephrol.* **11**, 497–506.

31. Griffin, K. A., Churchill, P. C., Picken, M., et al. (2001) Differential salt-sensitivity in the pathogenesis of renal damage in SHR and stroke prone SHR. *Am. J. Hypertens.* **14,** 311–320.

32. Churchill, P. C., Churchill, M. C., Griffin, K. A., Picken, M., Webb, R. C., Kurtz, T. W., et al. (2002) Increased genetic susceptibility to renal damage in the stroke prone spontaneously hypertensive rat. *Kidney Int.* (in press).

33. Carlson, S. H., Oparil, S., Chen, Y-F, and Wyss, J. M. (2002) Blood pressure and NaCl-sensitive hypertension are influenced by angiotensin-converting enzyme gene expression in transgenic mice. *Hypertension* **39,** 214–218.

34. Carlson, S. H. and Wyss, J. M. (2000) Long-term telemetric recording of arterial pressure and heart rate in mice fed basal and high NaCl diets. *Hypertension* **35,** e1–e5.

35. Griffin, K. A., Hacioglu, R., Abu-Amarah, I., Williamson, G. A., and Bidani, A. K. (2000) The effects of diabetes and reduced renal mass on blood pressure power spectra. *Am. J. Hypertens.* **13,** 216A.

36. Griffin, K. A., Abu-Amarah, I., Hacioglu, R., Williamson, G., Loutzenhiser, R., and Bidani, A. K. (2000) Effects of calcium channel blockade on dynamic renal autoregulation: implications for current interpretations of admittance gain parameters. *JASN* **11,** 359A.

23

In Vitro Studies on Renin Release

Boye L. Jensen, Ulla G. Friis, and Ole Skøtt

1. Introduction

Renin is an aspartyl peptidase that is synthesized, stored, and released from juxtaglomerular (JG) granular cells in the lamina media of the afferent arteriole. Each afferent arteriole contains 5–20 JG cells. Renin catalyzes the cleavage of angiotensin I (ANG I) from renin substrate; angiotensin I is further converted to the physiologically active form angiotensin II by angiotensin-converting enzyme (ACE). Angiotensin II (ANG II) is an important vasoconstrictor, and it promotes release of aldosterone from the adrenal gland. Thus, the renin-angiotensin-aldosterone system is important in the regulation of salt and water homeostasis and blood pressure. In keeping with its complex homeostatic roles, the regulation of renin secretion is under the control of a number of systemic factors. Release is stimulated by decreases in arterial pressure, increases in sympathetic nervous activity, and by a decrease in the tubular NaCl concentration at the macula densa (MD).

The application of cellular methods to the study of renin release from JG cells in the kidney has been hampered by difficulties in obtaining pure preparations of these cells. Furthermore, when cultured, they rapidly lose their ability to store renin. Thus, native JG cells can only be studied in partially pure primary cultures. A cell line (As4.1) that is derived from a renin-producing tumor may circumvent some of these problems, but the applicability of the results derived from this cell line to native JG cells remains an open question.

Here, we describe methods for isolation of JG cells from rats and mice, and their subsequent use for study of secretion from incubated JG cells and for single-cell patch-clamp on JG cells.

2. Materials

1. Isolation buffer: (in mmol/L) NaCl 130; KCl 5; $CaCl_2$ 2; D-glucose 10; sucrose 20; HEPES 10, pH 7.4 (KOH, 37°C).

From: *Methods in Molecular Medicine, vol. 86: Renal Disease: Techniques and Protocols*
Edited by: M. S. Goligorsky © Humana Press Inc., Totowa, NJ

2. Incubation buffer: RPMI1640 with $NaHCO_3$ 2.2 g/L, fetal calf serum (2%), insulin 0.66 U/mL, Penicillin (100) + streptomycin (100 μg/mL) 10 mL; equilibrated with 95% O_2 and 5% CO_2, pH 7.2.

3. 0.1 M Phosphate buffer: 2.76 g $NaH_2PO_4 \cdot H_2O$, 3.0 mL 20% human albumin. Dissolve and mix ingredients with distilled water. Set pH to 6.5 with 2 N NaOH (about 5 mL). Fill up to 200 mL with distilled water. Aliquot 5 mL into vials and freeze.

4. Barbital buffer (pH 8,6): 0,1 g thiomersal (sodium salt), 16 g sodium barbitol, 1.6133 g (EDTA) ethylenediaminetetraacetic acid (titriplex III), 6.25 mL 20% human albumin solution. Dissolve and mix substances with distilled water. Set pH to 8.6 with 2 N HCl (about 5 mL). Fill to 1000 mL with distilled water. Aliquot into 250- and 100-mL containers and freeze at –20°C.

5. Tracer: Amersham's [125]I Angiotensin I (ANGI) tracer works well.

6. Renin standards: Renin is expressed in terms of Goldblatt units (GU) compared with renin standards (MRC Reagent no. 65/119) obtained from the National Institute for Biological Standards and Control (Potters Bar, Hertsfordshire, UK). Prepare stock solution with 0.02 GU/mL. Aliquot 75 μL/vial.

7. Charcoal used for separation in RIA: 0.1 g thiomersal, 16 g sodium barbital. Dissolve in distilled water. Set pH to 8.6 with 2 N HCl before adding distilled water to 1000 mL. This solution is called solution A. Weigh 30 g active charcoal and mix with 400 mL solution A. Weigh 6 g Dextran-70 and mix with solution A. When the dextran is completely dissolved, it is added slowly to the charcoal solution while stirring. The stock solution of charcoal is kept at 4°C. Constant stirring of the charcoal solution is necessary when it is aliquotted into the stoppers.

8. 20% human albumin: We get human albumin as 20% infusion solution for human use from the Danish Statens Serum Institute, but any source would probably work. The pH of the human albumin solution is set to 3.6 with 2 M phosphoric acid and returned to pH 7.5 with 5 N NaOH (*see* **Note 1**).

9. Rabbit ANGI Antibody (20 μL/vial). We use in-house made rabbit angI antibody, but it is possible to obtain ANGI antibody from commercial sources.

10. "Internal" solution for patch clamp (in mmol/L). Control: 135 mM K-glutamate, 10 mM NaCl, 10 mM KCl, 1 mM $MgCl_2$, 10 mM HEPES-NaOH, 0.5 mM Mg-ATP, 0.3 mM Na_2GTP, osmolality was 307 mOsm/kg; pH 7.00 (adjusted with KOH, 22°C). The osmolality was measured by an osmometer (model 3D3 from Advanced Instruments, Inc.). Osmolality is important, because the renin secretory process is osmo-sensitive.

11. "External" solution for patch clamp: 10 mM HEPES, 140 mM NaCl, 2.8 mM KCl, 1 mM $MgCl_2$, 2 mM $CaCl_2$, 11 mM glucose, 10 mM sucrose, osmolality was approx 300 mOsm/kg (range 296–314 mOsm/kg); pH 7.25 (adjusted with KOH, 25°C).

12. Both external and internal solutions are prepared in larger quantities (e.g., 50 mL of internal solution and 1000 mL of external solution) and then stored at –20°C in appropriate volumes (1–2 mL for internal solutions, and 40–50 mL for external solutions).

3. Methods

3.1. Isolation of Juxtaglomerular Cells from Mice and Rats

3.1.1. Isolation of Mouse JG Cells

JG-cells are isolated essentially as described by Della Bruna et al. (*1*).

1. We use male mice (C57Bl/6bg, 4–6-wk-old—size matters!) with free access to tap water and standard rodent chow. The mice are sacrificed by cervical dislocation.
2. The kidneys are removed and decapsulated, and then minced carefully with scalpel blades in a plastic Petri dish.
3. The tissue paste is transferred to 30 mL sterile isolation buffer supplemented with 0.1% (w/v) collagenase (0.5 U/mL) and 0.25% (w/v) trypsin (1300 BAEE U/mg).
4. The tissue is incubated in a 100–mL flask and gently shaken (not stirred) in a horizontal position for 70 min at 37°C (*see* **Note 2**). Following digestion, the cell suspension is filtered through a sterile 22-μm nylon mesh. This takes place in a sterile bench. First, the filter is flushed with buffer, then the cells are filtered, and finally the flask is flushed with buffer to recover all cells.
5. The cell suspension is transferred to sterile 50 mL-tubes. The filtered cells are washed twice to remove enzymes with isolation buffer by centrifugation (1000*g* for 7 min). The cell pellet is then resuspended in 4 mL isolation buffer and is ready for gradient centrifugation.
6. Alternatively, the cells are suspended in RPMI medium with 2% FCS and seeded onto glass plates in cell-culture dishes for patch-clamp investigations.

3.1.2. Isolation of Rat JG Cells

Male Sprague-Dawley rats (50–80 g) with free access to tap water and standard rodent chow are used.

1. The rat is sacrificed by cervical dislocation, and the kidneys are removed. The kidney cortex is separated from the medulla by dissection with a scalpel blade.
2. The cortex is cut into small pieces with scalpel blades and digested by modest shaking for 90 min at 37°C with an enzyme mixture as described for mice JG-cells.
3. Cells are filtered, washed, and resuspended as described for mice JG-cells. Cells are either used directly for patch-clamp or further separated.

3.1.3. Gradient Centrifugation

To obtain a relative enrichment in JG-cells, the isolated cells are subjected to centrifugation through isotonic Percoll gradients.

3.1.3.1. Gradient Centrifugation of Mouse JG Cells

The kidney-cell suspension from mice is separated using a 30% Percoll isotonic density gradient in isolation buffer and centrifuged for 30 min at 27,000*g* (4°C). Four cell layers with different specific renin activity are obtained. The cellular layer (equivalent to a density of 1.049 g/mL) with the highest renin concentration is used for the experiments. These cells are recovered from the gradient with sterile plastic pipets and are then washed 2× with isolation buffer and resuspended in RPMI cell-culture medium with 2% FCS, insulin, penicillin, and streptomycin as in **Subheading 2.2.**

3.1.3.2. Gradient Centrifugation of Rat JG Cells

Rat kidney cortical cells are also separated by a Percoll density gradient (26% isoosmotic Percoll) in isolation buffer and centrifuged at 27,000*g* for 30 min at 4°C (Sorvall). Band III cells corresponding to a density of 1.06 g/mL *(2)* are collected and washed twice as in **Subheading 3.1.3.1.** In our experience, this procedure increases specific renin activity 2–4× compared to a crude cortical-cell suspension.

3.1.4. Counting and Seeding of Cells

1. We routinely count samples of the final cell suspension for single-round "JG-like cells" (*see* **Note 3**).
2. The suspension is diluted to a concentration of 150,000 cells/mL and seeded in 100-μL aliquots for renin-secretion studies. This procedure results in fairly similar contents of renin per well between experiments.
3. When these plated cells are stained immunocytochemically for renin with a specific renin antibody, there are many renin-positive granular cells (*see* **Note 4**).

3.2. Renin Release from Incubated JG Cells

3.2.1. Renin Secretion Studies from Incubated Rat or Mouse JG Cells

1. Aliquots (100 μL) of the cell suspension are seeded in 96-multiwell plates (Sarstedt) for renin-secretion studies and incubated for 20 h (overnight). Culture medium is then removed, and the cells are washed once with 100 μL warm RPMI-1640 medium. Then, 100 μL fresh prewarmed RPMI-1640 medium with the agents to be tested is added.
2. Renin secretion can be studied after incubation for a variable time on the order of hours. For a better time resolution, the cells can be directly loaded to columns after isolation and superfused, or can be investigated by patch-clamp. In order to screen for the effects of substances, we routinely incubate the cells for 20 h, then medium is collected and centrifuged at 10,000*g* for 10 min at room temperature to remove floating-cells and debris. The supernatants are stored at –20°C until assayed for renin concentration. The pellets are also stored.
3. The cells remaining in the culture wells are lysed by addition of 100 μL phosphate-buffered saline (PBS) with 0.1% of Triton X-100 and 0.1% *human* serum albumin to each well. (Traces of human renin in the albumin do not disturb the renin assay because human renin does not generate ANGI from rat renin substrate.)
4. Next, the wells are shaken for 45 min at room temperature, and the lysates are collected and added to the pellets obtained by centrifugation of the cell-conditioned medium. This mixture is vortexed and then centrifuged at 10,000*g* for 10 min at room temperature. The supernatants are stored at –20°C until renin measurements.

3.3. Renin Assay

This assay uses the "antibody trapping" technique of Poulsen *(3,4)*. The renin-containing sample is incubated with excess renin substrate in the presence of ANGI antibody that "traps" ANGI and protects it from enzymatic breakdown. This is followed by RIA against ANG I. In the ultramicroassay, the rat renin substrate has been purified by affinity chromatography with renin antibody to remove residual renin, and the incubation time is extended to 24 (or 48) h. The advantage of this assay is its high sensitivity. The detection limit corresponds to less than the content of one single renin granule *(5)*, and allows measurement of renin concentration in nL samples of plasma or renal tubular fluid. The small amount of sample or plasma used in the assay makes repeat samples on mice possible.

3.3.1. Production of Rat Renin Substrate

Principle: rats are treated with estrogen to increase substrate production in the liver. Then the rats are nephrectomized to remove endogenous renin, and 24 h later the plasma is harvested.

1. Rats are injected subcutaneously (sc) with estrogen (2.5 mg/mL). Friday: 0.2 mL/200 g rat, Monday 0.1 mL/200 g rat, Tuesday 0.1 mL/200 g rat.
2. Wednesday: Anesthetize rats (Hypnorm 0.3 mL/kg, Dormicum 2 mg/kg), remove both kidneys through a dorsal approach, and close wound with agraffes. Inject estrogen 0.1 mL/200 g rat sc, and 0.1 mL Temgesic sc as analgesics.
3. Thursday: Anesthetize rats (Hypnorm 0.3 mL/kg, Dormicum 2 mg/kg). Laparatomize and bleed from abdominal aorta into 10-mL vacutainers with 340 mg EDTA. Centrifuge blood and pool plasma from all rats.
4. Removal of endogenenous angiotensinases: pH of the plasma is reduced to pH 3.6 with 2 M phosphoric acid. Leave for 20 min at 25°C. Set pH to 7.5 with 5 N NaOH: Add phosphoric acid at a slow rate to avoid clotting.
5. Test a standard curve against previous batch of rat renin-substrate. The resulting renin substrate concentration is usually in the order of 4–5000 ngANGI/mL.
6. This rat-renin substrate can be used in an ordinary renin assay. For use in the ultramicroassay, further purification is necessary.

3.3.2. Purified Rat Renin Substrate

1. 6 mL treated plasma from nephrectomized rats is mixed with 2 mL cyanogen bromide (CNBR)-activated sepharose beads coupled with anti-renin antibody. Mix well for 3 h at 4°C.
2. Centrifuge 2000g for 10 min at 4°C. Save supernatant, save beads too!
3. 15 mL 0.1 M phosphate buffer (pH 6.5) is mixed with the supernatant.
4. Aliquot 2 mL into vials, add 10 μL neomycin (80 mg/mL), and freeze.
5. The resulting renin substrate concentration is usually approx 1200 ng ANGI /mL.

6. After use, reconstitute sepharose beads by washing twice in 0.9% saline. Then wash 3× in the following week. After the last wash, add 100 µL neomycin (80 mg/mL) to the beads. Wash once a month with saline with neomycin. In our experience, one batch of beads has worked for over 10 yr when treated in this way.

3.3.3. Ultramicroassay for Renin

When working with single JG cells (*6,7*), release of renin from single afferent arterioles (AAs) or single juxtaglomerular apparatuses (JGAs) (*8*), there may not be enough sample to do serial dilutions, or to make measurements in duplicates. When working with plasma samples that contain native renin substrate, it is an advantage to make dilution series, and to accept only results with linearity in a dilution series (for example, 25×, 50×, and 100×). This is especially important in mouse plasma, in which the endogenous substrate concentration is high.

1. Make a renin-standards series from the renin standard by mixing 50 µL of the 0.02 GU/mL standard with 1950 ul buffer (yielding a concentration of 0.5×10^{-3} GU/mL). From this solution, take 80 µL and mix with 170 µL phosphate buffer (=16×10^{-5} GU/mL). Make a serial dilution from this to obtain 8, 4, 2, 1, 0.5, 0.25, 0.125, 0.0625 × 10^{-5} GU/mL.
2. Make serial dilutions of samples with phosphate buffer.
3. Make antibody/substrate mixture: Add 450 µL phosphate buffer to 20 µl angI antibody. Add about 12% of this mixture to 2000 µL plasma (*see* **Note 5**).
4. Aliquot 20 µL of the antibody/substrate mixture into all vials (except the ones for total counts). Add 5 µL standard or unknown sample into each vial.
5. Close all vials with stoppers and incubate for 24 h at 37°C in an incubator. Avoid evaporation by incubation in a moist atmosphere—for example, incubate in a plastic bag together with open water containers.
6. Stop incubation after 24 h by transfer to ice bath and add 1 mL barbital buffer with human albumin with ANGI tracer.
7. Make charcoal stoppers by adding 150 µ: charcoal (use a repeater pipet) into each hollow stopper and use one per vial. Be cautious when inserting the stoppers into the vials. If the charcoal drips into the solution, the sample is void.
8. Let the solution equilibrate for at least 18 h at 4°C.
9. Mix well with charcoal for 30 sec and centrifuge at 5800*g* for 13 min at 4°C (*see* **Note 6**).
10. The supernatant is decanted into vials for gamma counting. Usual counting time is 5 min per vial.

3.4. Patch-Clamp on JG Cells

Whole-cell patch-clamp has been modified for use on isolated mouse and rat JG cells (*6,7*).

3.4.1. Identification of Cells Used for Patch-Clamp

Because the isolated cells are not 100% JG cells, the identity of cells used for patch-clamp experiments must be confirmed as renin-containing JG cells by several approaches:

1. First, cells are selected by their appearance as large granular cells.
2. After establishing GΩ-seal and the whole-cell configuration, the current-voltage relation (*I*-V curve) is used as an inclusion criterion. Only cells, that have the characteristic appearance of JG cells, should be used: an outward rectification at positive membrane potentials and very limited net currents between –30 and 0 mV (*9*).
3. To further assure cell identity, presumed JG cells can be sampled through modified patch pipets, and the renin content of various numbers of sampled cells can then be measured. Cells are added directly to 50 μL lysis buffer (PBS with 0.1% of Triton X-100 and 0.1% human serum albumin) and 5 μL of this is used for radioimmunoassay of renin concentration (*see* **Subheading 3.3.**).
4. To assure that the granular cells express prepro-renin mRNA, single cells can be transferred via modified patch pipets to 50 μL guanidinium-thiocyanate solution, 10 μg yeast tRNA is added as a carrier, and total RNA is isolated using the Dynabead mRNA direct micro kit (Dynal, Oslo, Norway). All mRNAs are reverse-transcribed to cDNA with an oligo dT primer and renin cDNA (194 bp) is amplified by PCR. The renin sense primer spanned the exon 6/exon 7 border (5'-ATG AAG GGG GTG TCT GTG GGG TC-3') and the anti-sense primer is located on exon 8 of the renin gene (5'-ATG TCG GGG AGG GTG GGC ACC TG-3'). JG-cell mRNA quality and quantity is assured by amplification of β-actin. As positive control for the PCR, renin and actin are amplified from 1 μg total RNA isolated from the renal cortex.

3.4.2. Patch-Clamp Experiments

For the patch-clamp studies, the washed cells are resuspended in RPMI-1640 with 2% FCS and transferred (2–3-mL suspension) to a 12-well multidish with glass cover slips placed at the bottom of each well. Mouse JG cells are allowed to sediment for at least 45 min (rat JG cells should sediment for at least 90 min) at 37°C in a humidified atmosphere containing 5% CO_2 in air. Now the cells are ready for experiments:

1. One glass cover slip with juxtaglomerular cells is gently superfused with the *Isotonic bath solution*, then transferred to the recording chamber and supplemented with the same buffer to a volume of approx 250 μL (depending on the size of the recording chamber). All solutions (externals and internals) are filtered through Minisart filters (0.20 μm).
2. A (borosilicate glass) pipet (works best with resistances in the range of 3–7 MΩ, and should be carefully heat-polished and Sylgard-coated) is filled with internal solution, attached to the preamplifier, and positioned directly above the selected cell.

3. The tip of the pipet is pressed (very!) slowly to the membrane of the selected JG-cell, until the resistance is approximately doubled (e.g., from 4 to approximately 8 MΩ). It is best to touch the JG cell in the center, as this will prevent the cell from movement during the increase in pressure.

4. Next, a tiny suction is applied, and the negative pressure is maintained steadily until the GΩ-seal is obtained (sometimes gradually, at approx 30 s, sometimes suddenly) (*see* **Note 7**).

5. The experiments are performed at room temperature in the tight-seal whole-cell configuration of the patch-clamp technique using heat-polished, Sylgard-coated patch pipets with resistances of 3–7 MΩ. Series resistances are in the range of 6–25 MΩ and seal resistances are in the range of 1–15 GΩ.

6. High-resolution membrane currents are recorded with an EPC-9 patch-clamp amplifier (HEKA) controlled by PULSE v8.11 software on a Power Macintosh G3 computer. High-resolution currents are low-pass filtered at 2.9 kHz and acquired at a sampling rate of 20 kHz. The reference electrode is an Ag/AgCl pellet connected to the bath solution through a 150 mmol/L NaCl/agar bridge. All potentials are corrected for the liquid junction potential that develops at the tip of the pipet when it is immersed in the bath solution.

7. The current-voltage (*I*-V) relationship is monitored by the response to nine voltage steps of 30 mV (covering a range of −110 to + 130 mV) for 60 ms from a holding potential of −30 mV (the membrane potential of cells in the wall of pressurized AAs). The *I*-V pulses are applied immediately after establishment of the whole-cell configuration, and the shape of the *I*-V curve is used as an inclusion criterion.

8. The patch-clamp technique makes it possible to monitor secretory activity (exocytosis of renin granules) in a single cell by measurement of the cell-membrane capacitance, C_m, as an index of membrane-surface area. Low time resolution acquisition of membrane capacitance, C_m, is measured with the "sine+dc" method using the LockIn extension of the PULSE v8.11 software. The C_m measurements are started maximally 30 sec after the *I*-V recording. Data from an entire sweep are averaged to result in one C_m point per sweep, resulting in an acquisition rate of about 5 Hz using the Xchart extension of the PULSE software.

4. Notes

1. It is important to use human albumin. Human renin does not react with rat substrate, so human renin impurities will not harm the assay. Bovine renin does react with rat substrate, and therefore renin impurities in bovine albumin (or FCS) result in high background, and may ruin the assay.

2. Cell quality is significantly higher when the cells are shaken compared to stirring with a magnet.

3. Using hemocytometer counting, the cell numbers acquired with an ordinary Coulter counter are about 10× higher, and do not provide a good estimate of the JG cell number.

4. In our experience, these protocols do not result in cultures that consist of 80–90% renin-positive cells, as originally reported *(2)*. The renin-positive cells represent only a minor fraction, but the JG cell content is high enough to result in renin concentrations far above the detection limit of the radioimmunoassays.
5. The antibody concentration should be adjusted to provide maximal sensitivity in the range where the samples are. In standard recipes it is usually stated that the optimal antibody concentration is the one that yields a binding of about 50%, but the highest sensitivity is found with considerably lower binding (down to 25%).
6. Do not exceed the time indicated here. The charcoal swaps unbound tracer, and if left for too long, the tracer bound to antibody will begin dissociating again.
7. In order to obtain a successful whole-cell configuration, it is imperative that the pipet is completely stable. Be sure to tighten the holder firmly enough that the pipet does not move (on a scale of 1 µm) when you give suction. If the electrode/pipet is not absolutely stable, it is better to lift the pipet (together with the attached cell) from the bottom, and then give an additional suction until the whole-cell configuration is obtained. Having the JG-cell lifted from the bottom is also an advantage for other reasons: the whole-cell configuration can be maintained for long periods (up to 1 h), and is not so easily disrupted during external solution changes. Some patch-clamp setups have a "zap"-pulse-function to break the patch membrane. However, this function does not work on JG cells. In addition, Ag-ions are not tolerated by JG-cells, so it is also imperative that the pipet electrode is properly chlorided.

References

1. Della Bruna, R., Pinet, F., Corvol, P., and Kurtz, A. (1991) Regulation of renin secretion and renin synthesis by second messengers in isolated mouse juxtaglomerular cells. *Cell. Physiol. Biochem.* **1,** 98–110.
2. Kurtz, A., Della Bruna, R., Pfeilschifter, J., Taugner, R., and Bauer, C. (1986) Atrial natriuretic peptide inhibits renin release from juxtaglomerular cells by a cGMP-mediated process. *Proc. Natl. Acad. Sci. USA* **83,** 4769–4773.
3. Poulsen, K. and Jørgensen, J. (1974) An easy radioimmunological microassay of renin activity, concentration, and substrate in human and animal plasma and tissues based on angiotensin I trapping by antibody. *J. Clin. Endocrinol. Metab.* **39,** 816–825.
4. Lykkegaard, S. and Poulsen, K. (1976) Ultramicroassay for plasma renin concentration in the rat using the antibody trapping technique. *Anal. Biochem.* **75,** 250–259.
5. Skøtt, O. (1986) Episodic release of renin from single superfused rat afferent arterioles. *Pflügers Arch. Eur. J. Physiol.* **407,** 485–491.
6. Friis, U. G., Jensen, B. L., Aas, J., and Skøtt, O. (1999) Direct demonstration of exo- and endocytosis in single mouse juxtaglomerular cells. *Circ. Res.* **84,** 929–936.
7. Friis, U. G., Jensen, B. L., Sethi, S., Andreasen, D., Hansen, P. B., and Skøtt, O. (2002) Control of renin secretion from rat juxtaglomerular cells by cyclic AMP-specific phosphodiesterases. *Circ. Res.* **90,** 996–1003.

8. Skøtt, O. and Briggs, J. P. (1987) Direct demonstration of macula-densa mediated renin release. *Science* **237,** 1618–1620.

9. Kurtz, A. and Penner, R. (1989) Angiotensin II induces oscillations of intracellular calcium and blocks anomalous inward rectifying potassium current in mouse renal juxtaglomerular cells. *Proc. Natl. Acad. Sci. USA* **86,** 3423–3427.

24

Mitochondrial Function

Joel M. Weinberg and Pothana Saikumar

1. Introduction

Mitochondrial oxidative phosphorylation generates 20-fold greater amounts of adenosine triphosphate (ATP) through pyruvate oxidation to CO_2 than anaerobic glycolysis, which produces ATP by enzymatic reactions from glucose to pyruvate. In the kidney, proximal tubules are almost completely dependent on mitochondria for the generation of ATP. This bioenergetic function and its compromise during states of injury have long been recognized as major elements of cellular physiology and pathophysiology. During the past decade, it has also become evident that mitochondria are major regulators of apoptosis and the dynamics of intracellular calcium transients, and play important roles in signal transduction via their production of reactive oxygen species (ROS). Thus, interest in their function and in ways of evaluating it has grown, and has become relevant to an expanding range of research questions.

This chapter examines the measurement of respiratory function, ATP sampling and quantitation, and the evaluation of mitochondrial membrane potential and cytochrome c release as aspects and results of mitochondrial function that are of particular interest relative to contemporary questions with emphasis on approaches for evaluating the behavior of mitochondria in intact cells that we have extensively used and verified in our own laboratories.

Because of space considerations, this chapter does not cover procedures for evaluating matrix enzymes or matrix metabolites and their transporters—including the adenine nucleotide translocase and the Ca^{2+} uniporter, the proton ATPase, or individual components of the electron transport chain by methods other than measurements of respiration—but many excellent treatments of all these topics exist *(1,2)*.

From: *Methods in Molecular Medicine, vol. 86: Renal Disease: Techniques and Protocols*
Edited by: M. S. Goligorsky © Humana Press Inc., Totowa, NJ

2. Materials

2.1. Measurement of Respiration

1. Membranes for Clark electrode and other oximeter-specific items.
2. Carbonyl cyanide p-trifluoromethoxyphenylhydrazone (FCCP, Sigma, St. Louis, MO): 5 mM stock in ethanol, stable refrigerated for prolonged periods. Use at final concentration of 5 μM.
3. Ouabain (Sigma): 500 mM in dimethyl sulfoxide (DMSO, Sigma) made fresh daily. Use at final concentration of 1 mM.
4. Nystatin (Sigma): 40 mg/mL made fresh the day of use. Use at a final concentration of 40 μg/mg protein.
5. 150 mM KCl for calibration of the oximeter.
6. Intracellular buffer: 110 mM KCl, 30 mM Tris-HEPES, pH 7.4, 5 mM potassium phosphate, 2 mM EGTA, 1 mM ADP, and 50 μg/mg protein digitonin (Calbiochem, San Diego, CA).
7. 400 mM stock solutions of glutamate, malate, succinate, and ascorbate as potassium salts neutralized to pH 7.0–7.4, stable at –20°C for prolonged periods. Use at final concentrations of 4 mM.
8. 10 mM stock of rotenone (Sigma) in ethanol, stable refrigerated for prolonged periods. Use at final concentration of 10 μM.
9. 1 mM stock of antimycin-A (Sigma) in ethanol, stable refrigerated for prolonged periods. Use at final concentration of 1 μM.
10. 30 mM N,N,N'N'-tetramethyl-p-phenylenediamine (TMPD) in water prepared fresh the day of the experiment. Use at final concentration of 0.3 mM.

2.2. Collection of Samples of Cellular Nucleotides and Other Metabolites

2.2.1. Perchloric Acid Method for Cells Growing as Monolayers

1. Perchloric acid (PCA-ACS grade). Make up to 6% w/v in deionized water (5 mL of 70% chloroform brought up to 100 mL).
2. Potassium carbonate (K_2CO_3, ACS grade). Make up to 5 M in deionized water.
3. Sodium hydroxide (ACS grade). Make up to 0.5 N. Stable refrigerated indefinitely.

2.2.2. Trichloracetic Acid Method for Cells and Tubules in Suspension or Growing as Monolayers

1. Trichloroacetic acid (TCA-ACS grade). Make up to 6% or 12% (w/v) in deionized water. Stable refrigerated indefinitely.
2. Trioctylamine (98% solution, Aldrich).
3. 1,1,2-trichlorotrifluoroethane (CFC-113, HPLC grade, Aldrich).
4. Chloroform (HPLC grade, Aldrich).
5. Sodium hydroxide (ACS grade). Make up to 0.5 N. Stable refrigerated indefinitely.

2.3. Luciferase Assay

1. ATP Bioluminescence kit (Sigma or Roche Applied Science). The ATP bioluminescence reagent is supplied as a lyophilized powder. Reconstituted reagent is stable for 2 wk at 0–4°C and longer at –20°C without repeated freezing and thawing.
2. Adenosine-5'-triphosphate (Sigma) 1 mM stock in deionized water. Store in aliquots at –20°C.

2.4. HPLC

1. C_{18} reversed-phase ion pairing columns: 150-mm main column, 45-mm guard column (Beckman, Fullerton, CA).
2. Acetonitrile (high-performance liquid chromatography [HPLC] grade, Fisher Scientific).
3. KH_2PO_4 (HPLC grade, Fisher Scientific).
4. Tetrabutylammonium dihydrogen phosphate (TBAP): 1.0 M solution in water (Aldrich, Milwaukee, WI) (*see* **Note 10**).

2.5. Measurement of Changes
in Mitochondrial Membrane Potential ($\Delta\psi_m$)

1. 5,5',6,6'-tetrachloro-1,1'3,3'-tetraethylbenzimidazocarbocyanine iodide (JC-1, Molecular Probes, Eugene, OR or R&D Systems Inc., Minneapolis, MN). Subaliquot a storage stock solution of 2 mg/mL in DMSO and keep at –20°C. The solution will be stable for months stored in this fashion. Avoid repeated freeze/thaw of the aliquots. Prepare working stock solution of 200 μg/mL JC-1 fresh the day of use by mixing one part of the storage stock with four parts calf serum or 5% bovine serum albumin, then dispersing into PBS to provide the desired volume of the working stock. This working stock is stable for at least 8 h when kept on ice and used the day of preparation (*see* **Note 13**).
2. Rinse and resuspend solution (Solution A) prepared and used at 4°C: 100 mM NaCl, 25 mM Na-HEPES, pH 7.2, 1.25 mM CaCl$_2$, 1.0 mM MgCl$_2$, 1.0 mM KH$_2$PO$_4$, 3.5 mM KCl, 5.0 mM glycine, 5% polyethylene glycol (average mW 8000). This solution is stable for weeks when kept refrigerated.

2.6. Cell Fractionation

1. Mitochondria isolation medium: 20 mM K-HEPES, pH 7.4, 250 mM sucrose, 10 mM KCl, 1.5 mM MgCl$_2$, 5 mM EGTA, and 5 mg/mL fatty acid-free bovine serum albumin (BSA).
2. Detergent lysis buffer: 20 mM Na-HEPES, pH 7.4, 150 mM NaCl, 1.5 mM MgCl$_2$, 1 mM EGTA, and protease inhibitors: 1 mM 4-(2-aminoethyl) benzenesulfonyl fluoride hydrochloride, 0.8 μM aprotinin, 50 μM bestatin, 15 μM E-64, 20 μM leupeptin, 10 μM pepstatin A (Protease Inhibitor Cocktail Set III, Calbiochem, San Diego, CA.)
3. Digitonin (high purity, Calbiochem, 5% stock in DMSO).

4. Dounce tissue grinder with tight pestle (B-type; Kontes, Vineland, NJ, or Wheaton, Millville, NJ).
5. Potter-Elvehjem homogenizer (Thomas Scientific, Swedesboro, NJ).
6. Nitrogen bomb (Parr Instrument, Moline, IL, or Kontes).

2.7. Detection of Cytochrome c Release

1. Anti-cytochrome c antibodies (mouse monoclonal, Pharmingen, San Diego, CA, or rabbit polyclonal, Santa Cruz Biotechnology, Santa Cruz, CA).
2. NuPAGE polyacrylamide gels (4–12% or 10%, Invitrogen, Carlsbad, CA).
3. Sample buffer: 62.5 mM Tris-HCl pH 6.8, 10% glycerol, 4% sodium dodecyl sulfate (SDS), 25 mM dithiothreitol (DTT).
4. NuPAGE SDS sample buffer (Invitrogen, Carlsbad, CA).
5. Horseradish peroxidase-conjugated anti-mouse or anti-rabbit IgG (Jackson ImmunoResearch, West Grove, PA).
6. PBS, pH 7.4.
7. PBS containing 0.05% Tween-20 (PBST).
8. Polyvinylidene fluoride (PVDF) or nitrocellulose membranes (0.2–0.45-μm pore size).
9. Chemiluminescence detection kit (Pierce, Rockford, IL, or Amersham, Piscataway, NJ).
10. Modified Zamboni's fixative: 4% paraformaldehyde and 0.19% picric acid in PBS, pH 7.4 (*see* **Subheading 3.6.6.2**).
11. Prolong Anti-fade Kit (Molecular Probes).
12. Cy3 or fluorescein isothiocyanate (FITC) conjugated anti-mouse or anti-rabbit IgG (Jackson ImmunoResearch).

3. Methods

3.1. Measurement of Respiration

Mitochondria are the main oxygen consumers of cells, since oxygen is the ultimate electron acceptor for the mitochondrial respiratory chain. A full reduction of oxygen during normal transit of electrons through the entire respiratory chain produces water. Incomplete reduction of oxygen at intermediate points in the electron transport chain is a major intracellular source of ROS.

Respiratory rates are usually measured polarographically with a Clark electrode on either intact cells or isolated mitochondria by following oxygen consumption in a sealed, temperature-controlled chamber. A number of such devices are on the market, and new hardware has appeared as interest in these measurements has increased again. This section focuses on the approaches used for reaching conclusions about mitochondrial behavior within intact cells rather than on hardware-specific issues.

1. Calibrate the Clark electrode using air-saturated 150 mM KCl (**Note 1**).
2. Assay respiration of intact cells or isolated tubules in suspension at 37°C.

3. For studies of intact cells, keep the suspension in its complete experimental medium and obtain a basal rate of oxygen consumption. Then add either ouabain, nystatin, or FCCP to produce a modified rate to provide additional information, as described in **Note 4**.

4. For studies of permeabilized cells to allow evaluation of parts of the electron transport chain, pellet cells and resuspend in 37°C intracellular buffer with the desired substrates (*see* **Note 5**). Then immediately transfer to the oximeter chamber for measurement of the respiratory rate.

3.2. Collection of Samples of Cellular Nucleotides and Other Metabolites

An accurate estimation of ATP relies on good extraction procedure. The procedure should provide for both quick release of ATP and instant inactivation of all ATP-consuming enzymes. An extraction method involving boiling, for example, is less efficient because of the lag in inactivation of ATP-degrading enzymes. Traditionally, cellular metabolites and other small solutes have been extracted and separated from cell protein by treatment with PCA or TCA followed by neutralization with alkaline salts *(3,4)*. Although well-established and highly effective, this method requires adjustment of pH and leaves a solution with additional salts in it that must then be removed before analysis. Organic extraction using a water-insoluble amine *(5)* is an alternative approach to neutralization that can be scaled for a very wide range of sample sizes, including very small ones, and does not require any stepwise additions or pH determinations. Here, we present the procedures and the methods that are used most extensively and fully verified in our labs, but variations on them (e.g., use of perchloric acid with suspended cells or tubules) are readily extrapolated (*see* **Notes 6** and **8**).

3.2.1. Procedure for Cells Growing in Monolayers (see **Notes 6** and **8**)

1. Wash cells with 3× with PBS after medium is aspirated from the culture dishes.

2. Add 1, 2, or 3 mL of PCA for 35-mm, 60-mm or 100-mm plates, respectively. Keep dishes at 4°C for 15 min swirling periodically.

3. Collect PCA extract into a 12 × 75-mm test tube.

4. Transfer 1 mL of the PCA extract into a fresh 12 × 75-mm test tube on ice. Add 80 μL of ice-cold 5 M K_2CO_3 dropwise. Mix by vortexing immediately after each addition of K_2CO_3. Intersperse cooling periods on ice between each addition of the K_2CO_3. Alternatively, the PCA samples may be neutralized with either KOH or by organic extraction with trioctylamine:chloroform as described in **Subheading 3.2.2.**

5. Allow the salt precipitate to settle on ice for 15 min, then centrifuge at 500g for 5 min in a tabletop centrifuge.

6. The supernatant sample can be stored for later use for maximum of 3 wk at 4°C or at –20°C for longer periods of time.
7. The cell protein left on the plate is scraped into 0.5 N NaOH to dissolve it for assay.
8. TCA with trioctylamine: CFC-113 neutralization as described in **Subheading 3.2.2.** can be substituted for PCA in this procedure.

3.2.2. Procedure for Suspensions of Isolated Tubules or Individual Cells

1. Dissolve trioctylamine in either CFC-113 (1:3.44, v/v) or in chloroform (1:1.72, v/v) the day of use and keep at room temperature.
2. To sample cells and medium together, mix equal volumes of cell/tubule suspension and 12% TCA by vortexing in a plastic centrifuge tube. Microcentrifuge tubes are most convenient when total volumes do not exceed their 1.7-2-mL capacities.
3. Pellet the precipitated protein by centrifugation. If the volumes of sample fit into 1.7-mL. microcentrifuge tubes, they are spun at 12,000g for 30–45 sec. Larger volumes are spun for 5 min at 500g in a tabletop centrifuge.
4. Remove the entire supernatant and immediately mix well by vortexing with an equal volume of trioctylamine:CFC-113 or trioctylamine:chloroform in a 12 × 75 mm glass tube.
5. Separate the aqueous and organic phases by centrifugation for 5 min at 500g in a tabletop centrifuge.
6. Aspirate and save the upper aqueous layer for analysis. Leave some of the aqueous layer behind to avoid including any of the organic phase material in the sample.
7. The original protein pellet is dissolved overnight at room temperature in 0.5 N NaOH for analysis by the Lowry or bicinchoninic acid assays.
8. To sample cells and medium separately, the two components are separated by centrifugation. The medium is combined with an equal volume of 12% TCA as used for whole suspension samples. The cells are mixed into 6% TCA.

3.3. Assay of ATP and Other Purine and Related Metabolites

The quickest, simplest, and most widely accessible method for assaying ATP content is the luciferase assay. HPLC provides much additional relevant information about other adenine nucleotides and nucleoside breakdown products, as well as guanine nucleotides and some pyridine nucleotides.

3.3.1. Luciferase Assay

1. Mix 50–100 µL of sample or ATP standard with an equal volume of luciferase reagent.
2. Follow luciferase activity in a luminometer or luminescence reader for 10 sec.
3. Determine the concentration of ATP in the supernatant from a standard curve of log-log plot of luminescence and ATP concentration. A calibration curve must be done every time the stored reagent is used, because a slight loss of activity occurs during storage.

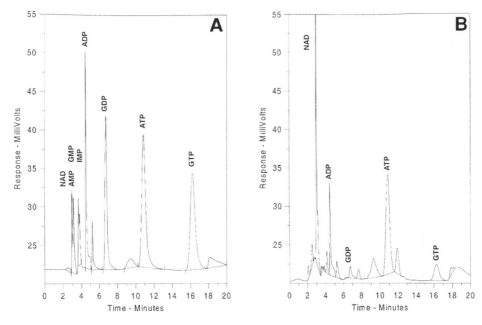

Fig. 1. Measurement of nucleotides by isocratic elution. **(A)** Standard containing (in μ*M*): 2 nicotinamide adenine dinucleotide (NAD), 2 adenosine monophosphate (AMP), 2 guanosine monophosphate (GMP), 2 inosine monophosphate (IMP), 10 adenosine monophosphate (ADP), 10 guanosine diphosphate (GDP), 20 ATP, and 20 guanosine triphosphate (GTP). **(B)** Trioctylamine/CFC-113-processed TCA extract of freshly isolated rabbit proximal tubules.

3.3.2. HPLC

3.3.2.1. Isocratic Method (similar to ref. *6*)

1. The mobile phase consists of 18.5% acetonitrile, 40 m*M* KH$_2$PO$_4$, 10 m*M* tetra-butylammonium dihydrogen phosphate, pH 3.25 (*see* **Note 11**).
2. Sample volume is typically 20 μL.
3. The column is eluted at a flow rate of 1 mL/min, and peaks are detected at an absorbance of 254 nm. Major temperature fluctuations in the room can shift retention times, so we keep the column temperature controlled at 25°C. The total run time for each sample injection is 24 min.
4. The procedure separates nicotinamide adenine dinucleotide (NAD), adenosine monophosphate (AMP), guanosine monophosphate (GMP), inosine monophosphate (IMP), adenosine diphosphate (ADP), guanosine diphosphate (GDP), ATP, and guanosine triphosphate (GTP) (**Fig. 1**). In experimental samples, some peaks can be obscured when adjacent peaks are very large or by overlap from other solutes in the sample or artifacts, but these problems virtually never limit mea-

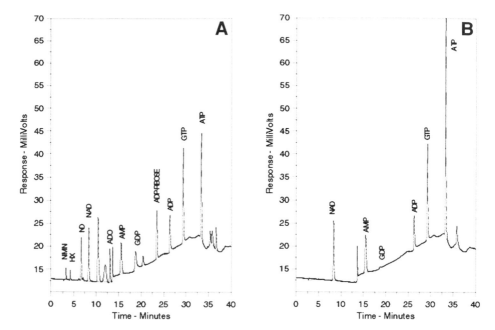

Fig. 2. Measurement of nucleotides and their metabolites by gradient elution.
(**A**) Standard containing (in μ*M*): 2.5 nicotinamide mononucleotide (NMN), 0.5 hypoxanthine (HX), 5 inosine (INO), 5 NAD, 2.5 adenosine (ADO), 5 AMP, 5 GMP,
5 GDP, 2.5 ADP-ribose, 5 ADP, 10 GTP, and 10 ATP. (**B**) Trioctylamine/CFC-113-
processed TCA extract of freshly isolated rabbit proximal tubules.

surement of the later eluting ATP and GTP peaks. Concentrations in samples are
determined by comparison of peak heights with those in mixtures of pure nucleotides at known concentration.

3.3.2.2. Gradient Method (similar to ref. 7)

1. Solution A of the mobile phase consists of 100 m*M* KH_2PO_4, 5 m*M* TBAP,
   2.5% (v/v) acetonitrile, pH 6.0. Buffer B consists of 100 m*M* KH_2PO_4, 5 m*M*
   TBAP, 25% acetonitrile, pH 5.5.
2. Sample volume is typically 20 μL.
3. The column is eluted at 25°C for 1 min with 100% Solution A at 0.1 mL/min then
   for 10 min with Solution A at 1.0 mL/min, then for 2 min with Solution A plus
   Solution B increasing to 11%, and then for a further 25 min with solution B
   progressively increasing to 100%. The column is then re-equilibrated for 20 min
   with 100% solution A before the next injection.
4. This procedure cleanly separates nicotinamide mononucleotide, hypoxanthine,
   inosine, NAD, adenosine, AMP, GMP, GDP, ADP-ribose, ADP, GTP, and ATP
   in cell samples (**Fig. 2**) under virtually all conditions.

3.4. Measurement of Changes in Mitochondrial Membrane Potential ($\Delta\psi_m$)

$\Delta\psi_m$ is a marker of mitochondrial function and integrity as well as a regulator of mitochondrial processes that mediate their critical role in programmed cell-death mechanisms. The precise quantitation of $\Delta\psi_m$ is complex and a matter of some continuing debate (2). Useful estimates of how it is changing during experimental conditions can be obtained by following the uptake and retention of membrane-permeant cationic fluorophores that are trapped in the matrix as a function of their negative charge. Although superficially simple, there are multiple complexities involved in these measurements related to self-quenching of the probes, effects of plasma-membrane potential on uptake, and perturbation by the probes of mitochondrial function (2). Based on these considerations and the need to compare multiple separate samples at the end of prolonged experimental periods as opposed to following changes within single samples after preloading, we have found the probe 5,5',6,6'-tetrachloro-1,1'3,3'-tetraethylbenzimidazocarbocyanine iodide (JC-1) to be most useful (8–12). At high $\Delta\psi_m$, this probe displays an emission shift from green to red due to the formation of aggregates (*see* **Notes 20–22**).

3.4.1. Cell and Tubule Suspensions

1. At the end of the desired experimental maneuvers, add enough of the working stock of JC-1 to the experimental medium to produce a final concentration of 5–10 µg/mL, and continue incubation for another 15 min at 37°C (*see* **Note 14**).
2. Pellet the cells gently and remove and discard the supernatant.
3. Resuspend the cells in ice-cold Solution A, then wash twice more in ice-cold Solution A.
4. For measurements of fluorescence or microscopic viewing, resuspend the cells to a final concentration of 1–3 mg protein/mL in Solution A. Keep on ice (*see* **Note 15**).
5. Suspensions of individual cells can be analyzed by fluorescence-activated cell sorting (FACS) if available. Population behavior of suspensions of individual cells and tubules is readily quantitated on a standard fluorometer with a stirring attachment.
6. For analysis of population behavior, add 300 µL of the cell suspension in Solution A to an additional 2.2 mL. of ice-cold solution A in a disposable polystyrene fluorometer cuvet with a stir bar and run an emission scan from 500–610 nm at 488-nm excitation. The green peak from the monomeric form of the dye in cells is at 536 nm, and the red peak is at 595 nm (**Fig. 3**). These measurements are best made immediately (*see* **Note 16**).
7. For viewing on a conventional fluorescence microscope, a sample is placed under a cover slip and observed using FITC and tetramethylrhodamine isothiocyanate filter sets for the green and red signal respectively (*see* **Notes 16–18**).

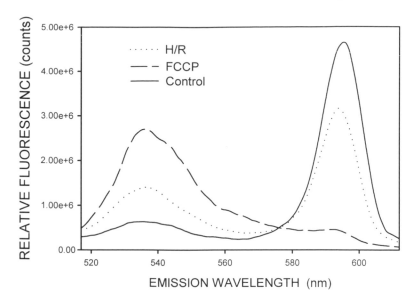

Fig. 3. Emission scan of JC-1-loaded, freshly isolated rabbit tubules after incubation under control conditions, 60 min hypoxia followed by 60 min reoxygenation (H/R), or with the uncoupler, FCCP. Excitation was at 488 nm. Emission wavelengths are as shown. The green peaks are at 535–537 nm. The red peaks are at 595–597 nm.

3.4.2. Cells in Monolayer

1. Load cells grown on glass cover slips with JC-1 for 15 min following the same procedures as for cells in suspension.
2. At the end of the loading period, rinse cover slips with ice-cold Solution A and keep in Solution A until viewing by conventional or confocal microscopy, as described for cell suspensions. Detailed considerations for optimal viewing of cells appear in **Notes 16–18**.

3.5. Release of Proteins
from the Mitochondrial Intermembrane Space

During the past several years, studies have revealed that mitochondria play a central role in cell death caused by apoptosis via release of cytochrome c as well as other injury-promoting proteins from the space between the inner and outer mitochondrial membranes *(1,12,13)*. Cellular redistribution of cytochrome c and other intermembrane-space proteins may be examined by cell fractionation or by immunocytochemistry techniques. Cell fractionation can be achieved by physical disruption of the plasma membrane by homogenization or nitrogen cavitation, or by chemical disruption with detergents such as digitonin. Digitonin can be used to selectively permeabilize cell plasma membrane to collect cytosol, but leaves mitochondrial membrane intact because of the differing contents of cholesterol in the plasma and mitochondrial membranes (*14*; *see* **Note 23**).

3.5.1. Homogenization of Tissues for Preparation of Isolated Mitochondria

1. To isolate mitochondria from soft tissues such as the liver and kidney, rapidly remove, wash, and mince fresh tissue in ice-cold mitochondria isolation medium.
2. Homogenize the minced tissue using 10 mL of mitochondrial isolation medium per 1 g tissue, using a precooled Potter-Elvehjem glass-teflon homogenizer. Generally, mitochondria with a high respiratory-control index are obtained when complete homogenization is achieved with a minimum number of strokes.

3.5.2. Homogenization of Cell or Tubule Suspensions

1. Collect cultured cells by scraping in medium on ice. Centrifuge cells at 600*g* for 2 min at 4°C. Remove supernatant and wash cells in ice-cold PBS with resuspension and centrifugation.
2. Remove PBS and resuspend cells in 0.8 mL ice-cold mitochondria isolation medium (5×10^7–10^8 cells/mL medium). Isolated tubules are pelleted from their medium and resuspended to a final concentration of 20–30 mg/mL in mitochondrial isolation medium.
3. Homogenize suspended cells or tubules in an ice-cold Dounce (glass pestle) homogenizer with 40–50 passes. Check cell breakage under the microscope. If less than 80% cells are broken, subject cells to 10 more passes until >80% cells are lysed.

3.5.3. Cell Disruption by Nitrogen Cavitation

1. Collect, wash, and suspend cells in mitochondria isolation buffer as described for homogenization. All steps are carried out at 4°C.
2. Transfer the cell slurry to the cell-disruption chamber of the nitrogen bomb. Pressurized nitrogen (300–1500 psi for 5–30 min) is then introduced, which diffuses into cells and, upon pressure reduction during lysate recovery, nitrogen bubbles rupture the cells.

3.5.4. Differential Centrifugation to Separate Mitochondria After Cell Disruption

1. Spin the cell homogenate at 600*g* for 10 min in a refrigerated high-speed centrifuge to remove unbroken cells and nuclei as the resulting pellet.
2. Spin the 600*g* supernatant at 10,000*g* for 10 min to separate a mitochondrial pellet from the supernatant that contains cytosol and microsomes.
3. Pour off the supernatant and replace with fresh mitochondrial isolation medium.
4. Gently resuspend the pellet using a Pasteur pipet to spray medium across its surface. Avoid resuspending the dark brown center of the pellet, which contains lysosomes.

5. Spin again at 10,000g for 10 min
6. Discard the supernatant. Resuspend the pellet in the desired study or holding medium.

3.5.5. Cell Fractionation by Digitonin Permeabilization

1. Pellet cells or isolated tubules, then resuspend for 5 min in room temperature detergent lysis buffer (3–5 mg/mL protein) containing 0.02% digitonin with periodic gentle mixing by inversion. Then cool the suspension on ice to 4°C until further processing (*see* **Note 24**).
2. For cells growing as monolayers in dishes, remove the experimental medium and wash with PBS. Then add room-temperature detergent lysis buffer (1 mL/ 10^7 cells) containing 0.02% digitonin. Swirl the dish periodically during lysis for 5 min (*see* **Note 24**).
3. Immediately scrape the cells into the medium and transfer to centrifuge tubes at 4°C. Keep the time of lysis to a maximum of 5 min from the addition of digitonin to collecting the lysate.
4. Centrifuge the lysates at 12,000–15,000g for 10 min at 4°C to separate supernatants (medium + cytosol) from pellets (mitochondria and other cell membranes).
5. The pellet can be further extracted with ice-cold detergent (1% Nonidet P-40 or Triton X-100 or CHAPS) in lysis buffer containing protease inhibitors for 60 min at 4°C on a rocker to release membrane- and organelle-bound proteins including mitochondrial cytochrome c. Alternatively, the pellet can be directly extracted with SDS containing sample buffer after digitonin lysis.
6. Measure proteins content of all fractions. Store samples frozen at –80°C until ready for electrophoresis.

3.5.6. Detection of Cytochrome c Release

3.5.6.1. IMMUNOBLOTTING (*SEE* NOTE 25)

1. Mix samples (3 vol) to be analyzed with 1 vol of 4X SDS-sample buffer and heat for 10 min at 70°C, if sample buffer contained sucrose, or boil for 10 min if sample buffer contains glycerol.
2. Centrifuge the heated samples for 10 min at room temperature in a microfuge (15,000g) and load on an SDS-PAGE gel for electrophoresis.
3. After proteins are resolved on SDS-PAGE gel, transfer to PVDF or nitrocellulose membranes by electroblotting.
4. After blotting, block the membranes by incubating with 2% bovine serum albumin (BSA) in PBST, for 1 h at room temperature.
5. Wash the membranes for 10 min with PBST three times.
6. Incubate the membranes with anti-cytochrome c antibody diluted in 5% nonfat dry milk solution in PBST for 1 h at room temperature or overnight at 4°C.
7. Wash the membranes for 10 min with PBST three times.
8. Incubate the membranes with horseradish peroxidase-conjugated secondary anti-mouse or anti-rabbit antibody in 5% nonfat milk in PBST for 1 h at room temperature.
9. Wash the membranes for 10 min with PBST three times.

10. Treat with chemiluminescent substrates for 1 min according to manufacturer's directions.
11. Visualize by exposing the blot to X-ray film.

3.5.6.2. PREPARATION OF MODIFIED ZAMBONI'S FIXATIVE FOR IMMUNOCYTOCHEMISTRY (*SEE* **NOTE 26**)

1. All steps are performed under a fume hood.
2. Add 0.8 g of paraformaldehyde (EM grade) to 15 mL of hot (~60°C) 0.1 M sodium phosphate buffer, pH 7.5, with stirring.
3. Add NaOH (1 N; 40 μL) dropwise until solids are dissolved.
4. Cool the solution in a water bath at room temperature.
5. Add 180 mg of NaCl with stirring.
6. After NaCl is completely dissolved, add 3 mL of saturated picric acid and adjust the pH to 7.4 with 1 N NaOH.
7. Make up volume to 20 mL with 0.1 M sodium phosphate buffer, pH 7.5, then filter.
8. Prepare fresh each day of use.

3.5.6.3. IMMUNOCYTOCHEMISTRY (*SEE* **NOTE 26**)

1. Use monolayers of cells plated on glass-cover slips (1 mm thick) coated with either collagen or poly-lysine.
2. After experimental treatment, wash cells 3× with PBS.
3. Fix by adding modified Zamboni's fixative for 1 h at room temperature.
4. Wash for 5 min 3× with PBS.
5. Incubate with PBS containing 100 mM glycine for 10 min to quench excessive formaldehyde. At this point, the cover slips can be stored in PBS at 4°C overnight.
6. Permeabilize the cells by incubation with 0.1% SDS in PBS at room temperature for 5 min.
7. Wash three times for 5 min with PBS.
8. Block with 5% normal goat serum in PBS at room temperature for 1 h.
9. Wash three times for 5 min with PBS.
10. Treat with primary antibody (1–5 μg/mL) diluted in PBS-2% BSA for 1 h at room temperature in a covered plastic container with moist towels placed at the bottom.
11. Wash three times for 5 min with PBS.
12. Treat with 5% normal goat serum in PBS for 30 min.
13. Wash three times for 5 min with PBS.
14. Treat with goat anti-mouse or anti-rabbit antibody (FITC or CY3- labeled, freshly diluted 1:100 or 1:200 in PBS-2% BSA) at room temperature for 1 h.
15. Rinse 4× with PBS.
16. Mount on microscope slide using an anti-fade mounting medium (e.g., Prolong Anti-fade Kit, Molecular Probes).
17. Slides are ready for viewing after they dry overnight. They can be kept in the dark at room temperature for several months with no significant deterioration.

4. Notes

4.1. Measurement of Respiration

1. In calibrating the Clark electrode with 150 mM KCl, keep in mind that the oxygen content of the solution will vary with its temperature. If used at room temperature, that temperature should be known, or the solution should be prewarmed to a defined temperature. Oxygen solubilities in 150 mM KCl and in 0.25 M sucrose at temperatures ranging from 5–4°C are given in **ref. 15**.

2. The amounts of cell protein required for good measurements will vary with the capabilities and configuration of the specific oximeter apparatus being used. In our system, using a 1.8-mL. chamber and a YSI Model 5331 Clark electrode (YSI, Inc., Yellow Springs, OH), 4–5 mg/mL protein of fresh proximal tubules provides sensitivity that allows decreases to 10–15% of normal basal respiratory rates (35 nmol O_2/min/mg protein) to be accurately quantitated. Cultured cells have fewer mitochondria and substantially lower respiratory rates.

3. Respiratory rates will depend on the available substrates in a cell-specific manner. In proximal tubules, maximal rates are seen in the presence of exogenous short-chain fatty acids because of a combination of their preferential metabolism and the lower efficiency of phosphorylation relative to oxygen consumption that results from delivery of most of their reducing equivalents to complex II of the respiratory chain rather than to complex I *(16,17)*.

4. A number of agents can be used to elicit changes in respiration of intact cells that are informative with respect to the state of mitochondrial function and the nature of energy demands in the cell. Ouabain inhibits the Na^+-pump, eliminating its contribution to ATP utilization and to the oxygen consumption required to maintain that ATP. Nystatin maximally stimulates the Na^+ pump and respiration to meet the demand of the increased Na^+ turnover *(16)*. FCCP and other similar protonophoric uncouplers maximally increase respiration by providing an alternate path for proton reentry into the mitochondrial matrix *(12,16)*. In isolated mitochondria, the maximal rates of respiration driven by ADP (State 3) are similar to uncoupled rates *(18)*. In intact tubules, however, nystatin-stimulated rates, though often considered to produce a condition equivalent to State 3, are consistently less than uncoupled rates. With both nystatin and uncouplers, the stimulated rates trail off progressively over time because of the subsequent changes of cellular electrolytes and substrate uptake caused by the agents, so initial rates after addition are most useful.

5. Permeabilized cells are used to assure that plasma-membrane transport processes are not limiting for delivery of substrates that allow analysis of different portions of the electron transport chain *(12,16)*. Oxygen consumption in the presence of glutamate + malate requires the entire electron transport chain including complex I, but it should be kept in mind that it also reflects the behavior of the citric acid cycle and glutamate metabolism reactions. Succinate is used in combination with the complex I inhibitor, rotenone, to test complexes II-IV. TMPD plus ascorbate, in combination with the complex III inhibitor antimycin, tests cytochrome c and cytochrome oxidase (complex IV). Other than TMPD-ascorbate, these sub-

strate approaches do not provide information about a single complex, but, together they can localize the likely areas of abnormality that can then guide more complex-specific assays *(1)*, which require more extensive cell disruption or isolated mitochondria.

4.2. Cellular Nucleotides and Other Metabolites

6. The samples obtained by extraction with either PCA or TCA are suitable for measurement of ATP by either the luciferase assay or HPLC without further processing other than filtration if they are to be used for HPLC. Although additional reagents are required for it, the trioctylamine method allows more rapid, consistent processing of larger numbers of samples in our experience. The aqueous phase after neutralization with trioctylamine has a pH of 5.8–6.0. The samples can easily be screened immediately or later for proper handling by checking the pH on 1-μl aliquots using nitrazine paper. If samples are checked immediately and there has been an error in the extraction, the pH will be lower. Trioctylamine treatment can be repeated without degradation of metabolites if it is done promptly. ATP and other adenine nucleotides processed in this fashion and stored at –20°C are stable for years, and can be used readily for HPLC determination of nucleotides, regardless of whether samples were initially processed with perchloric acid or trichloroacetic acid.

7. If monolayer cells detach during experiments, the cells that remain on the plates can be scraped into the medium, and it can then be treated as a suspension. Alternatively, to avoid disrupting the cells still on the plate or to measure metabolites separately in adherent and attached cells, the medium containing the detached cells is removed. These cells are pelleted and then treated with 6% TCA or PCA. The remaining adherent cells can then either be treated separately with TCA or PCA, or if only a combined value is desired, the TCA or PCA used to extract the pellet can then be transferred to the plate.

8. Acid extraction followed by either trioctylamine, K_2CO_3, or KOH neutralization can also be used in the same fashion as detailed here to process samples of intact kidney tissue from in vivo studies. Because of the rapid ATP degradation known to occur during sampling of the intact kidney, these samples should be collected by snap-freezing *(3,4)*. When fresh tubules are being studied, substantial decreases of ATP occur, even during brief centrifugation procedures to separate pellet from medium. This problem can be circumvented by centrifuging them directly into 12% TCA under a layer of bromododecane or dibutyl phthalate: dioctyl phthalate (2:1 v/v) *(19–21)*.

4.3. Assay of ATP and Other Purine and Related Metabolites

9. The standard luciferase assay is sensitive to ATP concentrations as low as 10 nm (10^{-12} moles). The ATP concentration is constant with time and gives an almost constant light signal at a defined ATP concentration because of low luciferase activity present in the assay. Therefore, during the assay, there is sufficient time for addition of the reagent, placing the sample into the luminometer,

and measurement. At high luciferase enzyme concentrations, the sensitivity can be increased to 10 pm (10^{-15} moles). During the high sensitivity assay, the ATP concentration of the sample decreases with time, and the light output declines rapidly from the start of the reaction. To guarantee accuracy, the reagent volume, the injection conditions, and the start of measurements must be absolute and reproducibly constant. For these reasons, ATP estimations using high-sensitivity reagent are not suitable for manual injections.

10. HPLC-grade TBAP can be purchased from Beckman/Coulter at high cost. We find that we can use virtually all lots of the Aldrich product with minimum adjustments to the mobile-phase pHs to achieve equivalent results from different lots. They are stable for years at room temperature, and consistent results are obtained for all bottles of a given lot.

11. Two major factors that influence the consistency of behavior of these mobile phases are their pH and the removal of acetonitrile by evaporation during degassing. The acceptable pH range for optimal results with the isocratic procedure mobile phase is relatively narrow—3.22–3.26. Degassing is limited to 7 min to avoid excessive loss of acetonitrile.

12. The HPLC methods readily detect concentrations as low as 100 nm. ATP levels for fresh isolated proximal tubules incubated at 37°C are 7–10 nmol/mg protein. Cultured tubule cells have 20–30 nmol/mg protein. At the cell densities used in most studies, either the HPLC or luciferase methods can readily quantitate decreases of ATP to 1% of these values.

4.4. Measurement of Changes in Mitochondrial Membrane Potential

13. JC-1 does not disperse well directly into protein-free media. It can be added to medium with 10% fetal calf serum (FCS), but if the serum is not otherwise needed for the experiments, the protein content complicates measurement of cell protein. Mixing the concentrated storage stock of JC-1 with calf serum or 5% bovine serum albumin allows it to readily disperse while adding a negligible amount of protein to the experimental medium.

14. In the literature, JC-1 has generally been loaded at concentrations of 5–10 µg/mL for 10–20 min. We have increased the loading concentration for isolated proximal tubules from 5 µg/mL to 9 µg/mL because of recent variation in the probe that we have received from the supplier. In freshly isolated control tubules, loading within 15 min is about 80% of the levels that will be occur over 60 min. We limit our loading period to 15 min so as not to move too far from the original experimental conditions that preceded the loading. A 15-min uptake of JC-1 does not affect tubule-cell ATP levels.

15. In cold, washed samples, the red signal is highly stable in samples kept on ice for over 60 min. The green signal decreases by 2–4% every 10 min in samples kept on ice, so measurements are best made immediately or at short durations after sampling that are kept constant between samples.

16. JC-1 exhibits relatively high photosensitivity, which is worse when exciting in the green range (515–560 nm) with TRITC filter sets when viewing cells. Since the dye emits both green and red when excited in the blue range (450–490 nm in conventional FITC filter sets), it is preferable to excite at 450–490 and view the green and red emissions using appropriate emission filters. This can be accomplished using either custom filter sets, filter wheels, or by long-pass FITC filter (emission >520 nm) and a camera such as the SPOT (Diagnostic Instruments Inc., Sterling Heights, MI) with internal filters that allow collection of the green and red signals separately. Simple viewing of the both red and green signals combined using a long-pass filter is also very useful for qualitatively following changes because cells exhibit a range of colors from complete green to orange, resulting from overlap of the signals and depending on their relative intensities.

17. The decay of the green signal described for the suspension determinations also affects the microscopic appearance of the cells, but ample fluorescence is present for >60–90 min after sampling to allow enough time for observation and pictures that can be used to compare conditions as long as the delay before viewing is kept constant. Overall cellular structure is very stable over this period of time in ice-cold solution A with no cell swelling, blebbing, or redistribution of mitochondria within the cells because of the presence of glycine and polyethylene glycol.

18. JC-1 can be visualized by confocal microscopy using the same approaches as described for the conventional fluorescence microscope, except that photobleaching is worse. Thus, speed and not exciting with green light until absolutely necessary are essential, and all results must be interpreted based on the unavoidable contribution of some photobleaching. Quantitation of the data in the images is done with standard image-analysis software.

19. Data can be analyzed as red/green ratios or by changes in the absolute red and green signals for either constant numbers of cells or factored for cell number or protein. Protein can be quantitated on washed JC-1-loaded cells by the Lowry assay without interference.

20. Several important issues should be considered with respect to the interpretation of results using JC-1 and other $\Delta\psi_m$ probes. Complete de-energization and complete energization can usually be inferred with confidence. Intermediate changes can be usefully quantitated, but not as directly proportional to the actual $\Delta\psi_m$ *(17)*. When intermediate values are obtained in population studies, it must be determined whether these represent partial de-energization of individual mitochondria within cells or shifts between proportions of fully de-energized vs fully energized mitochondria, either within cells or between cells. This is done by microfluorometry and cell-sorting procedures. Plasma-membrane effects on probe entry into cells vary with cell type, and experimental conditions and must be considered in the specific context of the work. The effects of plasma-membrane potential on probe uptake by mitochondria can be evaluated using digitonin permeabilization in intracellular buffer as in Section I for studying

mitochondrial respiration. Retention of $\Delta\psi_m$ during injury states can result from continued electron transport or by action of the mitochondrial proton ATPase in reverse mode using ATP generated by glycolysis in the cytosol. To help discriminate between these possibilities, oligomycin can be used to inhibit the proton ATPase (22).

21. Mitotracker Red (Molecular Probes) is an alternative to JC-1 for "end of experiment" assessment of membrane potential that is fixable because its chloromethyl moiety binds to protein thiols. However, the thiol binding is irreversible and toxic to mitochondria, with effects that include inhibition electron-transport complex I, which limits its applicability to experiments in which continued exposure to the probe during the experiment is necessary. In our experience with freshly isolated proximal tubules, Mitotracker Red does not reliably remain intramitochondrial after fixation with paraformaldehyde. A companion probe, Mitotracker Green (Molecular Probes), can be used as a $\Delta\psi_m$-independent marker to simply localize mitochondria.

22. For following dynamic changes of mitochondrial membrane potential in living cells over prolonged periods, the currently favored probes are the methyl and ethyl esters of tetramethylrhodamine (TMRM and TMRE) at low concentrations (<50 nm) in which intramitochondrial quenching is less of an issue, but such low concentrations can also be limiting for uptake. **Reference 2** contains a detailed treatment of the complexities of evaluating dynamic changes in living cells.

4.5. Release of Proteins
from the Mitochondrial Intermembrane Space

23. For simply following cytochrome c release *in situ* as a function of experimental maneuvers, cell fractionation with digitonin is preferable to the physical disruption methods because during the mechanical procedures, mitochondria can be damaged and cytochrome c can be found in cytosol fractions from normal cells. Moreover, after cell injury, mitochondrial membranes may be more sensitive to mechanical damage, so that mechanical disruption methods further perturb integrity of the outer membrane during isolation and magnify any release that has occurred prior to the isolation procedure. Nitrogen cavitation, which is considered gentler than homogenization for mitochondrial isolation, requires individual determination of the times and pressures required to lyse cells, with minimum damage to organelles for the cell type being studied. The inclusion of $MgCl_2$ and bovine serum albumin in homogenization buffers is optional if only cytochrome c release is being assessed. They are useful when mitochondrial function is being analyzed. A calcium chelator is used to prevent uptake of calcium during isolation, which occurs even at 4°C. EGTA is preferable to EDTA for this purpose because EDTA depletes mitochondrial Mg^{2+}. Some methods reported in the literature—which use gradients of sucrose or Ficoll or Percoll to isolate mitochondria—provide increased purity of mitochondria but do not recover the entire population of mitochondria.

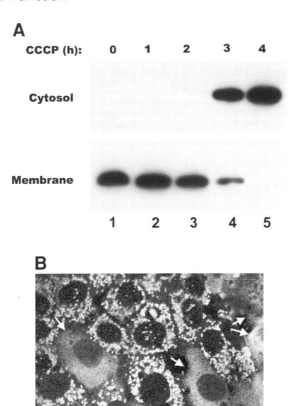

Fig. 4. Immunoblotting and immunocytochemistry of cytochrome c in normal and ATP-depleted, cultured rat kidney proximal tubule cells. (**A**) Immunoblot analysis of release of cytochrome c into cytosol during 5 h of ATP depletion induced by a mitochondrial uncoupler (carbonyl cyanide m-chlorophenolhydrazone—CCCP). (**B**) Immunocytochemistry of cytochrome c in rat kidney proximal tubule cells during 3 h of hypoxia. Cells after fixation with modified Zamboni's fixative, were treated with anti-cytochrome c monoclonal antibody (clone 6H2.B4, Pharmingen) followed by FITC-conjugated goat anti-mouse IgG. Cytochrome c has a diffuse distribution in the cytosol after release from mitochondria (arrows), as opposed to the punctate distribution in cells that have not yet been affected.

24. For cells in monolayers, digitonin permeabilization can be monitored microscopically using a phase-contrast lens as progressively decreased density of the cytosol. For both monolayer and suspended cells, effective permeabilization should be confirmed by documenting complete release of lactate dehydrogenase to the medium.

4.6. Detection of Cytochrome c Release

25. Immunoblotting is the most common method used to detect cytochrome c, regardless of technique used to isolate cell fractions. The amount of protein to be used for immunoblotting depends on the source of sample being analyzed (10–50 µg).

26. Immunocytochemistry allows localization of proteins both in normal and injured cells. Using this technique, the distribution of cytochrome c is punctate in normal cells and diffuse after its release to the cytosol (**Fig. 4**). For immunocytochemistry of cytochrome c, we have tested several fixatives, and found Zamboni's fixative was superior and worth the effort to prepare it. Use of 4% paraformaldehyde in PBS as a fixative is also acceptable as long as the fixation time does not exceed 1 h. Paraformaldehyde-lysine-periodate-fixation, which works well for many other proteins, is not optimal for cytochrome c.

References

1. Trounce, I. A., Kim, Y. L., Jun, A. S., and Wallace, D. C. (1996) Assessment of mitochondrial oxidative phosphorylation in patient muscle biopsies, lymphoblasts, and transmitochondrial cell lines. *Methods Enzymol.* **264,** 484–509.
2. Nicholls, D. G. and Ward, M. W. (2000) Mitochondrial membrane potential and neuronal glutamate excitotoxicity: mortality and millivolts. *Trends Neurosci.* **23,** 166–174.
3. Williamson, J. R. and Corkey, B. E. (1969) Assays of intermediates of the citric acid cycle and related compounds by fluorometric enzyme methods. *Methods Enzymol.* **13,** 434–513.
4. Williamson, J. R. and Corkey, B. E. (1979) Assay of citric acid cycle intermediates and related compounds—update with tissue metabolite levels and intracellular distribution. *Methods Enzymol.* **55,** 200–222.
5. Khym, J. X. (1975) An analytical system for rapid separation of tissue nucleotides at low pressures on conventional anion exchangers. *Clin. Chem.* **21,** 1245–1252.
6. Juengling, E. and Kammermeier, H. (1980) Rapid assay of adenine nucleotides or creatine compounds in extracts of cardiac tissue by paired-ion reverse-phase high-performance liquid chromatography. *Anal. Biochem.* **102,** 358–361.
7. Bernocchi, P., Ceconi, C., Cargnoni, A., Pedersini, P., Curello, S., and Ferrari, R. (1994) Extraction and assay of creatine phosphate, purine, and pyridine nucleotides in cardiac tissue by reversed-phase high-performance liquid chromatography. *Anal. Biochem.* **222,** 374–379.

8. Reers, M., Smith, T. W., and Chen, L. B. (1991) J-Aggregate formation of a carbocyanine as a quantitative fluorescent indicator of membrane potential. *Biochemistry* **30,** 4480–4486.
9. Smiley, S. T., Reers, M., Mottola-Hartshorn, C., Lin, M., Chen, A., Smith, T. W., et al. (1991) Intracellular heterogeneity in mitochondrial membrane potentials revealed by a J-aggregate-forming lipophilic cation JC-1. *Proc. Natl. Acad. Sci. USA* **88,** 3671–3675.
10. Di Lisa, F., Blank, P. S., Colonna, R., Gambassi, G., Silverman, H. S., Stern, M. D., et al. (1995) Mitochondrial membrane potential in single living adult rat cardiac myocytes exposed to anoxia or metabolic inhibition. *J. Physiol. (Lond.)* **486,** 1–13.
11. Weinberg, J. M., Venkatachalam, M. A., Roeser, N. F., Saikumar, P., Dong, Z., Senter, R. A., et al. (2000) Anaerobic and aerobic pathways for salvage of proximal tubules from hypoxia-induced mitochondrial injury. *Am. J. Physiol. Renal Physiol.* **279,** F927–F943.
12. Weinberg, J. M., Venkatachalam, M. A., Roeser, N. F., and Nissim, I. (2000) Mitochondrial dysfunction during hypoxia/reoxygenation and its correction by anaerobic metabolism of citric acid cycle intermediates. *Proc. Natl. Acad. Sci USA* **97,** 2826–2831.
13. Saikumar, P., Dong, Z., Patel, Y., Hall, K., Hopfer, U., Weinberg, J. M., et al. (1998) Role of hypoxia-induced Bax translocation and cytochrome c release in reoxygenation injury. *Oncogene* **17,** 3401–3415.
14. Fiskum, G., Craig, S. W., Decker, G. L., and Lehninger, A. L. (1980) The cytoskeleton of digitonin-treated rat hepatocytes. *Proc. Natl. Acad. Sci. USA* **77,** 3430–3434.
15. Reynafarje, B., Costa, L. E., and Lehninger, A. L. (1985) O_2 solubility in aqueous media determined by a kinetic method. *Anal. Biochem.* **145,** 406–418.
16. Harris, S. I., Balaban, R. S., Barrett, L., and Mandel, L. J. (1981) Mitochondrial respiratory capacity and Na+- and K+-dependent adenosine triphosphatase-mediated ion transport in the intact renal cell. *J. Biol. Chem.* **256,** 10,319–10,328.
17. Balaban, R. S. and Mandel, L. J. (1988) Metabolic substrate utilization by rabbit proximal tubule. An NADH fluorescence study. *Am. J. Physiol.* **254,** F407–F416.
18. Weinberg, J. M., Harding, P. G., and Humes, H. D. (1982) Mitochondrial bioenergetics during the initiation of mercuric chloride-induced renal injury. I. Direct effects of in vitro mercuric chloride on renal mitochondrial function. *J. Biol. Chem.* **257,** 60–67.
19. Cornell, N. W. (1980) Rapid fractionation of cell suspensions with the use of brominated hydrocarbons. *Anal. Biochem.* **102,** 326–331.
20. Weinberg, J. M. (1985) Oxygen deprivation-induced injury to isolated rabbit kidney tubules. *J. Clin. Invest.* **76,** 1193–1208.
21. Dickman, K. G. and Mandel, L. J. (1989) Glycolytic and oxidative metabolism in primary renal proximal tubule cultures. *Am. J. Physiol.* **257,** C333–C340.
22. Nieminen, A.-L., Saylor, A. K., Tesfai, S. A., Herman, B., and Lemasters, J. J. (1995) Contribution of the mitochondrial permeability transition to lethal injury after exposure of hepatocytes to t-butylhydroperoxide. *Biochem. J.* **307,** 99–106.

25

Detection of Cysteine S-Nitrosylation and Tyrosine 3-Nitration in Kidney Proteins

Mark Crabtree, Gang Hao, and Steven S. Gross

1. Introduction and Background

Nitric oxide (NO) is a diatomic free-radical product of mammalian cells that has diverse and important physiological functions, including the regulation of renal, cardiovascular, pulmonary, gastrointestinal, neuronal, inflammatory, and immune systems. At the cellular level, NO is a pivotal modulator of proliferation, differentiation, migration, and programmed cell death. These actions of NO are engendered by covalent chemical addition of NO (or NO-derived species) to protein targets.

In this chapter, we describe procedures to quantify two distinct chemical reaction products of NO and NO-derived species with proteins—these are S-nitrosylation of cysteine residues and 3-nitration of tyrosine residues. These NO-dependent post-translational modifications of proteins have each been shown to mediate cell signaling by NO, although cysteine-nitrosylation has generally been considered in the context of physiology (*1*) and tyrosine-nitration has most often been implicated in pathophysiology (*2*). In any event, NO excess and insufficiency have each been linked to disease pathogenesis (including diseases of the kidney), and resulting perturbation in the levels of protein S-nitrosylation and nitration can serve as either an effector mechanism or hallmark of disease. Accordingly, measurement of the changing extent of protein S-nitrosylation and nitration (along with identification of relevant target proteins, their sites of modification, and functional consequences) will undoubtedly advance our understanding of the molecular processes that are fundamental to renal health and disease.

1.1. S-Nitrosylation of Cysteine

The importance of NO-mediated regulation of vascular tone has been widely appreciated, and received worldwide recognition with award of the 1998 Nobel

From: *Methods in Molecular Medicine, vol. 86: Renal Disease: Techniques and Protocols*
Edited by: M. S. Goligorsky © Humana Press Inc., Totowa, NJ

Prize in Physiology or Medicine for pioneering discoveries. In mediating vasorelaxation, NO was believed to exclusively bind ferrous-iron in the heme cofactor of soluble guanylyl cyclase, resulting in a conformational change that accelerates enzymatic activity, thereby relaxing smooth muscle by augmenting levels of 3',5'-cyclic guanosine monophosphate (cGMP). Nonetheless, the vasorelaxant effect of NO is not fully blocked by drugs that inhibit guanylyl cyclase, suggesting that a significant component of NO-induced relaxation is cGMP-independent (3). In fact, many of the known effects of NO now appear to be completely independent of intracellular cGMP accumulation.

An emerging mechanism by which NO modulates the activity of numerous effector proteins is by the chemical addition of NO to sulfur on cysteine residues of proteins, a modification known as S-nitrosylation. The NO adduct of cysteine is termed a nitrosothiol, and accounts for NO-dependent alteration of numerous protein activities in vivo, including caspases-3 and -8, olfactory cyclic nucleotide-gated channels, NMDA-receptor subunits, hemoglobin β-chains, and glyceraldehyde-3-phosphate dehydrogenase (for review, see ref. 4).

The reversible regulation of protein function by S-nitrosylation has led to the suggestion that this post-translational protein modification may have global importance, analogous to phosphorylation (5). Nonetheless, testing of the ubiquity of protein S-nitrosylation as a cell-signaling modality has been hampered by methodological limitations. Nitrosothiols are labile because of their reactivity with intracellular reducing agents such as ascorbic acid and glutathione (6), as well as reduced metal ions, especially $Cu(I)$ (7), resulting in tissue half-lives of seconds to minutes (8). The existing methods available to study phosphorylation utilize radiolabeled precursors, such as $[^{32}P]ATP$. However, in the case of S-nitrosylation, radioactive isotopes of nitrogen or oxygen are not available, necessitating the development of novel sensitive methods to detect the nitrosothiol moiety. Stamler and associates have utilized a method based on photolysis followed by ozone-chemiluminescence (9), and this approach has demonstrated and quantified endogenous nitrosothiol presence in several cellular proteins, including hemoglobin, albumin, and ryanodine receptors. Despite efficacy, this methodology has two significant limitations. First, the necessary equipment is highly specialized and expensive, precluding widespread application. Second, this method can only be useful to test if a particular purified protein possesses a nitrosothiol, but is not applicable for unbiased identification of S-nitrosylated proteins (SNO-proteins) in complex biological mixtures. In an attempt to overcome these methodological limitations, Jaffrey et al. have developed a chemical method to identify S-nitrosylated proteins based on covalent introduction of biotin in place of NO on nitrosothiols (10). This "biotin-swap" method is described in the following paragraph. It can be used to both identify proteins that are S-nitrosylated under physiological conditions and detect proteins that become S-nitrosylated under pathophysiological conditions of NO excess.

In the first step of the *biotin-swap* method, free thiols are blocked by incubation with the thiol-specific methylthiolating agent, methyl methanethiosulfonate (MMTS). Sodium dodecyl sulfate (SDS) is used as a protein denaturant to ensure access of MMTS to buried cysteines. Under the conditions used, MMTS reacts with free SH-groups, but not nitrosothiols or disulfide bonds. In a second step, nitrosothiols are selectively reduced by incubation with ascorbate, resulting in conversion of nitrosothiols to free SH-groups. In the final step, the newly formed thiols are reacted with N-[6-(biotinamido)hexyl]-3'-(2'-pyridyldithio)propionamide (biotin-HPDP), a sulfhydryl-specific biotinylating reagent. Because MMTS can compete with biotin-HPDP for reaction with SH-groups, it is necessary to remove MMTS prior to biotin-HPDP addition. This can be accomplished by acetone-induced protein precipitation and subsequent dissolution of the precipitate in a buffer that is suitable for biotinylation. Biotinylated proteins can then be affinity-purified by chromatography on immobilized streptavidin, eluted with β-mercaptoethanol and resolved using either one- or two-dimensional (2D) SDS polyacrylamide gel electrophoresis (SDS/PAGE). Using this method and suitable controls, bands representing S-nitrosylated proteins in the starting sample can be visualized using standard protein staining methods (e.g., with Coomassie blue or colloidal-silver). Identification of proteins can be performed by either Western blotting or using mass fingerprint analysis (MFA) of extracted peptides following in-gel proteolysis.

1.2. 3-Nitration of Tyrosine

NO reacts at near diffusion-limited rate with other free radicals. An important reaction of NO in many biological systems is with superoxide radical. This reaction is often considered to limit the bioactive lifetime of NO *per se* and result in generation of a highly reactive species with its own unique chemistry and biology, peroxynitrite ($OONO^-$). Formation and reactions of $OONO^-$ have been implicated in the pathogenesis of numerous diseases, including acute and chronic inflammatory conditions, ischemia-reperfusion injury, and neurodegeneration *(11)*. Peroxynitrite was first appreciated as a biological product of NO in pathophysiological settings by Beckman and Freemen, *(12)*, and accumulation in proteins of a reaction product of peroxynitrite, 3-nitro-L-tyrosine (3-NT), has served as a hallmark of $OONO^-$ formation. It is now apparent that in addition to $OONO^-$, other NO-derived species can similarly lead to 3-NT production (e.g., the products of reactions involving CO_2 *[13]* and HOCl *[14]*) and may be more relevant precursors to 3-NT in biological systems. Whatever the precise chemical origin, it is clear that free and protein-

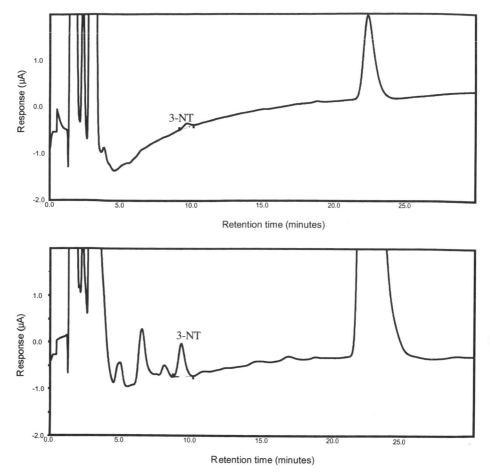

Fig. 1. Typical HPLC trace showing elution and electrochemical detection of 3-NT in a mouse kidney extract, following the 3-NT analytical procedure described herein. Upper panel: free 3-NT. Lower panel: protein-incorporated 3-NT.

incorporated 3-NT are indicative of NO production in the setting of significant oxidative stress. Accordingly, accumulation of 3-NT (free and in proteins) has been widely utilized as a pathophysiological marker. Identification of specific proteins that undergo tyrosine-nitration has been accomplished in many cases, including a proteomic approach *(15)*, however, the extent to which this modification of proteins is important for cell signaling or is merely a footprint that is of diagnostic use for nitrosative/oxidative stress reactions remains unclear.

Here we describe two alternative procedures for detection of 3-NT. One is a quantitative HPLC method based on that described by Muruyama et al. *(16)*

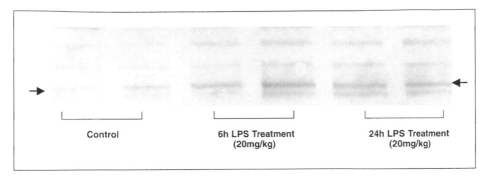

Control | 6h LPS Treatment (20mg/kg) | 24h LPS Treatment (20mg/kg)

Fig. 2. Western blot depicting 3-NT-containing proteins in rat kidney extract. Paired sample lanes show 3-NT in kidney protein from control and LPS-treated mice (6 h and 24 h). Male C57BL/6 mice, 7–9 wk old, were divided into three groups. Two groups received 20 mg/kg of LPS intraperitoneally (serotype O111:B4) and a control group received saline vehicle. The LPS-treated groups were sacrificed by CO_2 asphyxiation at 6 and 24 h after treatment, respectively. Note that LPS-treatment increases 3-NT expression in proteins in excess over control levels. Arrows indicate a protein of apparent 55-kDa mass whose expression level was analyzed by densitometry (shown in **Fig. 3**). 3-NT detection was conducted according to the described procedure.

that utilizes electrochemical (EC) detection for measuring amounts of free 3-NT and protein-incorporated 3-NT in biological extracts (*see* **Fig. 1**). The second method is a more commonly used and semi-quantitative—it relies on Western blotting for detection of 3-NT in proteins from a biological extract, following resolution of the proteins by SDS/PAGE (*see* **Figs. 2** and **3**).

2. Materials

2.1. SNO-Protein Analysis by "Biotin-Swap"

N-[6-(biotinamido)hexyl]-3'-(2'-pyridyldithio) propionamide (Biotin-HPDP) can be purchased from Amphotech Inc. (Beverly, MA) or Pierce (Rockford, IL). MMTS, neocuproine, β-mercaptoethanol, *N*,*N*-dimethylformamide (DMF), SDS, ascorbic acid, ethylenediamine tetraacetic acid (EDTA), S-nitrosoglutathione, streptavidin-agarose gel, and all other reagents may be purchased from Sigma Chemical Co.

1. MMTS stock solution: 2 mL MMTS is dissolved in 8 mL DMF to give a 2 *M* stock solution. This can be stored indefinitely at –20°C.
2. Biotin-HPDP stock solution: 50 mg biotin-HPDP are dissolved in DMF to make a 20 m*M* stock solution. This can be stored for at least 3 mo at –70°C.
3. 100 m*M* ascorbate stock solution: 200 mg of ascorbic acid is dissolved in 10 mL water to make a 100 m*M* stock solution. This is best freshly prepared, but aliquots may be stored at –70°C and thawed once.

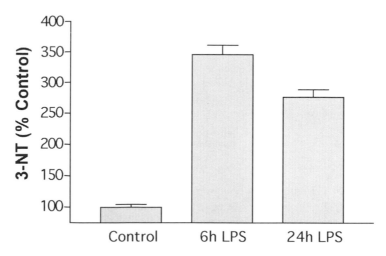

Fig. 3. Summary data, showing LPS-elicited accumulation of protein-incorporated 3-NT in mouse kidney. Mice were treated as described in **Fig. 2**, and kidneys were processed for Western blot analysis of 3-NT using the described protocol. Results are mean densitometric values for the apparent 55-kDa protein indicated by arrows in **Fig. 2**. Expression of this 55-kDa protein is quantified as percentage of control.

4. Lysis buffer: 50 mM Tris-HCl, pH 7.6, 150 mM NaCl, 1 mM EDTA, 0.1 mM neocuproine, 0.5% Triton X-100.
5. Blocking buffer: 50 mM Tris-HCl, pH 7.6, 5% SDS, 1 mM EDTA, 0.1 mM neocuproine, 20 mM MMTS.
6. Resuspension buffer: 50 mM Tris-HCl, pH 7.6, 1% SDS, 1 mM EDTA, 0.1 mM neocuproine.
7. Biotinylation buffer: Resuspension buffer with 2 mM Biotin-HPDP and 4 mM ascorbic acid.
8. Neutralization buffer: 50 mM Tris-HCl, pH 7.6, 0.5% Triton X-100 and 100 mM NaCl.
9. Washing buffer: Neutralization buffer with 600 mM NaCl.

2.2. HPLC Analysis of 3-Nitrotyrosine in Proteins

3-Nitrotyrosine, acetonitrile, proteinase K, sodium acetate, citric acid, EDTA, sodium octanosulfonate, and all other chemicals are available from Sigma Chemical Co (St. Louis, MO). Centrifugal mol-wt cut-off filters (10 kDa) are available from Millipore (Microcon; Bedford, MA) and other vendors.

1. HPLC Analysis: An isocratic HPLC system is needed that includes a pump with all plumbing and fittings of nonmetallic composition (for compatibility with EC detection). The EC detector is preferably of the coulometric type (e.g., Coulochem or CoulArray; ESA, Inc.) The optimal potential for detection of 3-NT was found to be +700 mV. 3-NT is effectively resolved from background species using a

100-mm C-18 column (Microsorb-MV, Varian Instrum.) running the mobile phase below, at a flow rate of 0.75 mL/min. A column heater with temperature set above ambient (e.g., 30°C) is necessary for reproducible column retention time and resolution of 3-NT. Quantitation of 3-NT is performed by comparison of peak area with that of external standards.

2. HPLC Mobile Phase: Sodium acetate (90 mM), citric acid (35 mM), EDTA (130 µM) and sodium octane sulfonate (460 µM) are dissolved in 18 megaohm resistance water (e.g., "MilliQ", Waters Inc.) and stored at room temperature. Mobile phase is vacuum-filtered through 0.2 µm nylon membranes to remove microparticles and degassed prior to use.

2.3. Western Blot Analysis of 3-Nitrotyrosine in Proteins

The protocol described is based on SDS/PAGE performed in the mini-gel format. Polyclonal 3-NT antibody (raised in rabbit), horseradish peroxidase (HRP)-conjugated anti-rabbit IgG, and *LumiGLO* chemiluminescent substrate may be purchased from Cell Signaling Technology, Inc., MA. All other chemicals are available from Sigma Chemical Co.

1. Transfer Buffer: 25 mM Tris-base, 0.2 M glycine, 20% methanol made up to 1 L water, pH 8.5.
2. Blocking Buffer: 10 mM Tris-HCl, 150 mM NaCl, 0.05% Tween 20, 5% nonfat milk, pH 7.4.
3. 10 X TBS: 100 mM Tris-HCl, 1.5 M NaCl, pH 7.4.
4. Primary antibody: 1:1000 dilution—10 µL of rabbit polyclonal 3-NT antibody is diluted in 10 mL of blocking buffer.
5. Secondary antibody: 1:1000 dilution—10 µL of HRP-conjugated anti-rabbit IgG is diluted in 10 mL of blocking buffer.

3. Methods
3.1. SNO-Protein Detection by "Biotin-Swap"

1. Tissue (e.g., 1 g of kidney) is rinsed of blood using iced phosphate-buffered saline (PBS) solution or other physiological buffer (pH 7.2–7.4), minced with a scissors, and then disrupted in 20 vol of iced lysis buffer using a hand-held homogenizer, Brinkman polytron, or sonicater (e.g., Branson Instrum.). Cell homogenates are centrifuged at 10,000g for 30 min, and the supernatant is retained (*see* **Notes 1** and **2**).
2. Protein is precipitated by addition of 2 vol of iced-acetone, followed by centrifugation at 1000g for 30 min.
3. The protein pellet is resuspended in 100 mL of blocking buffer and incubated at 50°C for 40 min (*see* **Notes 3** and **4**).
4. Proteins are reprecipitated with 200 mL of iced-acetone, followed by centrifugation at 10,000g for 5 min.
5. The protein pellet is resuspended in 5 mL of biotinylation buffer and vortexed, and then incubated at room temperature for 2 h.

6. Proteins are precipitated with 10 mL of iced-acetone, followed by centrifugation at 10,000g for 5 min.
7. Precipitated proteins are resuspended in 5 mL of neutralization buffer and incubated at room temperature for 1 h with 100 µL of a 1:1 suspension of streptavidin-agarose (in buffer as supplied by Sigma).
8. Samples are centrifuged for 5 min at 1000g and the supernantant is removed with a glass Pasteur pipet. Beads are resuspended in 1 mL of washing buffer and recentrifuged—washing is repeated 4x more.
9. For 1D SDS/PAGE bound proteins are eluted for 10 min at 95°C in 100 µL SDS-PAGE loading buffer, containing freshly added 100 mM β-mercaptoethanol (*see* **Note 5**).
10. For 2D SDS/PAGE, protein-beads are washed 3x with 1 mL of 20 mM ammonium bicarbonate buffer. Bound proteins are eluted with 100 µL of 20 mM ammonium bicarbonate buffer containing 100 mM β-mercaptoethanol.
11. Proteins from **steps 9** and **10** are resolved by conventional 1D or 2D SDS-PAGE, respectively.
12. Total SNO-protein is visualized using a high-sensitivity gel-staining method—e.g., colloidal-silver, sypro-ruby (*see* **Note 6**).
13. When desired, specific proteins are identified using Western blot analysis (after protein electroelution to nitrocellulose or PVDF membranes) or after in-gel digestion using mass spectrometric (MS) analysis of peptide fingerprints, possibly confirmed by MS-based amino acid sequencing of one or more peptides. Suitable programs for searching a database of *in silico* digested peptides of all known proteins includes PROWL, Protein Prospector (*see* **Note 7**).

3.2. Detection of Free and Protein-Incorporated 3-Nitrotyrosine by HPLC-EC

1. Tissues or cells (50 mg or more) are rinsed of blood using iced PBS solution or other physiological buffer (pH 7.2–7.4), minced with a scissors, and then disrupted in 5 mL per g wet wt of tissue in a buffer consisting of 50 mM Tris-HCl, 150 mM NaCl, 0.1 mM EDTA, and 20 mM CHAPS (pH 7.4). Tissue disruption may be accomplished using a hand-held homogenizer, Brinkman polytron or sonicater (e.g., Branson Instrum.).
2. Homogenates are centrifuged at 100,000g for 60 min, and supernatants are retained for analysis of 3-NT. Each sample may be divided in half for independent analysis of free and protein-incorporated 3-NT, and a sample is retained for protein assay (*see* **Note 1**).
3. For analysis of protein-incorporated 3-NT, 1 µL of proteinase K solution (40 U/mL) is added to 100-µL samples and incubated for 8 h at 55°C. For analysis of free 3-NT, the proteinase K treatment step is omitted, and the method proceeds to **step 4**.
4. To 100 µL vols of sample, 300 µL of iced-acetonitrile is added. Samples are vortexed briefly and then incubated on ice for 5 min.
5. Samples are centrifuged at 12,000g for 15 min in a microfuge at 4°C.

6. Supernatants are retained and concentrated to dryness in a rotary evaporator (SpeedVac, Savant Instruments, Farmington, NY).
7. Dried samples are reconstituted in 400 μL of HPLC mobile phase and centrifuged through a 10,000 mol-wt cut-off filter to remove high mol-wt species.
8. HPLC-EC quantification of 3-NT is performed on 100-μL sample vols, injected manually or preferably using an autoinjector (*see* **Notes 2–4**).

3.3. Detection of Free and Protein-Incorporated 3-Nitrotyrosine by HPLC-EC

1. Sample protein (10 μg per well, prepared as described in **Subheading 3.2.**, **steps 1–2**) is resolved by 10–20%, gradient SDS/PAGE 10–20%, and proteins are electrotransferred to nitrocellulose or PVDF membranes using standard methods.
2. Endogenous peroxidase activity is blocked by incubating membranes in 20 mL 30% H_2O_2 for 5 min at room temperature.
3. Membranes are washed 3× (5 min each) with 1X TBS.
4. Nonspecific protein binding to membranes is blocked by incubation in blocking buffer for 1 h at room temperature.
5. Membranes are washed 3× (5 min each) with 1X TBS.
6. Membranes are incubated at 4°C overnight in 10 mL of 1:1000 polyclonal 3-NT antibody (diluted with blocking buffer).
7. Membranes are washed 3× (5 min each) with 1X TBS.
8. Membranes are incubated for 60 min at room temp with 1:1000 HRP-conjugated anti-rabbit IgG (diluted with blocking buffer).
9. Membranes are washed 3× (5 min each) with 1X TBS.
10. TBS is removed and membranes are incubated for 1 min in 10 mL of LumiGLO chemiluminescent substrate, drip-dried, and exposed to film.
11. Film is typically developed after 2–10 min, depending on 3-NT expression level.

4. Notes

4.1. SNO-Protein Detection by "Biotin-Swap"

1. S-nitrosothiols are photolabile. All steps prior to the biotinylation reaction should be performed in a darkened room. Tubes containing solutions may be wrapped in foil to avoid photocleavage of nitrosothiols prior to visualization. Care should be taken to avoid overheating the tissue by working on ice and using multiple short bursts of homogenization.
2. A sample of cell supernatant may be pretreated for 30 min with 100 μ*M* S-nitroso-glutathione to optimally S-nitrosylate proteins, and serve as a positive control. Cells or animals pretreated with a selective NO synthase inhibitor, such as N^{ω}-methyl-L-arginine (L-NMA), can serve as a negative control to confirm that detection of a given SNO-protein indeed depends on arginine-derived NO production.
3. Some precipitated proteins are difficult to dissolve, even in solutions containing 1% SDS. If protein resuspension proves to be problematic, a syringe with 22–26-gauge needle can be used to forcibly agitate the suspension to facilitate dissolution.

4. For optimal results, protein concentration should not exceed 1 mg/mL. If protein levels are significantly lower than this, incomplete precipitation of protein will result, and detection of SNO-proteins will be diminished. However, if protein concentration is significantly greater (>1 mg/mL), false-positive detection of SNO-proteins may arise from incomplete blocking with MMTS. If blocking of free SH-groups is incomplete, negative control samples will produce a relatively large signal, and the difference between positive and negative controls will be attenuated. In this case, reduce the protein concentration of test samples, use freshly prepared MMTS and/or block for a longer duration. It should be noted, however, that longer blocking duration will result in greater degradation of protein nitrosothiols, and thus a reduced level of detection. Therefore, with samples containing SNO-protein levels approaching the detection limit, it is best to experimentally determine the optimal incubation time that yields maximal signal strength in positive control samples and minimal background in negative control samples.

5. Washing with 20 mM ammonium bicarbonate buffer (pH 8.0) serves to remove salts that would otherwise interfere with first-dimension electrofocusing during the 2D SDS/PAGE procedure.

6. If mass spectrometry is to be performed on protein in gel slices, it is necessary to use a protein staining procedure that is compatible with subsequent MS analysis. This is not the case for all silver-stain procedures.

7. Experiments in which MS-based identification of SNO-proteins is intended are best performed with tissue from man, mouse, or other organisms from which the entire genomic sequence is available.

4.2. Detection of Free and Protein-Incorporated 3-Nitrotyrosine by HPLC-EC

8. An aliquot (25–50 µL) of each sample should be retained for protein determination using a microassay method (e.g., Bradford or dye-binding assay; Bio-Rad). Quantification of 3-NT should be normalized to protein content and expressed in terms of pmol · mg^{-1} protein.

9. Reverse-phase HPLC analysis should be performed isocratically, using a C18 column and flow rate of 0.75 mL/min. Using this system, the retention time of 3-NT will be approx 9.5 min. Detection of 3-NT is based on the amplitude of current as the column eluate undergoes oxidation in an electrochemical cell set to + 700 mV. Quantitation is performed by comparing the area of 3-NT peaks in samples with that of external standard injections consisting of pure 3-NT. Standards may range from 1 to 100 pmol of 3-NT injected; this is the anticipated range of 3-NT in biological samples, prepared as described. The limit of detection by this assay is <0.5 pmol.

10. Confirmation that the 9.5-min peak is indeed 3-NT, can be provided by demonstrating that the peak disappears after brief exposure of an unknown sample to 10 mM sodium hydrosulphite (final concentration). This treatment chemically reduces 3-nitro- to 3-amino-tyrosine, silencing the electrochemical signal.

11. Water used for composing the mobile phase should be 18 MΩ for minimal background electrode currents. Mobile phase should be passed through a Nylon 0.2-μm filter (Whatman, UK) prior to running through the column to degass the solvent and remove microparticulate matter. For preservation of the electrochemical cells, do not apply potential when the mobile phase is not flowing.

References

1. Stamler, J. S., Lamas, S., and Fang, F. C. (2001) Nitrosylation: the prototypic redox-based signaling mechanism. *Cell* **106,** 675–683.
2. Greenacre, S. A. and Ischiropoulos, H. (2001) Tyrosine nitration: localisation, quantification, consequences for protein function and signal transduction. *Free Radic. Res.* **34,** 541–581.
3. Denninger, J. W. and Marletta, M. A. (1999) Guanylate cyclase and the NO/cGMP signaling pathway. *Biochem. Biophys. Acta* **1411,** 334–350.
4. Hess, D. T., Matsumoto, A., Nudelman, R., and Stamler, J. S. (2001) S-nitrosylation: spectrum and specificity. *Nat. Cell Biol.* **3,** E46–E49.
5. Lane, P., Hao, G., and Gross, S. S. (2001) S-Nitrosylation is emerging as a specific and fundamental posttranslational protein modification: head-to-head comparison with O-phosphorylation. *Science's STKE* www.stke.org/cgi/content/full/OC sigtrans;2001/86/re1.
6. Kashiba-Iwatsuki, M., Kitoh, K., Kasahara, E., Yu, H., Nisikawa, M., Matsuo, M., and Inoue, M. (1997) Ascorbic acid and reducing agents regulate the fates and functions of S-nitrosothiols. *J. Biochem. Tokyo* **122,** 1208–1214.
7. Dicks, A. P. and Williams, D. L. (1996) Generation of nitric oxide from S-nitrosothiols using protein-bound Cu2+ sources. *Chem. Biol.* **3,** 655–659.
8. Stubauer, G., Giuffre, A., and Sarti, P. (1999) Mechanism of S-nitrosothiol formation and degradation mediated by copper ions. *J. Biol. Chem.* **274,** 28,128–28,133.
9. Simon, D. I., Mullins, M. E., Jia, L., Gaston, B., Singel, D. J., and Stamler, J. S. (1996) Polynitrosylated proteins: characterization, bioactivity, and functional consequences. *Proc. Natl. Acad. Sci. USA* **93,** 4736–4741.
10. Jaffrey, S. R., Erdjument-Bromage, H., Ferris, C. D., Tempst, P., and Snyder, S. H. (2001) Protein S-nitrosylation: a physiological signal for neuronal nitric oxide. *Nat. Cell Biol.* **3,** 193–197.
11. Radi, R., Peluffo, G., Alvarez, M. N., Naviliat, M., and Cayota, A. (2001) Unraveling peroxynitrite formation in biological systems. *Free Radic. Biol. Med.* **30,** 463–488.
12. Beckman, J. S., Beckman, T. W., Chen, J., Marshall, P. A., and Freeman, B. A. (1990) Apparent hydroxyl radical production by peroxynitrite: implications for endothelial injury from nitric oxide and superoxide. *Proc. Natl. Acad. Sci. USA* **87,** 1620–1624.
13. Berlett, B. S., Levine, R. L., and Stadtman, E. R. (1998) Carbon dioxide stimulates peroxynitrite-mediated nitration of tyrosine residues and inhibits oxidation of methionine residues of glutamine synthetase: both modifications mimic effects of adenylylation. *Proc. Natl. Acad. Sci. USA* **95,** 2784–2789.

14. Eiserich, J. P., Cross, C. E., Jones, A. D., Halliwell, B., and van der Vliet, A. (1996) Formation of nitrating and chlorinating species by reaction of nitrite with hypochlorous acid. A novel mechanism for nitric oxide-mediated protein modification. *J. Biol. Chem.* **271,** 19,199–19,208.
15. Aulak, K. S., Miyagi, M., Yan, L., West, K. A., Massillon, D., Crabb, J. W., and Stuehr, D. J. (2001) Proteomic method identifies proteins nitrated in vivo during inflammatory challenge. *Proc. Natl. Acad. Sci. USA* **98,** 12,056–12,061.
16. Maruyama, W., Hashizume, Y., Matsubara, K., and Naoi, M. (1996) Identification of 3-nitro-L-tyrosine, a product of nitric oxide and superoxide, as an indicator of oxidative stress in the human brain. *J. Chromatogr. B Biomed. Appl.* **676,** 153–158.

26

Products of Arachidonic Acid Metabolism

Mairead A. Carroll, John C. McGiff, and Nicholas R. Ferreri

1. Introduction

Segmentation of the nephron relative to transport mechanisms and secretory activity has been recognized for decades, beginning with the pioneering studies of Alfred Newton Richards *(1)*. Nephron segmentation regarding transcellular sodium and water movement has been subjected to a "comprehensive analysis of sodium transporter and water-channel protein abundance along the renal tubule" by Knepper and Masilamani *(2)*. This experimental approach, based on targeted proteomics, uses an "ensemble of rabbit polyclonal antibodies directed to the major sodium transporters and water channels expressed in each renal tubule segment." It allows and facilitates characterization and analysis of tubular functional differences that define individual nephron segments. However, individual tubular segments can be further subdivided according to secretory activity and transport mechanisms as, for example, the proximal tubules which have three portions (S_1, S_2, S_3) distinguished by morphological differences and exhibiting multiple segregated functions such as the organic and anion secretory system *(3)* housed primarily in the straight segment (S_2), and angiotensin II (ANGII) regulated reabsorptive function, localized primarily in the first few mm of the proximal tubules S_1 segment *(4)*.

Similarly, the renal microcirculation has well-defined anatomical features that facilitate demarcation of preglomerular segments: moving toward the glomerulus from the interlobar artery to the arcuate then interlobular artery and finally afferent glomerular arterioles. For our purposes, the definition of the distribution of cytochrome P450 (CYP) monooxygenases and their isoforms within both the renal vasculature and nephron *(5–7)* has mandated characterization of the CYP metabolic/catabolic machinery within tubular and vascular segments. The importance of these projects is evident in mapping the distribution of ω hydroxylase isoforms (four in rats) in the nephron and renal vasculature, as their activity is individually regulated *(7)*. Furthermore, their localization in

From: *Methods in Molecular Medicine, vol. 86: Renal Disease: Techniques and Protocols*
Edited by: M. S. Goligorsky © Humana Press Inc., Totowa, NJ

key renal structures, microvessels *(6)* and medullary thick ascending limb (mTAL) *(8,9)* and proximal tubules *(10)*, indicates essential contributions to renal circulatory and excretory function. The greatest activity and enzyme concentrations of ω hydroxylases are in the proximal segments, whereas epoxygenases are concentrated in the distal segments *(5)*. However, notable exceptions are evident—as for example, the production of 5,6-epoxyeicosatrienoic acid (EET) by the proximal tubules at which site, it acts as a modulator of the actions of high-dose ANGII on sodium reabsorption *(11)*. It should be noted that cultured cells quickly lose their ability to metabolize arachidonic acid (AA) via CYP, at least within several passages *(12)*.

Our entry into segmental analysis of the nephron—previously known as the province of micropuncture methods—necessarily bypassed this experimental approach, as we were obliged to obtain sufficient tissue for biochemical analysis. A successful attempt was mounted to isolate the mTAL tubules/cells in 80% or greater homogeneity because this segment is invested with critical transport functions, including the establishment of the medullary osmotic gradient. The initial study by Ferreri et al. *(8)* pointed the way for isolation of tubular segments in sufficient abundance to conduct biochemical and functional studies on the pathways of AA metabolism. The isolation of a cell suspension of mTAL tubules, the first and crucial step, was followed by biochemical and functional studies on the AA metabolizing machinery, its products, and the definition of its major attributes *(8)*. Examination of the biological properties of the mTAL-CYP pathway, disclosed AA products that were vasoactive and inhibited Na^+-K^+-ATPase (the Na^+ pump) *(13)*. It instigated an extraordinary parade of findings on CYP-related mechanisms: autoregulation, tubuloglomerular feedback, modulation and mediation of the actions of renal hormones—ANGII, endothelin-1 (ET-1), parathyroid hormone (PTH), dopamine, epidermal growth factor (EGF) *(5,7,14)*. A key study in this succession was based on identifying the action of CYP products, particularly 20-hydroxyeicosatetraenoic acid (HETE) on transport mechanisms in the mTAL: 20-HETE was shown to inhibit the Na^+-K^+-$2Cl^-$ symporter *(15)* and to reduce the open-state probability of the intermediate-conductance luminal K^+ channel *(16)*. This study provided the impetus and conceptual framework for inquiries into abnormalities of 20-HETE-dependent transport mechanisms in salt-sensitive (SS) hypertensive rats (Dahl SS strains) *(17)*. Finally, the definitive study by Carroll et al. on identification of CYP-AA products and their biological characteristics, proved to be an impetus to a series of studies that dissected pathways of AA metabolism in the mTAL and the functional consequences of either deleting 20-HETE or stimulating its production *(13)*. The initial study on isolation of mTAL cells/tubules conducted by Ferreri et al. *(8)* was thus seminal, in view of the attention that CYP-AA products now command.

In a similar fashion, exploration of the CYP pathway of AA metabolism in preglomerular microvessels (PGMV) revealed key mechanisms governing the renal circulation and glomerular hemodynamics, and required a reliable method for isolating renal microvessels (*18*). Thus, the procedures to be described address the issues enveloping the crucial experiments that isolate and recover the mTAL and PGMV. These studies on renal tubular and vascular segments converge on the identity of biochemical pathways of AA metabolism housed in the various anatomical segments of the renal vasculature and the nephron.

1.1. mTAL

The mTAL reabsorbs approx 25% of filtered NaCl and is the site of action of "loop" diuretics. This water-impermeable nephron segment dilutes the tubular fluid and generates a hypertonic medullary interstitium because of its ability to reabsorb NaCl without accompanying water (*19*). The energy for this process is provided by Na^+-K^+-ATPase (Na^+ pump) on the basolateral membrane of the mTAL. Na^+, K^+, and Cl^- are reabsorbed from the tubular fluid via the Na^+/K^+/$2Cl^-$ cotransporter on the apical membrane, and K^+ is recycled back to the tubular fluid via apical K^+ channels. The K^+ recycling and transcellular movement of Cl^- establishes a lumen-positive electrical potential that provides the driving force for reabsorption of Ca^{2+} and Mg^{2+} via the paracellular pathway (*20*).

The study of cellular mechanisms in renal tubules is complicated by the heterogeneity of the cell types along the nephron. Compared to the large number of studies conducted in proximal tubules, relatively few studies have been performed in the mTAL, primarily because of the difficulty in obtaining a sufficient number of cells with high purity (*21*). In some instances, the use of isolated cells from different nephron segments is an attractive alternative to studies using renal slices or intact kidneys. However, the use of primary cell cultures has several limitations, including the relatively small number of cells available for study and a limited lifespan in culture.

Several approaches have been used to isolate mTAL cells, including immunodissection (*22*), growth of cultures from explants of microdissected mTAL segments (*23*), centrifugal elutriation (*12*), and enzymatic dissociation of outer medullary tissue with subsequent density-gradient separation (*24*). The latter technique was modified by Trinh-Trang-Tan and colleagues, and further modified in our laboratory to establish mTAL cells in primary culture with a purity of approx 90–95% (*25*). This technique, which can be performed in approx 3 h, takes advantage of the anatomical arrangement in the inner stripe of the outer medulla so that a careful dissection of this region yields renal tissue that is more than 70% mTAL tubules. The inherent resistance to enzymatic digestion of the mTAL compared to potential contaminating cell types in the inner stripe, permits a simple size-exclusion step, performed after the enzymatic digestion step, to yield a highly purified tubule suspension that is then placed in culture and results in the growth of mTAL cells in primary culture.

1.2. PGMV

The "complex control mechanisms" governing the renal circulation are funneled into the PGMV. PGMV are the effector component of key renal regulatory mechanisms: autoregulation of renal blood flow and TGF (26). Multiple signals arising from diverse sources (endocrine, paracrine, autocrine)—the autonomic nervous system, circulating hormones, the nephron, and renal microvessels—act on PGMV where they are transduced, forming lipid mediators/modulators. 20-HETE, as noted, is the principal eicosanoid in PGMV (27), and is the dominant arachidonate metabolite in crucial sites intrarenally: the afferent arterioles and contiguous microvessels, proximal tubules, and the mTAL (5,13,28). ANGII has been shown to increase renal efflux of 20-HETE (29) as well as its release from PGMV (27).

The kidney possesses a large capacity to generate CYP-AA products, chiefly the ω and ω-1 hydroxylase-derived metabolites, 19- and 20-HETEs, and lesser amounts of epoxides, primarily 11,12 EETs (30,31). However, studies of whole kidney capacity cannot distinguish localization of CYP enzymes in specialized renal tissues, nor can they assign to CYP enzymes and their products their relative importance in the regulation of renal function. Thus, the findings of high concentrations of ω hydroxylase in the mTAL and epoxygenase in the medullary collecting ducts have directed studies to elaborate transport mechanisms in which 20-HETE and the EETs function in these tubular segments (32,33). In order to localize critical sites of hormonal interactions intrarenally, we studied HETE release in response to ANGII from PGMV, the vascular segments governing changes in renal vascular resistance (34).

2. Materials

2.1. Preparation of mTAL

1. Anesthetics: Pentobarbital (50 mg/mL) is given at a dose of 5 mg/100 g body wt.
2. Nylon Mesh: 53 μm (Spectrum Laboratories Inc.; Catalog #08670201).
3. Rats: Male Sprague-Dawley rats (Charles River Lab, Wilmington, MA) weighing 100–110 g are maintained on standard rat chow (Ralston-Purina, Chicago, IL) and given tap water *ad libitum*. The procedure is typically performed using two rats for experiments in which cells are cultured in 6-well plates, and one rat for establishing cultures in 24-well plates.
4. Hank's Balanced Salt Solution (HBSS; Gibco #12455-010) is supplemented by the addition of HEPES (2.38 gm/L; Gibco #11344-033) and $NaHCO_3$ (0.35 gm/L; Sigma #S5761) and the pH adjusted to 7.2.

5. The HBSS solution is oxygenated (95% O_2/5% CO_2) for 30 min on ice and the pH is adjusted to 7.4 before use.

6. HBSS containing 2% bovine serum albumin (BSA; Sigma# A4503) is prepared using the oxygenated HBSS in **step 1**. The pH is adjusted to 7.2.

7. 0.1% collagenase (Sigma C9891) in HBSS- Collagenase from *Clostridium histolyticum* is dissolved in an appropriate volume of HBSS and gassed as described in **step 1**.

8. The solutions described in **steps 1–4** are filtered before use. All solutions are kept on ice and capped to prevent diffusion of oxygen.

9. 6-well plates (Corning #07-200-83).

10. 24-well plates (Fisher #08-772-1).

11. Growth media is composed of: 100 mL Dulbecco's Modified Eagle's Medium (DMEM)/F12 (Gibco #12441-010), containing 10 mL fetal bovine serum (FBS; Gemini #100-106), 1 mL of 200 m*M* l-glutamine (Gibco #12381-018), 70 µL gentamycin (Gemini #400-108), 1 mL penicillin-streptomycin (Gibco #15140-122), 1 mL fungizone (Gemini #400-104), and 50 µL murine EGF (Gibco #53003-018).

12. Quiescing media is composed of: 100 mL RPMI-1640 (Gibco #22400-071), containing 0.5 mL FBS (Gemini #100-106), 1 mL 200 m*M* l-glutamine (Gibco #12381-018), 1 mL penicillin-streptomycin (Gibco #15140-122), 1 mL MEM-non-essential amino acid solution (Gibco #11140-050), 1 mL 100 m*M* MEM sodium pyruvate solution (Gibco #11360-070), and 0.4 µL 2-mercaptoethanol (Sigma #M3148).

2.2. Preparation of PGMV

Dulbecco's phosphate-buffered saline (PBS, Sigma #D-5773), Tyrode's salt solution (Sigma #T-2145), NADPH (Sigma #N-7505) and indomethacin (Sigma #I-7378). Indomethacin is dissolved in 4.2% $NaHCO_3$.

2.3. Preparation for AA Metabolism

AA [1-^{14}C], 1.868 Bq/mmol in ethanol is obtained from New England Nuclear. All organic solvents are high-performance liquid chromatography (HPLC)-grade.

3. Methods

3.1. Preparation of mTAL Cell Culture

3.1.1. Surgical Procedure and Preparation of Kidneys for Removal

After anesthesia has been induced by intraperitoneal (ip) injection of pento-barbital, the peritoneal cavity is opened and the kidneys are perfused through the renal artery with 20 mL of sterile 0.9% sodium chloride.

3.1.2. Removal of Kidneys

After the kidneys have been flushed so that they are devoid of circulating blood elements, they are removed from the peritoneal cavity and placed on ice in a 50 mL conical test tube containing 15 mL of ice-cold oxygenated HBSS, following removal of the renal capsule.

3.1.3. Dissection and Preparation of the Inner Stripe of the Outer Medulla

1. Each kidney is midsagitally sectioned, and the inner stripe of the outer medulla is carefully dissected free of cortical and inner medullary tissue with a pair of small dissection scissors.
2. The excised tissue is placed in a 60-mm Petri dish on ice containing 4 mL of collagenase in HBSS, chopped to a paste-like consistency using a brand new razor blade and transferred to a 50-mL conical centrifuge tube.

3.1.4. Enzymatic Digestion of Outer Medullary Tubules

The digestion procedure is started by adding 4 mL of collagenase solution to the inner stripe tissue that was previously chopped into small pieces as indicated above. Gentle agitation may be employed by an up-and-down motion using a 5 mL pipet.

1. The tissue is sequentially digested 3× for 10 min at 37°C to obtain the maximum possible number of viable tubules.
2. After each incubation period, the suspension is placed on ice for 30 s to allow sedimentation of the tubules by gravity.
3. After 30 s, the supernatant is aspirated with a 5 mL pipet and transferred to a 50 mL centrifuge tube containing HBSS + 2% BSA.
4. A fresh aliquot (4 mL) of collagenase is then added to the sedimented, partially digested tissue, and a second incubation for 10 min at 37°C is performed. **Steps 2–4** should be repeated 2–4×, depending on the amount of tissue being digested and the efficiency of the digestion process.
5. Twenty mL (3 vol) of HBSS containing 2% BSA is added to the recovered supernatants, which contain the harvested tubular fragments, and the suspension is centrifuged (500g) for 10 min at room temperature.
6. The supernatant is discarded and the pellet resuspended in 5 mL of oxygenated HBSS.

3.1.5. Size Exclusion Using a Nylon Mesh

1. A piece of 53-μm nylon mesh large enough to fit over the opening of a 50 mL conical centrifuge tube is cut and saturated with oxygenated HBSS.
2. The tubular suspension is then pipetted onto the surface of the mesh and washed with oxygenated HBSS. Repeat twice.
3. The tubule fragments are collected into a 50 mL conical centrifuge tube and centrifuged (500g) for 10 min at room temperature.

3.1.6. Preparation of Cells for Primary Culture

The final pellet containing tubular fragments digested from the mTAL is resuspended in the appropriate amount of growth medium and placed in culture as follows:

1. One rat, one 24-well plate: The final cell pellet is resuspended in 15–20 mL of growth media, and 0.4 mL is added to each well of a 24-well plate.
2. Two rats, 2–3 6-well plate system: The final cell pellet is resuspended in 30–40 mL of growth media and 2 mL are added to each well of a 6-well plate.

3.1.7. Culturing of mTAL Cells

Cells are cultured in a tissue-culture incubator maintained at 37°C and saturated with 95% air/5% CO_2.

1. The media are replaced every 48–72 h. After 3 d, monolayers of cells are approx 80–90% confluent.
2. The cells are quiesced (see media composition) for 18–24 h prior to their use.

3.2. Isolation of PGMV

Rat PGMV can be isolated by either the magnetized iron oxide method, based on the procedure of Chatziantoniou and Arendshorst *(35)*, or by microdissection techniques.

3.2.1. Isolation of PGMV Using the Magnetized Iron Oxide Method

1. Male Sprague-Dawley rats (300–320 g) are anesthetized with sodium pentobarbital (100 mg/Kg, ip). After midline laparotomy, the abdominal aorta above (between the celiac and mesenteric arteries) and below the kidneys, is cleaned from connective tissue, and silk ties are loosely threaded around the vessel. The kidneys are isolated, and renal arteries and veins are cleaned.
2. All subsequent isolation procedures are performed at 4°C. A butterfly needle (23 G), which has been slightly blunted, and an attached 20 mL syringe are filled with saline (0.9% NaCl). The upper aorta thread is tied, and a small incision is made in the lower aorta in which the butterfly is inserted and tied, and the kidneys are immediately flushed with 20 mL saline to remove blood elements. During this procedure the renal veins, which are prominently expanded, are carefully cut. The kidneys are then immediately perfused with a 1% solution of magnetized iron oxide for 15 s (approx 20 mL), via the aorta.
3. The kidneys are removed and hemisected along the corticopapillary axis. The cortex is excised and finely diced in 1 mL PBS in a Petri dish with a razor blade at 4°C. The minced cortex is transferred to a 50 mL conical tube to which approx 20 mL PBS is added and homogenized using an electric homogenizer for two bursts of 15 s. The iron-laden PGMV are separated from other cortical tissues—e.g., tubules, by magnetic separation, using a special-

ized test tube rank (Advanced Magnetics, Inc.). A strong magnet can be used as an alternative. The non-magnetized elements fall to the bottom of the tube and can be gently removed, thus retaining the magnetized tissues adherent to the side of the tube.

4. The iron-laden tissue is washed from the side of the tube with 20 mL PBS. This procedure is repeated twice, and the retained magnetic tissue is further purified by several magnetic isolations.

5. The iron oxide-containing tissue is resuspended in 2 mL PBS and passed through an 18-g needle and subsequently through 21-g and 23-g needles, in order to remove attached tubules and glomeruli, and the resultant suspension is subjected to a final magnetic separation.

6. The suspension is viewed using a light microscope. This procedure results in an isolate, which is devoid of glomeruli, but remnants of proximal tubules are present. The PGMV are washed 3× in Tyrode's solution (pH 7.4) oxygenated with 95% O_2 and 5% CO_2.

3.2.2. Isolation of PGMV Using Microdissection Techniques

1. As described previously, the kidneys of male Sprague-Dawley rats (150–175 g) are isolated and flushed, via the abdominal aorta, with 20 mL ice-cold saline to remove blood elements (iron oxide is not perfused). The kidneys are removed and cut in half along the corticopapillary axis. After hemisection, the kidney halves are pinned on a Petri dish coated with a silicon-gel (184 silicone elastomer kit, Sylgard Brand) and bathed with ice-cold PBS. The interlobar arteries (200–250 µm), and arcuate (100–150 µm)/interlobular (60–80 µm) arteries are isolated by using a fine straight-spring scissors and forceps and visualized with a dissection microscope (Zeiss, 475002-9902), set at 20X. Care is taken not to touch or stretch the vessels. The isolated arteries are cut into small sections approx 1–2 mm in length and transferred to 6 × 100-mm test tubes, and washed 3× with Tyrode's solution.

3.3. Metabolism of AA by Isolated mTAL and PGMV

1. Tubules and microvessels (0.5 mg/mL protein) can be preincubated for 15 min with inhibitors (e.g., arachidonic acid [AA] oxygenases such as indomethacin, 2.8 µ*M*). Samples are then preincubated with NADPH (1 m*M*) for 5 min with the exception of NADPH-free control, before addition of hormones and 7 µ*M* [14]C- AA. The final incubation volume of each sample is brought up to 1 mL with oxygenated Tyrode's solution.

2. The sodium salt of ^{14}C-AA is prepared by removing the ethanol under a stream of N_2 and adding 100 µL of 0.01 *N* NaOH vortexing and making up the remaining volume with Tyrode's solution. The ^{14}C-AA is added to each sample in a volume of 100 µL with vortexing between each addition.

3. The uncapped samples are incubated in an orbital shaking water bath (160 rpm) for 5–30 min at 37°C.

4. The incubations are stopped with the addition of one drop of 0.9% formic acid and vortexing the samples. The pH is checked (pH 4.0), and 2 vol of ethyl acetate are added and the samples vortexed. The upper organic layer of the samples is pipetted into clean test tubes, and the extraction with ethyl acetate is repeated.
5. The samples are evaporated to dryness either in a concentrator or under a stream of nitrogen. The dried, extracted samples are resuspended in methanol, capped under nitrogen and stored at –20°C.
6. The samples are analyzed by reverse-phase (RP)-HPLC on a C18 μ Bondapak column (4.6 × 24 mm) using a linear gradient of 50% pump A (acetonitrile: water:acetic acid [25%:75%:0.05%]): 50% pump B (100% acetonitrile) to acetonitrile (100%) over 20 min at a flow rate of 1 mL/min.
7. Radiolabeled samples are monitored by an online radiodetector (β-RAM: INUS Systems) and peak areas calculated as percentage of conversion of AA. The identity of the peaks is based on the elution profile of authentic standards monitored by UV absorbance (205 nm) and formation of radioactive peaks corresponding to known AA metabolites may be converted to pmol/mg protein/30 min.
8. Microvascular protein of the individual samples is determined by resuspending arteries in 100 μL of 1N NaOH for 2 d to digest the protein. Protein concentration is measured by transferring the solubilized samples to a 1-mL ground glass homogenizer and manually disrupting any remaining tissue. Protein concentration is then determined using the Bradford method (*36*).

4. Notes
4.1. mTAL Cell Culture

The entire procedure is performed from start to finish without stopping. Aseptic technique is used throughout; thus, all surgical instruments should be autoclaved and solutions filtered before use.

1. The percentage of collagenase used may be reduced to between 0.075% and 0.1% if problems with viability arise. In some instances, the percentage of collagenase required is related to the age of the enzyme preparation. The longer the enzyme has been stored, the more likely that a higher percentage will be required to achieve satisfactory digestion of the tissue. However, our most recent experience has utilized 0.1% collagenase with no detrimental effects on cell viability.

   The mTAL is extremely sensitive to anoxic damage because of the high metabolic activity required to sustain active salt transport (*37*). Accordingly, gassing the solutions and keeping them on ice helps to maintain tissue viability throughout the isolation procedure. The pH must be adjusted because the constant bubbling of 5% CO_2 will acidify the solutions.

   It is critical that during the dissection of the inner stripe of the outer medulla, contamination with cortical and inner medullary (papilla) tissue is kept to a minimum. Careful dissection will ensure that the starting tissue preparation is rich in mTAL, with some contamination by thin limbs and collecting duct.
2. The growth of mTAL cells is more vigorous when the starting outer medullary tubule suspension is prepared from young (100–110 g) rats.

3. A small volume of the tubule suspension may be checked under a light micro-scope to monitor the progress of the digestion protocol.
4. It is important not to aspirate the sedimented tissue after the digestion of the tubule suspension with collagenase, as there are large undigested tissue frag-ments that require further digestion in the material that has become sedimented at the bottom of the tube.
5. The BSA should be checked periodically for precipitation that may have occurred because of denaturation of the protein during the pH steps.
6. The wash of the recovered tubule fragments with HBSS containing 2% BSA is done to help inactivate any remaining collagenase, to remove any cellular debris, and to help prevent sticking of the tubular tissue to the sides of the centrifuge tubes.
7. The washing of the tubule suspension on the nylon mesh reduces any cellular contamination, including red blood cells, tubular cells, and small tubular frag-ments (<53 μm), to pass through the mesh while the mTAL tubular fragments are suspended on the surface.

   The cells should exhibit dome formation, which is indicative of vectorial ion transport. This can be detected by visual inspection using a light microscope, and suggests that the isolation procedure yielded a highly purified preparation of renal tubular epithelial cells. Further confirmation of mTAL purity should be done by immunofluorescent staining for the Tamm-Horsfall protein, as well as determi-nation of other mTAL markers as described previously *(38,39)*.

4.2. PGMV

8. The purity and measurement of PGMV diameters (using an eyepiece linear reticle; 0.05-mm divisions, Fischer Scientific) of each microvascular preparation can be examined using light microscopy (100X magnification).
9. There are distinct advantages and disadvantages of the iron oxide and microdis-section methods:

   The time to isolate and the amount of PGMV obtained varies considerably between the iron oxide and microdissection method. The entire time of procedure from excising the kidneys to obtaining PGMV takes 45 min using the iron oxide method, and results in approx 10 mg protein, sufficient for 20 samples, whereas it takes 2 h by microdissection to obtain sufficient ves-sels for 4–8 samples.
10. Isolation of PGMV using the iron oxide method results in a mixture of interlobar (135 ± 9 μm) and arcuate arteries (74 ± 5 μm) and interlobular (42 ± 1 μm) and afferent arterioles (14 ± 1 μm). Based on the number and size of each vessel, we have assessed the relative contribution of larger PGMV (interlobar and arcuate arteries) to smaller PGMV (interlobular and afferent arterioles) as approx 50:50%. However, this technique results in PGMV suspensions that are contami-nated with residual proximal tubules. Only preparations that have minimal proxi-mal tubular contamination (less than 5%) are used for the experiments. A marker for proximal tubules, alkaline phosphatase activity, should be measured routinely as described *(39)*.

11. The microdissection method results in PGMV of high purity that are devoid of proximal tubular contamination. It is also possible to separate individual interlobar, arcuate, and interlobular arteries. However, it is not feasible to isolate afferent arteries which are essential to autoregulation and TGF.

12. Vascular segments ranging from interlobar arteries to afferent arterioles differ in terms of receptor distribution, reactivity, and localization of oxygenases; the latter generates a different mix of eicosanoids. Therefore, analyses of findings obtained from different renal vascular preparations require cautious interpretation and are rarely, if ever, strictly comparable.

4.3. AA Metabolites

13. The HPLC gradient described will allow for separation of metabolites of major AA oxygenase pathways: COX, lipoxygenases, and CYP. The gradient system can be modified to separate and identify individual eicosanoids—e.g., CYP and COX metabolites from PGMV samples and COX metabolites from cultured mTAL samples.

14. Definitive identification and quantitation of HPLC-purified eicosanoids can be obtained by subsequent analyses by immunoassays and by gas chromatography-mass spectrometry.

Acknowledgments

This work was supported by NIH grants: PPG-HL34300 (MAC, NRF, JCM); RO1-HL25394 (MAC, JCM); and RO1-HL56423 (NRF). The authors thank Melody Steinberg for preparation of this manuscript and editorial assistance.

References

1. Fishman, A. P. and Richards, D. W. (eds.) (1964) *Circulation of the Blood.* Oxford University Press, New York, p. 591.
2. Knepper, M. A. and Masilamani S. (2001) Targeted proteomics in the kidney using ensembles of antibodies. *Acta Physiol. Scand.* **173**, 11–21.
3. Brenner, B. M. and Rector, F. C. (eds.) (1991) *The Kidney*, 4th ed., Vol. 1., W.B. Saunders Company, Philadelphia, PA, p. 486.
4. Cogan, M. (1990) Angiotensin II: a powerful controller of sodium transport in the early proximal tubule. *Hypertension* **15**, 451–458.
5. Omata, K., Abraham, N. G., and Schwartzman, M. L. (1992) Renal cytochrome P-450 arachidonic acid metabolism: intrarenal localization and hormonal regulation in SHR. *Am. J. Physiol.* **262**, F591-F599.
6. McGiff, J. C. and Quilley, J. (1999) 20-HETE and the kidney: resolution of old problems and new beginnings. *Am. J. Physiol.* **277**, R607–R623.
7. Roman, R. J. (2001) P-450 metabolites of arachidonic acid in the control of cardiovascular function. *Physiol. Rev.* **82**, 131–185.
8. Ferreri, N. R., Schwartzman, M., Ibraham, N. G., Chander, P. N., and McGiff, J. C. (1984) Arachidonic acid metabolism in a cell suspension isolated from rabbit renal outer medulla. *J. Pharmacol. Exper. Ther.* **231**, 441–448.

9. Schwartzman, M., Ferreri, N. R., Carroll, M. A., Songu-Mize, E., and McGiff, J. C. (1985) Renal cytochrome P450-related arachidonate metabolite inhibits (Na^+-K^+) ATPase. *Nature* **314,** 620–622.

10. Escalante, B. A., McGiff, J. C., and Oyekan, A. O. (2002) Role of cytochrome P-450 arachidonate metabolites in endothelin signaling in rat proximal tubule. *Am. J. Physiol.* **282,** F144–F150.

11. Romero, M. F., Madhun, Z. T., Hopfer, U., and Douglas. J. G. (1991) An epoxygenase metabolite of arachidonic acid 5,6-epoxy-eicosatrienoic acid mediates angiotensin-induced natriuresis in proximal tubular epithelium. *Adv. Prostaglandin Thromboxane Leukotriene Res.* **21,** 205–208.

12. Drugge, E. D., Carroll, M. A., and McGiff, J. C. (1989) Cells in culture from rabbit medullary thick ascending limb of Henle's loop. *Am. J. Physiol.* **256,** C1070–C1081.

13. Carroll, M. A., Sala, A., Dunn, C. E., McGiff, J. C., and Murphy, R. C. (1991) Structural identification of cytochrome P450-dependent arachidonate metabolites formed by rabbit medullary thick ascending limb cells. *J. Biol. Chem.* **266,** 12,306–12,312.

14. Imig, J. D. (2000) Eicosanoid regulation of the renal vasculature. *Am. J. Physiol.* **279,** F965–F981.

15. Escalante, B., Erlij, D., Falck, J. R., and McGiff, J. C. (1991) Effect of cytochrome P450 arachidonate metabolites on ion transport in rabbit kidney loop of Henle. *Science* **251,** 799–802.

16. Wang, W., Lu, M., and Hebert, S. C. (1996) Cytochrome P-450 metabolites mediate extracellular Ca^{2+}-induced inhibition of apical K^+ channels in the TAL. *Am. J. Physiol.* **271,** C103–C111.

17. Ma, Y.-H., Schwartzman, M. L., and Roman, R. J. (1994) Altered renal P-450 metabolism of arachidonic acid in Dahl salt-sensitive rats. *Am. J. Physiol.* **267,** R579–F589.

18. Carroll, M. A., Kemp, R., Cheng, M. K., and McGiff, J. C. (2001) Regulation of preglomerular microvascular 20-hydroxyeicosatetraenoic acid levels by salt depletion. *Med. Sci. Monit.* **7,** 567–572.

19. Burg, M. B. (1982) Thick ascending limb of Henle's loop. *Kidney Int.* **22,** 454–464.

20. Hebert, S. C., Culpepper, R. M., and Andreoli, T. E. (1981) NaCl transport in mouse medullary thick ascending limb. I. Functional nephron heterogeneity and ADH-stimulated NaCl cotransport. *Am. J. Physiol.* **241,** F412–F431.

21. Scott, D. M. (1987) Differentiation in vitro of primary cultures and transfected cell lines of epithelial cells derived from the thick ascending limb of Henle's loop. *Differentiation* **36,** 35–46.

22. Allen, M. L., Nakao, A., Sonnenburg, W. K., Burnatowska-Hledin, M., Spielman, W. S., and Smith, W. L. (1988) Immunodissection of cortical and medullary thick ascending limb cells from rabbit kidney. *Am. J. Physiol.* **255,** F704–F710.

23. Burg, M., Green, N., Sohraby, S., Steele, R., and Handler, J. (1982) Differentiated in cultured epithelia derived from thick ascending limbs. *Am. J. Physiol.* **242,** C229–C233.

24. Eveloff, J., Haase, W., and Kinne, R. (1980) Separation of renal medullary cells: isolation of cells from the thick ascending limb of Henle's loop. *J. Cell Biol.* **87,** 672–681.

25. Trinh-Trang-Tan, M.-M., Bouby, N., Coutaud, C., and Bankir, L. (1986) Quick isolation of rat medullary thick ascending limbs: Enzymatic and metabolic characterization. *Pflugers Arch.* **407,** 228–234.

26. Navar, L. G. (1998) Integrating multiple paracrine regulators of renal microvascular dynamics. *Am. J. Physiol.* **274,** F433–F444.

27. Croft, K. D., McGiff, J. C., Sanchez-Mendoza, A., and Carroll, M. A. (2000) Angiotensin II releases 20-HETE from rat renal microvessels. *Am. J. Physiol.* **279,** F544–F551.

28. Imig, J. D., Zou, A. P., Stec, D. E., Harder, D. R., Falck, J. R., and Roman, R. J. (1996) Formation and actions of 20-hydroxyeicosatetraenoic acid in rat renal arterioles. *Am. J. Physiol.* **270,** R217–R227.

29. Carroll, M. A., Balazy, M., Huang, D. D., Rybalova, S., Falck, J. R., and McGiff, J. C. (1997) Cytochrome P450-derived renal HETEs: storage and release. *Kidney Int.* **51,** 1696–1702.

30. McGiff, J. C. and Carroll, M. A. (1987) Cytochrome P-450-related arachidonic acid metabolites. *Am. Rev. Respir. Dis.* **136,** 488–491.

31. Morrison, A. R. and Pascoe, N. (1981) Metabolism of arachidonate through NADPH-dependent oxygenase of renal cortex. *Proc. Natl. Acad. Sci. USA* **78,** 7375–7378.

32. McGiff, J. C. (1991) Cytochrome P-450 metabolism of arachidonic acid. *Annu. Rev. Pharmacol. Toxicol.* **31,** 339–369.

33. Schwartzman, M. L. and McGiff, J. C. (1995) Renal cytochrome P450. *J. Lipid Mediat. Cell Signal.* **12,** 229–242.

34. Tobian, L. (1987) Does essential hypertension lead to renal failure? *Am. J. Cardiol.* **60,** 42I–46I.

35. Chatziantoniou, C. and Arendshorst, W. J. (1993) Angiotensin receptor sites in renal vasculature of rats developing genetic hypertension. *Am. J. Physiol.* **265,** F853–F862.

36. Bradford, M. M. (1976) A rapid and sensitive method for the quantitation of microgram quantities of protein utilizing the principle of protein-dye binding. *Anal. Biochem.* **72,** 248–254.

37. Brezis, M., Rosen, S., Silva, P., and Epstein, F. H. (1984) Selective vulnerability of the medullary thick ascending limb to anoxia in the isolated perfused rat kidney. *J. Clin. Invest.* **73,** 182–190.

38. Escalante, B. A., Ferreri, N. R., Dunn, C. E., and McGiff, J. C. (1994) Cytokines affect ion transport in primary cultured thick ascending limb of Henle's loop cells. *Am. J. Physiol.* **266,** C1568–C1576.

39. Macica, C., Escalante, B. A., Conners, M. S., and Ferreri, N. R. (1994) TNF production by the medullary thick ascending limb of Henle's loop. *Kidney Int.* **46,** 113–121.

27

Methods for Measurements of Heme Oxygenase (HO) Isoforms-Mediated Synthesis of Carbon Monoxide and HO-1 and HO-2 Proteins

Nader G. Abraham, Houli Jiang, Michael Balazy, and Alvin I. Goodman

1. Introduction

As the key enzyme in heme degradation, heme oxygenase activity governs cellular heme concentration. Heme oxygenase catalyzes the conversion of heme to carbon monoxide and bilirubin with the release of iron, which can drive the synthesis of ferritin for iron sequestration *(1,2)*. This is the major pathway of heme degradation, and it plays a critical role in the regulation of cellular heme levels *(1)*. Heme functions as a prosthetic group in hemoprotein enzymes involved in endothelial-cell function—e.g., nitric oxide synthase, soluble guanylate cyclase, cytochrome P450, peroxidase, and catalase. To date, two heme oxygenase isoforms have been characterized, each encoded by a different gene *(3–5)*. Heme oxygenase-1 is expressed under basal conditions at low levels in endothelial cells *(6–11)* and kidney, liver, and spleen, and can be induced in these and other tissues by oxidative stress, heme, cytokines, hypoxia, nitric oxide, and heavy metals *(1,3,12,13)*. Heme oxygenase-2 is constitutively expressed in the blood vessels, endothelium, testis, and most other tissues, where its levels are relatively unaffected by factors inducing heme oxygenase-1 *(1,3)*. All heme oxygenase isoforms are inhibited by heme analogs in which the central iron atom is replaced by tin, zinc, or chromium *(1,3,14)*. Heme oxygenase-dependent metabolism of heme to biliverdin-bilirubin and carbon monoxide has been demonstrated in homogenates of several endothelial-cell types and in arteries *(15–20)*.

Heme oxygenase-1 is considered one of the most sensitive and reliable indicators of cellular oxidative stress. Heme oxygenase-1 is usually difficult to detect

From: *Methods in Molecular Medicine, vol. 86: Renal Disease: Techniques and Protocols*
Edited by: M. S. Goligorsky © Humana Press Inc., Totowa, NJ

in cells other than macrophages, but it is activated in virtually all cell types by initiators of stress, such as hyperthermia, oxidized lipoproteins *(21)*, inflammatory cytokines *(10,22)*, and hypoxia *(23)*, and it is found to be upregulated in disease models such as ischemia in rodents *(24)*, Alzheimer's disease in humans *(25)*, and diabetes in rats *(26)*. Recently, we reported that the endothelial cells of various caliber vessels manufacture bilirubin and carbon monoxide (CO) via a pathway that is downregulated by pretreatment of the endothelial cells or the vessels with heme oxygenase-1 or -2 anti-sense oligodeoxynucleotides *(9,27,28)*. Most of the evidence suggests that under basal conditions, the expression of heme oxygenase-2 is more prominent than that of heme oxygenase-1, whereas in stressful settings, the latter becomes dominant.

Evidence of the cytoprotective role of heme oxygenase-1 is based on the following findings: heme oxygenase-1 in vivo suppresses a variety of inflammatory responses, including endotoxic shock and hypoxia *(29)*, acute pleurisy *(30)*, ocular inflammation *(31)*, ischemia-reperfusion injury *(32)*, and graft rejection *(33,34)*. Under the inhibition of heme oxygenase activity by tin protoporphyrin, exogenous carbon monoxide suppressed graft rejection and restored the potential for long-term graft survival. This effect of carbon monoxide was associated with the inhibition of platelet aggregation, thrombosis, and apoptosis *(35)*. We have previously shown that upregulation of heme oxygenase-1 in endothelial cells, via delivery of the human heme oxygenase-1 gene, enhances cell proliferation and angiogenesis *(36)*. More recently, we have shown that delivery of human heme oxygenase-1 into spontaneously hypertensive rats lowers blood pressure, the effect attributed to endogenous elevation of carbon monoxide *(37)*. It has also been shown that carbon monoxide generated by heme oxygenase-1 prevented endothelial-cell apoptosis *(38)*. When heme oxygenase activity is blocked by tin protoporphyrin or the action of carbon monoxide is inhibited by hemoglobin, heme oxygenase activity no longer prevents endothelial-cell apoptosis *(7,38–40)*. The anti-apoptotic effect of heme oxygenase-1 mediated carbon monoxide in endothelial cells has been shown to the mediated via the activation of p38 mitogen-activated protein kinase *(38,41)*. Peroxynitrate (ONOO⁻) produced a concentration-dependent increase in cell cytotoxicity. Increased heme oxygenase-derived carbon monoxide caused a significant shift to the left in the concentration-cell death curve, but this effect could be reversed by inhibition of heme oxygenase *(42)*.

CO generated by the heme oxygenase (HO) system has been proposed to function as an intracellular messenger, partially regulating cyclic guanosine monophosphate (cGMP) levels. HO-catalyzed CO release is widely reported in brain, testes, liver, and cardiovascular tissues. CO has been found to regulate smooth-muscle cell function and modulate platelet activity. The physiological function of CO in the nervous, circulatory, and immune systems has been the focus of recent studies. Techniques for CO measurement are summarized in **Subheading 2**.

2. Materials

2.1. For CO Measurements

1. Gas chromatography/mass spectrometry (GC/MS).
2. Saturated CO (99.0+%, Aldrich Chemical Co., WI).
3. Internal standard solution of ^{13}C-carbon monoxide (99.0 + % ^{13}C and 12% ^{18}O, Isotec, Inc., OH).
4. HP5989A mass spectrometer interfaced to a HP 5890 gas chromatograph (Hewlett-Packard). GC analysis.
5. GS-Molesieve capillary column (30 m, 0.53 mm internal diameter (ID), J&W Scientific, Folsom, CA).
6. Helium gas.
7. Teflon/silicon septum.

2.2. For Western Blot Analysis

1. T75 flasks.
2. Cells homogenate or tissues.
3. Cells washed with PBS and trypsinized (0.05% trypsin w/v with 0.02% ethylenediaminetetraaceticacid [EDTA]).
4. Buffer: Tris-Cl 50 mM, EDTA 10 mM, Triton X-100 1% v/v, PMSF 1%, pepstatin A 0.05 mM, and leupeptin 0.2 mM.
5. Sodiumdodecyl sulfate (SDS) 10% w/v.
6. Glycerol 10% v/v.
7. 2-mercaptoethanol 10% v/v.
8. Bromophenol blue 0.04%) in a ratio of 4:1.
9. 12% gels.
10. Electrophoresis (150 V, 80 min).
11. Nitrocellulose membranes (Bio-Rad, Hercules, CA; 1 h, 200 mA per gel).
12. 5% nonfat milk.
13. Primary antibody; the polyclonal rabbit antibodies, directed against the human HO-1, rat HO-1, or rat HO-2 (from Stressgen Biotechnologies Corp., Victoria, BC, Canada).
14. Secondary antibody (1:5000).
15. Alkaline phosphatase.
16. Solution buffer 0.56 mM 5-bromo-4-chloro-3-indolyl phosphate and 0.48 mM nitro blue tetrazolium.
17. Scion Image software (Scion Corp., New York, NY).

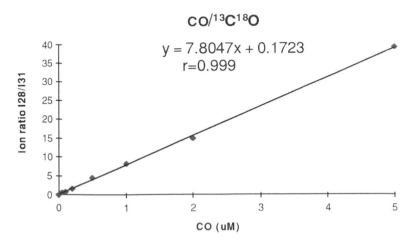

Fig. 1. Correlation standard curve of CO and $^{13}C^{18}O$.

3. Methods

3.1. CO Measurements

3.1.1. Standard Curve

The standard curve of GC/MS correlation ($CO/^{13}CO$ and $CO/^{13}C^{18}O$) is measured by mixing different micro-volumes of saturated CO with 1 μL saturated isotope-labeled carbon monoxide in 1 ml of distilled water in a vial with a total vol of 2 mL. The mixture is vortexed for 10 s, and then 100 μL of the head space gas is injected to the GC/MS for detection. The standard curve of $CO/^{13}C^{18}O$ ($r = 0.999$) is used to calculate the sample CO concentration, as it has a bigger mass difference and better linear correlation than $CO/^{13}CO$. The correlation standard curve is shown in **Fig. 1**.

3.1.2. Carbon Monoxide Detection by GC/MS

Gas chromatography (GC) is a good starting point for CO separation, but thus far, the reported detection methods since GC have encountered serious problems. The thermal conductivity detector (TCD) does not have sufficiently high sensitivity, and CO reduction to methane or reaction with mercuric oxide is a questionable indirect method. Some research groups detect CO through biological coincubation assay, which actually measures the cGMP level. Here, we report the sensitive method for direct detection of CO from biological samples using GC/MS *(43)*.

Saturated CO solution is made by bubbling CO (99.0+ %, Aldrich Chemical Co., WI) through a syringe needle in 5 mL of distilled water at a rate of about 5 bubbles per s for 15 min. Internal standard solution of ^{13}C-carbon monoxide

(99.0+ % ^{13}C and 12% ^{18}O, Isotec, Inc., OH) is prepared in the same way. The concentration of saturated CO in water is taken as 1 mM at room temperature. The ratio of CO/$^{13}C^{18}O$ from the solution is measured, and a constant value is considered to be an indication of CO saturation in water.

GC/MS is performed on a HP5989A mass spectrometer interfaced to a HP 5890 gas chromatograph (Hewlett-Packard). GC analysis is carried out on a GS-Molesieve capillary column (30 m, 0.53 mm ID, J & W Scientific, Folsom, CA). The column temperature is kept constant at 40°C, and 100 μL of headspace gas is injected using the splitless mode at the injector temperature of 120°C. Helium is used as the carrier gas with a linear velocity of 0.3 m/s. The other mass spectrometer parameters are as follows: ion source temperature, 120°C; electron energy 21 ev; transfer line temperature 120°C. Selected ion monitoring is used to record ion abundances at m/z 28, 29, and 31 corresponding to CO, ^{13}CO and $^{13}C^{18}O$, respectively. For the measurement of CO concentration, the sample in 1 mL buffer is prepared in an amber glass vial (total vol 2 mL) and capped tightly with Teflon/silicon septum. Then, 1 μL of the ^{13}C-carbon monoxide saturated solution (1 mM) is added into the sample, resulting in the internal standard concentration of 1 μM. After sample equilibration, 100 μL of the headspace gas is taken from the vial and injected to the GC injector. The amount of CO from samples is calculated from the standard curve according to the ratio of the peak areas of m/z 28 and m/z 31. The accuracy and sensitivity of this method are discussed in **Notes**.

3.1.3. Application of CO Micro-Assay Methods to Cells or Tissues Using Retroviral HHO-1 Sense (S) and Anti-Sense (AS) Constructs the Rate of Cellular Heme Catabolism and CO Production

Cells expressing HO-1 sense (S) and anti-sense (AS) orientations metabolize heme and generate CO at a different rates. We applied the GC/MS to measure the levels of CO following exogenous heme addition in HO-1 S- and AS-transduced human endothelial cells (HMEC-1). Cells were cultured in the presence of 10 μM heme for 24 h; heme content was then determined. As shown in **Table 1**, in cells transduced with HO-1-AS, heme content was increased to 265 ± 92-pmol/mg protein as compared to 159 ± 78-pmol/mg proteins in control cells. Control cells were able to catabolize heme at a higher rate than HO-1-AS-transduced cells, reflecting the decrease in HO activity following HO-1 AS expression. In contrast, HMEC-1 transduced with HO-1-S exhibited a 5.6-fold increase in HO activity and a decrease in cellular heme content by 65%, as compared to cells transduced with HO-1-AS. These results further indicate that the exogenous heme was degraded primarily by HO-1 but not HO-2, because in the HO-1-transduced cells, the rate of heme catabolism was diminished significantly with no change in HO-2 protein content. Because HO

Table 1
Effect of Retroviral Human HO-1 S and AS Transfer on Heme Content
and HO Activity in Human Microvessel Endothelial Cells (HMEC-1)

Cell types	Heme content (pmol/mg microsomal protein)	HO activity (nmol/mg/30 min)
HMEC-1	159 ± 78	0.54 ± 0.08
HMEC-1/HO-1-AS	265 ± 92*	0.30 ± 0.12*
HMEC-1/HO-1	92 ± 63*	1.69 ± 0.13*

HMEC-1 cells nontransduced or transduced with HOP-driven HO-1 S (HMEC-1/HHO-1) and HOP-driven HO-1-AS (HMEC-1/HO-1-AS) were treated with heme (10 μM) for 24-h. Heme content and heme oxygenase activity were measured as described in Methods. *$p < 0.05$ vs nontransduced HMEC-1 cells. Values expressed as means ± SD of three experiments *(43)*.

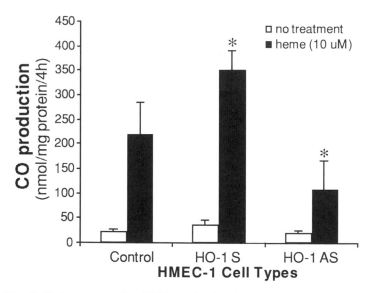

Fig. 2. Carbon monoxide (CO) production in HMEC-1 cells nontransduced or transduced with HO-1 S (LSN-HOP-HO-1) or HO-1 AS (LSN-HOP-HO-1-AS). Measurement of CO production is described in **Subheading 3**. CO production is expressed as means ± SD of four experiments. *$p < 0.05$ vs control HMEC-1 cells *(43)*.

is the sole enzyme involved in physiologic heme degradation and generation of CO, we measured the levels of CO in HMEC-1 endothelial cells transduced with human HO-1 S and HO-1 AS. CO production in cells transduced with HO-1 S and AS after exposure to heme was 350 ± 39 and 109 ± 58 nmol/mg protein/4 h, respectively, as compared to the control HMEC-1 cells ($220 \pm$ 64 nmol/mg protein/4 h) (**Fig. 2**). The levels of CO generated in cells transduced with HO-1 S and AS were significantly different ($p < 0.05$). These results conform with the decrease in heme degradation observed following HO-1 AS gene delivery.

3.2. Methods for HO-1 and HO-2 Protein Measurements by Western Blot Analysis

Cells are incubated with stimulants in T75 flasks for 24 h, washed with PBS, and trypsinized (0.05% trypsin w/v with 0.02% EDTA). The pellets are lysed in buffer (Tris-Cl 50 m*M*, EDTA 10 m*M*, Triton X-100 1% v/v, PMSF 1%, pepstatin A, 0.05 m*M*, and leupeptin 0.2 m*M*), and after mixing with sample loading buffer (Tris-Cl 50 m*M*, SDS 10% w/v, glycerol 10% v/v, 2-mercaptoethanol 10% v/v, and bromophenol blue 0.04%) in a ratio 4:1, are boiled for 5 min. Samples (10 µg protein) are loaded onto 12% gels and subjected to electrophoresis (150 V, 80 min). The separated proteins are electrotransferred to nitrocellulose membranes (Bio-Rad, Hercules, CA; 1 h, 200 mA per gel). After transfer, the blots are incubated overnight with 5% nonfat milk in TTBS) followed by incubation with 1:1000 dilution of the primary antibody for 3 h. After washing with TTBS, the blots are incubated for 2 h with secondary antibody (1:5000) conjugated to alkaline phosphatase. Finally, the blots are developed using a premixed solution containing 0.56 m*M* 5-bromo-4-chloro-3-indolyl phosphate (BCIP) and 0.48 m*M* nitro blue tetrazolium (NBT) in buffer (Tris-HCl 10 m*M*, NaCl 100 m*M*, $MgCl_2$ 59.3 µ*M*, pH 9.5). The blots are scanned, and the optical density of the bands is measured using Scion Image software (Scion Corp., New York, NY).

3.3. Examples of Measurements of HO-1 /-2 in Human Cells Overexpressing HO-1

We used retroviral vector to deliver human HO-1 gene to infect endothelial cells, and measured the effect of gene transfer on CO production and HO-1/HO-2 proteins expression (Quan et al., 2001). Experiments were carried out to examine the effect of delivery of HO-1 under the control of the human HO-1 promoter. We selected a +19 to –1500 human HO-1 promoter in which heme response elements are present *(44)*. Cells transduced with control vector (LSN-HOP) and cells transduced with HO-1 promoter-driven HO-1 gene (S and AS) were examined by Western blot analysis. The results of three representative experiments are shown in **Figs. 3** and **4**. Western blot analysis revealed that the HO-1 protein expression was increased by 14.2-fold in HMEC-1 cells transduced with HOP-driven HO-1-S as compared to control HMEC-1 cells. The addition of heme (10 µ*M*, 24 h) further increased HO-1 expression by twofold.

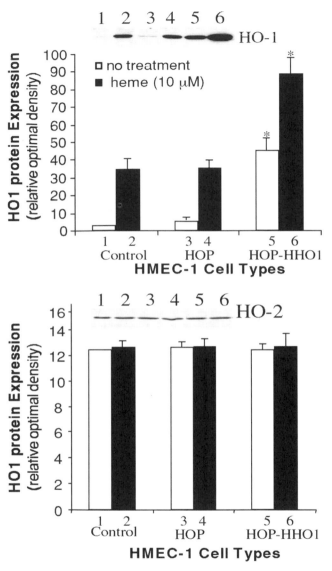

Fig. 3. Western blot analysis of HMEC-1 cells nontransduced or transduced with retroviral vector LSN-HOP (HOP) or LSN-HOP-HO-1 (HOP-HO-1). Some cells were treated with heme (10 μ*M*) for 24 h. The HO-1 protein expression in nontreated or heme-treated HO-1-transduced cells (HOP-HO-1) was increased by 14.2-fold and 2.6-fold, respectively, compared with their corresponding control HMEC-1 cells (*$p < 0.05$). However, there was no significant difference in HO-1 protein expression among three groups of HMEC-1 cells *(43)*.

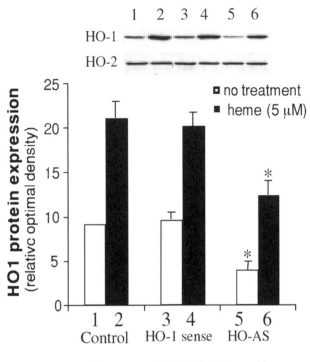

Fig. 4. Western blot analysis of HMEC-1 cells nontransduced or transduced with retroviral vector LSN-HOP (HOP) or LSN-HOP-HO-1-AS (HOP-HO-AS). HOP, human HO-1 promoter. Some cells were treated with heme (5 μM) for 24 h. The HO-1 protein expression in nontreated or heme-treated HO-1-AS transduced cells (HOP-HO-1-AS) was decreased by 55% and 45%, respectively, as compared to their corresponding control cells *(43)*.

As shown in **Fig. 4**, HO-1 AS substantially inhibited HO-1 protein expression in both heme-induced and non-induced cells. Addition of heme (5 μM/24 h) increased the levels of HO-1 protein by twofold in both the nontransduced cells and the cells transduced with control retroviral vector (LSN-HOP; empty vector). In contrast, endothelial cells transduced with retrovirus-mediated HO-1 anti-sense displayed diminished levels of HO-1 protein by 55% and 45% in both nontreated cells and in cells treated with heme for 24 h, respectively. There were no changes in HO-2 protein levels in nontransduced cells or cells transduced with retroviral mediated HO-1 S and AS. These data demonstrate the applicability of methods for western blot analysis, CO measurements, and HO activity in small samples of cells or tissues.

4. Notes

1. The precision and accuracy of this method was tested by measuring a 0.5-μM CO sample 4–6× in 2 d. In each case the measured value was calculated to be 0.50 ± 0.02 μM, which indicates a ±4% variation. (The 0.5-μM CO sample is prepared by adding 0.5 μL saturated CO to 1 mL water in a vial of 2-mL capacity.)

2. 1.0 μM CO solution can be easily made by adding 1 μL saturated CO water solution to 1 mL water. The same type of vial with a 2-mL capacity is used. Injection of 100 μL top space gas resulted in a peak (ion 28) with a signal-to-noise ratio of approx 50/L. This indicates that a CO sample with a concentration of 100 nM may have a peak with a signal-to-noise ratio of 5/1. In actual measurement, a CO sample of 40 nm concentration can get a peak of 2/1 signal-to-noise ratio. It represents the absolute amount of 4 pmol CO (40 nm × 100 μL).

Acknowledgments

This work was supported by NIH grant RO1 DK56601 and PO1 HL34300 and by AHA 50948T and Westchester Artificial Kidney Center, Inc.

References

1. Abraham, N. G., Drummond, G. S., Lutton, J. D., and Kappas, A. (1996) The biological significance and physiological role of heme oxygenase. *Cell. Physiol. Biochem.* **6,** 129–168.

2. Eisenstein, R. S., Garcia-Mayol, D., Pettingell, W., and Munro, H. N. (1991) Regulation of ferritin and heme oxygenase synthesis in rat fibroblasts by different forms of iron. *Proc. Natl. Acad. Sci. USA* **88,** 688–692.

3. Maines, M. D. (1988) Heme oxygenase: function, multiplicity, regulatory mechanisms and clinical applications. *FASEB J.* **2,** 2557–2568.

4. McCoubrey, W. K., Jr., Huang, T. J., and Maines, M. D. (1997) Isolation and characterization of a cDNA from the rat brain that encodes hemoprotein heme oxygenase-3. *Eur. J. Biochem.* **247,** 725–732.

5. Shibahara, S., Yoshizawa, M., Suzuki, H., Takeda, K., Meguro, K., and Endo, K. (1993) Functional analysis of cDNAs for two types of human heme oxygenase and evidence for their separate regulation. *J. Biochem. Tokyo* **113,** 214–218.

6. Balla, J., Jacob, H. S., Balla, G., Nath, K., Eaton, J. W., and Vercelloti, J. M. (1993) Endothelial-cell heme uptake from heme proteins: Induction of sensitization and desensitization to oxidant damage. *Proc. Natl. Acad. Sci. USA* **90,** 9285–9289.

7. Deramaudt, B. M., Braunstein, S., Remy, P., Abraham, B. G. (1998) Gene transfer of human heme oxygenase into coronary endothelial cells potentially promotes angiogenesis. *J. Cell. Biochem.* **68,** 121–127.

8. Nath, K. A., Balla, J., Croatt, A. J., and Vercellotti, G. M. (1995) Heme protein-mediated renal injury: a protective role for 21-aminosteroids in vitro and in vivo. *Kidney Int.* **47,** 592–602.

9. Wagener, F. A. D. T. G., da Silva, J.-L., Farley, T., de Witte, T., Kappas, A., and Abraham N. G. (1999) Differential effects of heme oxygenase isoforms on heme

mediation of endothelial intracellular adhesion molecule 1 expression. *J. Pharmacol. Exp. Ther.* **291**, 416–423.

10. Wagener, F. A. D. T. G., Feldman, E., de-Witte, T., and Abraham, N. G. (1997) Heme induces the expression of adhesion molecules ICAM-1, VCAM-1, and E selectin in vascular endothelial cells. *Proc. Soc. Exp. Biol. Med.* **216**, 456–463.

11. Yachie, A., Niida, Y., Wada, T., Igarashi, N., Kaneda, H., Toma, T., et al. (1999) Oxidative stress causes enhanced endothelial cell injury in human heme oxygenase-1 deficiency. *J. Clin. Investig.* **103**, 129–135.

12. Foresti, R., Clark, J. E., Green, C. J., and Motterlini, R. (1997) Thiol compounds interact with nitric oxide in regulating heme oxygenase-1 induction in endothelial cells. Involvement of superoxide and peroxynitrite anions. *J. Biol. Chem.* **272**, 18,411–18,417.

13. Ignarro, L. J., Bush, P. A., Buga, G. M., Wood, K. S., Fukuto, J. M., and Rajfer, J. (1990) Nitric oxide and cyclic GMP formation upon electrical field stimulation cause relaxation of corpus cavernosum smooth muscle. *Biochem. Biophys. Res. Commun.* **170**, 843–850.

14. Durante, W., Kroll, M. H., Christodoulides, N., Peyton, K. J., and Schafer, A. I. (1997) Nitric oxide induces heme oxygenase-1 gene expression and carbon monoxide production in vascular smooth cells. *Circ. Res.* **80**, 557–564.

15. Coceani, F., Kelsey, L., Seidlitz, E., Marks, G. S., McLaughlin, B. E., Vreman, H. J., et al. (1997) Carbon monoxide formation in the ductus arteriosus in the lamb: implications for the regulation of muscle tone. *Br. J. Pharmacol.* **120**, 599–608.

16. Haider, A., Olszanecki, R., Gryglewski, R., Schwartzman, M. L., Lianos, E., Nasjletti, A., et al. (2001) Regulation of cyclooxygenase by the heme-heme oxygenase system in microvessel endothelial cells. *J. Pharm. Exp. Ther.* **300**, 188–194.

17. Ishizaka, N., De Leon, H., Laursen, J. B., Fukui, T., Wilcox, J. N., De Keulenaer, G., et al. (1994) Angiotensin II-induced hypertension increases heme oxygenase-1 expression in rat aorta. *Circulation* **96**, 1923–1929.

18. Kozma, F., Johnson, R. A., Zhang, F., Yu, C., Tong, X., and Nasjletti, A. (1999) Contribution of endogenous carbon monoxide to regulation of diameter in resistance vessels. *Am. J. Physiol.* **276**, R1087–R1094.

19. Neil, T. K., Abraham, N. G., Levere, R. D., and Kappas, A. (1995) Differential heme oxygenase induction by stannous and stannic ions in the heart. *J. Cell. Biochem.* **57**, 409–414.

20. Sammut, I. A., Foresti, R., Clarck, J. E., Exon, D. J., Vesely, M. J. J., Sarathchandra, P., et al. (1998) Carbon monoxide is a major contributor to the regulation of vascular tone in aortas expressing high levels of haeme oxygenase-1. *Br. J. Pharmacol.* **125**, 1437–1444.

21. Tsao, P. S., Aoki, N., Lefere, D. J., Johnson, G., and Lefer, A. M. (1990) Time course of endothelial dysfunction and myocardial injury during myocardial ischemia and reperfusion in the cat. *Circulation* **82**, 1402–1412.

22. Kadoya, C., Domino, E. F., Yang, G. Y., Stern, J. D., and Betz A. L. (1995) Preischemic but not post ischemic zinc protoporphyrin treatment reduces infarct size and edema post ischemic zinc protoporphyrin treatment reduces infarct size and edema accumulation after temporary focal cerebral ischemia in rats. *Stroke* **26**, 1035–1038.

23. Morita, T. and Kourembanas, S. (1995) Endothelial cell expression of vasoconstrictors and growth factors is regulated by smooth muscle cell-derived carbon monoxide. *J. Clin. Investig.* **96**, 2676–2682.

24. Hibbs, J. B., Westenfelder, C., Taintor, R., Vavrin, Z., Kablitz, C., Babanowski, J. P., et al. (1992) Evidence for cytokine-inducible nitric oxide synthesis from L-arginine in patients, receiving interleukin-2 therapy. *J. Clin. Investig.* **89**, 867–877.

25. Yan, S. D., Chen, X., Fu, J., Chen, M., Zhu, H., Roher, A., et al. (1996) RAGE and amyloid-beta peptide neurotoxicity in Alzheimer's disease. *Nature* **382**, 685–691.

26. Wang, R., Wang, Z., Wu, L., Hanna, S. T., and Peterson-Wakeman, R. (2001) Reduced vasorelaxant effect of carbon monoxide in diabetes and the underlying mechanisms. *Diabetes* **50**, 166–174.

27. Kaide, J.-I., Zhang, F., Yu, C., Abraham, N. G., and Nasjletti, A. (1999) Heme oxygenase (HO)-2-derived carbon monoxide (CO) is an inhibitory regulator of small renal artery reactivity to phenylephrine (PE). *Hypertension* **34**, P151.

28. Zhang, F., Kaide, J.-I., Yu, C., Abraham, N. G., and Nasjletti, A. (1999) Heme oxygenase (HO)-2-derived carbon monoxide (CO) inhibits myogenic responses in rat gracilis muscle arterioles (GA). *Hypertension* **34**, P152.

29. Minamino, T., Christou, H., Hsieh, C. M., Liu, Y., Dhawan, V., Abraham, N. G., et al. (2001) Targeted expression of heme oxygenase-1 prevents the pulmonary inflammatory and vascular responses to hypoxia. *Proc. Natl. Acad. Sci. USA* **98**, 8798–8803.

30. Willis, D., Moore, A. R., Frederick, R., and Willoughby, D. A. (1996) Heme oxygenase: a novel target for the modulation of the inflammatory response. *Nat. Med.* **2**, 87–90.

31. Laniado-Schwartzman, M., Abraham, N. G., Conners, M., Dunn, M. W., Levere, R. D., and Kappas, A. (1997) Heme oxygenase induction with attenuation of experimentally induced corneal inflammation. *Biochem. Pharmacol.* **53**, 1069–1075.

32. Amersi, F., Buelow, R., Kato, H., Ke, B., Coito, A. J., Shen, X. D., et al. (1999) Upregulation of heme oxygenase-1 protects genetically fat Zucker rat livers from ischemia/reperfusion injury. *J. Clin. Investig.* **104**, 1631–1639.

33. Hancock, W. W., Buelow, R., Sayegh, M. H., and Turka, L. A. (1998) Antibody-induced transplant arteriosclerosis is prevented by graft expression of anti-oxidant and anti-apoptotic genes. *Nat. Med.* **4**, 1392–1396.

34. Soares, M. P., Lin, Y., Anrather, J., Csizmadia, E., Takigami, K., Sato, K., et al. (1998) Expression of heme oxygenase-1 (HO-1) can determine cardiac xenograft survival. *Nat. Med.* **4**, 1073–1077.

35. Sato, K., Balla, J., Otterbein, L., Smith, R. N., Brouard, S., Lin, Y., et al. (2001) Carbon monoxide generated by heme oxygenase-1 suppresses the rejection of mouse-to-rat cardiac transplants. *J. Immunol.* **166**, 4185–4194.

36. Abraham, N. G., Lavrovsky, Y., Schwartzman, M. L., Stoltz, R. A., Levere, R. D., Gerritsen, M. E., et al. (1995) Transfection of the human heme oxygenase gene into rabbit coronary microvessel endothelial cells: protective effect against heme and hemoglobin toxicity. *Proc. Natl. Acad. Sci. USA* **92,** 6798–6802.

37. Sabaawy, H. E., Zhang, F., Nguyen, X., Elhosseiny, A., Nasjletti, A., Schwartzman, M., et al. (2001) Human heme oxygenase-1 gene transfer lowers blood pressure and promotes growth in spontaneously hypertensive rats. *Hypertension* **38,** 210–215.

38. Brouard, S., Otterbein, L. E., Anrather, J., Tobiasch, E., Bach, F. H., Choi, A. M., et al. (2000) Carbon monoxide generated by heme oxygenase 1 suppresses endothelial cell apoptosis. *J. Exp. Med.* **192,** 1015–1026.

39. Otterbein, L. E., Bach, F. H., Alam, J., Soares, M., Tao, L. H., Wysk, M., et al. (2000) Carbon monoxide has anti-inflammatory effects involving the mitogen-activated protein kinase pathway. *Nat. Med.* **6,** 422–428.

40. Wiseman, H. and Halliwell, B. (1996) Damage to DNA by reactive oxygen and nitrogen species: role in inflammatory disease and progression to cancer. *Biochem. J.* **313,** 17–29.

41. Clark, J. E., Foresti, R., Sarathchandra, P., Kaur, H., Green, C. J., Motterlini, R. (2000) Heme oxygenase-1-derived bilirubin ameliorates postischemic myocardial dysfunction. *Am. J. Physiol. Heart Circ. Physiol.* **278,** H643–H651.

42. Foresti, R., Sarathchandra, P., Clark, J. E., Green, C. J., and Motterlini, R. (1999) Peroxynitrite induces haem oxygenase-1 in vascular endothelia to apoptosis. *Biochem. J.* **339,** 729–736.

43. Quan, S., Yang, L., Abraham, N. G., and Kappas, A. (2001) Regulation of human heme oxygenase in endothelial cells by using sense and antisense retroviral constructs. *Proc. Natl. Acad. Sci. USA* **98,** 12,203–12,208.

44. Lavrovsky, Y., Schwartzman, M. L., Levere, R. D., Kappas, A., and Abraham, N. G. (1994) Identification of binding sites for transcription factors NF-kappa B and AP-2 in the promoter region of the human heme oxygenase 1 gene. *Proc. Natl. Acad. Sci. USA* **91,** 5987–5991.

28

The Juxtamedullary Nephron Preparation

Daniel Casellas and Leon C. Moore

1. Introduction

1.1. Why and How to Directly Study the Renal Microcirculation

Major aspects of renal function such as glomerular filtration, blood flow autoregulation, tubular reabsorption, and medullary concentrating ability rely on an exquisite paracrine-autocrine control of renal microvascular resistances, and on the coordinated network behavior of the vasculature (*1,2*). However, vascular and microvascular networks of mammalian kidneys are mostly inaccessible to microscopic observation, which greatly limits the direct study of renal microcirculation. There have been ongoing efforts to overcome this technical difficulty. In the seventies, glomerular microcirculation was observed in adult renal tissue grafted into a chamber in the rabbit ear (*3*), and in neonatal renal tissue grafted into a chamber in the hamster cheek pouch (*4,5*). At the same time, micropuncture techniques were applied to the Munich-Wistar rat, which is endowed with surface glomeruli. This greatly increased our knowledge of single-nephron dynamics and filtration (*6,7*). By the mid-eighties, three additional techniques were implemented for real-time microscopic evaluation of single renal arteriolar dynamics (*8*). Steinhausen et al. (*9*) took advantage of the tubular destruction provoked by hydronephrosis to visualize all segments of the renal microvasculature. Using an adaptation of the tubular microperfusion techniques (*10*), Edwards (*11*) and Osgood et al. (*6*) perfused single glomerular arterioles of rabbits and dogs in vitro. Peti-Peterdi (Chapter 8) and Pallone (Chapter 30) present further refinements of this elegant technique elsewhere in this book.

In 1984, Casellas and Navar (*12*) described the "in vitro blood-perfused juxtamedullary nephron preparation" (designated here as the juxtamedullary nephron preparation; JMN preparation). This approach is based on the unique anatomy of the inside surface of the renal cortex. Although it requires extensive

From: *Methods in Molecular Medicine, vol. 86: Renal Disease: Techniques and Protocols*
Edited by: M. S. Goligorsky © Humana Press Inc., Totowa, NJ

surgery and dissection, it does not involve tissue grafting, chronic pathology, or the complete isolation of a single, viable microvessel. The JMN technique gives direct microscopic access to the tubules and the complete vasculature of a population of JMNs. Many articles from several groups are based on the JMN preparation, and its validity as a method for assessing single arteriolar reactivity and glomerular autoregulation in the rat has been firmly established. **Ref. *1*** lists a number of studies conducted in the JMN preparation.

1.2. Anatomic Basis of the JMN Preparation

Figure 1 illustrates the tubular-vascular anatomy of the inside cortical surface that lines the pelvic cavity, after removal of the pelvic mucosa, connective tissue, and large arcuate veins. In this area, vessels and tubules, including the macula densa segment, are superficial (**Fig. 1**). Most nephrons, although located at the surface, are anatomically similar to other JMNs *(13)*. These nephrons are fully developed at birth *(14)*, they possess long loops of Henle, and their efferent arterioles break into vasa recta *(12)*. Therefore, normal renal development generates a population of "superficial" JMNs in which vessels lay on top of an essentially two-dimensional (2D) tubular topology. This anatomy contrasts with that of most cortical nephrons, in which proximal and distal tubular loops adopt a compact three-dimensional (3D) arrangement around the glomerulus *(16)*. The anatomy of the inside cortical surface illustrated in **Fig. 1** is not unique to rodents, as it is also present in the human kidney (Casellas and Moore, unpublished observations).

Implementation of the JMN preparation therefore requires a dissection procedure that permits an *en face* microscopic view of the inside cortical surface. At the same time, tubular and vascular function is maintained by perfusion of a blood substitute. This chapter describes the materials, methods, and technical tips currently used in our laboratory; other useful information can be found in a recent account of the JMN preparation from a different laboratory *(15)*.

2. Materials

2.1. Solutions

1. Modified Krebs-bicarbonate-Ringer (KBR): 105.1 mM NaCl, 16 mM Na acetate, 0.6 mM Na$_2$HPO$_4$, 1.19 mM MgSO$_4$, 4.84 mM KCl, 2.22 mM CaCl$_2$, 5.55 mM glucose, 4.99 mM urea, 24.99 mM NaHCO$_3$, 0.13 mM NaH$_2$PO$_4$, and 5 mM N,2-hydroxyethylpiperazine-N',2-ethanesulfonic acid (HEPES); pH adjusted to 7.4. HEPES was found to greatly stabilize pH of KBR. A mixture of L-amino acids is prepared separately, and added to KBR to yield the following concentrations: 0.33 mM methionine, 0.3 mM isoleucine, 2 mM alanine, 2.3 mM glycine, 0.5 mM arginine, 0.31 mM proline, 0.2 mM aspartate, 0.5 mM glutamate, 1 mM serine. All compounds are from Sigma.

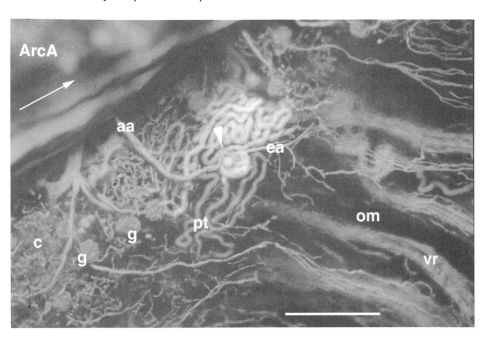

Fig. 1. Microscopic view of the tubular-vascular anatomy of the inside cortical surface of the rat kidney. The vasculature was partially filled with red silicone rubber (Microfil, Flow Tech Inc., Carver, MA, www.flowtech-inc.com/), and a single tubule was filled from the proximal to the connecting tubule with yellow silicone rubber using a micropipet inserted into Bowman's capsule, as described previously *(12)*. c, cortex; om, outer medulla; vr, vasa recta; ArcA, arcuate artery; Arrow, direction of blood flow; aa, afferent arteriole; ea, efferent arteriole; g, glomeruli; pt, proximal tubule; arrowhead, macula densa; Bar: 500 μm.

2. Fraction V bovine serum albumin (BSA, Sigma, Ref. A-4503); dissolved in distilled water (no stirring to avoid foam), dialyzed overnight (4°C) against a large volume of distilled water, using dialysis tubing with a molecular cut-off of 12–14,000 (Spectra/Por 2, Ref. P02900-20, Cole-Parmer Instrument Company, Vernon Hills, IL (www.coleparmer.com). Albuminated KBR is prefiltered by gravity (to avoid foam) on glass microfiber filters (GF/D, 2.7 μm exclusion, ref. 1823 090; Wathman Inc., Clifton NJ), and is further filtered to either 0.7 μm exclusion (GF/F, ref. 1825 090, Wathman Inc.) for superfusate, or to 0.22 μm exclusion (Millex-GS syringe filter, Millipore Corporation, Bedford, MA) for perfusates. Albuminated KBR can be kept for 1–2 days at 4°C.
3. Superfusate: filtered KBR (no amino acids) containing 1% dialyzed BSA.
4. Dissection perfusate: filtered KBR with amino acids and 4% dialyzed BSA.
5. Blood perfusate: filtered KBR with amino acids, and 6% dialyzed BSA. Washed erythrocytes added to a hematocrit of ~ 30%, (*see* **Subheading 3.1.**).

6. Anesthetic: sodium pentobarbital.
7. Heparin: 5000 UI / mL.
8. Lidocain (xylocaine 2%, Astra).
9. Agar (Sigma) 5% warm aqueous solution (*see* **Subheading 3.3., step 3**).
10. Phenol (Sigma) 10% solution in absolute ethanol (*see* **Subheading 3.2., step 2**).

2.2. Dissection and Blood Collection

1. Dissection stereomicroscope on boom stand.
2. Fiberoptic illumination (*see* **Note 2**).
3. Tracheal cannula.
4. Blood collection line, jugular line.
5. Adson tissue forceps with opposed teeth (Ref. 11027-12, Fine Science Tools Inc., Foster City, CA, http://www.finescience.com/).
6. Curved eye-dressing forceps (Ref. 11051-10, FST).
7. Large surgical scissors.
8. 4-0 and 6-0 surgical silk (Ethicon Inc., Somerville, NJ).
9. Bulldog clamps.
10. Castroviejo scissors, curved and blunt tips for fine dissection (Ref 9921, Moria, Paris, France, E-mail: clientel@worldnet.fr).
11. Moria extra fine spring scissors, curved (Ref. 9601, Moria). Has extremely fine tips, should be used exclusively during the finest dissection steps.
12. Dumont no. 5 forceps straight and 45° tips (Ref. 11253-20, 11253-25, FST) (*see* **Note 1**).
13. Micro needle holder Castroviejo (Ref. 12060-02, FST).
14. Microsutures, 25 μm (10-0) and 35 μm (9-0) nylon monofilament (Ethicon).
15. Customized needle guide for 35-μm nylon monofilament (*see* **Note 3**).
16. Wicks: 4 × 12-mm strips of Kimwipes, strips of surgical gauze (*see* **Note 4**).
17. External filter tips, 45-μm exclusion, (Ref. FT 2002, Centaur West).
18. Acid-washed glass microbeads (150–212 μm, Ref. G-1145, Sigma) (*see* **Note 5**).
19. Stainless steel insect pins 000 cut to 15 mm (Ref. 26001-25, FST).
20. 22–18-gauge stainless-steel tubing (Small Parts Inc., Miami, FL).
21. A 50-mm bottom of a glass Petri dish with a 4-mm layer of silicone rubber (ref. Sylg 184, World Precision Instruments, Saratosa, FL, http://www.wpiinc.com/).
22. Silicone rubber tubings of various diameters with thick or thin walls (e.g., Silastic tubing, Dow Corning Corporation, Midland, MI), C-Flex tubing (Cole-Parmer Instrument Company), Tygon tubing (Cole-Parmer).
23. Razor blades (Gillette type).
24. Refrigerated centrifuge with low speed (≈2500*g*).

2.3. Dissection and Perfusion-Superfusion Setup

1. The dissection chamber is a rectangle of polycarbonate sheet (Small Parts Inc.; 19 × 14 × 0.7 cm), in the middle of which the top of a glass Petri dish is glued upside down. The bottom of the dish is covered with Sylgard. Two miniature Prior micromanipulators (Ref. 55122, Stoelting) are fixed on opposite sides of

the Petri dish and hold the perfusion line, and a siphon (PE 250 polyethylene catheter) connected to the vacuum line. A fiberoptic light probe provides separate lighting (*see* **Note 2**).

2. The perfusion vial provides 4% albuminated KBR during the entire dissection/microdissection period. It consists of a large glass vial (250 mL of perfusate); head pressure is obtained by compressing air with a 50-mL syringe connected to a 3-way stopcock; a bubble trap (glass scintillation vial), and a 0.45-μm filter are placed along the perfusate line. Perfusate flow is controlled with a fine screw clamp.

3. The blood-perfusion vial permits oxygenation of reconstituted blood. It filters and provides pressure-controlled blood perfusate, and allows refill of blood perfusate. It is a wide-mouth borosilicate glass vial with rubber-lined screw caps (40-mL vial Ref. P-08918-24, Cole-Parmer). Three 5-mm holes are drilled through cap and gasket. Thick-wall Silastic tubing (Dow Corning) are threaded through the holes, and 18-gauge stainless-steel tubings are forced through the Silastic tubing to provide pressure-proof seals. The tubing of the perfusion line goes to the bottom of the vial and is fitted to a 45-μm filter tip. The compressed gas line stops near the top of the vial, as does the tube for blood refill. We do not stir the blood, as even low-speed stirring with a stir bar may induce hemolysis. Instead, the vial is shaken by hand from time to time to avoid erythrocyte sedimentation.

4. Superfusion vial(s) are similar to the perfusion vial (*see* **step 2**). Head pressure is provided by a tank of compressed gas. Depending on the experimental protocol, one or several superfusion vials are connected to the same head pressure, and are connected to the superfusion cannula via miniature manifolds (Small Parts, Inc.) allowing rapid switching from one superfusate to another.

5. The perfusion cannula is illustrated in **Fig. 2**.

6. The superfusion cannula is illustrated in **Fig. 3**.

7. The perfusion chamber is illustrated in **Fig. 4**.

8. Two cylinders of compressed gas, (97% O_2 / 3% CO_2) with two-stage regulators, are used to separately drive superfusate and perfusion blood. Pressure lines are connected to in-line gas filters (Wathman), pressure gauges (0–300 mmHg), and to leak-valves for easy changes of the pressure head.

9. Vacuum line.

10. Low-compliance pressure transducer (e.g., Model P50, Gould Inc., Oxnard, CA) and recorder. The water-filled transducer is connected to the saline-filled pressure line of the perfusion cannula.

2.4. Microscopy and Video Microscopy

1. Upright microscope with fixed stage (Laborlux D-FS, Leitz), trinocular microscope head with erect image, and camera c-mount adaptor. Two dry objectives are used, a 4× (EF 4/0.12, 25 mm working distance, Leitz) for wide-field observation, and a 25× (NPL Fluotar L25/0.35, Leitz) for fine observation. Its 18-mm working distance provides adequate clearance for papilla, superfusion cannula, micropipets, and avoids condensation on the front lens.

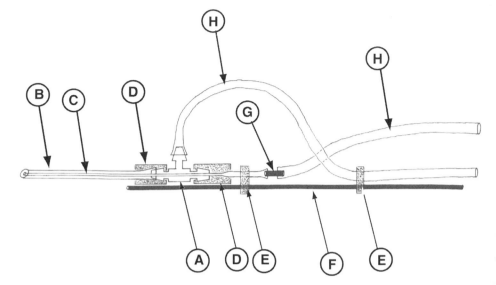

Fig. 2. The perfusion cannula provides blood perfusate, and allows continuous monitoring of blood-perfusion pressure from the tip of the cannula. (**A**) miniature barbed polypropylene "Tee" fitting (Cole-Parmer, Ref # 6365-90). (**B**) pulled-out polyethylene catheter, overall tip length is ~35 mm, tip outer diameter is ~1 mm. (**C**) pressure line is a pulled-out polyethylene catheter; it goes all the way to the tip of the perfusion line (**B**). (**D**) seals are provided by two 7-mm-long pieces of Silastic tubing (Cole-Parmer, Ref. #6411-62). (**E**) Silastic holders. (**F**) 10-cm-long 18-gauge post (Small Parts Inc.). (**G**) 18 gauge connector. (**H**) Tygon tubing.

2. Black-and-white CCD camera (4710 series CCIR, Cohu Inc., San Diego, CA). Removing the front infrared filter substantially increases light sensitivity.
3. ARGUS 10-image processor (Hamamatsu Photonic Systems, Bridgewater, NJ). This is used for on-line image processing, including background substraction (e.g., eliminates the strong light gradient caused by lateral illumination), contrast enhancement, and frame averaging. It generates a 1/100 s lock display on every frame, and permits on-line or off-line measurements (length, perimeter, surface area).
4. Video recorder: experimental details are recorded on the sound track.
5. Video printer.
6. Video monitor.
7. Stage micrometer (for length-calibration routine).

3. Methods

3.1. Blood Collection, Preparation of Blood Perfusate

1. Two aged male rats (weighing 400–600 g) are used as blood donors. Under pentobarbital anesthesia (50 mg/kg iv), both kidneys are removed (to limit renin secre-

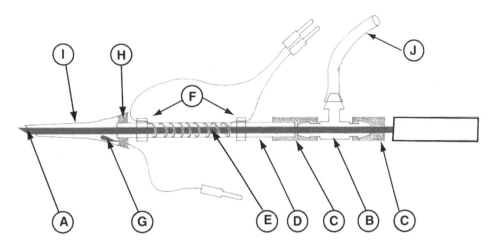

Fig. 3. Superfusion cannula. (**A**) the cannula is built around a 0.8-mm-diameter straight light probe, beveled and polished, and connected to the light source via a fiberoptic cable (*see* **Note 2**). (**B**) miniature "Tee" fitting (*see* **Fig. 2**). (**C**) Silastic seals (*see* **Fig. 2**). (**D**) superfusate heating unit is a piece (0.2-cm-diameter, 5.5-cm-long, fire-polished ends) of wiretrol 100-µL hematocrit tube (Drummond Scientific Company, Broomall, PA). (**E**) 22 cm of tungsten wire (Magnetic Wire Inc., 25 Wahler St., New York, NY; wire size 32, electrical resistance 10 Ω/foot). Tungsten spiral with non-touching loops is fixed on the glass tube with 5-min epoxy glue. (**F**) wire free extremities maintained with Tygon tubing, and soldered to male gold clips. Tungsten wire is heated by 12 V D.C. source via a temperature controller (Cell Microcontrols, Norfolk, VA, www.cellmc.com). (**G**) miniature temperature probe (TH-1 thermistor probe; Ref. #331-9623, (Cell Microcontrols, Norfolk, VA, www.cellmc.com) threaded through a 2-mm-thick silastic seal (**H**). The temperature probe provides temperature monitoring and feedback via a YSI-43T series Telethermometer (YSI Precision Temperature Group, Dayton, OH). (**I**) cannula tip made with a pulled disposable polyethylene pipet tip (15 mm in length). Cannula tip is sealed to the glass tubing (**D**) with a piece of silastic tubing (**H**, Cole-Parmer, Ref. #6411-62). (**J**) superfusate input, Silastic tubing (Cole-Parmer, Ref. #406411-60).

tion) through an abdominal incision. Left carotid arteries and right jugular veins are cannulated, the animals are heparinized, and blood is gently aspirated through the carotid line until exsanguination. The typical yield is 30–35 mL of blood.

2. Blood is centrifuged at low speed ($\approx 2500g$), plasma and white cells are discarded and packed erythrocytes are resuspended in 6% albuminated KBR containing amino acids. The red-blood-cell suspension is centrifuged again and the supernatant is discarded. This operation is repeated 2–3×. Before the last centrifugation, the red-blood-cell suspension is passed through a glass bead filter (*see* **Note 5**).

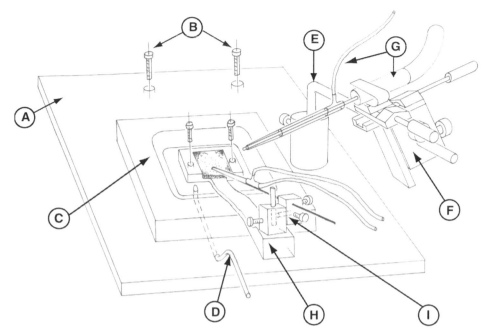

Fig. 4. Perfusion chamber. (**A**) rectangular sheet of polycarbonate (Small Parts Inc.; 22 × 19 × 0.6 cm). (**B**) Mounting to the x-y movement of the microscope stage. (**C**) 5 × 5-cm central well made of three superposed layers of 4-mm-thick polycarbonate. (**D**) aspiration line opening at the bottom of the well. (**E**): L-shaped metallic post fixed with screw clamp on an aluminum stub (2-cm diameter, 3 cm high). It holds a miniature Prior manipulator (**F**), and allows broad swinging movements. (**G**) Superfusion line; it can be moved with 6 degrees of freedom. The heating wire and temperature probe are not represented for clarity (*see* **Fig. 3**). (**H**) Preparation holder made of polycarbonate is attached with nylon screws to the bottom of the well. The "spoon" part has a layer of Sylgard (dotted area) to allow pinning of kidney preparations. The "tail" part holds the perfusion cannula via a micropositioner (**I**; 5 degrees of freedom) made with two blocks of polycarbonate, two metallic posts and three nylon screws.

Packed erythrocytes are resuspended in 6% albuminated KBR containing amino acids. Hematocrit is adjusted to ~30% as an optimal trade-off between oxygen transport capacity and viscosity.

3. Reconstituted blood is kept in the refrigerator and shaken regularly until its introduction into the blood-perfusion vial. Blood is prepared fresh for every experiment and should keep a bright red color. If blood leaks are appropriately controlled in the JMN preparation (*see* **Subheading 3.2.**, **step 5**), 30–35 mL of blood perfusate will allow a 3.5–4 h perfusion.

3.2. Kidney Perfusion and Isolation

1. A third male rat (same strain as blood donors) is used as kidney donor and is anesthetized. Young animals are preferable, as they have less fat and interstitial connective tissue. A tracheal and jugular cannula are inserted, laparotomy is performed (from sternum to bladder), and the right kidney is removed after ligating its vascular pedicle (to limit renin secretion).

2. The colon is cut distally between two ligatures (4-0 silk) near the bladder. The entire intestine, stomach, and spleen are covered with saline-soaked gauze and reflected on the right side of the animal. The left adrenal vein is cut near the renal vein between two ligatures (6-0 silk), and the left renal artery is carefully separated from its vein. The left kidney is denervated by brushing the renal artery with a cotton swab soaked in phenol solution. Denervation prevents renal vascular spasms.

3. A loose ligature (4-0 silk) is placed around the aorta between the renal arteries, a second is placed downstream close to the iliac bifurcation, a third ligature 2–3 cm downstream from the left renal artery, and a fourth around the left renal vein close to the vena cava.

4. Fifteen minutes after denervation, the animal is heparinized, the aorta is clamped immediately downstream from the left renal artery, and the iliac ligature is tightened. The perfusion cannula with free-flowing perfusate (1 mL/min, room temperature) is introduced retrogradely into the aorta via an incision made near the iliac ligature (*see* **Note 6**). The perfusion line is secured by gently tightening the ligature downstream from the renal artery, and pushed toward the left renal artery. The aortic clamp is removed, perfusate flow is rapidly increased to 3–4 mL/min, and the aortic ligature between renal arteries is tightened. Rapid and homogeneous blanching of the kidney surface indicates appropriate perfusion. Kidneys showing patchy perfusion are discarded. The ligature around the renal vein is tightened, and the vein is vented to allow free escape of the blood/perfusate mixture. Fluid flow to the kidney is never interrupted during the entire procedure, as vascular collapse may damage the endothelium (*17*).

5. The renal artery is exposed up to its entrance into the kidney by removing the renal vein, connective tissue, and adipose tissues. The ureter is sectioned. The left adrenal artery, which branches from the renal artery, is cut between tightened ligatures (6-0 silk). The tip of the perfusion cannula is advanced until it reaches the main bifurcation of the renal artery and is secured with a gently tightened ligature (6-0 silk). This avoids perfusate leaks through aortic branches. The main branch of the renal artery supplying the ventral half-kidney is ligated (35-μm suture) to limit perfusate leaks during subsequent dissection steps. The kidney is decapsulated, freed from attachments, and removed from the abdominal cavity.

6. As shown in **Fig. 5A**, the ventral half-kidney is resected with a razor blade in a para-sagittal plane so that the papilla is left attached to the remaining dorsal half-kidney. Two incisions are made along the lateral fornices with Castroviejo scissors (to facilitate tilting of the papilla), and renal tissue is excised laterally with a razor blade. The final preparation (**Fig. 5B**) corresponds to 20–30% of the initial total kidney mass. The entire dissection procedure is done at room temperature.

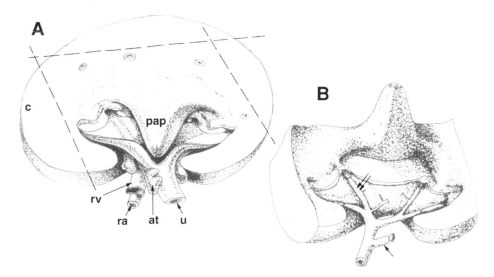

Fig. 5. Kidney dissection. Perfusion cannula is not represented for clarity. (**A**) Appearance of the kidney after removing its ventral half with a razor blade; papilla (pap) is left *in situ*. c, cortex; ra, renal artery; rv, renal vein; at, adipose tissue; u, ureter that continues into pelvic mucosa. Dotted lines: lines of resection of excess renal tissue. (**B**) Appearance of the preparation after removal of pelvic mucosa, opening of major veins, and ligating major arcuate arteries downstream. Insect pins are not represented. Arrow: first branch of the renal artery feeding the ventral half-kidney. The most frequent arterial pattern is represented here. Only the arcuate artery indicated by a double arrow is used for an experiment, and others are ligated to limit blood losses.

7. The renal preparation, attached to the perfusion cannula, is transferred to the Petri dish. It is fixed to the layer of Sylgard with insect pins, and the papilla is reflected upwards and fixed in position with insect pins. The Petri dish is transferred to the dissection chamber, and the siphon is set up to keep the preparation slightly bathed with perfusate. The papilla tip is kept moist with a wick folded over it. The perfusion line is secured to its manipulator, avoiding traction on vessels, and the surface of the preparation is illuminated laterally with a light probe (*see* **Note 2**).

3.3. Kidney Dissection and Exposure of the Inside Cortical Surface

1. The pelvic mucosa, which exhibits slow regular peristaltic activity, is resected back to the point of insertion into the renal cortex. The major arcuate veins are cut open, revealing the underlying arcuate arteries. Using the microsuture guide (*see* **Note 3**) arcuate arteries are closed distally with tight ligatures (35 μm). This step increases intravascular pressure, and perfusate flow must be readjusted to avoid ballooning or spasming of the vasculature.

2. Using fine Moria scissors and no. 5 forceps, the interstitial tissue that covers the inside cortical surface is carefully removed (*see* **Note 7**). Usually, a single arcuate artery (**Fig. 5B**, double arrow) is connected to enough arteries and arterioles to perform an experiment. The remaining arcuate arteries may then be ligated, reducing total flow to the preparation.

3. The preparation is unpinned from the Petri dish and transferred to the perfusion chamber, and is pinned to the Sylgard layer of the preparation holder (**Fig. 4**), papilla facing up. The perfusion line is adjusted on its micromanipulator to avoid traction on the vessels. Liquid agar is delivered around the preparation with 2-mL syringe/18-gauge needle, and a wick is folded on the papilla tip. The superfusion cannula is installed until it slightly touches the surface of the preparation at a low angle. Wicks are positioned around the observation field to establish a high-capillarity pathway to the aspiration line (*see* **Note 4**), and the vacuum is switched on. Superfusate flow rate is adjusted to maintain a thin layer of liquid on the preparation and to establish a stable meniscus around the tip of the superfusion cannula.

4. The perfusion is switched from cell-free media to blood substitute at low pressure (30–40 mmHg). The filling of the vasculature with blood perfusate is observed under the dissecting microscope. Blood leaks become rapidly visible. They must be corrected by vascular ligations or by adjusting the wicks. Concealed vascular leaks must be suspected when the blood perfusion pressure (at the tip of perfusion cannula) does not parallel changes imposed to the head pressure of the blood perfusion vial via the gas tank. Blood leaks must be found and corrected, or the preparation must be discarded.

5. The perfusion chamber is mounted with screws on the microscope x-y stage. Fine adjustments of the wicks and the light are performed using a 4× objective. Superfusate heating is turned on, and temperature control is set at 37°C. Blood-perfusion pressure is set at 80–100 mmHg, and preparation is left for stabilization for 15–30 min. During that time, a complete map of the available vasculature is made.

3.4. Videomicroscopy and Assessment of Autoregulatory Vascular Responses

1. Using the 25× long working distance objective, lateral fiberoptic illumination allows the observer to optically "cut" through the remaining superficial connective tissue and sharply delineate arteriolar walls by adjusting the focal plane (**Fig. 6**). Blood-perfused preglomerular vessels of the JMN preparation develop spontaneous, calcium-dependent basal tone, and both myogenic responses and tubuloglomerular feedback mechanism are operative at perfusion pressures >60 mmHg *(18)*.

2. Robust autoregulatory vascular responses can be elicited by step changes in blood-perfusion pressure, as illustrated in **Fig. 7**. Spatial organization *(19)* as well as pathologic alterations (e.g., during hypertension; *see* **ref. 20**) of vascular autoregulatory responses have been documented by the JMN preparation.

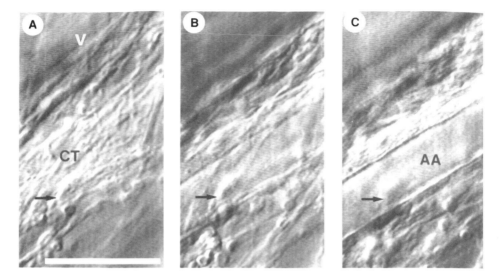

Fig. 6. Blood-perfused JMN preparation. Photos taken from the screen of the video monitor illustrating the optical "cutting" capability of low-angle lateral illumination. Direction of light is vertical from bottom to top. (**A**) focusing on the surface reveals a superficial vein (V) and abundant connective tissue (CT). Arrows point to the same spot on the three pictures. (**B**) Focusing down reveals a better image of the vein margin. (**C**) Focusing down again reveals clearly the margins of an afferent arteriole (AA) running parallel to the vein. Bar: 50 μm.

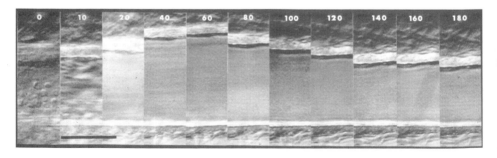

Fig. 7. Typical autoregulatory responses of an arcuate arterial branch of a blood-perfused JMN preparation. Blood-perfusion pressure was varied stepwise from 0 to 180 mmHg (11 steps), and the same vascular segment was photographed after stabilization of its diameter. The composite view is made of 11 pictures, in which one vessel wall was lined up to reveal diameter changes. Individual erythrocytes are visible at zero perfusion pressure (zero flow), and their image is blurred at higher pressures (flows). From 0–60 mmHg, diameter increases with pressure, whereas an active constriction (myogenic response) appears at pressures >60 mmHg. Bar: 50 μm.

4. Notes

1. Microdissection instruments are polished to reduce tissue adhesion. Sharp edges of #5 forceps act as scissors on fine nylon sutures. Furthermore, sharp tips easily puncture renal tissue or vessels during dissection, and both should be blunted and polished. Lapping films with embedded diamond particles ranging from 15–0.1 μm (Electron Microscopy Sciences, Fort Washington, PA, www.emsdiasum.com/) permit coarse abrasion and fine polishing of metallic instruments. Additional practical tips can be found in **ref. *10***.

2. Miniature fiberoptic light guides (Miniprobe set, Ref. P-09742-40, Cole-Parmer). During dissection, the surface of the kidney is illuminated with a straight 1-mm-diameter light probe mounted on a Prior manipulator (Ref. 55023, Stoelting, Wood Dale, IL, www.stoeltingco.com/physio). The JMN preparation itself is illuminated with a 0.8-mm-diameter straight light probe. Its tip is beveled at a 30–40° angle and polished (*see* **Note 1**) to permit low-angle epi-illumination. It is fixed on a miniature Prior micromanipulator (Ref. 55122, Stoelting) attached to the perfusion chamber. Both probes are connected via a flexible fiberoptic cable to a variable-intensity 150W illuminator (Fiber-Lite series 180, Dolan-Jenner Industries, Lawrence, MA). Usually, the lowest illumination intensity is sufficient to properly visualize structures. Green illumination may further help to generate contrast.

3. Microsutures have sharp, soft microneedles that are difficult to guide around arcuate arteries without puncture. To lead a 9-0 nylon monofilament around arteries, a convenient instrument was made from a 5–7-mm piece of 32-gauge hypodermic needle with a blunted and polished tip (*see* **Note 1**). The cut end of the needle is ground on a fine Arkansas stone, polished, and reamed with insect pins. The needle is curved, like a fishing hook, and attached at the flattened end of a length of 22-gauge tubing (Small Parts) with fine copper wire and fixed with a drop of crazy glue. A piece of 35-μm nylon monofilament can now be threaded through the needle and guided around the artery by rotating the instrument's handle.

4. Wicks are placed on the papilla and renal surfaces that are not protected by agar to keep them moist. They are also positioned like overlapping tiles around the field of observation to direct blood leaks away (originating from the zone of insertion of the pelvic mucosa, or from open veins) and to establish a continuous capillary contact between superfusate overflow and aspiration line. At a given aspiration rate, the thickness of the fluid layer on top of the JMN preparation can be finely tuned by adjusting superfusate flow (1–3 mL/min).

5. Glass-bead filters are prepared by pouring 1.5-mL of glass beads into a piece of silicone rubber tubing (5 cm, 6-mm lumen). Both ends are plugged with filter tips held in place with miniature plastic hose clamps (Cole-Parmer). Erythrocytes suspended in albuminated KBR are slowly flushed through the filter to eliminate residual platelets, white blood cells, cell debris and aggregates. A similar filter is also placed upstream along the blood-perfusion line.

6. Great care must be exercised to avoid bubbles in the perfusion line, as even tiny air bubbles may destroy the endothelium. Air bubbles should also be avoided in the superfusion line, as they interfere with microscopic observation.

7. The safest procedure is to pick up superficial collagenous strands, pull them up, and cut them horizontally with the curved microscissors. It is usually better not to peel off all connective tissue as arterioles are easily damaged by simple contact with the tweezers tips, and the low-angle illumination procedure provides the ability to optically cut through connective tissue (*see* **Fig. 6**). Connective tissue also tends to accumulate in the vicinity of the glomerular vascular pole, and Bowman's capsules can be easily damaged, as they bulge at the surface. A trade-off must thus be made between visibility and functional status. The cell-free perfused renal tissue has very low contrast. To obtain optimal visualization of the vessels, tubules, and glomeruli, the light probe is placed below the superfusate layer (to avoid light reflection), and approaches the tissue at a 10–15° angle. The superficial anatomy is explored by rotating the dissection chamber, as only arterioles or tubules that are perpendicular to the light path will show up. If lighting is properly performed, a complete map of the superficial vasculature can be drawn at this stage. Care must be exercised not to cut open superficial veins that usually parallel or partially cover arteries (**Fig. 6**). Similarly, if even a single arteriole is cut, the emerging blood can obscure the entire visual field. Inadvertently cut arterioles should be ligated with 10-0 or 11-0 monofilaments, or covered with a wick.

Acknowledgments

We are grateful to Annie Artuso and Aija Brizgalis for their technical assistance. Image processing was performed by Patrick Schuman (ISIS 24, Montpellier).

References

1. Navar, L. G., Inscho, E. W., Majid, D. S. A., Imig, J. D., Harrison-Bernard, L. M., and Mitchell, K. D. (1996) Paracrine regulation of the renal microcirculation. *Physiol. Rev.* **76,** 425–536.
2. Casellas, D. and Carmines, P. K. (1996) Control of the renal microcirculation: cellular and integrative perspectives. *Curr. Opin. Nephrol. Hypertens.* **5,** 57–63.
3. Hobbs, J. B. and Cliff, W. J. (1971) Observations on tissue grafts established in rabbit ear chambers. *J. Exp. Med.* **134,** 963–985.
4. Oestermeyer, C. F. and Bloch, E. (1977) In vivo microscopy of hamster renal allografts. *Microvasc. Res.* **13,** 153–180.
5. Gilmore, J. P., Cornish, K. G., Rogers, S. D., and Joyner W. L. (1980) Direct evidence for myogenic autoregulation of the renal microcirculation in the hamster. *Circ. Res.* **47,** 226–230.
6. Osgood, R. W., Reineck, H. J., and Stein, J. H. (1982) Methodologic considerations in the study of glomerular ultrafiltration. *Am J. Physiol.* **242,** F1–F7.
7. Arendshorst, W. J. and Gottschalk C. W. (1985) Glomerular ultrafiltration dynamics: historical perspective. *Am. J. Physiol.* **248,** F163–F174.
8. Navar, L. G., Gilmore, J. P., Joyner, W. L., Steinhausen, M., Edwards, R. M., Casellas, D., et al. (1986) Direct assessment of renal microcirculatory dynamics. *Fed. Proc.* **45,** 2851–2861.

9. Steinhausen, M., Snoei, H., Parekh, N., Baker, R., and Johnson, P., C. (1983) Hydronephrosis: A new method to visualize vas afferens, efferens, and glomerular network. *Kidney Int.* **23**, 794–806.

10. Duling, B. R., Gore, R. W., Dacey, R. G. Jr., and Damon, D. N. (1981) Methods for isolation, cannulation, and in vitro study of single microvessels. *Am. J. Physiol.* **241**, H108–H116.

11. Edwards, R. M. (1983) Segmental effects of norepinephrine and angiotensin II on isolated renal microvessels. *Am. J. Physiol.* **244**, F526–F534.

12. Casellas, D. and Navar, L. G. (1984) In vitro perfusion of juxtamedullary nephrons in rats. *Am. J. Physiol.* **246**, F349–F358.

13. Casellas, D. and Taugner, R. (1986) Renin status of the afferent arteriole and ultrastructure of the juxtaglomerular apparatus in "superficial" juxtamedullary nephrons from rats. *Renal Physiol.* **9**, 348–356.

14. Liu, L. and Barajas, L. (1993) The rat renal nerves during development. *Anat. Embryol.* **188**, 345–361.

15. Inscho, E. W. (2001) The in vitro blood-perfused juxtamedullary nephron technique, in *Methods in Molecular Medicine, Vol. 51: Angiotensin Protocols* (Wang, D. H., ed.), Humana Press, Totowa, NJ, pp. 435–449.

16. Beeuwkes, R., III. (1971) Efferent vascular patterns and early vascular-tubular relations in the dog kidney. *Am. J. Physiol.* **221**, 1361–1374.

17. Lewis, D. A., Loomis, J. L., and Segal, S. S. (1991) Preservation of endothelial cells in excised rat carotid arteries. Effects of transmural pressure and segment length. *Circ. Res.* **69**, 997–1002.

18. Casellas, D. and Moore, L. C. (1990) Autoregulation and tubuloglomerular feedback in juxtamedullary glomerular arterioles. *Am. J. Physiol.* **258**, F660–F669.

19. Casellas, D., Bouriquet, N., and Moore, L. C. (1997) Branching patterns and autoregulatory responses of juxtamedullary afferent arterioles. *Am. J. Physiol.* **272**, F416–F421.

20. Casellas, D., Bouriquet, N., and Herizi, A. (1997) Bosentan prevents preglomerular alterations during angiotensin II hypertension. *Hypertension* **30**, 1613–1620.

29

Tubuloglomerular Feedback

Volker Vallon and Jurgen Schnermann

1. Introduction

As originally described by Golgi, one consistent anatomical feature of all mammalian and many vertebrate kidneys is that a segment of the distal tubule is firmly attached to the vascular pole of its own glomerulum (*1*). This attachment is formed early in development, and is maintained throughout the elongation of the proximal convoluted tubule and the descending and ascending limbs of the loops of Henle. In mammalian kidneys, the tubular epithelium at the point of contact is differentiated into a specialized plaque of cells known as the macula densa (MD) cells. The MD cells, together with underlying interstitial cells and glomerular arteriolar smooth-muscle cells, form the juxtaglomerular apparatus (JGA). Another cell type in the JGA are the juxtaglomerular granular cells, modified smooth-muscle cells that are responsible for the synthesis and secretion of renin. The connection between tubule and glomerulum is the structural basis of a functional interaction known as tubuloglomerular feedback (TGF) (*2*). Whenever NaCl concentration at the MD deviates from its normal value, a signaling cascade is initiated that results in a dilatation of the vessel when the NaCl concentration decreases, and a constriction of the vessel when the NaCl concentration increases. Dilatation and constriction of afferent arterioles (AAs) is associated with increases or decreases in the single-nephron glomerular filtration rate (SNGFR) respectively, and these changes usually return MD NaCl toward normal. Thus, the importance of TGF lies in the stabilization of distal NaCl concentration, and thus in the stabilization of NaCl excretion. A second mechanism that serves to stabilize distal NaCl concentration is the mechanism of glomerulotubular balance (GTB), the direct relationship between tubular flow and tubular fluid reabsorption.

TGF has been described as a system with two variables, SNGFR and late proximal flow rate (V_{LP}), and by the two functions that describe their inter-

From: *Methods in Molecular Medicine, vol. 86: Renal Disease: Techniques and Protocols*
Edited by: M. S. Goligorsky © Humana Press Inc., Totowa, NJ

relationships *(3)*. The *feedback function* (TGF) describes the inverse relationship between SNGFR and V_{LP}, and the *transport* or *feedforward function* (GTB) describes how SNGFR affects V_{LP}. The operating point of the feedback loop, defined as the steady-state values of SNGFR and V_{LP}, can be graphically determined as the point of intersection of these two functions when they are plotted on the same coordinates. Description of the TGF system in terms of these two variables is advantageous because it reduces TGF to two quantities that can be experimentally determined as well as manipulated.

To explore the TGF mechanism, one must produce a predictable change in NaCl concentration at the MD, and measure the alteration in glomerular arteriolar vasomotor tone resulting from this change *(2,4)*. SNGFR is the ideal index of the overall result of TGF-induced vasomotor changes, but other indices of glomerular arteriolar tone may be substituted (glomerular capillary pressure, single-nephron blood flow, arteriolar vessel diameter). Since the TGF mechanism is a single-nephron event, the study of TGF requires the use of techniques with single-nephron resolution.

2. Materials

Equipment needed for standard micropuncture:

1. Micromanipulator (three manipulators are needed for orthograde perfusion, four for retrograde perfusion) (*see* **Note 1**).
2. Stereomicroscope with magnification to at least 150× (working distance of 2–3 cm is important for introduction of micropipets).
3. Fiberoptic light guide.
4. Small animal operating table with servo-controlled heating plate or heating pad (Vestavia Scientific; web site: www.microperfusion.com).
5. Microperfusion pump for 0–40 nL/min range (Vestavia Scientific).
6. Servo null pressure device (System 900A; WPI, Sarasota FL) (*see* **Note 2**).
7. Analog-Digital converter and data analysis software (PowerLab).
8. Capillary grinder (Vestavia Scientific).
9. Capillary puller (Vestavia Scientific).
10. Capillary holder.
11. Glass capillaries (WPI, Sarasota FL; Corning).
12. Lucite kidney cups (Vestavia Scientific).
13. Wax injection apparatus (modification of Wells microdrive; Vestavia Scientific).

Equipment for closed-loop analysis:

1. Pneumatic microinjection pump (WPI, Sarasota, FL).
2. Neon green laser (Melles Griot #05-LGR-171, 543.5 nm).
3. Videocamera (Cohu model #5100, SID camera modified to a framing rate of 60 Hz).
4. Tape recorder.
5. Videometric analyzer (IPM, model 204AH).

6. Video frame grabber (Data Translation 3851).
7. Image analysis software (Global Lab Image®).

3. Methods

3.1. In Situ *Techniques to Study TGF*

3.1.1. Animal Preparation

Most of the original studies on TGF have been done in single nephrons on the surface of the rat kidney, although the existence of the TGF mechanism has been confirmed in dogs and two amphibian species *(4)*. In recent years, the availability of transgenic mice has motivated work in this species. For *in situ* studies of TGF, rats are usually anesthetized with thiobutabarbital (Inactin®, 120 mg/kg intraperitoneally), providing adequate relaxation for the course of an entire experiment. In mice, we have found that inactin is not sufficient as a single anesthetic, but requires combination with ketamine (100 mg/kg). Gas anesthesia using halothane or isoflurane is another option that may interfere less with vascular reactivity *(5)*. Body temperature must be monitored and regulated by heat application, since both rats and mice rapidly cool off during anesthesia. To replace surgical fluid losses, animals typically receive an electrolyte-maintenance infusion, but the exact protocol to achieve "euvolemia" varies between laboratories. Infusion rates are in the order of 0.5–1 mL/h/100 g in rats and 1–1.5 mL/h/100 g in mice, and infusion solutions are electrolyte solutions with the addition of a colloid (for example, 4 g/dL albumin). Kidneys are most commonly accessed by flank incision, using mineral oil to prevent dissemination of animal hair and cautery to cut the muscle layer. Kidneys are then freed of tissue connections and perirenal fat, and placed in a lucite cup for immobilization. In rats and mice, the kidney capsule should not be removed, as it provides protection and stabilizes inserted micropuncture pipets. For kidney immobilization, pieces of cotton balls soaked in 0.85% NaCl are packed between the kidney and the Lucite cup. The kidney surface must be kept moist, and this is best achieved by covering it with a layer of mineral oil. 2% agar in 0.85% NaCl can be used to cover the cotton and prevent leakage of the superfused mineral oil. Ureteral catherization is standard in most rat studies, but less useful in mice because of the tendency of catheters to become obstructed. Such a preparation is stable for several hours in the rat, but limited to only 1–2 h in mice.

3.1.2. Open-Loop Approach (see **Note 3**)

3.1.2.1. Input Variation by Orthograde Perfusion

In many studies the TGF input—e.g., NaCl concentration at the MD—was varied by changing V_{LP} by means of orthograde microperfusion (**Fig. 1A**). Set-

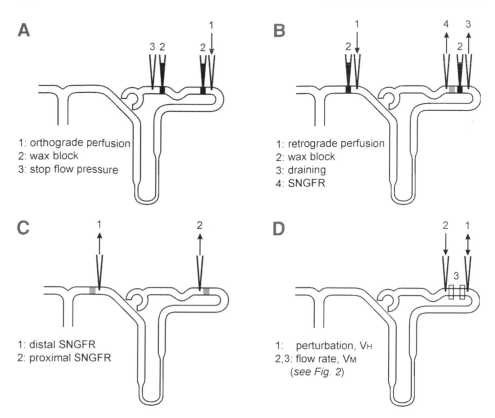

Fig. 1. Schematic drawing showing different approaches to study TGF. Gray boxes downstream from the collection pipet in (**B**) and (**C**) indicate short columns of water-saturated oil that are introduced from the collection pipet into the tubule before the collection is started to prevent downstream loss of tubular fluid.

ting up a nephron for orthograde loop of Henle microperfusion consists of the following steps:

1. Finding: a nephron is identified by puncturing a long proximal tubule segment with a pipet containing stained Ringer solution (often called artificial tubular fluid, ATF), and observing staining of downstream loops. A nephron is usable only when several loops stain. It is important to memorize the layout of the nephron, especially to recall the injection site and last superficial segment of the proximal tubule, before the finding pipet is withdrawn.

2. Blocking: a paraffin wax block is injected at the site of insertion of the finding puncture, and swelling of upstream segments is noted (*see* **Note 4**). This is no problem in normal kidneys at normal SNGFR, but can be difficult when SNGFR is low. Alternatively, the downstream portion of a long segment can be blocked, providing unambiguous definition of an upstream segment.

3. Perfusing: a microperfusion pipet is inserted into the last superficial segment with the perfusion set at a low flow rate. The perfusion fluid used in our laboratory has the following composition (mM): 136 NaCl, 4 NaHCO$_3$, 4 KCl, 2 CaCl$_2$, 7.5 urea, and 100 mg/dL FD&C green for staining. Overall, the exact composition of artificial perfusion fluids used during orthograde perfusion is not especially critical because of the equilibration taking place en route to the MD site. However, under some circumstances, native tubular fluid may include constituents that are missing in artificial fluid, which may have an impact on the TGF response. The collection of tubular fluid into a perfusion pipet by reversing the direction of the perfusion pump, and the use of this fluid for microperfusion in a different tubule or even in a different animal is feasible (*6*). Generally, the need for this somewhat tedious maneuver is not especially compelling.

3.1.2.2. INPUT VARIATION BY RETROGRADE PERFUSION (*SEE* **NOTE 5**)

Setting up a nephron for retrograde loop of Henle microperfusion (**Fig. 1B**) consists of the following steps:

1. Finding: a proximal tubule segment is punctured with a pipet containing stained Ringer solution, and staining of downstream loops is observed. Several downstream proximal segments are required, but the appearance of two distal surface segments is essential. One may accept a single extended distal segment, but it is not always easy to determine its flow direction.
2. Blocking: paraffin wax is injected into the proximal tubule at the site of the exploring puncture, and into the second distal loop (or into the distal-most portion of a single loop).
3. Perfusing: a perfusion pipet is inserted into the first distal loop, and the tubule is perfused at a rate of 15–20 nL/min. This relatively high flow rate diminishes the risk of alterations in perfusate fluid composition.
4. Draining: a collection pipet (10 µm diameter) is inserted into the last superficial proximal segment, and the perfusate is collected and discarded.

3.1.2.3. OUTPUT MEASUREMENT: SNGFR OR STOP FLOW PRESSURE (P_{SF})

Once a tubule is set up for orthograde or retrograde perfusion of the MD segment, it can be used for either measurement of SNGFR or P_{SF} (**Fig. 1A,B**). P_{SF} is a correlate of glomerular capillary pressure (P_{GC}), and its changes are identical to those in P_{GC} (*see* **Note 6**).

1. Measurement of P_{SF}: a pressure-measuring pipet connected to a servo null pressure device is inserted into a conveniently located proximal tubular segment upstream of the wax block avoiding punctures at 90° angles. The recorded pressure should rapidly settle at an elevated level, typically between 30 and 45 mmHg. Since arterial blood pressure is a major determinant of P_{SF}, it is mandatory to simultaneously record arterial blood pressure so that changes in P_{SF} resulting from pressure variations can be recognized. One can directly deter-

mine the glomerular capillary pressure responses by puncturing capillaries in rats with superficial glomeruli, but this is technically difficult and unsuitable as a screening method *(7)*.

2. Measurement of SNGFR: When measuring SNGFR, animals must be infused with a marker substance such as inulin or iothalamate. Inulin is usually given as H^3-inulin, but it can also be determined chemically. H^3-inulin is relatively unstable, requiring occasional dialysis to remove free H^3. Before starting a fluid collection, the nephron must be vented upstream from the wax block to avoid collection of accumulated marker substance. Fluid collections are made for timed periods after injection of a small indicator oil block. Collections times should be at least 2 min or longer. Repeat measurements, at different rates of loop perfusion, are best done by moving each collection site slightly upstream. We have made up to six collections in the rat without noticing leakage, but find repetitive collections more difficult in the mouse. Since collection sites are located in the first half of the proximal tubule, TGF responses can be reliably evaluated by simply measuring flow rate without correction for water absorption.

3.1.3. Proximal Distal SNGFR Difference (see **Note 7**)

TGF input can be acutely reduced by collecting fluid at a proximal site, and SNGFR derived from these collections can be compared with measurements in the distal tubule—e.g., without a change in TGF input *(4)*. Distal and proximal segments of the same nephron can be identified by insertion of a small (4–5 μm) finding pipet into the proximal tubule, and following the course of dye injections. The finding pipet can be left in place during the subsequent fluid collections, and it can actually serve to control proximal intratubular pressure during the collections. Timed collections are first performed from the distal tubule and then from the proximal tubule (**Fig. 1C**). Fluid volumes are determined in a constant bore glass capillary, and SNGFR is calculated by single-nephron inulin or iothalamate clearance.

3.1.4. Closed-Loop Approach (see **Note 9**)

Closed-loop perturbation analysis permits determining the "homeostatic efficiency" of the TGF system, the ability of the TGF system to stabilize V_{LP} *(8)*. In this approach V_{LP} is perturbed in free-flowing nephrons by applying small positive or negative perturbations (V_H). Simultaneously, the response in tubular flow rate just upstream from the perturbation (V_M) is measured by a noninvasive optical method called videometric flow velocimetry *(9)* (**Figs. 1D, 2**).

3.1.4.1. PERTURBATION OF TUBULAR FLOW (V_H)

After mapping a proximal tubule (*see* **Subheading 3.1.2.1.**), a microperfusion pipet filled with late proximal ATF (for composition *see* **Subheading**

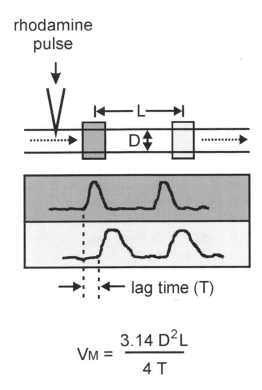

rhodamine
pulse

$$V_M = \frac{3.14\, D^2 L}{4\, T}$$

Fig. 2. Determination of flow rate (V_M) by videometric flow velocitometry for closed-loop analysis of TGF. Simultaneously to flow perturbation (not shown) pulses of rhodamine-labeled dextran as a fluorescent marker are serially injected upstream from the site of flow measurement. Illustrated are sample recordings of image intensity vs time for the two video windows for two applied pulses. D and L are the diameter of the nephron segment and the distance between video windows. T is the lag time required for a fluorescent bolus to traverse the interval between the two windows.

3.1.2.1.) and connected to a nanoliter pump is introduced into the last superficial loop of a free-flowing proximal tubule (**Fig. 1D**). Only nephrons with a long last or second-to-last superficial proximal tubular segment can be used because flow rate will be measured immediately upstream from the microperfusion pipet. V_{LP} is perturbed by the addition or withdrawal of fluid. To add mostly original late proximal tubular fluid in the perfusion mode, the nanoliter pump is started in withdrawal mode. The perfusion rate may be varied in the following order: 0, –4, +4, –8, +8, 0, –12, and +12 nL/min. The first 0 nl/min perfusion interval allows the measurement of ambient flow rate. The second 0 nL/min interval also helps to prevent TGF from resetting.

3.1.4.2. MEASUREMENT OF TUBULAR FLOW RATE (V$_M$)
BY VIDEOMETRIC FLOW VELOCITOMETRY

The system is allowed 2 min at each level of flow perturbation, and V$_M$ is determined over the last 30 s. As illustrated in **Fig. 2**, small boluses (10–15 pl) of ATF containing 1–2% rhodamine B-labeled dextran (Sigma) as a fluorescent marker are injected into the very proximal portion of the long proximal tubular segment upstream to the perturbation site using pressure pulses (frequency 0.3– 0.5 Hz and duration 5–15 ms) applied to a micropipet by a pneumatic microinjection pump. The light of a neon green laser is reflected onto the kidney surface to excite the rhodamine B-labeled dextran. The image of the kidney surface is magnified (×100), filtered (<570 nm) to maximize resolution of the emitted fluorescence (584 nm), and monitored videomicroscopically. The images are recorded using a tape recorder, and are analyzed after finishing the in vivo experiment. At that time, a videometric analyzer is used to place two video windows at two points along the superficial proximal tubular segment—one window just distal to the injection pipet, the other further downstream—and the intensity of the video images at these points are measured simultaneously. After digitizing (Data Translation Model 2801), detrending, and smoothing the images by a technique of weighted (.25, .50, .25) running means, the filtered data are segmented to permit separate calculations for each pulse. The lag time, T$_{max}$, of the fluorescent bolus between the proximal and distal video window can be calculated as the value of T maximizing a cross-correlation *(8)*. Images of the tubular segment are digitized using a video frame grabber, and are used to determine the length (L) and diameter (D) of the tubular segment between the two video windows employing proprietary computer software (Global Lab Image®). V$_M$ is calculated from the lag time and nephron geometry as shown in **Fig. 2**.

3.2. In Vitro Techniques to Study TGF

3.2.1. Isolated Double-Perfused Nephron

Using microdissection, specimens are isolated from kidney slices taken from New Zealand white rabbits or mice, which consist of glomerulum with adherent afferent and efferent arterioles, and with the tubule attached at the site of the MD. Both the AA and the thick ascending limb are cannulated and perfused using two microperfusion systems *(10)*. The pressure in the AA can be controlled through a concentric pressure pipet advanced through the arteriolarperfusion pipet using the Landis dye compensation method. Although the vessel is perfused at constant pressure, the composition of the tubular perfusate can be altered. The output measured as index of TGF regulation is the diameter of the glomerular arterioles determined from video recordings with the help of an image-analysis system.

3.2.2. Juxtamedullary Nephron Preparation

TGF responses are evaluated in this preparation by changing NaCl at the MD, and determining the change in glomerular arteriolar diameter. This approach is outlined in this book in detail in the contribution by Casellas and Moore (Isolated perfused kidney and juxtaglomerular nephron [JMN] preparation).

3.3. TGF in Intact Animals

Several approaches have been used to activate or inhibit the TGF mechanism in all nephrons simultaneously. These techniques are experimentally simple, and are therefore suited to study TGF whenever micropuncture methods are not feasible.

3.3.1. Hypertonic NaCl Infusion

Infusion of hypertonic NaCl into the renal artery of dogs causes an anomalous vasoconstriction that is caused by TGF activation in all nephrons *(11)*. When renal artery infusion is difficult, as it is in small animal species, this technique is less useful because the concomitant extracellular volume expansion alters TGF responsiveness.

3.3.2. Carbonic Anhydrase (CA) Inhibition

Inhibition of CA inhibits proximal tubule $NaHCO_3$ absorption and leads to an increase in $NaHCO_3$ concentration at the MD. The increased $NaHCO_3$ delivery to the MD is believed to activate TGF, and to be responsible for the well-known effect of CA inhibition to reduce GFR *(12)*. CA inhibitors (acetazolamide, benzolamide) have been used as general activators of TGF. The usefulness of this approach is doubtful because of our recent observation that CA inhibitors also reduce GFR and RBF in A1AR knockout mice that do not have a functional TGF (S. Hashimoto and J. Schnermann, unpublished results.)

3.3.3. Administration of Loop Diuretics

Studies in single nephrons have shown that loop diuretics can completely inhibit TGF. Thus, the intravenous (iv) administration of furosemide or bumetanide can be used to examine the consequences of an absence of TGF control. In general, the iv doses required to achieve full TGF inhibition are much higher than therapeutic doses.

3.3.4. Adenosine 1-Receptor Knockout Mice

Targeted deletion of the adenosine 1-receptor gene in mice has been shown to be associated with the complete absence of TGF responsiveness *(13)*. These chronically TGF-less mice, which otherwise appear to do well, would seem to be the ideal model to determine the long-term effects of TGF deficiency.

4. Notes

1. Several manipulators with either mechanical or pneumatic pipet advancement are on the market, but not all are suitable. Mechanical micromanipulators proven to be highly dependable are manufactured by Leitz (Leica Vertrieb GmbH, Bensheim, Germany).

2. Evaluation of TGF responsiveness on the basis of stop-flow pressure requires availability of a servo-null pressure device, the only method that permits continuous intratubular pressure measurements. User-friendliness is the most important aspect in choosing a device, since the requirements for "stiffness" and response time are not particularly demanding in this application. The most convenient of the commercially available instruments uses an air-filled tube connected to a bellows system to generate the pressure for servo control of resistance, but this machine is unfortunately not being manufactured anymore (WPI, Sarasota, FL). The successor model (System 900A, WPI) although technically superior and faster, is less convenient.

3. Since the feedback loop is physically interrupted or opened during both orthograde and retrograde microperfusion, these techniques are referred to as "open-loop" approaches. With open-loop approaches the *TGF function* can be determined with great precision, but the *feedforward* or *GTB function* is disregarded. As a consequence, the operating point and the compensatory power of the system around the operating point are indeterminate. Compensatory potential can only be estimated from the slope of the TGF function.

4. Paraffin wax for histology with a melting point between 42 and 44°C is used. Filling a pipet (12 μm tip) with liquefied wax is done on a hot plate through a long steel cannula. It is important not to overfill. The deposited wax is driven toward the tip with the microdrive piston. A good wax pipet can last a long time if handled with care.

5. Orthograde vs retrograde microperfusion: Although changes in V_{LP} are the physiological way to manipulate NaCl concentration at the MD, this approach is not well-suited to define the luminal signal perceived at the sensor site because the composition of the fluid after passage of descending and ascending limbs is unknown. To test the effect of compositional changes in the perfusate on TGF, the retrograde approach is preferable (**Fig. 1B**). In this case, the distance between infusion site and MD is greatly shortened, and as a reasonable approximation one can assume that the perfusion fluid reaches the sensing site largely unaltered. Perfusion fluid changes are possible, but not as easy as with the orthograde perfusion technique.

6. The use of P_{SF} as index of TGF activity is an ideal screening method to detect changes in TGF characteristics. Furthermore, TGF responses can be examined over the entire range of flow rates. However, P_{SF} changes can be dissociated from changes in SNGFR under some conditions (*14*). Most notably, non-parallel changes in SNGFR and P_{SF} are seen at subnormal flow rates caused by asymmetry of TGF-effector mechanisms; thus, it is advisable to verify parallel changes of both TGF indices.

7. Distal and proximal fluid collections must be made in the same nephron in order to reduce the impact of SNGFR scatter. The advantage of this approach is its ease. Furthermore, it is a good indication of the degree to which SNGFR is restrained by TGF at any given moment. Finally, there is no risk that the artificial perfusion fluid differs in its effects on TGF from native tubule fluid.

8. A change in the perfusion fluid can be done most easily by making a pump exchange with a second pump prepared ahead of time. Withdrawal and reinsertion of pumps can be done several times in the same nephron without leakage if care is taken to utilize the same insertion site. Another way to alter the perfusion fluid is to insert two pumps at the same time, and alternate between them. With this arrangement it is also possible to achieve a range of compositional changes— for example, in the concentration of a drug, by changing the rates of the drug-containing and drug-free pumps simultaneously and in an opposite direction.

9. The fractional compensation, $C=-V_M / V_H$ reflects the ability of the "TGF system" to stabilize V_{LP} *(8)*. Furthermore, the fractional compensation of the system for a perturbation in V_{LP} is equivalent to the fractional compensation for a perturbation imposed anywhere along the system. Thus, the fractional compensation for a perturbation in V_{LP} is equivalent to the fractional compensation for a perturbation in SNGFR. Because the feedback loop is intact, this approach also considers the feedforward or GTB function. The role of the TGF process *per se* can be derived from perturbation analysis by subtracting the effects on GTB. This approach has only been applied to the rat because flow rates in mice appear too low to apply reliably small enough perturbations (1–2 nL/min) and to perceive the upstream changes in flow rate with sufficient precision. There are three major differences between the information provided by this approach as compared with the open-loop approach described previously. First, by adding or subtracting fluid under free-flow conditions, the technique permits manipulation of the dependent variable (V_{LP}) in known reference to the natural operating point of the system. This is useful for studying the operational characteristics of the TGF system, which depend on its behavior around the operating point. Second, when V_{LP} is perturbed under closed loop conditions, the resulting changes in V_{LP} are constituted by an error signal representing the fraction of the perturbation not compensated by the TGF system. As a consequence, most of the data are concentrated to within ± 5 nL/min of the operating point *(15)*. Third, this technique measures the integrated effects of the TGF system consisting of TGF and GTB. To delineate the role of the TGF process *per se*, effects of GTB can be subtracted from the overall efficiency of the TGF system *(15)*.

10. Administration of drugs: To test the effect of drugs, agonists, or antagonists on the TGF system, drugs can be included in the perfusion fluid. In this case, the drug target must be on the luminal membrane (for example, NKCC2), or the drug must be able to cross the epithelial barrier (for example, adenosine receptor antagonists). In the closed-loop approach a drug can be employed by a second-perfusion pipet inserted immediately downstream to the perturbation pipet, and adjustment of the perturbation rate to employ the appropriate net flow perturba-

tion *(16)*. With orthograde perfusion, the exact drug concentration at the MD is unknown, yet this uncertainty is less obvious during retrograde perfusion. To interfere with extraluminal targets, drugs can be administered by peritubular perfusion in the general region of the nephron under study. In a few instances drugs have also been administered through the lumen of a neighboring nephron. Finally, iv application is possible, but this is limited to substances with no major systemic actions, and therefore excludes many substances of interest.

11. The use of in vitro preparations is ideally suited to study the effect of changing the extraluminal composition, and to examine the effect of agents that cannot be used in vivo for toxicity reasons. Furthermore, in the isolated perfused JGA preparation, the MD is visible and accessible, potentially permitting concomitant evaluation of MD-cell function and TGF responses. This approach can also be applied to the mouse in principle *(17)*.

References

1. Golgi, C. (1889) Annotazioni intorno all'istologia dei reni dell'uomo e di altri mammiferi e sull'istogenesi dei canalicoli oriniferi. *Atti della Reale Accademia dei Lincei* **5**, 334–342.
2. Schnermann, J., Wright, F. S., Davis, J. M., Stackelberg, W. V., and Grill, G. (1970) Regulation of superficial nephron filtration rate by tubulo-glomerular feedback. *Pflugers Arch* **318**, 147–175.
3. Briggs, J. (1982) A simple steady-state model for feedback control of glomerular filtration rate. *Kidney Int.* **22**, Suppl. 12, S143–S150.
4. Schnermann, J. and Briggs, J. P. (2000) Function of the juxtaglomerular apparatus: control of glomerular hemodynamics and renin secretion, in *The Kidney Physiology and Pathophysiology* (Seldin, D. W. and Giebisch, G., eds.), Vol. 1, 2 vols. Lippincott, Williams &Wilkins, Philadelphia, PA, pp. 945–980.
5. Leyssac, P. P. and Baumbach, L. (1983) An oscillating intratubular pressure response to alterations in Henle loop flow in the rat kidney. *Acta Physiol. Scand.* **117**, 415–419.
6. Haberle, D. A. and Davis, J. M. (1984) Resetting of tubuloglomerular feedback: evidence for a humoral factor in tubular fluid. *Am. J. Physiol. Renal Physiol.* **246**, F495–F500.
7. Briggs, J. P. (1984) Effect of loop of Henle flow rate on glomerular capillary pressure. *Ren. Physiol.* **7**, 311–320.
8. Thomson, S. C. and Blantz, R. C. (1993) Homeostatic efficiency of tubuloglomerular feedback in hydropenia, euvolemia, and acute volume expansion. *Am. J. Physiol. Renal Physiol.* **264**, F930–F936.
9. Chou, C. L. and Marsh, D. J. (1987) Measurement of flow rate in rat proximal tubules with a nonobstructing optical method. *Am. J. Physiol.* **253**, F366–F371.
10. Ito, S. and Carretero, O. A. (1990) An in vitro approach to the study of macula densa-mediated glomerular hemodynamics. *Kidney Int.* **38**, 1206–1210.
11. Nashat, F. S., Tappin, J. W., and Wilcox, C. S. (1976) The renal blood flow and the glomerular filtration rate of anaesthetized dogs during acute changes in plasma sodium concentration. *J. Physiol.* **256**, 731–745.

12. Tucker, B. J., Steiner, R. W., Gushwa, L. C., and Blantz, R. C. (1978) Studies on the tubulo-glomerular feedback system in the rat. The mechanism of reduction in filtration rate with benzolamide. *J. Clin. Investig.* **62,** 993–1004.
13. Sun, D., Samuelson, L. C., Yang, T., Huang, Y., Paliege, A., Saunders, T., et al. (2001) Mediation of tubuloglomerular feedback by adenosine: Evidence from mice lacking adenosine 1 receptors. *Proc. Natl. Acad. Sci. USA* **98,** 9983–9988.
14. Persson, A. E., Gushwa, L. C., and Blantz, R. C. (1984) Feedback pressure-flow responses in normal and angiotensin- prostaglandin-blocked rats. *Am. J. Physiol. Renal Physiol.* **247,** F925–F931.
15. Vallon, V., Blantz, R. C., and Thomson, S. (1995) Homeostatic efficiency of tubuloglomerular feedback is reduced in established diabetes mellitus in rats. *Am. J. Physiol. Renal Physiol.* **269,** F876–F883.
16. Vallon, V. and Thomson, S. (1995) Inhibition of local nitric oxide synthase increases homeostatic efficiency of tubuloglomerular feedback. *Am. J. Physiol. Renal Physiol.* **269,** F892–F899.
17. Ren, Y. L., Garvin, J. L., Ito, S., and Carretero, O. A. (2001) Role of neuronal nitric oxide synthase in the macula densa. *Kidney Int.* **60,** 1676–1683.

30

Microdissected Perfused Vessels

Thomas L. Pallone

1. Introduction

In vitro microperfusion was developed in order to study the transport of solutes and water across nephrons *(1,2)*. The approach was later extended to renal microvessels for the purpose of measuring vasomotion of glomerular arterioles *(3)*. The purpose of this chapter is to provide a general description of the use of in vitro microperfusion techniques to study the physiological functions of microvessels. The investigator must create a series of micropipets to be mounted on specialized holders so that they can be concentrically aligned to cannulate, perfuse, and in some cases, collect effluent from the microvessel under study. In vitro perfusion of renal arteriolar segments is generally performed either to quantify the transport of solutes or to examine vasomotion.

2. Materials
2.1. Micropipets for In Vitro Perfusion

Microperfusion of vessels in vitro requires four separate types of micropipets: holding pipets, perfusion pipets, exchange pipets, and collection pipets. Construction of any of these is a two-step process. First, glass tubing of appropriate diameter and wall thickness is mounted on a coarse pipet puller that rotates the glass within the coils of a nichrome wire. The wire is heated to the melting temperature so that, under gravity, the glass separates to yield a tapered region that can be further worked under a microscope to form the desired shape. Once this "first pull" has been completed, the tapered pipet glass is remounted on a microforge. The microforge permits observation of the tapered region of the glass tubing with a horizontal stereomicroscope. The taper of the glass is placed within the loop of a platinum wire. The platinum wire is heated in a controlled fashion to shape the tip to yield the final pipet. Here, we consider each style of pipet separately.

From: *Methods in Molecular Medicine, vol. 86: Renal Disease: Techniques and Protocols*
Edited by: M. S. Goligorsky © Humana Press Inc., Totowa, NJ

2.2. Holding Pipets

Glass tubing 0.084" × 0.064"; outside diameter (OD) × internal diameter (ID) is used (Drummond, Broomall, PA, N51A glass capillaries) for construction of holding pipet. The purpose of a holding pipet is to aspirate the end of the microdissected vessel into a holding area so that a second concentric microperfusion pipet can be advanced into the microvessel lumen to perfuse and pressurize its interior (**Fig. 1**). Of the various types of pipets required for perfusion, the construction of the tip of the holding pipet requires the most complex sequence of maneuvers. The first step is to form a hook on the end of the glass. This is accomplished by touching the end of the pipet to the platinum wire while heating to anneal the glass to the wire. In a single rapid motion, the filament is heated and moved outward and upward to bend the glass into a hook. When the heat is turned off by decompressing a foot switch, the glass hook cools and hardens. Because of the outward and upward motion of the filament, the glass remains within the interior of the wire loop for subsequent operations. We place a weight (a metal washer or nut on a wire, 675 mg) onto the hook and then lower the pipet within the heating filament so that another brief application of heat bends and relieves any torque on the glass. Subsequently, the pipet is lowered until the region of the taper on which the holding area will be formed lies within the loop of the heating filament. Heat is again applied so that, under the force of the weight, the glass melts and pulls to form a region with dimensions of 500–1000-μm long and 20–30-μm wide. During the last step, some movement of the glass up and down within the loop is needed to obtain a uniform diameter. Care must be taken to lower the level of the heat so that the pipet does not completely separate. Subsequently, a smaller weight (a tiny piece of thin wire formed into a loop, ~5 mg) must be substituted onto the hook. With the smaller weight, further heating has a greater effect to thicken than to pull and narrow the region of the pipet under construction. At this stage, simply to avoid undesired lateral deformation of the pipet tip, it is necessary to shield the pipet from breezes in the room. This can be done by shrouding the entire microforge or by cupping one's hands around the area of the filament.

To complete construction of the holding pipet, several sequential maneuvers must be performed. First, gradual heating, generally slightly above the narrow area of the pipet, creates a constriction against which the microvessel will be stopped when aspirated into the pipet. Next, the pipet is raised within the filament so that the area just below the constriction can be thickened and narrowed to provide an entrance region with the desired diameter. Finally, the pipet is raised until the filament is well below the holding area, and after this the 675-mg weight is repositioned onto the glass hook. A burst of high heat is applied to the filament until the pipet completely separates.

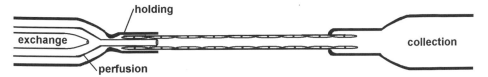

Fig. 1. Microperfusion. Microperfusion requires assembly of three concentric pipets mounted into acrylic holders (not shown). The outermost "holding pipet" allows the microvessel to be aspirated into an entrance region. The "perfusion" pipet is advanced into the lumen and pressurized to induce flow. The "exchange" pipet allows the investigator to rapidly change the buffer that flows into the perfusion pipet. The far end of the vessel is drawn into a collection pipet. The "collectate" that flows from the structure can be sampled and analyzed to measure rates of solute and water transport.

To complete the construction of the holding pipet, the tip must be broken free to open the entrance area. This is best accomplished by the "anneal and break" method. The pipet is rotated through a 90° angle to lie parallel rather than perpendicular to the floor. The heating filament positioned just below the desired holding area of the pipet. As the filament is heated to a low level that barely melts the glass, the pipet entrance area is lowered onto the filament so that the pipet glass just begins to melt. Immediately, as the glass starts to deform, heating is stopped by decompression of the microforge footswitch. As the filament cools, it shortens and withdraws, pulling the entrance region apart and breaking it into two halves. Finally, the very tip of the entrance region is slightly heat-polished with the pipet in a vertical position just above the filament. Heat-polishing should make the end smooth without visibly narrowing the entrance.

2.3. Collection Pipet

Glass tubing 0.084" × 0.064"; OD × ID is used for the collection pipet. Construction of collection pipets is identical to holding pipets, except that no constriction is created above the entrance region and the tip is heavily heat-polished in order to achieve a narrowing that provides a snug fit for the end of the microperfused vessel. When a tight seal is needed to avoid inflow of bath solution, the entrance area can be coated with Sylgard polymer (Dow Corning), a hydrophobic silicone resin that cures onto the glass. Prior to use, the collection pipet is dipped into liquid Sylgard to coat it with a hydrophobic fluid. An alternate approach is to enclose the collection pipet in a separate concentric pipet that contains Sylgard. In this case, after aspirating the collection end of the vessel or tubule into the collection pipet, the collection pipet can be withdrawn into the Sylgard pipet to seal the entrance from bath inflow. Sylgard seals are important for transport experiments in which collectate must undergo chemical or radioisotope analysis. It is not needed for vasomotion experiments, for which the only goal is to pressurize the vessel lumen.

2.4. Perfusion Pipet

Glass tubing 0.047" × 0.040"; OD × ID is used for the perfusion pipet. Perfusion pipets are constructed from thin-walled glass of smaller diameter. As with the holding and collection pipets, construction begins by completing the coarse "first pull," transfer to the microforge, and completion of hook formation to hang a weight on the end of the tapered region. A much smaller weight is used to complete the formation of the perfusion pipet (165 mg) than is used for creation of the larger holding and collection pipets (675 mg). The taper formed during the first pull is heated on the microforge to form a section of glass 500–1000 microns long of appropriate diameter to pass through the constriction of the holding pipet and cannulate the vessel. We finish construction by manually breaking the glass at the end of the perfusion area with fine forceps. Because resistance to fluid flow is inversely proportional to ID raised to the fourth power, the diameter of the region that will cannulate the vessel will have a major influence on the pressure required to drive perfusion of buffer through the pipet. When ID is ≥10 μm, a few mmHg is enough. In contrast, when the ID falls to only a few microns, >100 mmHg may be needed to achieve perfusion rates of ~10 nL/min.

2.5. Exchange Pipet

Glass tubing 0.020" × 0.012"; OD × ID is used for the exchange pipet. The exchange pipet is the third inner concentric pipet that fits within the perfusion pipet to enable rapid change of solutions that perfuse the lumen (**Fig. 1**). We subject the glass to a first pull to create a taper on the end. The glass is then placed into the microforge for easy visualization, and the tip is broken off along the taper at a location in which the diameter is small enough to permit the tip to fit near the entrance of the fine region of the perfusion pipet tip.

2.6. Sampling, Volumetric Constriction Pipets

Glass tubing 0.020" × 0.012"; OD × ID is used for sampling pipets. The purpose of the sampling pipet is to aspirate controlled volumes of fluid from the collection end of the vessel (**Fig. 2**). These are constructed by forming a constriction above the area of interest at a diameter along the taper that will determine the final volume that lies beyond the constriction. The glass has a thick wall, and requires high heat with a small weight to form the constriction. Once the constriction is formed, it is raised above the heating filament, and a larger weight is attached so that the region of the tapered opening can be pulled to its final shape. The tip opening can be created by breaking it off with forceps

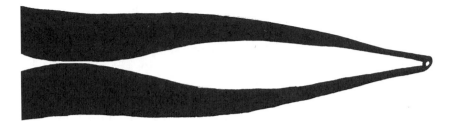

Fig. 2. The volumetric sampling pipet. The tip of a volumetric construction pipet used to sample microvessel effluent is shown. In order to determine the rate that collectate leaves the vessel, the constriction delimits a region of fixed volume. The time required for collectate to fill the tip of the sampling pipet to its constriction yields the collection rate. Collected fluid can be retrieved for chemical or radioisotopic analysis. The length of the volumetric region is typically 100–1000 μm and the maximal internal diameter, typically 10–200 μm. The constriction point is reduced to an internal diameter as small as 10 μm.

or by using the "anneal and break" approach. Volume of the constriction pipet can be estimated as approximately one-half of the volume of a cylinder of height equal to the distance from the tip to the constriction and diameter equal to the largest ID of the sample area. Final calibration must be performed using chemical assays with dilutions or with radioisotopes. One generally seeks target volumes of 5–100 nL, depending on the collection rate and type of microanalysis anticipated.

3. Methods

3.1. Tissue Isolation, Microdissection, and Transfer

To harvest renal tissue, we anesthetize rodents (thiopental, 50 mg/kg body wt, intraperitoneal), open the abdomen, and cut out the kidneys with scissors. The kidneys are decapsulated and cut into thin slices with a sharp razor blade. The slices are placed for storage into cooled buffer (in mM): HEPES 5, NaCl 140, NaAcetate 10, KCl 5, MgCl$_2$ 1.2, Na$_2$HPO$_4$ 1.71, NaH$_2$PO$_4$ 0.29, CaCl$_2$ 1, alanine 5, glucose 5, and albumin 0.5 g/dL, pH = 7.4. During stereoscopic observation at 10–50x, Dumont number 5, fine-tipped forceps are used to peel small tissue wedges along the corticomedullary axis. Once a wedge several hundred microns in width has been isolated, a sharpened stainless-steel needle is used to peel away and isolate nephrons and microvessels. The stainless-steel needle is sharpened to the shape of a flat-head screwdriver with successive grits of fine sandpaper (Thomas Scientific). On a daily basis, prior to dissection, the tip is polished to a mirror finish by successive use of 5- and 0.3-μm grit paper.

Once a structure of interest (e.g., microvessel or nephron segment) has been isolated, it is raised off the bottom of the glass Petri dish by waving the needle near the structure in an upward direction. A Pasteur pipet is used to aspirate the structure along with a minimum of buffer into the tip. The pipet tip is rapidly moved to the perfusion chamber on an inverted microscope. Under continuous observation using a low-power (2×) scanning objective with the microscope field diaphragm set for high contrast, buffer is slowly expelled from the tip to deposit the structure within the chamber. As soon as the structure leaves the Pasteur pipet, the pipet is lifted vertically out of the buffer so that it settles to the bottom of the chamber. Microdissected structures can be easily lost during the transfer process. To avoid this, it is important that the perfusion chamber be prefilled to a low level and that the structure being transferred remain close to the inlet of the Pasteur pipet. The chamber cannot be heated during the transfer process because convection currents otherwise tend to sweep the deposited microvessel away from the field of view.

3.2. Cannulation, Collection, and Perfusion

To cannulate the microvessel, it is first drawn into the holding pipet to the constriction (**Fig. 1**). Next, we advance the perfusion pipet through the constriction of the holding pipet to the entrance point of the microvessel and then pressurize the perfusion pipet to initiate flow of buffer. This has the effect of "blowing open" the microvessel so that the perfusion pipet can be advanced further into the lumen to stabilize the vessel between the perfusion and holding pipet. We find it advantageous to make subtle adjustments of alignment as the perfusion pipet is advanced. Once perfusion has commenced, the opposite end of the microvessel is drawn into the opening of the collection pipet. At that point, the pipets and structure are relocated to the desired focal plane above the bottom of the chamber, the chamber is repositioned to place the perfused structure into the desired location downstream of the bath inlet, and bath flow is initiated.

3.3. Measurement of Permeability to Solutes

Transport properties of perfused microvessels can be examined by measuring efflux or influx of solutes and water. To measure diffusional permeability to a solute by quantifying lumen to bath efflux, a tracer such as a radioisotope or fluorescent compound is included in the perfusate. As the tracer diffuses from the lumen to the bath, its concentration falls between the perfusion and collection pipets. Making the assumption that the efflux (J) is given by the product of permeability (P) and lumen-to-bath concentration difference, $J = P(C - C_B)$, integrating and solving the appropriate differential equation yields the result:

$$P = (Qo / \pi DL) \ln [(C_P - C_B) / (C_C - C_B)] \tag{1}$$

where D and L are vessel diameter and length, and C_P, C_C, and C_B are the tracer concentrations in the perfusate, collectate, and bath, respectively. Permeability can also be measured from the rate of bath-to-lumen influx, and in this case a similar analysis yields:

$$P = (Qo / \pi DL) \ln [(C_B - C_C) / (C_B - C_P)] \tag{2}$$

Thus, one must measure the rate of perfusion Q and the concentration of the tracer in the perfusate, bath, and collectate. In practice, lumen-to-bath tracer fluxes are most practical to use, and tracer concentration in the bath will be zero. **Equations 1** and **2** are only correct when transport is only by diffusion so that solvent drag (transport of solute across the vessel wall by convection) is zero or negligible. When volume flux (Jv) also occurs across the vessel wall, more complex analysis is needed to account for convectional transport and molecular sieving.

3.4. Measurement of Water Transport

The methods required for quantification of the rate of water transport across a perfused vessel or nephron segment are straightforward. Water transport from the lumen of the perfused microvessel to the bath can be calculated from measurement of the collection rate (Qc) and the concentration of an impermeant tracer in the perfusate and collectate. Designating Qo as perfusion rate and Qv as the rate of efflux across the vessel wall, mass balance yields:

$$Qv = Qc [(Cc / Co) - 1] \tag{3}$$

It is most conventional to normalize Qv by dividing by the vessel length or surface area. When this has been done, the final parameter is often dubbed "Jv," meaning volume flux, with units of either $nL/(min \cdot mm)$ or cm/s, respectively. Rigorously, Jv should represent a vector quantity equal to the velocity of fluid at a single point perpendicular to the membrane surface. In practice, this is seldom the connotation used in the literature because transport experiments can only measure overall water transport averaged over the entire preparation.

Radiolabeled inulin is the tracer most commonly used as a "volume marker" to measure water flux across nephron segments. In a microvessel, this ~5000 mol wt substance is too small to reliably satisfy the need for an impermeant tracer. As a substitute, we have used a 2×10^6 mol-wt fluorescein isothiocyanate (FITC)-labeled dextran as our "volume marker." Fluorescence of FITC dextran is correlated with concentration with excellent linearity, and can be measured by microanalysis from the collectate (*4*). Alternately, we have used real-time measurements of fluorescence in the collectate during the experiment to continuously monitor water flux across the microvessel wall (*5,6*) (**Fig. 3**).

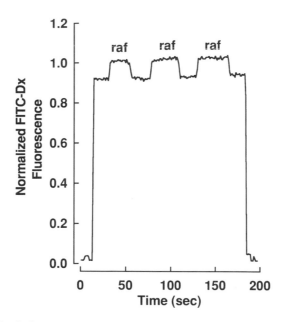

Fig. 3. Real-time measurement of collectate-volume-marker fluorescence. A convenient method for measuring the rate at which water is transported across a microvessel wall is to include an impermeant high mol-wt fluorescein isothiocyanate-labeled dextran (FITCDx) to the perfusate. When raffinose is present, water flows from the lumen to the bath and concentrates the dextran so that collectate fluorescence rises. The graph shows an experiment during which collectate fluorescence (ordinate) was monitored continuously in the entrance region of the collection pipet. The bath was exchanged from one that was isosmolar with the perfusate to one made hypertonic by addition of 200 mM raffinose. Three bath exchanges are shown.

3.5. Measurement of Vasomotion by Videomicroscopy

It is more common for investigators to employ microperfusion of arteriolar segments to measure vasomotion than it is to examine transport properties. To quantify vasomotion, the microvessel is cannulated and perfused to pressurize its lumen, and then videomicroscopy is performed so that changes in vessel diameter can be measured as agents of interest are applied to the luminal or abluminal surfaces of the vessel from the perfusate and bath, respectively. This method was first adapted to the study of renal glomerular arterioles. Since then, both large- and small-generation renal microvessels including intralobular arterioles (~25-μm diameter), afferent and efferent glomerular arterioles (20 μm), and the small-generation descending vasa recta (15 μm) have been extensively studied by this method (*3,7*). In the case of larger arterioles with diameters that are hundreds of microns, perfusion can be accomplished by

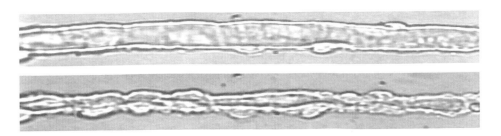

Fig. 4. Vasoconstriction of a descending vas rectum by Angiotensin II. Descending vasa recta (DVR) are examples of a type of contractile microvessel. In the top panel, a vessel is microperfused to pressurize the lumen. The cell bodies of smooth-muscle-like pericytes can be seen to protrude from the abluminal surface. In the bottom panel, the same vessel has been exposed to 10 n*M* angiotensin II, causing constriction to occur at various foci along its length.

tying them onto glass pipets with very fine suture. An example of a microperfused descending vas rectum constricted by abluminal application of angiotensin II (ANGII) is shown in **Fig. 4**.

The most sophisticated use of this technique in the kidney has been by investigators interested in tubuloglomerular feedback. Measurement of afferent arteriolar diameter has been performed at controlled pressure while perfusing the macula densa (MD) via the cortical thick ascending limb of Henle *(8)*. Since simultaneous perfusion of the thick ascending limb and afferent arteriole is required, two systems of concentric pipets for microperfusion must be employed. Control of perfusion pressure within the cannulated afferent arteriole has been achieved by inserting a pressure measurement pipet through the vessel entrance beyond the holding pipet tip.

The microvessel constriction that occurs in response to the experimental maneuver of interest is recorded on videotape, and later quantified as a change in diameter. As such, the measurement is a bioassay that reveals the ability of a particular hormone, pharmaceutical agent, or maneuver to induce vasoconstriction or relaxation. Once the recording is obtained, the actual quantification of diameter poses an additional methodological problem. In its simplest form, a set of calipers can be used along with calibration of the video screen to sequentially measure either ID or OD of the vessel at the point of interest. Automated "videocalipers" are commercially available to make this process most efficient. Unless the investigator is blinded to the events of the experiment, this approach risks the introduction of bias. Methods that employ edge detection schemes can also be used to measure vasomotion in real time, and decrease the risk of investigator bias.

3.6. Measurement of Fluorescent Probes During Microperfusion Experiments

The capabilities of the inverted microscope can be expanded considerably to examine physiologically relevant questions by quantitative fluorescent microscopy. Once a microdissected vessel has been immobilized within a perfusion chamber on an inverted microscope, fluorescent probes can be loaded into the membranes or cytoplasm of smooth muscle and endothelial cells. Fluorescent probes are available to measure various properties such as intracellular concentration of ions (Ca^{2+}, Mg^{2+}, Na^+, K^+, Cl^-, H^+), membrane potential, membrane fluidity, nitric oxide (NO) generation, and generation of reactive oxygen species (ROS). Three broad categories of fluorescent probes exist. Some are excited at a single wavelength, and emission is monitored at a single wavelength (e.g., fluorescein or rhodamine). Others are excited at a single wavelength with measurement of emission at two wavelengths (e.g., Indo-1 for Ca^{2+}, SNARF-1 for pH). Finally, another group (e.g., fura2 for Ca^{2+}, BCECF for pH) is alternately excited at two wavelengths while emission is monitored at one wavelength. Commercially available computer-controlled and synchronized systems are available to select excitation wavelengths and monitor emitted fluorescence with photomultiplier(s) or intensified video cameras.

3.7. Measurement of Solute Generation by Microvessels

Another notable extension of microperfusion methods is to measure solute generated by the vessel. As an example, renin generation by superfused tubules and juxtaglomerular cells has been assayed *(9,10)*, and NO generation by microvessels has been measured by microelectrodes *(11)*.

4. Notes

1. There are limitations to the use of microperfusion for the measurement of solute permeability. If the transport rate of the solute is too low, very low perfusion rates and long vessels must be used in order to attain a measurable difference in tracer concentration between perfusate and collectate. This becomes difficult because very long collection times are required to obtain sufficient sample volumes for microanalysis. Conversely, if permeability and tracer fluxes are too high, then very rapid perfusion of short segments must be used to avoid near equilibration along the vessel axis.

    The limitations of permeability measurements are illustrated in **Fig. 5**, where **Equation 1** has been solved for lumen to bath tracer efflux with $C_B = 0$. The graphs show the perfusion rate (Qo) required to achieve a collectate to perfusate tracer concentration ratio of 0.75, 0.5, or 0.25 to allow for low, intermediate, and high permeability measurements, respectively. On each graph, results are shown for vessels between 100 and 1000 μm in length. **Figure 5A** shows that a 1000-μm vessel would have to be perfused at 1 nL/min if permeability is as low as

10^{-5} cm/s. If 20 nL of fluid is required for tracer measurement by microanalysis, a 20-min collection time would be required for only one replicate. Given that permeabilities to large solutes can be lower than 10^{-5} cm/s, it is apparent that microperfusion methods will be inadequate to obtain single-vessel measurements for macromolecules. Conversely, if permeability to a small hydrophilic solute such as urea or tritiated water is very high (~500×10^{-5} cm/s), even vessels as short as 200 μm will have to be perfused rapidly to achieve the marginally acceptable collectate-to-perfusate ratio of 0.25 (**Fig. 5C**).

An alternative to microperfusion for the purpose of measuring transport of macromolecules has been described for measuring albumin transport across glomerular capillaries. Fluorescently labeled albumin is loaded into the capillary lumen by prolonged incubation. Subsequently, the bath is exchanged to buffer free of the labeled albumin, and the decline in fluorescent signal is measured as the labeled albumin is transported, largely by diffusion, across the capillary wall (*12,13*). The approach is a zero-flow rate adaptation of the methods described in this section.

2. Computation of the conductance of the vessel wall to transport of water is generally expressed as hydraulic conductivity (Lp) or, equivalently, osmotic water permeability:

$$Jv = Lp \left[(P_L - P_B) - \Sigma \, \sigma i (\Pi_L - \Pi_B) \right] \qquad (4)$$

where P_B and P_L are hydraulic pressure in the bath and lumen, respectively. Π_B and Π_L are osmotic pressure resulting from the ith solute in the bath and lumen, and σi is the reflection coefficient of the vessel wall to the ith solute.

Experiments to compute Lp or σi are difficult because a number of variables including hydraulic pressure and solute concentrations must be controlled and measured. Rigorous determination of these parameters is also rendered difficult because transport of water can occur via a number of pathways such as paracellular convection, via aquaporins and by solubility/diffusion through lipid membranes. Each of these pathways has separate and potentially very different properties. For example, aquaporins impart a hydraulic conductivity roughly 1/10 that of the paracellular pathway, but have a reflection coefficient to small hydrophilic solutes of unity. In contrast, the paracellular route may have a low or zero reflection coefficient to small solutes with near-unity reflection coefficient to macromolecules. Because of these many considerations, design and analysis of in vitro microperfusion experiments for the purpose of measuring Lp or σi is fraught with difficulties. Simple formulae like **Equations 1** and **2** cannot always be readily derived to describe an experiment. Instead, numerical integration of systems of differential equations may be needed so that an iterative search for the parameters can be performed. Examples of the use of in vitro microperfusion of microvessels to measure water permeability of paracellular and aquaporin water-channel pathways are available in the literature. Rigorous analyses of the types of problems posed by the experimental designs have been given (*5,6*).

3. Fluorescent probes have tremendous power, but also numerous pitfalls. Calibration of probe fluorescence is often difficult, and fluorescent emission is frequently

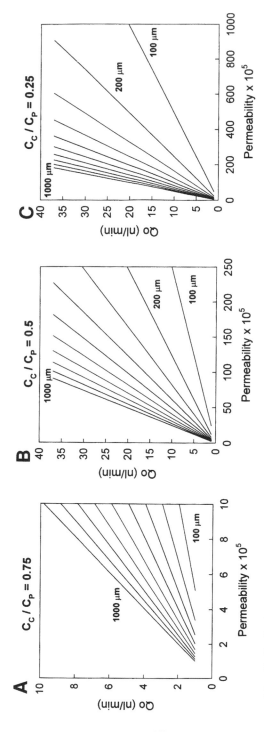

Fig. 5. Perfusion rates required to measure diffusional permeability. The graphs show the rate at which perfusion must be performed (ordinate, Qo) to achieve a collectate to perfusate concentration ratio (Cc / Cp) of 0.75 (**panel A**), 0.5 (**panel B**) or 0.25 (**panel C**) when permeability is as specified on the abscissa. Each panel shows results for vessels 100–1000 µm long.

454

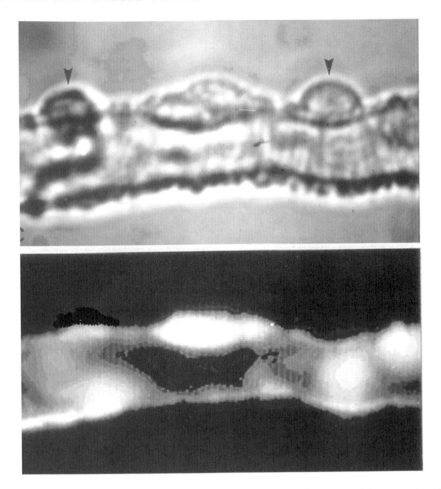

Fig. 6. Loading of fura2 into descending vasa recta. The top and bottom panels show white light and fluorescent images of a vessel loaded with the Ca²⁺ sensitive fluorescent probe, fura2. The abluminal pericytes (arrows) are absent in the fluorescent image indicating that fura2 loads largely into endothelial cells.

influenced by several factors. Additional problems with photobleaching and leak of the probe from the cell can reduce fluorescence, and finally, distribution of the probe between endothelia and smooth muscle must be understood for proper interpretation of experimental results (**Fig. 6**). On first use of a fluorescent probe in our laboratory, we compare white light and fluorescent images to determine cellular distribution and study their spectral characteristics to determine the optimal excitation wavelength(s) for quantification. More extensive discussion of this topic is beyond the scope of this chapter, but authoritative reviews exist (*14*).

References

1. Burg, M., Grantham, J., Abramow, M., and Orloff, J. (1966) Preparation and study of fragments of single rabbit nephrons. *Am. J. Physiol.* **210,** 1293–1298.
2. Burg, M. B. (1982) Isolated perfused tubule. Introduction: background and development of microperfusion technique. *Kidney Int.* **22,** 417–424.
3. Edwards, R. M. (1983) Segmental effects of norepinephrine and angiotensin II on isolated renal microvessels. *Am. J. Physiol.* **244,** F526–F534.
4. Pallone, T. L., Work, J., and Jamison, R. L. (1990) Resistance of descending vasa recta to the transport of water. *Am. J. Physiol.* **259,** F688–F697.
5. Pallone, T. L., Kishore, B. K., Nielsen, S., Agre, P., and Knepper, M. A. (1997) Evidence that aquaporin-1 mediates NaCl-induced water flux across descending vasa recta. *Am. J. Physiol.* **272,** F587–F596.
6. Pallone, T. L. and Turner, M. R. (1997) Molecular sieving of small solutes by outer medullary descending vasa recta. *Am. J. Physiol.* **272,** F579–F586.
7. Pallone, T. L. (1994) Vasoconstriction of outer medullary vasa recta by angiotensin II is modulated by prostaglandin E2. *Am. J. Physiol.* **266,** F850–F857.
8. Ito, S. and Carretero, O. A. (1990) An in vitro approach to the study of macula densa-mediated glomerular hemodynamics. *Kidney Int.* **38,** 1206–1210.
9. Greenberg, S. G., He, X. R., Schnermann, J. B., and Briggs, J. P. (1995) Effect of nitric oxide on renin secretion. I. Studies in isolated juxtaglomerular granular cells. *Am. J. Physiol.* **268,** F948–F952.
10. Skott, O. and Briggs, J. P. (1988) A method for superfusion of the isolated perfused tubule. *Kidney Int.* **33,** 1009–1012.
11. Thorup, C., Kornfeld, M., Winaver, J. M., Goligorsky, M. S., and Moore, L. C. (1998) Angiotensin-II stimulates nitric oxide release in isolated perfused renal resistance arteries. *Pflugers Arch.* **435,** 432–434.
12. Savin, V. J., Sharma, R., Lovell, H. B., and Welling, D. J. (1992) Measurement of albumin reflection coefficient with isolated rat glomeruli. *J. Am. Soc. Nephrol.* **3,** 1260–1269.
13. Daniels, B. S. (1994) Increased albumin permeability in vitro following alterations of glomerular charge is mediated by the cells of the filtration barrier. *J. Lab Clin. Med.* **124,** 224–230.
14. Takahashi, A., Camacho, P., Lechleiter, J. D., and Herman, B. (1999) Measurement of intracellular calcium. *Physiol. Rev.* **79,** 1089–1125.

31

Renal Microperfusion Techniques

Charles S. Wingo, I. David Weiner, and Shen-Ling Xia

1. Introduction

The advent of the technique of the isolated perfused tubule allowed renal physiologists to examine the transport characteristics of all portions of the nephron for the first time. The understanding of renal function prior to the advent of in vitro microperfusion rested on the integrative understanding drawn from clearance techniques and renal micropuncture experiments. Historically, clearance techniques were one of the first physiological tests of renal function. These studies were complemented and extended by the pioneering work of Richards, who developed the technique of micropuncture between 1925 and 1937, although the first reports of this technique in the mammalian nephron occurred later.

Micropuncture provided considerably more insight into what had previously been only understood on the basis of whole-kidney clearance experiments with a clearer definition of the function of the superficial proximal tubule, but it was hampered by the inability to measure transport in nephron segments located deep within the substance of the kidney. The advent of the isolated perfused tubule technique dramatically expanded our understanding of renal physiology by allowing investigators to study segments that were previously inaccessible by micropuncture. However, both microperfusion and micropuncture have their strengths and their limitations. With regard to microperfusion, the strengths include the ability to examine all aspects of the nephron and to study them under precisely defined conditions in which the composition of the solution can be completely defined. Yet, certain limitations must be acknowledged. First, the transport characteristics of the perfused tubule may only partially mimic the transport characteristics exhibited in vivo as a result of the absence of hormonal stimuli that may modulate the transport properties to be studied. The strengths and weaknesses of microperfusion complement those of

From: *Methods in Molecular Medicine, vol. 86: Renal Disease: Techniques and Protocols*
Edited by: M. S. Goligorsky © Humana Press Inc., Totowa, NJ

micropuncture, in which the tubule is studied in its native environment but numerous hormonal factors may influence transport, and many cannot be controlled rigorously.

2. Materials

2.1. Animal Studies

Several animals have been used in microperfusion. The most commonly studied animal for this technique is the New Zealand White rabbit, because of the ease of dissection. Studies have also been performed in rats, mice, and reptile kidneys, and there are isolated reports of perfusion of human kidneys harvested for transplantation that were not suitable for transplantation.

2.2. Equipment

This section examines the use of dissecting forceps, stereoscopic microscopes, pipet pullers and microforge, capillary glass, syringes and tubing, vacuum equipment, micromanipulators, microperfusion pumps, heating apparatus, electrometers and voltage measurement equipment, chart recorders, microanalysis equipment, volume flux and inulin measurements, osmolality, alkali and alkali earth measurements, chloride and halide analysis, measurements of total CO_2, and bicarbonate concentration and measurements of ammonium.

2.2.1. General Microperfusion Equipment

The preparation of a microperfusion rig involves modification of an inverted microscope, such as a Nikon Diophot or Olympus IMT microscope with micromanipulators. Several companies provide this modification (ITM, Roger Rick, White Scientific). This allows the mounting of concentric glass pipets. The outer pipet is usually made of 0.084 soft glass, and the inner pipet 0.047 soft glass. These pipets are first pulled on an instrument such as a Stolting vertical puller, and then the final manufacture is constructed with a microforge (Defondrunne). Typically, two outer holding pipets of .084 glass are utilized, and an inner perfusing pipet 0.047 glass is used for introduction of luminal fluid. Diffusion pressure is typically regulated by the height of the hydrostatic pressure column, although motor-driven pumps are available. The bath solution (vol ≈ 0.2 mL in our case) for transepithelial flux measurements may be of a slow exchange (<0.5 mL/min) or fast exchange (>1 mL/min) system, depending on the need for rapid changes in the composition of the basolateral solution. A heater unit with nichrome wire embedded in the heating unit will allow maintenance of 37°C when bath flow rates are less than 2 mL/min. Transepithelial voltage can be measured by means of the high impedance electrometer (WPI, FT 223, or a KS 700) using silver silver-chloride electrodes in a series of agarous bridges connected to the perfusion solution and the bath solution. Typical electrode resistances are less than 1 MΩ tip resistance completed for a microperfusion circuit prior to introduction of the tubule. Luminal diameters of both the outer holding pipets and inner perfusion pipets vary greatly depending on the segment and species studied, but are generally between 10 and 40 μm in diameter. Input impedance for typical transepithelial voltage measurements should be 10^{12} ohms. The electrometers can be connected to a chart recorder or to a computer to record events during the experiment. For transepithelial volume flux, ^{3}H-inulin methoxy extensively dialyzed according the method of Schafer et al. *(1)*, provides a highly accurate measure of volume flux because of its high specific activity, and detection of small leaks in the tubule.

3. Methods

3.1. General Methods of Microperfusion

3.1.1. Animal Sacrifice

The method of animal sacrifice is usually by cervical decapitation after light anesthesia. Sodium pentathol (50 mg/mL) may be used for anesthesia administered by an ear vein for rabbits (30 mg/kg). For mice, intraperitoneal (ip) injection of approx 0.1 mL for a 20–25 gm mouse is sufficient to induce anesthesia. After sacrifice, the abdominal cavity is opened, the intestines are displaced, and a kidney is rapidly removed. The kidney capsule is removed, and thin coronal slices (approx 1 mm) are obtained and then placed into a Ringers bicarbonate solution that is iso-osmotic to plasma (approx 290 mOsm/kg.) Alternatively, we have found that placing tissue slices into Dulbecco's Modified Eagle's Medium (DMEM) provides better preservation of the tissue, which can be grown in tissue culture.

3.1.2. Tubule Isolation

Tissues are microdissected using #5 stainless-steel forceps that have been hand-polished to a pyrimidal tip of approx 10 microns. For cortical slices, dissection proceeds from the papilla to the surface of the cortex with wedge-shaped segments of the renal parenchyma. Care should be taken to avoid touching or damaging any of the structures intended for perfusion. This dissection can be performed at 4°C or at room temperature.

For straight structures that run parallel to the collecting ducts, such as the pars recta, thin descending limbs, and thin ascending limbs, dissection can proceed by pulling thin strips of tubular bundles and progressively dividing these tubular bundles until individual nephron segments can be identified. Proximal tubules and the pars recta are readily identified by their refractile nature of the basolateral surface, whereas collecting ducts and thick ascending limbs have a less refractile appearance. In the dissection of proximal tubules, it is usually best to proceed from the cortico-medullary junction or superficially from the cortex in regions between medullary rays. Dissection of medullary structures, such as the medullary thick ascending limb and outer medullary collecting ducts, are usually most easily approached from strips of parallel bundles of tubules that are dissected from the corticomedullary junction toward the inner medulla. In all cases, careful delineation of landmarks prior to obtaining small tubular bundles is essential to establish the region of the nephron to be perfused unambiguously (*see* **Note 1**).

3.1.3. Microperfusion Cannulation and Setup

After microdissection of an appropriate tubule segment, it is transferred to the bath chamber, where it can be aspirated into the holding pipet (A pipet) and the perfusion pipet advanced into the lumen of the tubule. If net or isotopic flux methods are to be used, the ends of the holding pipet are generally sealed with Sylgard to allow electrical and mechanical isolation of the tubule. This requires the first application of Sylgard mixed with hardener, which is then heated to polymerize the Sylgard in the holding pipets. Non-polymerized Sylgard can then be applied to the tips of each of the pipets, which makes a good mechanical seal of the tubule.

After aspiration of the tubule into the holding pipet and advancement of the perfusion pipet into the lumen, the voltage across the epithelium can be determined as an initial index of viability. The distal end of the tubule is then aspirated into a collection pipet (C pipet) of 0.084 glass and behind this is a reservoir containing water-equilibrated mineral oil. Perfusate is then allowed to flow through the lumen of the tubule and into the collection pipet from which the collected fluid (collectate) can be removed at periodic intervals by an inner pipet that is concentrically mounted inside the C-pipet. The most common collecting pipet is a microscopic constriction pipet referred to as a constant volume pipet (CVP). This pipet, hand forged to have a small constriction distal to the tip, can accurately measure volumes of 10–40 nL with an accuracy of 1%. Samples of the collected fluid can then be transferred from the CVP to a scintillation vial for measurement of ^{22}Na, ^{24}Na, ^{36}Cl, ^{42}K, or ^{3}H-inulin. Quantitative transfer for the contents of the CVP to a liquid scintillation vial allows simultaneous measurement of net lumen-to-bath volume flux in nLs quantities of tubular fluid. In most cases, biodegradable scintillation solution should be used.

3.1.4. Flux Equations

Volume flux can be calculated by the following equation:

$$J_v = (CPM_o / CPM_i - 1) \cdot (V_o / L) \tag{1}$$

where J_v is net volume reabsorption, CPM_o and CPM_i are the respective [^{3}H]inulin counts per min (CPM) per nanoliter in collected and perfused fluid, V_o is the collected fluid rate in nL per min, and L is the tubular length in mm (*see* **ref. 2–4**).

The net flux of X ion ($J_{net\,[X]}$) from lumen to bath can be determined by use of the following equation:

$$J_{net\,[X]} = \frac{[X]_i \cdot V_i - [X]_o \cdot V_o}{L} \qquad (2)$$

where $[X]_i$ and $[X]_o$ are the activity of ion X in the perfusate and collected fluid, respectively, in milliequivalents per L. V_o and L are as before, and V_i is the perfusion rate. X ion concentration can be determined by picomole analysis with flameless atomic absorption spectrophotometry (**5**).

In experiments examining the isotopic flux of ion X (e.g., ^{22}Na, ^{24}Na, ^{36}Cl, or ^{42}K), lumen-to-bath ion flux (using the trace flux rate coefficient from lumen to bath, J_{x1b} as a marker) can be determined by the disappearance of ion X from the luminal fluid according to the following equation:

$$J_{xlb} = \frac{X_i^* \cdot V_i - X_o^* \cdot V_o}{L \cdot \rho} \qquad (3)$$

where X_i^* and X_o^* are the isotopic X cpm per nL in the perfused and collected fluid, respectively. V_o, V_i, and L are as before. ρ is the specific activity of the isotope X in cpm per picoequivalent.

For transepithelial flux experiments, flow rates typically reflect the luminal flow rates that are present in these segments in vivo—for example, for early proximal tubules, 15–25 nL per min, whereas for more distal segments such as the cortical collecting duct, flow rates are typically 1–4 nL per min.

3.1.5. Criteria for Acceptance of Microperfusion Experiment

Prior to performing a transepithelial flux experiment, several criteria should be met to ensure that the epithelium is intact. First, transepithelial voltage may provide an assessment of viability, particularly in tubule segments with substantial spontaneous transepithelial voltages such as in the proximal tubule, thick ascending limb of Henle, and the cortical and medullary collecting duct. Second, many microperfusionists utilize a supravital stain such as FD&C green, which will stain dead or damaged cells intensely blue-green (since this stain requires active extrusion by an adenosine triphosphate (ATP)-dependent process.) This provides indirect evidence of tubular viability when no staining is present. Third, in most cases we have made it a routine procedure to collect 5-min bath collection after cannulation of both the perfusion and holding pipets and allowing the temperature to equilibrate to 37°C. Typical leak rates in the

healthy tubule are less than 2%, and if greater than 5% of the perfusate is collected in the bath, the tubule should be discarded. Typically, during this period
the tubule is carefully inspected under 400× magnification or higher to ensure
that all cells have a normal morphological appearance and there is no evidence
of flattened or vacuolated cells.

If these criteria are acceptable for perfusion, flux collections may proceed.
Since most segments exhibit time-dependent changes, comparison of a treatment effect must randomize treatment and control periods to the first period,
examine a three-period protocol (control-treatment-control), or for two drug
treatments, utilize a Latin-square design to consider both time-dependent and
treatment effects.

3.1.6. Microanalytic Techniques

Net flux across the tubule epithelium can be measured either isotopically by
the equal isotope dilution method or by the measurement of net chemical flux
(2–4). Common net chemical flux methods include measurement of alkali and
alkali earth cations, chloride, or other halide anions, ammonia, carbon dioxide
and bicarbonate, osmolality, and urea.

Many alkali and alkali earth cations can be measured by flameless atomic
absorption spectrophotometry, utilizing a graphite furnace that can be used
to measure sodium, potassium, and calcium. A convenient method utilizes a
large-fold dilution of the analyte from the CVP into a fixed volume of ultra
high-purity water *(5)*. Another method for measurement of sodium and
potassium is the helium glow photometer *(6)*. Other more sensitive methods
include X-ray micronanalysis, but the expense of the equipment and the high
level of technical support that is required for the maintenance limit its wide
use *(7,8)*.

Chloride and halide anions can be measured by the method of Ramsay et
al. *(9)*. A convenient instrument is commercially available (WPI). The chloride concentration is measured potentiometrically. Electrical current is passed
through a silver wire, which causes oxidation of metallic silver to silver ions
with subsequent precipitation of AgCl from solution. The reduction in chloride concentration in the solution is measured potentiometrically. As the potential exceeds a preset value, this end point measures the total chloride
concentration in the solution, which yields a linear relationship between chloride concentration of the solution, and the total current with an accuracy of
plus or minus 1%.

Ammonia can be measured fluorometrically *(10)* or by the use of nicotinamide adenosine dinucleotide (NAD)-specific bacterial luciferase *(11)*. Total
CO_2 concentration can be measured by microcalorimetry *(12)*, which utilizes
the conversion of bicarbonate to CO_2 in the presence of a strong mineral acid

and the subsequent exothermic reaction with solid LiOH, which is detected by the heat liberated in the reaction of carbon dioxide with a hydrated lithium hydroxide crystal and amplified. The integral of temperature vs time output is proportional to carbon dioxide concentration.

Osmolality can be measured by freezing-point depression with a Clifton nL osmometer *(13)*. Urea may be measured by meta-flow methodology.

3.2. Measurement of Intracellular pH Using Fluorescent Dyes

The development of fluorescent pH-sensitive dyes that are easily loaded into living cells has revolutionized the ability to examine acid and base transport across plasma membranes. In the sections following, we review general principles of the use of these dyes and important considerations in their use and methods to evaluate the functional characteristics of transport activity. For complete discussion of intracellular pH regulation, the reader is referred to detailed reviews *(14,15)*.

3.2.1. Usefulness

In some conditions, an experimental stimuli alters cellular function, and as a consequence, intracellular pH *(16,17)*. In other cases, the functional presence of an acid-base transporter can be identified by intracellular pH measurements *(18,19)*. Lastly, the regulation of known acid-base transporters activity by specific stimuli can be studied *(20)*. Although alternative methods to measure intracellular pH are available, such as intracellular pH electrodes, the small size of most mammalian cells makes these techniques less feasible than fluorescent intracellular pH measurements.

3.2.2. Dye Compounds

Fluorescent pH-sensitive dyes are characterized by local pH-sensitive fluorescence. Fluorescein and its derivatives are the most commonly used compounds, and fluorescence following excitation at specific wavelengths increases as local pH increases (e.g., proton concentration decreases) *(21)*. The changes in emission are relatively large, making their detection relatively easy to quantify. However, changes in emission following excitation at a pH-sensitive wavelength can reflect changes in pH, or changes in cell volume or geometry, which may alter the concentration of the dye inside the cell. As a result, dual-excitation-ratio measurements are commonly utilized, involving excitation of the dye at both pH-sensitive and pH-insensitive wavelengths. The ratio of emission at the pH-sensitive wavelength to emission following excitation at the pH-insensitive wavelength assesses pH, independent of dye concentration and cell geometry.

3.2.3. Loading of Dyes into Cells

In order to use these compounds, they must be both loaded into cells and retained in the cytoplasm throughout the duration of the experiment. The majority of compounds are loaded into cells as a precursor compound that is relatively soluble in aqueous solution, yet is also permeable across plasma membranes. For example, BCECF is usually loaded into cells as the acetoxymethyl ester of BCECF, BCECF-AM. BCECF-AM diffuses rapidly across plasma membranes into the cell. Once intracellular, nonspecific esterases hydrolyze the acetoxymethyl ester group, yielding the final compound, BCECF. BCECF has a net charge of –4, making it poorly permeable across plasma membranes. We have observed less than 10% change in cytoplasmic BCECF over experimental durations of 1 h and more. However, in some cases specific transporters can export these dyes, complicating their use *(22)*.

3.2.4. Quantifying Dye Emission

Fluorescent emission of the dye can be quantified using a wide variety of techniques. Photometer-based systems are the most common, the least expensive, and generally, the easiest to use. Their primary limitation is that they measure emission from multiple cells, yielding a measurement of average intracellular pH in the field imaged. In heterogeneous tissues, this may be an important limitation. One technique that can be useful to minimize this concern is to narrow the field excited to the smallest size possible using the microscope's field diaphragm, and to narrow the field from which emission is being quantified to the smallest possible size using the emission diaphragm. Using these techniques, one can image only a few cells, which in some cases can allow measurement of intracellular pH in a single cell *(23,24)*.

Another method used to quantify emission is to use digital video microscopy. In this case, emission is measured using a highly light-sensitive digital camera, typically an intensified CCD camera *(25,26)*. Individual images are obtained with excitation at the pH-sensitive and pH-insensitive wavelengths. Computer software then calculates the ratio of intensity at each pixel of the image and generates a two-dimensional (2D) map of intracellular pH in the field imaged. Further computer processing allows determination of changes in intracellular pH in multiple regions of interest that are user-defined, and can be studied over time.

Confocal laser-scanning microscopy can also be used for intracellular pH measurements. It offers the advantage of improved spatial resolution over both photometer- and digital video-based systems *(22,27)*. Typically, this equipment is substantially more expensive, limiting its availability for widespread use. It is also limited by lower detection sensitivities than either of the other techniques, which results in the need for increased excitation intensities.

Because fluorescent dyes undergo excitation intensity-dependent phototoxicity and cause excitation intensity-dependent cellular damage *(23,28)*, minimizing excitation intensity is important when designing experiments.

3.2.5. Calibration of Emission to Intracellular pH

In order to convert pH-sensitive dye emission to changes in intracellular pH, one must perform a calibration procedure. In general, this should be performed at the end of most, if not all, experiments. Calibration involves clamping intracellular pH to known levels, measuring the fluorescence ratio, and then creating a calibration curve to convert measured fluorescence ratios to actual pH. The most commonly used technique is the high K^+-nigericin method *(21)*. In this process, nigericin, a K^+/H^+ exchanging compound, is added to the extracellular fluid (ECF) at concentrations of ~10–20 μM. This compound then inserts into the plasma membrane of the cells, and, by virtue of its ability to exchange K^+ for H^+, sets the intracellular H^+ (H^+_i)-to-extracellular H^+ (H^+_o) ratio equal to the intracellular K^+ (K^+_i)-to-extracellular K^+ (K^+_o) ratio. By using an extracellular solution with a potassium concentration similar to intracellular potassium, generally ~120 mEq/L, this process "fixes" intracellular pH to extracellular pH. A series of fluorescence ratio measurements are made over a range of pH that encompasses the intracellular pH range for the experiment. A calibration curve is then created and used to convert the fluorescence ratio to actual pH.

It is important to avoid the temptation of determining a calibration curve using a cell-free system. Binding of BCECF and many other fluorescent compounds to intracellular proteins results in pH-sensitivity characteristics which may be different inside cells than in a cell-free system. As a result, erroneous results may be obtained if intracellular calibration is not performed (**Note 3**).

3.2.6. Conversion of Intracellular pH Changes to Acid-Base Flux

BCECF and the other fluorescent pH-sensitive dyes only measure free proton concentration. There is substantial buffering of intracellular protons, so that less than 0.001% of protons transported across plasma membranes are unbuffered, causing changes in intracellular free proton concentration and, thus, intracellular pH. Accordingly, in order to determine rates of proton (or its equivalents) flux across plasma membranes, one must also consider the buffer capacity of the cell. Buffer capacity (β_T) reflects the ratio between protons added to or transported out of a cell and changes in intracellular pH, according to the formula: $\beta_T = \Delta acid/\Delta pH_i$, and results are typically reported as mmol H^+ per L cell vol per pH unit. Buffer capacity is intracellular pH-dependent, differs between different cell types, and can be substantially altered by differing extracellular solutions. Buffer capacity generally increases with intracellular acidosis when studied in CO_2-HCO_3^--free solutions. In contrast, the relationship between buffer capacity and intracellular pH is the opposite when studied in CO_2-HCO_3^--buffered solutions, increasing with intracellular alkalosis. Thus, when studying the activity of acid-base transporters under differing experimental conditions, measurement of buffer capacity is essential for the interpretation of pH_i changes.

3.2.7. Specific Examples of Use

The combination of intracellular pH measurement with the isolated in vitro microperfused tubule technique provides many important advantages in the evaluation of renal tubular acid-base transport. The major uses of these combined techniques are to identify ion transporters and their regulation and to determine whether intracellular pH is involved in the regulation of other cellular processes.

One of the most common uses of intracellular pH measurement is to identify the presence of specific acid-base transport mechanisms. Typically, intracellular pH is displaced from baseline, and the presence or absence of mechanisms to return intracellular pH back to baseline is identified. If present, the ionic requirements and inhibitor characteristics of this process are determined and used to characterize the acid-base transporter(s) involved in this process. In some cases, it is possible to identify transport simply by removing an ion that is transported by the protein being examined. For example, removal of extracellular Cl^- is sufficient to induce functional reversal of transport by many Cl^-/HCO_3^- exchangers, resulting in HCO_3^- movement into cells and intracellular alkalinization.

By specifically adding or removing ions and/or inhibitors from the luminal or peritubular solutions, one can determine whether the transporters involved are present at the apical or basolateral membrane, or both. It is important to emphasize that these techniques only provide a functional characterization of the transporter, and cannot identify with absolute certainty the molecular identify of the transporter(s) involved.

Once transport mechanisms have been identified, one can then examine their regulation. This involves evaluating the rate of proton or base equivalents transported in the absence and the presence of the experimental stimuli. It is important to recognize that intracellular pH measures only the "free" proton concentration and that the majority of acid-base equivalents transported are buffered in the cytoplasm. Accordingly, one should also determine buffer capacity in both the absence and the presence of the experimental stimuli in order to allow consideration of the relationship between changes in intracellular pH and changes in acid-base equivalent movement across plasma membranes *(20)*. In rare cases, it may also become necessary to measure cell volume *(23)*.

A third reason to measure intracellular pH is to determine whether intracellular pH is a mechanism that enables an experimental stimulus to alter cellular function. In this case, intracellular pH is measured in both the absence and the presence of the stimulus. If changes in intracellular pH are identified, then one must determine whether these changes are responsible for the change in cellular function *(16)*. This can be accomplished by adding weak acids or bases to the extracellular solutions or by inhibiting the normally constitutively active proton transporter, Na^+/H^+ exchange. Once experimental conditions have been identified that cause similar changes in intracellular pH as the stimulus under consideration, one can determine whether these conditions cause similar changes in cellular function as the stimulus being studied.

3.3. Techniques for Studying Cellular Calcium Signals

3.3.1. Calcium-Sensitive Fluorescent Indicators

Calcium-sensitive fluorescent indicators are powerful tools for measuring cytosolic free calcium ($[Ca^{2+}]_i$). In the early 1980s, a new generation of fluorescent indicators was introduced with quin2, fura-2, and indo-1 *(29–31)*. These tetracarboxylate fluorescent indicators contain a Ca^{2+}-selective binding site modeled on the well-known chelator EGTA (*see* **Note 4**). The technique has been widely used because these indicators allow monitoring of intracellular free calcium concentration in single cells, and even localized areas within cells, and also provide improvements in time resolution down to the ms range. However, these indicators require excitation at ultraviolet wavelengths (e.g., 340 nm/380 nm for fura-2) that is potentially injurious to cells *(32)*.

Recently, a group of new fluorescent indicators, with visible excitation and emission wavelengths such as fluo-3, have been synthesized for measuring cytosolic free Ca^{2+} *(32–34)*. These indicators increase their fluorescence intensity remarkably after binding Ca^{2+}, without a shift in excitation or emission (*see* **Note 4**). More recently, another indicator known as fluo-4 has been used widely because of its quantum yield properties and resistance to bleach (as compared to fluo-3). However, fluo-3 or fluo-4 are not as suitable for quantitative measurements of $[Ca^{2+}]_i$ as fura-2 or indo-1.

3.3.2. Loading of Indicators into Collecting-Duct Cells

The indicators can easily be loaded into the cell by either direct microinjection of the free salt form through a micropipet or via acetoxymethyl (AM) ester form from extracellular membrane *(35)*. The advantage of microinjection is that one can inject the indicators to a selected group of cells and deliver additional drugs with the indicators to study cellular signaling pathways. However, this requires additional microinjection instruments. The following sections focus mainly on the application of AM indicators, the "single-wavelength" indicator fluo-4/AM and "dual-wavelength" indicator fura-2/AM.

AM form loading is nondisruptive and can be loaded either from apical membrane via perfusion pipet to the lumen of the kidney tubule or from the basolateral membrane via bath solution directly (*see* **Note 5**). In the case of loading indicators from the lumen, the solution that contains the indicators must be filtered through a 0.4-μm filter to avoid possible blockade of the lumen of the collecting duct. The tubule will be loaded with a HEPES-based Ringer solution containing either 5 μM fluo-4/AM or 5 μM fura-2/AM indicator (Molecular Probes, Eugene, OR) at room temperature by 60-min incubation. The indicator will be diluted from the stock solution with a concentration of 10 mM in dimethyl sulfoxide (DMSO). The final concentration of DMSO in the loading solution must be always below 0.1% and should not have a major effect on cell activity. Before starting measurements, the tubule should be washed at least 3× with Ringer's solution and incubated in experimental solution for an additional 15–20 min to reduce the possibility of incomplete hydrolysis of the acetoxymethyl esters by intracellular esterases.

3.3.3. Fluorescence Image Analysis

3.3.3.1. [Ca^{2+}]$_i$ MEASUREMENT WITH FLUO-4/AM

The laser scanning confocal microscope (as an example, we use Zeiss LSM 510, Carl Zeiss, Thornwood) with fluorescent indicator fluo-4/AM is used to measure intracellular fluorescence intensity (as an index of [Ca^{2+}]$_i$) and is particularly studied to study how calcium signals are distributed in space and time within a single living cell (*see* **Note 6**). When the intact collecting duct is co-loaded with fluo-4/AM and Fura-red/AM (Fura-red/AM, 10 μM; Fluo-4/AM, 5 μM), the ratio signal can be achieved (*see* **Note 7**). When cells are excited with argon-ion laser light at 488 nm, fluo-4 exhibits an increase in green fluorescence (band-pass 515–530 nm) on Ca^{2+} binding, whereas Fura Red shows a decrease in red fluorescence (long-pass 590 nm). The emission ratio of fluo-4 to Fura Red can be then used as an index to monitor the changes in [Ca^{2+}]$_i$. Confocal fluorescence measurements are carried out using a Zeiss Axiovert 100M inverted microscope. The fluor 20× (N.A.=0.75) air, plan-neo 40× (N.A.=0.75) and plan-apo 100× (N.A.=1.4) oil objectives can be used according to need. Green and red fluorescence images are acquired simultaneously on two separate photomultiplier detectors. Mean fluorescence intensity from individual cells can be expressed as a percentage of change from the resting level before stimulation, and statistical significance can be examined off-line.

3.3.3.2. [Ca^{2+}]$_i$ MEASUREMENT WITH FURA-2/AM

[Ca^{2+}]$_i$ measurements are made with an imaging system (as an example, we use InCyt Im2, Intracellular Imaging, Inc., Cincinnati, OH), including a PC computer, a filter wheel of conventional design, a CCD camera, and a Nikon TE 300 microscope with either 100× oil objective (1.3 N.A.) or 40× air objective (0.65 N.A.). The fluorescence emitted at 510 nm from excitation at 340 nm and 380 nm can be measured and used for calculation of the emission ratio. The change in Ca^{2+} can be estimated after *in situ* calibration, using standard techniques *(31)*. The saturating level of fluorescence (F_{max}) is determined after perfusion with 5 μM or more ionomycin in HEPES Ringer (containing 1.5 mM or more calcium), and the minimum level (F_{min}) is determined after perfusion with low-calcium Ringer (0 mM calcium/2 mM EGTA).

The rate of image collection depends on the duration of the experiment, speed of the cell response, and degree of the bleaching. We have been able to use the rate of 3–10 s per image (515 × 512 pixels) for 45–90-min long experiments. The fluorescence of the region of the interest (either whole tubule or individual cells within the tubule) can be monitored using the software setting.

4. Notes

1. After a suitable collecting duct has been identified as a likely candidate for perfusion, several criteria should be established. First, the ends must be completely free so that cannulation of both ends in the pipet allows an adequate seal. The tubule should be carefully inspected to ensure that it has no evidence of damage. Tubules with high refractile characteristics are likely to be damaged and must be discarded. The tubule of interest should be examined under high magnification for this purpose. After examination, the tubule can be aspirated into a Pasture pipet or small capillary pipet and transferred to the microperfusion rig.

2. In all our experiments, the absolute magnitude of volume reabsorption was less than 0.1 nL·mm^{-1}·min^{-1}.

3. Two important limitations of all fluorescent dyes, including the pH-sensitive fluorescent dyes, are phototoxicity and photobleaching *(23,28,36)*. These refer to damage to the cell and a decrease in emission intensity, respectively, which result from excitation of the dye. In addition, excitation of these dyes, especially when excessive, can result in changes in their pH-sensitivity *(23)*. These adverse effects can be minimized by keeping the excitation duration and intensity as low as possible during the experiment.

4. Quin2, fura-2, and indo-1 have K_d of binding Ca^{2+} from 114–250 nm *(33,35)*. These indicators give very high binding selectivity (10^5:1) for Ca^{2+} over the most avidly competing ion, Mg^{2+}. The K_d of fluo-3 for binding Ca^{2+} is approx 400 nm at 22°C and 800 nm at 37°C, which allows more sensitive measurement at higher $[Ca^{2+}]_i$ *(32,37)*.

5. The AM ester form turns the indicators into lipophilic membrane-permeable derivatives that are cleaved by cytosolic esterases to generate free indicators trapped in the cytosol *(29,35)*. The AM esters are not water-soluble, and are usually introduced into the loading medium from DMSO. Pluronic F-127 is a non-

ionic, high mol-wt surfactant polyol that has been found to be useful for solubilization of water-insoluble indicators and other materials in physiological medium (Technical Support Material from Molecular Probes, Inc., Eugene, OR). It has been used to help disperse AM esters of fluo-3, fluo-4, and related ion indicators. In our experience, sonicating loading solution for 5 min usually helps the solubilization of indicators.

The available evidence suggests that the AM ester can accumulate in intracellular organelles (nucleus, sarcoplasmic reticulum, mitochondria, and others)—the so-called compartmentalization phenomenon *(32,34,35)*. Compartmentalization can give a false impression of a low $[Ca^{2+}]_i$ in one area and a high $[Ca^{2+}]_i$ in another area in some preparations. Loading at room temperature has been found to be favorable for reducing compartmentalization of the indicator. It seems to be advisable to use lower concentration of indicator with a longer loading time rather than to use a higher concentration of indicator for a shorter loading time (technical support material from Molecular Probes, Inc., Eugene, OR). However, indicators loaded into cytosol may leak out of cells *(35,37)*. In our experience, although it varies from cell to cell, an experiment of 90-min duration can be achieved without a significant loss of indicators.

6. Laser scanning confocal microscopy is commonly used in biomedical research *(38,39)*. The technique of confocal imaging optically filters out signals from regions outside the plane of focus. This provides increased image spatial resolution, and even more importantly, removal of out-of-focus information from two-dimensional (2D) images of three-dimensional (3D) structures. In a confocal imaging system, both the illumination and detection optics are focused on a single spot of the specimen (e.g., they are confocal). The detection optics incorporates an aperture (called the pinhole) in the optical path that is situated in a focal plane conjugate with the focal plane containing the spot under observation. In this way, only light emanating from the immediate vicinity of the illuminated spot passes through the pinhole to the detector (e.g., photomultiplier, or silicon photo diode). Further rejection of signals from out-of-focus spots occurs because of the nature of the illumination. In conventional microscopy, the whole of the volume of the specimen is bathed in a fairly uniform flux of illumination. In a confocal system, the illumination is focused on one spot of the volume at a time, so that the illumination beam diverges above and below the focal plane. Thus, spots away from the plane of focus receive a much lower flux of illumination and appear to be black *(40–42)*. A complete image is built up by sequentially sampling all the points within the focal plane (e.g., scanning). Since the scanning is carried out from point to point, the light source for illumination must be a point source, and therefore the single-mode laser is ideal for this purpose. All these properties make the resolution of imaging in a confocal microscope greater than ratiometric imaging in a conventional microscope.

7. It is advisable to use a high concentration of Fura-red because the fluorescence of fluo-4 is several-fold brighter than the Fura-Red signal *(43)*.

References

1. Schafer, J. A., Troutman, S. L., and Andreoli, T. E. (1974) Volume reabsorption, transepithelial potential differences, and ionic permeability properties in mammalian superficial proximal straight tubules. *J. Gen. Physiol.* **64(5)**, 582–607.
2. Wingo, C. S. (1987) Potassium transport by medullary collecting tubule of rabbit: effects of variation in K intake. *Am. J. Physiol.* **253(6 Pt 2)**, F1136–F1141.
3. Wingo, C. S. (1989) Active proton secretion and potassium absorption in the rabbit outer medullary collecting duct. Functional evidence for proton-potassium-activated adenosine triphosphatase. *J. Clin. Investig.* **84(1)**, 361–365.
4. Wingo, C. S. (1990) Active and passive chloride transport by the rabbit cortical collecting duct. *Am. J. Physiol.* **258(5 Pt 2)**, F1388–F1393.
5. Wingo, C. S., Bixler, G. B., Park, C. H., and Straub, S. G. (1987) Picomole analysis of alkali metals by flameless atomic absorption spectrophotometry. *Kidney Int.* **31(5)**, 1225–1228.
6. Vurek, G. G. and Bowman, R. L. (1965) Helium-glow photometer for picomole analysis of alkali metals. *Science* **149**, 448–450.
7. Ingram, M. J. and Hogden C. A. (1967) Electrolyte analysis of biological fluid with electron microprobe. *Anal. Biochem.* **18**, 54–61.
8. Morel, F. and Le Roineln Grimellec, C. (1969) Electron probe analysis of tubular fluid composition. *Nephron* **6**, 250–264.
9. Ramsay, J. A., Brown, R. H. J., and Croghan, P. C. (1955) Electrometric titration of chloride in small volumes. *J. Exp. Biol.* **32**, 822–829.
10. Good D. W. and Vurek G. G. (1983) Picomole quantification of ammonium ions by flow through fluorometry. *Anal. Biochem.* **130**, 199–202.
11. Nagami, G. T. and Kurokawa, K. (1985) Regulation of ammonia production by mouse proximal tubules perfused in vitro effective luminal perfusion. *J. Clin. Investig.* **75**, 844–849.
12. Vurek, G. G., Warnock, D. G., and Corsey, R. (1975) Measurement of picomole amounts of carbon dioxide by calorimetry. *Anal. Chem.* **47(4)**, 765–767.
13. Green, R. and Giebisch, G. (1984) Luminal hypotenicity: a driving force for fluid reabsorption from the proximal tubule. *Am. J. Physiol.* **246**, F167–F174.
14. Boron W. F. (1986) Intracellular pH regulation in epithelial cells. *Annu. Rev. Physiol.* **48**, 377–388.
15. Roos, A. and Boron, W. F. (1981) Intracellular pH. *Physiol. Rev.* **61**, 296–434.
16. Frank, A. E., Wingo, C. S., and Weiner, I. D. (2002) Effects of ammonia on bicarbonate transport in the cortical collecting duct. *Am. J. Physiol.* **278**, F219–F226.
17. Vehaskari, V. M., Hering-Smith, K. S., Moskowitz, D. W., Weiner, I. D., and Hamm, L. L. (1989) Effect of epidermal growth factor on sodium transport in the cortical collecting tubule. *Am. J. Physiol.* **256**, F803–F809.
18. Milton, A. E. and Weiner, I. D. (1997) Intracellular pH regulation in the rabbit cortical collecting duct A-type intercalated cell. *Am. J. Physiol.* **273**, F340–F347.
19. Weiner, I. D. and Milton, A. E. (1996) H^+-K^+-ATPase in rabbit cortical collecting duct B-type intercalated cell. *Am. J. Physiol.* **270**, F518–F530.
20. Milton, A. E. and Weiner, I. D. (1998) Regulation of B-type intercalated cell apical anion exchange activity by CO_2/HCO_3^-. *Am. J. Physiol.* **274**, F1086–F1094.

21. Thomas, J. A. (1986) Intracellularly trapped pH indicators. *Soc. Gen. Physiol. Ser.* **40**, 311–325.

22. Emmons, C. L. and Kurtz, I. (1990) Evidence for a basolateral organic anion transporter in principal cells studied with confocal fluorescence microscopy. *J. Am. Soc. Nephrol.* 1, 697 (Abstract).

23. Weiner, I. D. and Hamm, L. L. (1989) Use of fluorescent dye BCECF to measure intracellular pH in cortical collecting tubule. *Am. J. Physiol.* **256**, F957–F964.

24. Weiner, I. D. and Hamm, L. L. (1990) Regulation of intracellular pH in the rabbit cortical collecting tubule. *J. Clin. Invest.* **85**, 274–281.

25. Fay, F. S., Carrington, W., and Fogarty, K. E. (1989) Three-dimensional molecular distribution in single cells analysed using the digital imaging microscope. *J. Microscopy* **153**, 133–149.

26. Paradiso, A. M., Tsien, R. Y., and Machen, T. E. (1987) Digital image processing of intracellular pH in gastric oxyntic and chief cells. *Nature* **325**, 447–450.

27. Kurtz, I. and Emmons, C. (1993) Measurement of intracellular pH with a laser scanning confocal microscope. *Methods Cell Biol.* **38**, 183–193.

28. Becker, P. L. and Fay, F. S. (1987) Photobleaching of fura-2 and its effect on determination of calcium concentrations. *Am. J. Physiol.* **253**, C613–C618.

29. Tsien, R. Y. (1981) A non-disruptive technique for loading calcium buffers and indicators into cells. *Nature* **290**, 527–528.

30. Tsien, R. Y., Pozzan, T., and Rink, T. J. (1982) Calcium homeostasis in intact lymphocytes: cytoplasmic free calcium monitored with a new, intracellularly trapped fluorescent indicator. *J. Cell. Biol.* **94**, 325–334.

31. Grynkiewicz, G., Poenie, M., and Tsien, R. Y. (1985) A new generation of Ca^{2+} indicators with greatly improved fluorescence properties. *J. Biol. Chem.* **260**, 3440–3450.

32. Minta, A., Kao, J. P. Y., and Tsien, R. Y. (1989) Fluorescent indicators for cytosolic calcium based on rhodamine and fluorescein chromophores. *J. Biol. Chem.* **264**, 8171–8178.

33. Tsien, R. Y. (1988) Fluorescence measurement and photochemical manipulation of cytosolic free calcium. *TINS* **11**, 419–424.

34. Kao, J. P. Y., Harootunian, A. T., and Tsien, R. Y. (1989) Photochemically generated cytosolic calcium pulses and their detection by fluo-3. *J. Biol. Chem.* **264**, 8179–8184.

35. Cobbold, P. H. and Rink, T. J. (1987) Fluorescence and bioluminescence measurement of cytoplasmic free calcium. *Biochem. J.* **248**, 313–328.

36. Patterson, G. H., Knobel, S. M., Sharif, W. D., Kain, S. R., and Piston, D. W. (1997) Use of the green fluorescent protein and its mutants in quantitative fluorescence microscopy. *Biophys. J.* **73**, 2782–2790.

37. Merritt, J. E., McCarthy, S. A., Davies, M. P. A., and Moores, K. E. (1990) Use of fluo-3 to measure cytosolic Ca^{2+} in platelets and neutrophils. *Biochem. J.* **269**, 513–519.

38. Berridge, M. J. and Irvine, R. F. (1989) Inositol phosphates and cell signalling. *Nature* **341**, 197–205.

39. Williams, D. A. (1993) Mechanisms of calcium release and propagation in cardiac cells. Do studies with confocal microscopy add to our understanding? *Cell Calcium* **14,** 724–735.
40. Wilson, T. (1990) Confocal microscopy, in *Confocal Microscopy*. Wilson, T. (ed.), Academic Press, London, pp. 1–64.
41. White, J. G., Amos, W. B., Durbin, R., and Fordham, M. (1990) Development of a confocal imaging system for biological epifluorescence applications, in *Optical Microscopy for Biology*. Herman, B., and Jacobson, K. (eds.), Wiley-Liss, New York, pp. 1–18.
42. Kitagawa, H. (1994) Theory and principal technologies of the laser scanning confocal microscope, in *Multidimensional Microscopy*. Cheng, P.C., Lin, T.H., Wu, W.L., and Wu, J.L. (eds.), Springer-Verlag, New York, pp. 52–102.
43. Lipp, P. and Niggli, E. (1993) Ratiometric confocal Ca^{2+}-measurements with visible wavelength indicators in isolated cardiac myocytes. *Cell Calcium* **14,** 359–372.

32

How to Design a Clinical Trial

Bryan M. Curtis, Brendan J. Barrett, and Patrick S. Parfrey

1. Principles of Clinical Research

Clinical research, like all research, stems from curiosity. Although some research questions are harder to answer than others, the application of a well-designed trial coupled with the right question can yield valuable information. Indeed, a poorly designed randomized trial will not generate as much scientific information as a well-designed and well-executed prospective observational study. The success and applicability of a research trial depends on many factors. This chapter is not intended to be a treatise on clinical epidemiology or statistics, but instead will focus on some of these factors and other practical aspects of trial design specifically related to nephrology.

Epidemiology provides the scientific foundation by identifying risk factors and their distribution in the general population and establishing their role in poor outcomes, as well as quantifying the potential value of treating and preventing the risk in the general population *(1)*. The ultimate application of this epidemiological research is the clinical trial, and its rationale is to undertake safe human experiments and subsequently apply the premise that observation and interventions in groups are directly relevant to treatment and prevention of disease in individuals *(2)*. Although the randomized, controlled trial remains the gold standard to determine the efficacy of an intervention, determining clinical outcomes in very large trials is often unlikely in nephrology for logistical reasons. Therefore, observational studies remain necessary to complement the observations of a randomized control trial, generating hypotheses to be later tested with randomized control trials, or in some cases to provide answers that cannot be obtained in a randomized control trial *(3)*.

Although the randomized control trial may be the finest example of evidence generation in the evidenced-based medicine era, there is increasing concern that the interest of science and society should not prevail over the welfare

From: *Methods in Molecular Medicine, vol. 86: Renal Disease: Techniques and Protocols*
Edited by: M. S. Goligorsky © Humana Press Inc., Totowa, NJ

of individual patients *(3)*. Ethical Review Boards or Human Investigation Committees composed of medical professionals and non-medical members attempt to ensure the safety and welfare of the participants in clinical trials. Approval from these bodies is mandatory before undertaking any research involving human subjects. Participants must also enter into the research with free and informed consent.

Other challenges to clinical trials include modeling complex human behavior, concerns about generalizability, limitations in recognizing small treatment effects, and the inability to conduct trials of sufficient duration to mimic treatment of chronic disorders *(3)*. In providing examples for the issues discussed, we will examine trials that are performed or being planned in chronic kidney disease.

2. Asking the Question

2.1. Identifying the Problem

Clinical research questions arise from an identified problem in healthcare that requires study to provide evidence for change in clinical practice. Specific questions are asked, and trials are subsequently designed to obtain answers. However, in order to become a clinical trial research question, the identified problem must satisfy a number of requirements. The question must be a clinically important one from the perspective of patients, professionals, and society in general. Additionally, the answer must be generalizable and applicable to patients in a wide spectrum of medical practice. A good question will also help funding strategies and identify potential collaborators once colleagues are convinced the question is important. The issues in nephrology usually center around the medical, social, and financial burden posed by specific diseases and indeed chronic kidney disease as a whole. Thus, many opportunities exist to test interventions during earlier stages of disease, when treatable complications, if poorly managed, may reduce the length or quality of life.

The randomized control trial is specifically designed to test a hypothesis, and the research question must be amenable to the application of an experimental design. It must be logistically feasible, as one attempts to keep all other conditions the same while manipulating an aspect of care in the experimental group. As the outcome is measured after a predetermined period, this must also occur within a reasonable time period. For example, it would be very difficult to evaluate the effect of an intervention on an outcome if it is very rare or will not occur for 20–30 years.

Uncertainty must surround the answer to the question. Therefore, it is important to know whether the question has already been answered and how strong the evidence is to support the answer. Extensive reviews of the literature must be performed, using appropriate resources such as Medline or the

Cochrane Database to identify related prior work. This has implications when the research community is allocating scarce resources, and is a most relevant issue for ethical reasons. Investigators must not deny patients known treatment benefits for the sake of new knowledge. For example, it would now be unethical to knowingly treat a hypertensive patient with "placebo only" vs a new drug to investigate potential benefits. However, it may be necessary to repeat prior work for confirmation of results or with improvements on trial design. Of course, debate exists as to what constitutes prior evidence, or even the strength of evidence. For example, can a thorough meta-analysis replace a definitive randomized control trial? This question cannot be answered in general terms, and must be considered carefully for each case.

2.2. The Principal Research Question

Once investigators are satisfied that their research question is a valid one, they must outline a specific hypothesis to be tested—referred to statistically as the *alternate hypothesis*. The *null hypothesis*, or the negation of the hypothesis you want to establish, is then determined. It is the null hypothesis that is to be tested using statistical methods. Statistical purists believe that one can only reject or fail to reject (vs accept) a null hypothesis. It is convenient to discuss statistical error at this point. Because trials test a hypothesis on a subset of the whole population, it is possible to have results that are skewed because of chance, depending on the sample population. A type I error occurs when the results from the sample population permit investigators to reject a null hypothesis that in fact is true. Type II errors occur when investigators fail to reject the null hypothesis, when in fact the null hypothesis is false. Of course, the two possibilities for correct action include: i) rejecting a false null hypothesis—the probability of this is called power, and ii) failing to reject a true null hypothesis, sometimes called the confidence (**Fig. 1**). The risk of committing a type I error is denoted alpha, and the risk of committing a type II error is denoted beta. Power is thus equal to one minus beta and confidence is equal to one minus alpha. It has become customary to accept a 5% chance of committing a type I error.

3. Trial Design

3.1. Randomization

Randomization attempts to ensure that participants in different study groups are similar or comparable at baseline, and that the only difference will be the intervention. In clinical research, there is a mix of demographic and other attributes that investigators know about. Randomization attempts to ensure that the factors that the investigators are unaware of do not systematically affect

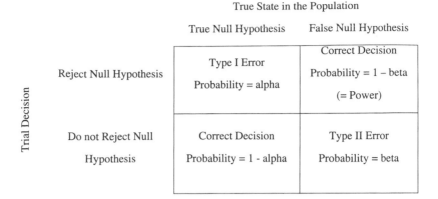

Fig. 1. Potential outcomes in a clinical trial.

results. Participants must have an equal chance of receiving either intervention *a priori*, ensuring no selection bias. The process is termed "allocation concealment," and prevents participants from being enrolled in a trial on the condition they only receive a pre-specified intervention. To increase validity in multicenter trials, the randomization and assignment should occur at a central location. This ensures consistency and decreases selection bias.

Other variants of randomization include "stratified randomization." This technique is used when investigators are concerned that one or more baseline factors are extremely important in determining outcome, and want to ensure equal representation in both arms—diabetics in chronic kidney disease, for example. When participants are screened, they are stratified according to whether the factor, like diabetes, is present or not before they are randomized from within these groups. "Cluster randomization" involves randomizing entire groups of participants *en block*, for example, by hospital or location. This method is particularly useful in the evaluation of non-therapeutic interventions such as education.

The principles of randomization discussed here are for two intervention arms with 1:1 representation in each arm. These principles are also applicable to other trial designs where there are three or more treatment arms such as placebo vs drug A vs drug B. Investigators may also wish to have more participants in one treatment arm vs the other. For example, 2:1 randomization has two-thirds of the participants randomized to one group and one-third to the other. This technique may be used to ensure adequate participant numbers in a treatment arm, for example, to evaluate side effects of a medication. Finally, a factorial design is one in which two or more independent interventions are tested simultaneously during the same trial (**Fig. 2**). The Heart Outcomes

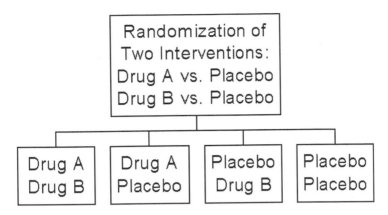

Fig. 2. Possible outcomes in a 2 × 2 factorial design. Each participant has an equal probability of receiving one of the four intervention combinations.

Prevention Evaluation (HOPE) trial is one example in which patients were randomized to receive either Ramipril vs Placebo or Vitamin E vs Placebo *(4,5)*. Therefore, participants had an equal probability of receiving one of four interventions: i) Ramipril and Vitamin E, ii) Ramipril and Placebo, iii) Placebo and Vitamin E, or iv) Placebo and Placebo. The benefits of this design include reducing costs and detecting interactions.

3.2. Blinding

Blinding is another technique utilized to decrease both participant and investigator bias. This means that participants and/or investigators do not know which treatment arm the participant is enrolled in. This is sometimes impossible or inappropriate, and thus, open-label trials are designed. If this is the case, then it is especially important to have objective outcomes and people blind to the intervention received in outcome adjudication or data analysis.

3.3. Crossover

Crossover occurs when participants assigned to one intervention receive the other intervention at some point. This can be a part of the trial design in which it is planned that each participant receives both interventions, preferably in random order. The advantage is that participants can serve as their own control. It is particularly suited for short-term interventions and outcomes in which time-related trends do not occur. The disadvantage is that one intervention may carry-over to affect the second intervention, requiring washout periods if possible. Loss resulting from follow-up can be particularly problematic when interpreting results.

3.4. Multicenter

Multicenter trials, although increasing in logistical complexity, allow for greater enrollment opportunities. They also have the advantage of diminished "center effect," making results of the trial more applicable to a wider spectrum of patients. It helps to include academic and non-academic centers when possible to further decrease case-mix bias.

3.5. Planned Trial Allocations and Interventions

It is important to precisely outline what the intervention will be and how both the treatment and the control groups will be managed. The goal is to decrease subjectivity in interpreting application of the trial protocol. Other details of dosing, co-therapy, and attainment of therapeutic targets should be clarified, as well as contingency plans for side-effects. It helps to have a flow diagram (**Fig. 3**) outlining the streaming of participants through the processes of screening, consent, further assessment of eligibility, contact to trial center, stratification, randomization, and follow-up. This will help to keep track of participants in the trial and account for them during interpretation and presentation of results.

3.6. Inclusion and Exclusion Criteria

Inclusion criteria are important to ensure that the study question is answered in a population of subjects similar to that in which the results must be applied. This may be difficult in chronic kidney disease because of the spectrum of different renal diseases with different natural histories. Investigators should strive to design trials that are representative of everyday clinical practice. For logistic reasons, participants must be residing in a location amenable to follow-up. People who are unable to give consent should be excluded. Furthermore, investigators should try to ensure that outliers do not contaminate the study population. In chronic kidney disease, this would include excluding participants with other diagnoses that confer poor prognosis. Finally, some people are excluded for general safety or ethical considerations, such as pregnant participants.

3.7. Primary and Secondary Outcome Measures

The primary outcome is the most important measure that provides an answer to the principal research question. Secondary outcome measures may be used to evaluate safety, such as mortality and co-morbidities, or additional effects of the intervention.

3.8. Measuring the Outcome Measures at Follow-Up

Investigators need a relevant, valid, precise, safe, practical, and inexpensive means of judging how a particular treatment affects the outcome of interest,

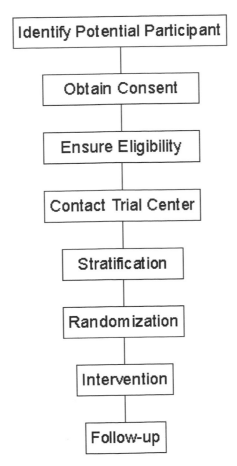

Fig. 3. Example of flow diagram for participants in multicenter randomized control trial.

such as progression of kidney disease *(6)*. In chronic kidney disease, hard end points such as death, dialysis, or transplantation are preferred because of their uniform definition and objectivity. However, it should be remembered that renal disease progresses at variable rates and the incidence of these advanced end points is too low to study in earlier kidney disease. Using surrogate markers, studies may be conducted with smaller sample sizes and over a shorter period of time. The principal drawback of surrogate markers is their imperfect relationship to hard end points. Nonetheless, for chronic kidney disease, it may be advisable to use "intermediate" end points such as doubling of serum creatinine and reduction in proteinuria by at least 30% from baseline *(6)*. Although less accurate, these measures are easy to evaluate, more practical than more cumbersome measures such as inulin clearance, and acceptable to the Food and Drug Administration.

Serum creatinine is perhaps the most widely used estimate of kidney function. It should be noted that laboratory differences in this measurement and within-person variation may affect interpretation of results *(7)*. This may be alleviated by the use of a central standardized laboratory and using repeated measures on subjects. There are two main ways to use creatinine in analysis: slope analysis using observed change in renal function over time as the outcome, and threshold analysis using a cutoff for all subjects to define the outcome of interest. Very different conclusions may be drawn from the same data, depending on the definition of outcome and the choice of slope vs threshold analysis. A slope analysis is probably more suitable when investigating risk factors for loss of renal function. A threshold analysis may be more informative from a public health perspective, since the adverse consequences of chronic kidney disease appear to be limited to those whose kidney function falls below a certain threshold *(7)*.

4. Size and Duration of Trial

4.1. Estimating Sample Size

Investigators need to know how many participants are required to provide results that are clinically and statistically significant from the expected outcomes. This allows for cost and time estimations for trials, and is a balance of event numbers and statistical precision. An estimate of the likely event rate in the control group from prior studies or from preliminary data is required to calculate sample size. Clinically relevant effects caused by the intervention are also chosen. The calculated estimation of the sample size has many other determinants, and the details of these are beyond the scope of this chapter: comparing means vs proportions, type I and type II error, one- vs two-tailed test, and underlying inherent variability in the outcome measurements or the standard deviation in the population. Computational programs are available to calculate the sample size. Sometimes overlooked, but very important, is underestimation of loss to follow-up, and dealing with missing or incomplete data when the trial ends. This must be anticipated beforehand and incorporated into sample-size estimation. A practical "rule-of-thumb" is to allow for a minimum of 20% loss. Finally, the sample size also depends on how the data is to be analyzed, whether by intention-to-treat or by treatment received.

4.2. Recruitment Rate

Again, experiences in prior studies, or preliminary data, are required to estimate recruitment rate. It must be emphasized that the number of participants who are practically willing or able to enroll will be lower than those who are eligible. Reasons such as participant location, eligible participants being overlooked, participants enrolled in other trials, participants unwilling or unable to consent, and other physicians hesitant to enter their patients in a particular trial all decrease the recruitment rate.

4.3. Duration of the Treatment Period

Along with time to recruit an adequate sample, the event rate of the primary outcome may affect the length of the trial. Additionally, the treatment or intervention may not begin when participants are enrolled in the trial. Depending on the protocol, there may be run-in periods when participants are monitored for further exclusion to ensure that applicability or time may be needed for wash-out periods of medications. Similarly, the treatment may end before the trial with time necessary to follow the participants for long-term outcomes, for example, Ponticelli's 10-yr membranous nephropathy follow-up *(8)*. In this trial, patients with idiopathic membranous nephropathy and nephrotic syndrome were randomly assigned to receive symptomatic therapy or a treatment with methylprednisolone and chlorambucil for 6 mo; clinical outcomes were then determined at 10 yr. Finally, treatment periods may end when certain outcomes are met, such as transplant, but participants need follow-up for other end points, such as death.

5. Trial Data

5.1. Data Management

Methods for easy-to-use data collection and collation must be decided. Data entry into databases is becoming more sophisticated, and may range from centralized entry by clerks using data collection forms to web-based entry at collection or clinical site. The database will need to be designed ahead of time, with original data secure. Methods to error check or clean the data must be dealt with.

5.2. Details of the Planned Analyses

Appropriate analysis and statistical methods to test the hypothesis depend on the question, and must be chosen during the planning phase. Intention-to-treat analysis is a method in which participants are analyzed according to their original group at randomization and attempts to recreate a real clinical setting. This technique attempts to analyze the data in a real-world fashion without adjusting for drop-out or drop-in effects. Per protocol analysis, or analysis by treatment received, attempts to analyze the groups according to what the actual treatments were. For example, if a participant drops out early in the trial, they are excluded from the analysis. Otherwise, the analysis depends on the type of variable, whether repeated measures are used, or whether "time to event" outcomes are important. The trial design will also affect analysis depending on confounders, stratification, multiple groups, or interactions with factorial design.

5.3. Planned Subgroup Analyses

Subgroup analysis is that done for comparison of groups within the main cohort—for example, diabetics vs non-diabetics in chronic kidney disease. Although not as rigorous as the main analysis on the primary outcome, important information may be obtained. It is better to decide upon limited subgroup analysis during trial design than after the data is collected. The problem in interpreting subgroup analysis is the higher risk of obtaining apparently statistically significant results that have actually arisen secondary to chance.

5.4. Frequency of Analyses

There may be reasons to analyze a trial while underway. Safety monitoring is probably the most common reason, although sometimes the outcomes may be significantly statistically robust (either much better or much worse) that the continuation of the trial is no longer necessary. These analyses examine the premise that differences between interventions may be greater than expected. In general, statistical stopping rules are used in this circumstance to preserve the originally chosen final alpha by requiring considerably smaller p-values to declare statistical significance before the planned end of the trial. Another reason to do interim analysis is if investigators are uncertain of likely event rates in the control group. Interim analyses that do not address the primary study question do not affect trial type I error rate. Combined event accumulation, or defined intervals or dates, may dictate the precise timing of the interim analysis. An example of a trial halted by the data safety committee is the Beserab erythropoietin trial *(9)*. This prospective study examined normalizing hematocrit in patients with cardiac disease who were undergoing hemodialysis by randomizing participants to receive erythropoietin to achieve hematocrit of 42% vs 30%. The study "was halted when differences in mortality between the groups were recognized as sufficient to make it very unlikely that continuation of the study would reveal a benefit for the normal-hematocrit group and the results were nearing the statistical boundary of a higher mortality rate in the normal-hematocrit group *(9)*."

5.5. Addressing Any Economic Issues

Economic issues are a reality when it comes to changing practice patterns and affecting health care policy. It helps if an intervention can be shown to be cost-effective. The methods can be quite complex, and are better reviewed elsewhere. It may be easier to acquire funding from government or hospital sources if it is in their financial interest in the long-term.

5.6. Audit Trail

For quality control and scientific merit, investigators must plan for ongoing record-keeping and an audit trail. Methods to check for and deal with errors may be done concurrently. Similarly, investigators will need to have a method of retaining records for future access if necessary. The length of time for retention may be determined by requirements of local or national regulatory agencies, Ethics Review Boards, or Sponsors.

6. Challenges to Trial Integrity

One goal of the clinical trial is to estimate the treatment effect, as even a well-executed trial is a model for the real-world setting. This section focuses on aspects of trials that will diminish the ability of the trial to detect the true treatment effect.

6.1. Rate of Loss to Follow-Up

Similar to the recruitment rate, in which it is not always possible to enroll eligible participants, it is not always possible to keep participants in trials once enrolled. People may "drop-out" because they become disinterested or disenchanted, or they maybe lost because of relocation or death. There are many strategies for dealing with this by first identifying the reason that participants are lost. Reminders, incentives, or regular contact with participants helps keep their interest, but this must be done without being too intrusive. Similarly, the trial team must be accessible, with efficient and effective measures in place to alleviate concerns that participants may have. To deal with relocation or death, it is advisable to have permission from participants to get collateral information from Vital Statistics Bureaus or from relatives.

Nephrology involves a number of particularly relevant problems with participant loss. Mortality can be very high in certain populations, such as that in hemodialysis. Predicting change in dialysis modality is tremendously difficult, and is a unique method of "drop-out," as is recovery or precipitous decline of renal function.

Another form of "drop-out" has been historically termed non-compliance. In this situation participants are still being followed; however, they do not adhere to the trial intervention. This particularly contaminates the active treatment group, and may decrease the effectiveness of an intervention. Strategies that have been utilized to reduce this include reinforcement, close monitoring, and pill counting. It is sometimes helpful to ensure attainment and stability in parameters influenced by treatment provided to aid compliance.

Similarly, participants in a placebo arm may inadvertently, or otherwise, receive the active treatment. This is termed "drop-in." These phenomena, when combined, act like a crossover design, in which the investigators are either unaware of its occurrence or may be aware but unable to control it. There is no easy way to deal with this, but most investigators will analyze the groups as they were originally assigned (e.g., intention-to-treat analysis). It is more important to identify areas in which this may occur during trial design and try to prevent it. Considering that some loss is inevitable, the importance of considering these issues when estimating sample size during trial planning is again emphasized.

Centers may affect trials in similar ways. They too may "drop-out," and this must be taken into consideration when planning. Prior and ongoing collaboration may decrease this occurrence, yet a different center case mix may dictate that some centers will not be able to continue in the trial. For example, they may not have enough potential participants. Otherwise, similar strategies to keep participants may be used to keep centers involved.

6.2. Methods for Protecting Against Other Sources of Bias

Standardization of training, methods, and protocol all must be considered to ensure rigor. Similarly, the use of a single laboratory in multicenter studies can lessen variability in results.

7. Funding

The research question must be answerable in a reasonable period of time for practical reasons. Cost, biological reasons (such as time for disease to manifest), time to recruit participants, and time for outcomes to accrue all affect the duration of a trial. A budget that encompasses these issues is essential.

7.1. Costs

The majority of today's clinical research is human resource-intensive, and funding is required for the expertise of research nurses and assistants. Similarly, money is needed to pay for research management, data entry, and other staffing necessary for administration of the trial. Employee benefits such as pensions and sick, compassionate, maternity/paternity leave, as well as jury duty and vacation must be factored into costs. Costs such as paper, fax, phone, travel, computers, and other consumables can be significant.

7.2. Licensing

Licensing involves establishing new indications for drugs or techniques. This increases costs for trials, as regulations for how these trials are conducted may be very strict, and for safety reasons, monitoring and quality control can be more intense. However, there is usually an increase in industry sponsorship to help alleviate the increased cost.

7.3. Funding Sources

Procuring funding is sometimes the major hurdle in clinical research. Fortunately, it is easier to find money to do topical research. For more expensive trials, it may be necessary to obtain shared or leveraged funding from more than one of the following limited sources. Public funding, as in foundations or institutes, is available. Examples that are specific to nephrology include The National Kidney Foundation and The National Institute of Health in the United States, as well as the Kidney Foundation of Canada and the Canadian Institute of Health Research. The advantage of these is that the applications are peer-reviewed. Government and hospital agencies have funds available for research, but they can be tied to quality improvement or research aimed at cost reduction. They may also contribute "in-kind" other than through direct funding by providing clinical space and nursing staff.

It is becoming increasingly difficult to conduct major clinical research without the aid of the private sector. Issues of data ownership must be addressed during the planning phase. It is usually preferable for the investigator to approach the private funding source first with the major planning of the trial already completed.

8. Details of the Trial Team

8.1. Steering Committee

Larger trials may need a steering committee for trial management. The main role is to refine design details, spearhead efforts to secure funding, and work out logistical problems. This may also include protocol organization and interim report writing. The committee may include experts in trial design, economic analysis, and data management, along with expertise in the various conditions being studied.

8.2. Endpoint Adjudication Committee

An endpoint adjudication committee may be used to judge clinical endpoints, and is required when there are subjective elements of decision-making or when decisions are complex or error-prone. Criteria for the clinical outcomes must be prespecified and applicable outside of a trial setting. In chronic kidney disease trials, the committee should include physicians and experts in nephrology and in specialties related to comorbid endpoints such as cardiology and neurology. They should not be otherwise involved in the trial, and should be blinded with respect to the participants' intervention.

8.3. Data Safety and Monitoring Committee

A data safety and monitoring committee is needed for trials if there is concern that there will be reason to stop a trial early, based on interim analysis, when sufficient data may exist to provide answers to the principal research question. This is especially relevant when outcomes of the trial are clinically important, such as mortality discrepancy between two interventions. Another reason would be because of the cost of continuing the trial. In chronic kidney disease trials, this committee, similar to the end point adjudication, should be made up of experts who are not otherwise involved in the trial and should include at least one nephrologist, statistician, and other relevant specialists. The committee may be blinded with respect to the intervention groups. Finally, they should consider external data that may arise during the trial in considering termination. For example, if an ongoing trial is testing Drug A vs Placebo and another trial is published showing conclusive evidence that Drug A, or withholding Drug A, is harmful, then the ongoing trial should be terminated (even before interim analysis). This occurred in The Reduction of Endpoints in NIDDM with the Angiotensin II Antagonist Losartan (RENAAL) trial (10) following publication of the HOPE study, after which it became unethical to withhold therapy aimed at blockade of the renin-angiotensin system to patients on conventional treatment.

8.4. Participating Centers

If multiple centers are required, then each center needs a responsible investigator to coordinate the trial at their center. This may include applying to local ethics boards, co-coordinating local staff, and screening, consenting, enrolling, and following participants. A letter of intent from each center's investigator is usually required to secure funding.

References

1. Whelton, P. K. (1994) Epidemiology of hypertension. *Lancet* **344**, 101–106.
2. Whelton, P. K. and Gordis, L. (2000) Epidemiology of clinical medicine. *Epidemiol. Rev.* **22**, 140–144.
3. Fuchs, F. D., Klag, M. J., and Whelton, P. K. (2000) The Classics: a tribute to the fiftieth anniversary of the randomized clinical trial. *J. Clin. Epidemiol.* **53**, 335–342.
4. Yusuf, S., Sleight, P., Pogue, J., Bosch, J., Davies, R., and Dagenais, G. (2000) Effects of an angiotensin-converting-enzyme inhibitor, ramipril, on cardiovascular events in high-risk patients. The Heart Outcomes Prevention Evaluation Study Investigators. *N. Engl. J. Med.* **20**, 145–153.
5. Yusuf, S., Dagenais, G., Pogue, J., Bosch, J., and Sleight, P. (2000) Vitamin E supplementation and cardiovascular events in high-risk patients. The Heart Outcomes Prevention Evaluation Study Investigators. *N. Engl. J. Med.* **20**, 154–160.

6. Bakris, G. L., Whelton, P., Weir, M., Mimran, A., Keane, W., and Schiffrin, E. for the Evaluation of Clinical Trial Endpoints in Chronic Renal Disease Study Group. (2000) The Future of Clinical Trials in Chronic Renal Disease: Outcome of an NIH/FDA/Physician Specialist Conference. *J. Clin. Pharmacol.* **40,** 815–825.
7. Hsu, C-Y., Chertow, G. M., and Curhan, G. C. (2002) Methodological issues in studying the epidemiology of mild to moderate chronic renal insufficiency. *Kidney Int.* **61,** 1567–1576.
8. Ponticelli, C., Zucchelli, P., Passerini, P., Cesana, B., Locatelli, F., Pasquali, S., et al. (1995) A 10-year follow-up of a randomized study with methylprednisolone and chlorambucil in membranous nephropathy. *Kidney Int.* **48,** 1600–1604.
9. Besarab, A., Bolton, W. K., Browne, J. K., Egrie, J. C., Nissenson, A. R., Okamoto, D. M., et al. (1998) The effects of normal as compared with low hematocrit values in patients with cardiac disease who are receiving hemodialysis and epoetin. *N. Engl. J. Med.* **339,** 584–590.
10. Brenner, B. M., Cooper, M. E., De Zeeuw, D., et al. (2001) Effects of losartan on renal and cardiovascular outcomes in patients with type 2 diabetes and nephropathy. *N. Engl. J. Med.* **345,** 861–869.

CONCLUSION

Mapping the Disease

Michael S. Goligorsky

"We have twelve that sail into foreign countries ... who bring us the books and abstracts... These we call Merchants of Light. We have three that collect the experiments, which are in all books. These we call the Depredators. We have three that collect the experiments of all mechanical arts, and also of liberal arts... Those we call Mystery Men. We have three that try new experiments... These we call Pioneers or Miners. We have three that draw the experiments of the former four into titles and tables... Those we call Compilers."

—Francis Bacon, *The New Atlantis*

Bacon's idealistic description of a research process, as naive and utopian as it sounds today, actually depicts the many functions of a single investigator, from literature search and collection of data to attempts of summing-up the investigation: the merchant, the miner, the depredator and the compiler in one face. All the better if some help could be furnished by *Renal Disease: Techniques and Protocols*, that would have replaced the need for the "merchant" and "depredator" and allowed more time to concentrate on the subject of investigation.

While the body of investigation is growing—whether it is of epithelial transport or renal disease—the investigators are entering areas of lesser familiarity, there is an increasing threat of "dilutional hypognosia." The similar situation was reflected upon by Erwin Chargraff: "The greater the circle of understanding becomes, the greater is the circumference of surrounding ignorance" *(1)*. With the experts in specific selected areas of renal physiology contributing to this volume and sharing their profound knowledge and innermost thoughts, it is hoped that such problems should be alleviated.

The utility of the toolbox provided in this volume is not self-evident, but depends on the larger, overarching investigational problems at hand. Toward

From: *Methods in Molecular Medicine, vol. 86: Renal Disease: Techniques and Protocols*
Edited by: M. S. Goligorsky © Humana Press Inc., Totowa, NJ

this end, the most frequently followed pathways for evolution of investigation into a disease process can be categorized by simple schematic sequences:

1) Search for unknown causal mechanism(s) of disease: suspected candidates (hypothetical or identified by gene/protein pool screening); use of experimental animals or cell culture systems to model the effect(s) of potential candidates; application of Koch's principles to confirm the causality of the particular mechanism.

2) Search for potential pharmacologic interventions: delineation of a mechanistic pathway leading to a certain disease, symptom, or syndrome; creation of an animal and/or cellular model; application of inhibitors of the particular pathway; if successful, initiation of a clinical trial.

3) Search for the role of genetic, habitual, or environmental factors of development/progression of the disease: comparative epidemiologic studies of representative populations overexpressing or underexpressing the particular phenotype; genetic, habitual or environmental screening; employment of animal or cellular models to mimic the particular phenotype; investigation into the outcomes of correcting the suspected genetic, habitual or environmental offender.

4) Search for function/dysfunction of a discovered molecule: expression systems of naïve cells; investigation of a phenotype of knockout or overexpressing animals; screening human disease processes for the particular molecular defect; application of techniques of gene therapy.

5) Search for the potential consequences of a dysregulated molecule: identification of the particular dysregulated molecule in the context of a pathological process (chance finding, hypothesis-driven observation or a result of high-throughput screening); pharmacological manipulation of the particular molecular suspect in a cell culture system and in whole animal model; morphologic and functional phenotyping; application of pharmacologic tools to correct the particular abnormality and determination of outcomes.

6) Investigation into the comparative chronological contribution of the known mechanistic pathways to the natural history of disease (mapping of disease): definition of key regulators of each implicated pathway; gene and protein profiling of these regulators throughout the course of disease (animal models and human disease); pharmacological manipulation of respective mutable mechanistic pathways at distinct stages of the pathological process; it successful, initiation of a clinical trial.

While many additional investigational paradigms can be encountered, the above sequences delineate the most common ones. It is easily observable that there are some common domains utilized in diverse investigational processes regardless of their initial purpose (**Fig. 1**). This commonality re-emphasizes the main philosophical tenets engraved in this volume: a) possession of a toolbox does not by itself translate into a successful investigation, b) requirement for carefully selecting tools of choice in pursuing specific tasks, c) permanency of interaction between unbiased screening processes and hypothesis-driven investigation, and d) contiguity of reductionistic and integrative approaches. There is

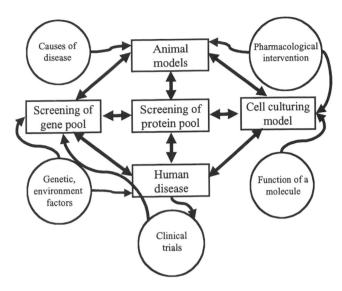

Fig. 1. Methodological algorithms of investigational processes.

not a single tool to solve the problem—tools should vary, as should the level of modeling—from molecules and cells to a living organism.

Emerging technologies like DNA and protein high-throughput screening, microsequencing, and laser-assisted microdissection, to name a few, should quite dramatically change the entire landscape of biomedical research in the next 5–10 years. These approaches will allow mapping of the molecular events governing the development of diverse physiologic and pathologic phenomena. Molecular charting of disease processes, from genes to proteins, represents the next frontier of biomedical research. Emerging technological platforms should uplift investigations to the field of molecular mapping of processes involved in the initiation and progression of disease and enable investigators to take the next challenge: focusing on the functional equivalents of thus disclosed molecular roadmaps. Development of technological tools for performing intravital videomicroscopy, an emerging substitute for the static biopsy of a pathologic specimen, should combine the benefits of morphologic and functional analyses. Though not supplanting traditional investigational tools and routes, these emerging technologies clearly supplement them with much stratified general strategies based on the above interactive principles of unbiased gene and protein screening with hypothesis-driven identification of functional correlates of the pathological process.

Putting aside the lucky chance, intuition, or other favorable circumstances driving research, it is, after all, the solid foundation of appropriate techniques, carefully selected from the plethora of choices that consolidate research efforts. The Tower of Babel was a failure in executing a daring architectural design not because the builders were multi-lingual, but as a result of a breakdown in communication. So it is with the most ingenuous ideas when they are not buttressed by adequate technological structures. Therefore, it is the sincere hope of all contributors to this volume that approaches, techniques, and strategies outlined herein will assist investigators in making correct choices in applying optimal research tools, avoiding their weaknesses and potential bottlenecks, assuring correct interpretation of results, and thus improving the overall strategic design and technical execution of the study.

Reference

1. Chargraff, E. (1963) First steps toward a chemistry of heredity, in: *Essays on Nucleic Acids* London, UK.

Index